Color Plate B. See page 206

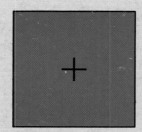

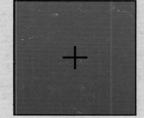

**Color Plate C.
See page 417**

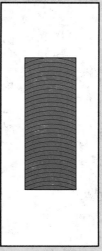

Color Plate D. See page 243

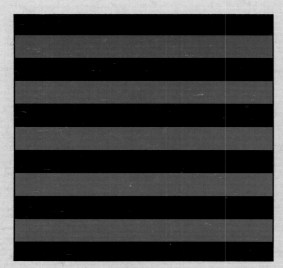

Color Plate G. See page 243

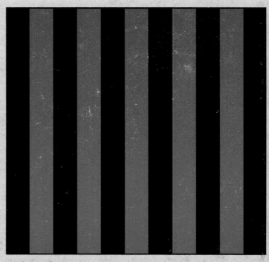

Color Plate G.

FUNDAMENTALS OF SENSATION
AND PERCEPTION

SECOND EDITION

FUNDAMENTALS OF SENSATION AND PERCEPTION

SECOND EDITION

Michael W. Levine

Department of Psychology
University of Illinois at Chicago

Jeremy M. Shefner

Division of Neurology
Brigham and Women's Hospital
&
Department of Neurology
Harvard Medical School

Brooks/Cole Publishing Company
Pacific Grove, California

Brooks/Cole Publishing Company
A Division of Wadsworth, Inc.

Printed in the United States of America

10 9 8 7 6 5 4 3 2

Library of Congress Cataloging-in-Publication Data

Levine, Michael W.,
    Fundamentals of sensation and perception / Michael W. Levine &
Jeremy M. Shefner. — 2nd ed.
        p.   cm.
    Includes bibliographical references and indexes.
    ISBN 0-534-14172-2
    1. Senses and sensation.   2. Perception.   I. Title.
BF233.L47   1990
    152.1—dc20   90-36562
                                                                                      CIP

Sponsoring Editor: *Vicki Knight*
Editorial Assistant: *Heather L. Riedl*
Production Editor: *Timothy A. Phillips*
Manuscript Editor: *Robert E. Baker*
Permissions Editor: *Marie DuBois*
Interior and Cover Design: *Roy R. Neuhaus*
Cover Photo: *Larry Hamill Stock Photography*
Art Coordinator: *Lisa Torri*
Interior Illustration: *Lotus Art, Cyndie Clark-Huegal, Wayne Clark*
Photo Editor: *Ruth Minerva*
Typesetting: *Shepard Poorman Communications Corp.*
Cover Printing: *Lehigh Press Lithographers*
Printing and Binding: *Arcata Graphics/Fairfield*

ABOUT THE AUTHORS

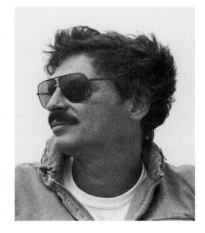

Dr. Michael W. Levine has been involved with researching vision and visual processes, especially the physiology of vision, for over twenty years. In addition to coauthoring the first edition of *Fundamentals of Sensation and Perception,* he has authored more than 30 technical articles, contributed two chapters to *Psychology: Themes and Variations* by W. Weiten, and has been invited to address several conventions. In 1987, he was awarded a Fogarty Senior International Fellowship. Dr. Levine is currently a professor of Psychology at the University of Illinois at Chicago, where he has been the Psychology Department director of undergraduate studies, a member of the Psychology Department Executive committee, and chair of the University Large Animal Welfare Subcommittee. He is also active in the University Committee on Neuroscience. Dr. Levine was born in New York City and currently lives with his wife and two children in Evanston, Illinois.

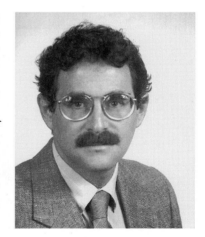

Dr. Jeremy M. Shefner has been involved with researching drug therapy and sensory abnormalities in lateral sclerosis, nerve regeneration, upper motor neuron diseases, and compound sensory action potentials for a number of years. In 1986 he spent a year as medical superintendent for the Ialibu District Hospital in Southern Highland Province, Papua New Guinea. In 1983 he was awarded an M.D. with distinction from Northwestern University. In addition to coauthoring the first edition of *Fundamentals of Sensation and Perception,* he has published more than a dozen technical articles. Dr. Shefner is currently Associate Physician in Neurology at Brigham and Women's Hospital in Boston and an instructor in Neurology at Harvard Medical School. Dr. Shefner was born in Chicago, Illinois, and currently lives with his wife in Brookline, Massachusetts.

PREFACE

RATIONALE

In our experiences in teaching courses in the psychology of sensation and perception, each of us has tried to integrate what we know about the physiology of sensory systems with the classical perceptual problems commonly discussed in psychology courses. Within this framework, students generally found the physiology sections of the course both interesting and useful in understanding the cognitive aspects of perception. Finding a textbook to accompany the lectures, however, proved to be a difficult task. The existing books discussed either the physiological aspects of sensation or the cognitive aspects of perception with little reference to their physiological bases. This book is our attempt to integrate these two complementary ways of studying perceptual processes.

In this book, we trace information about what happens to the physical stimulus as our sensory systems analyze it to produce complicated perceptions of the world around us. In tracing this pathway, we consider how anatomy and physiology allow us to extract the information upon which our perceptions are built. Perception is a very complex field, however, with many phenomena that cannot now be explained physiologically, and we draw upon explanations at the physiological, psychophysical, and cognitive levels.

In addition to a unique approach to perception, this book includes two topics that are not given detailed treatment in other sensation and perception texts. One active research area in the field of human visual perception today is spatial frequency analysis, an approach that may explain many complex perceptual phenomena in terms of a mathematical model of the visual system. We attempt to present this model in a way that will be understandable to students with little or no mathematical background. A second topic usually given little or no space in perception texts is speech perception. We devote a full chapter to this fascinating topic vital to understanding human communication.

FEATURES

In a few ways, this book may be different from other texts. Knowing about these features will help you get the most from this book.

Boxes

In each chapter are topics of interest and relevance to the subject at hand, but which are more advanced or specialized than the rest of the chapter. For example, in some cases, a few equations could make a point we have been discussing but would only confuse any reader who is not familiar with the mathematics. We have segregated this material into boxes. Other books have boxes with additional material that can be read or ignored, but these are usually placed to one side (like figures) where the reader has to interrupt the main text in order to stop and read each box. We have chosen to treat the boxes as if they were part of the text, but we indicate that this part can be bypassed with no loss of continuity. A proper name might be "alternate-pathway insertion modules," but boxes will do nicely.

Demonstrations

Many of the figures, particularly in Chapters 10 through 15, are intended to demonstrate a perceptual effect or illusion. In most cases, you can just look at the figure and say, "oh yes, that looks like (whatever)." In some cases, we have recommended a little more effort—looking at the figure from a greater distance, turning it upside down, or covering parts of it with another sheet of paper. We urge readers to take the trouble to do these things, for they will demonstrate the effect, or prove that it is real.

The most troublesome demonstrations are those in the chapter on color, Chapter 15. For the demonstrations of the trichromacy of vision, you must procure some colored cellophane and make a color wheel. Again, we urge you to expend the necessary effort; the difference between reading about a phenomenon and experiencing it makes the task well worth the trouble.

Stereograms

Stereograms (three-dimensional pictures) are among the demonstrations that will require a bit of work on your part. The perceptual effect of a three-dimensional scene justifies the effort you may make.

Printing stereograms in a book poses a special problem that is usually solved by one of two methods. One is direct and requires no extra equipment from the reader but is hard for many people to see; the other is easy for almost anyone to see, but requires having a small mirror, which often is not handy.

Stereograms consist of two pictures: one is to be seen by the right eye, and the other by the left. The small differences between the images in these two pictures (or frames) correspond to the differences in points of view of the two eyes; these differences lead to a strong perception of depth (see Chapter 12). In the direct-viewing method, the frames are printed side by side; the reader then must manage to look at each one with one eye (see the following box). In the mirror-viewing method, the frame on the right is printed as a mirror image of how it should appear to the right eye. A small mirror is held between the two frames so that the left eye views the left frame directly, while the right eye sees the right frame reflected in the mirror. Tilting the mirror makes it easy to position the images so that they overlap.

We have combined these methods so that the stereograms can either be viewed directly (if possible) or seen with the aid of a mirror. To our knowledge, this is the first book in which the reader is offered such an option; when you encounter stereograms in other books, you have to view them in the way the book says, or they will not work (unless by chance the right frame is mirror-symmetric). Here we have designed all the stereograms so that the right-hand frame is mirror-symmetric about its middle; it therefore looks the same whether viewed directly or in a mirror, and can be viewed by either method. The following box explains how to view our stereograms using each method.

BOX P–1

Before attempting to view a stereogram, check for stereoblindness—that is, that both eyes are used and the images fused to give a three-dimensional perception. A simple test for stereoscopic vision is shown in Figure I–1. Stare at a spot on a wall across the room (for example, the star in the figure). Bring your two hands in front of your face, about 1 foot in front of your eyes, with the pointer fingers aiming at each other. When the two pointers are about to touch (about $1/4$-inch apart), you should see what is shown on the top part of Figure I–1(b): the star (that you are focused on) should be sharp; in front of it, and blurred, should be a sausage-like blimp floating between your two fingers. If you focus on your fingers, the blimp vanishes and the fingers become sharp, and the star should split into two blurry stars (Figure I–1(b), lower). If you see either of the pictures shown in Figure I–1(b) you are not stereoblind, and should be able to see three-dimen-

sional stereograms (unless you also have double vision all the time). If you are stereoblind, you will see a single set of fingers (like the bottom illustration) *and* a single star (as in the top) *at the same time*. If you close one eye, there will be no change in the image; if you close the other, the star will jump to a different position relative to your fingers. If you are stereoblind, you will not see the three-dimensional effect in the stereograms, and will have to take our word for it. If you are not stereoblind, you should be able to achieve the effects by one of the following methods, practicing on the stereogram in Figure I–2.

Direct Method

The direct method requires no special equipment, but takes a bit of concentration. The idea is to look at the left frame with your left eye and the right frame with your right eye; the two

(continued)

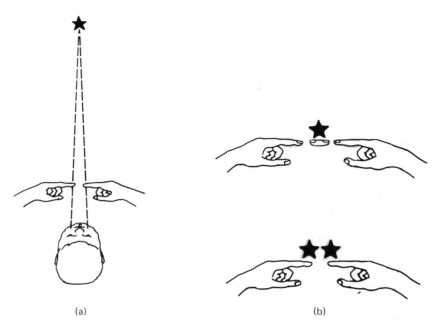

(a)   (b)

FIGURE I-1   Method for testing for stereoblindness. (a) Top view of subject. (b) Two ways the fingers and star should look to a normal (not stereoblind) person.

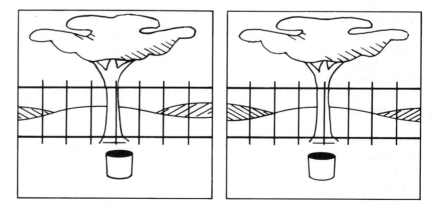

FIGURE I-2   Practice stereogram. The can should appear in front of the fence, and the tree behind. May be viewed by either the direct or mirror method.

(continued)

images then are superimposed (in your brain) and fuse into a single three-dimensional scene. The technique is shown in Figure I–3. Just look at the two frames directly, and concentrate on

2. Practice focusing for infinity by staring across the room, then try not to change focus as you bring the book into your field of view. Squinting may help.

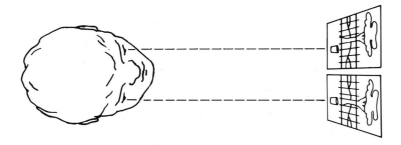

FIGURE I-3   Direct method of viewing stereograms; top view.

making the double images superimpose. When they do, it sometimes takes an extra moment or two for the three-dimensional effect to become obvious.

To view a stereogram by this method, you have to have your eyes looking apart, rather than converging. When you look at something close, like this book, your eyes automatically point inward so that both are aimed at the same point. They diverge when you look into the distance. Therefore you should relax your eyes as much as possible, as if you were looking into the distance, even though the book is still close to your eyes.

There are several tricks that can help you view stereograms by this method:

1. If you are nearsighted, and wear glasses to see in the distance (*not* for reading), take off the glasses. You will then have to focus for distance to see the book, and your eyes will diverge (see Chapter 4). If you wear reading glasses, you should keep them on.

3. When your eyes are diverging, you will see a pair of images of the stereogram, with the left frame of one image superimposed on the right frame of the other. Use the borders of the picture as a guide, and concentrate on bringing the corners of the overlapped frame into register. If one image is displaced upward relative to the other (instead of side to side) tilt your head slightly one way or the other. Tilting will also help you identify the two images you are trying to bring together.

4. If both of your eyes keep trying to look at the same frame, you can erect a barricade between them. Use a piece of paper and hold it between your nose and the division of the frames, like the mirror in Figure I–4. The barricade should prevent your left eye from seeing the right frame, and vice versa. Then you have only two images to try to bring together.

(continued)

5. You can help diverge your eyes slightly by pressing gently at the inside corners. Place your fingers on the sides of your nose, and press very gently into the corners of your eyes (do *not* do this if you have any kind of eye infection, glaucoma, or other eye ailments).

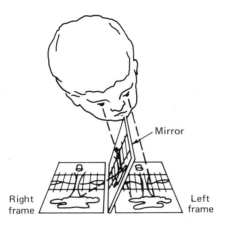

FIGURE I-4   Mirror method of viewing stereograms.

Mirror Method

Some people simply cannot see stereograms by the direct method, either because they cannot manage to diverge their eyes while seeing close up, or because their eyes are set too closely together in their heads. If you could not see the stereogram in Figure I–2 by the direct method and wish to see the effect, use the mirror method.

You will need a small hand mirror. The best is the rectangular kind that drugstores sell "for pocket or purse" that is about 3 or 4 inches square. The mirror built into a makeup kit will do, although the kit itself can get in the way. A shiny, smooth piece of metal will also work, but the image in it is not likely to be as good as that produced by mirror.

Place one edge of the mirror along the space between the frames of the stereogram, with the shiny side to the right (see Figure I–4). Bring your head down to the mirror, so that it divides your field of view; your left eye can look directly at the left frame, but cannot see the right frame because the view is blocked by the dull back of the mirror. Your right eye can see the right frame directly or reflected in the mirror, but cannot see the left frame.

Concentrate on the left frame, and change the tilt of the mirror until the right frame seen by the right eye (reflected in the mirror) lines up with it. As with the direct method, concentrate on aligning the corners of the frames. If there is a vertical misalignment, the mirror is not straight along the division between the frames. Left-to-right misalignment can be corrected by tilting the mirror or sliding it from left to right. The three-dimensional effect should appear moments after you align the two frames.

Suggested Readings

At the end of each chapter, we have a list of readings that you might wish to pursue. For the most part, these readings take you a little deeper into the subject than we have gone, but they are generally not at a very technical level. A brief description of each indicates roughly what to expect. You may wish to consult the readings for extra information, or to help you understand material that we did not make clear.

We have tried to find articles from *Scientific American* to suggest after each chapter. These articles are informative, interesting, and readable, with plentiful illustrations. The articles may be purchased as separate offprints (we have also given the offprint numbers[1]), and most of the ones we mention have been reprinted in one of the books of collected *Scientific American* readings, so they should be readily available.

Appendix

Many students in a perception course have little experience with science, and find the graphical presentation and mathematics unfamiliar. We have included an appendix that should help refresh your memory of graphs, equations, logarithms, and trigonometric functions.

Glossdex

Books have indexes so that the reader can find the pages where particular topics are discussed. They often also have glossaries, where the reader can find the definitions of terms. We have merged these functions in a "glossdex." Each word in the glossdex has a brief definition (unless it is a common term that requires none), followed by a list of the pages on which it is discussed in the text. Usually, the first page reference will be in bold type and will refer to the place where the term was introduced. When a term is first introduced, it is printed in italics and defined in the text.

   We think the glossdex is better than a separate index and glossary because it saves looking up each item twice. Looking up a word in a glossary locates its definition, but then it is necessary to go to the index to find the pages where more can be learned about it. Looking up words in an index does not indicate exactly what meaning of the term is indexed by the references given and may lead the reader to the wrong subject. In a glossdex the reader finds the meaning and the references in one place.

CHANGES FROM THE FIRST EDITION

There are a number of ways in which the second edition differs from the first edition of this text. First, of course, there have been many advances in the nearly ten years between editions, and all of the chapters have been extensively revised and updated. Some developments that seemed very exciting in 1980 have proven less fruitful than expected, and these topics have been pared down to a more appropriate size. In a few cases, beliefs current when the first edition went to press have proven misguided, and corrections have

---

[1]*Scientific American* offprints can be ordered by number from the W. H. Freeman Co., 4419 W. 1980 S., Salt Lake City, UT 84104. The current price is $1.25 each.

been made. Topics that were not generally discussed have taken a dominant position in our current thinking and have been added to this edition. We can only imagine what topics may be deemed important if a third edition is prepared at some future date.

One particular branch of research has undergone an information explosion in the last decade; this is the investigation of the role and functioning of visual areas of the cortex. Not long ago, we knew of cell types and a structural pattern in primary visual cortex but only made vague statements that the information must be processed in ''higher'' centers. We have now identified putative roles for many higher centers. In addition, we see parallel processing systems (identifiable at the lowest levels, but not noticed earlier) within the cortical pathways. We are just beginning to appreciate the ways in which these parallel systems interact and can hope one day to understand how a percept may emerge from the interplay of these regions. This explosion of information and understanding has so expanded the material about higher centers that we have now split what had been a single chapter, ''Higher Visual Centers,'' into two: ''The Primary Visual Areas of the Brain,'' and ''Architecture of Vision in the Cortex.''

The first edition of this text treated only two sensory systems: vision and audition. While these are still our primary emphases, we have added two new chapters discussing other sensory systems. Chapter 20 treats the ''body'' senses—the senses of body position, touch, and temperature. Closely related to these is an important though unpleasant sense: the sense of pain. Chapter 21 adds the ''chemical'' senses—taste and smell. While these additions are not intended to make this book an encyclopedia of sensory and perceptual processes, they do repair some serious omissions.

ACKNOWLEDGMENTS

An important contribution to this book was made by the reviewers who read and criticized the manuscript. Their valuable suggestions have altered and improved the manuscript in many ways, although any mistakes or misinterpretations that may remain are entirely our responsibility. For their assistance in shaping the first edition, we thank

Israel Abramov
Brooklyn College of the City
    University of New York
Brooklyn, New York

Charles E. Collyer
University of Rhode Island
Kingston, Rhode Island

Bruce Ambler
The University of Texas at
    Arlington
Arlington, Texas

Norma Graham
Columbia University in the City
    of New York
New York, New York

W. Lawrence Gulick
Hamilton College
Clinton, New York

Wayne Hershberger
Northern Illinois University
DeKalb, Illinois

Lloyd Kaufman
New York University
New York, New York

Frederick L. Kitterle
University of Toledo
Toledo, Ohio

Alvin Liberman
University of Connecticut
Storrs, Connecticut

Donald H. Mershon
North Carolina State University
    at Raleigh
Raleigh, North Carolina

J. Anthony Movshon
New York University
New York, New York

Joel Pokorny
University of Chicago
The Pritzher School of Medicine
Chicago, Illinois

Robert Shapley
New York University
New York, New York

Vivianne C. Smith
University of Chicago
The Pritzher School of Medicine
Chicago, Illinois

David M. Snuttjer
Calvin College
Grand Rapids, Michigan

After the first edition appeared, several professors who had adopted our text for use in their classes approached us with corrections or suggestions for improvement. Most of these suggestions have been incorporated into the second edition. We are particularly grateful to

Duane G. Albrecht
University of Texas
Austin, Texas

Russell L. DeValois
University of California
Berkeley, California

Daniel G. Green
University of Michigan
Ann Arbor, Michigan

John R. Schuck
Bowling Green State University
Bowling Green, Ohio

Leland Wilkinson
University of Illinois
Chicago, Illinois

Reviewers also assisted us in producing the second edition. Their advice about what areas should be developed guided the revision processs; their comments on the revisions further shaped this edition. We are grateful for the suggestions made by the following:

Richard Bowen
Loyola University
Chicago, Illinois

John Dowling
Harvard University Biolabs
Cambridge, Massachusetts

Sheldon Ebenholtz
State University of New York,
    College of Optometry
New York, New York

Daniel Green
University of Michigan
Ann Arbor, Michigan

Peter Kaiser
York University
North York, Ontario
CANADA

R. A. Kinchla
Princeton University
Princeton, New Jersey

William MacKavey
Boston University
Boston, Maryland

John Pittenger
University of Arkansas—Little
    Rock
Little Rock, Arkansas

We are especially grateful to Dr. Israel Abramov, Brooklyn College of the City University of New York, Brooklyn, New York, for his meticulous and valuable comments on our first revision. Some of the better analogies and arguments in this book were suggested or inspired by his review.

BRIEF CONTENTS

CONTENTS

FUNDAMENTALS OF SENSATION
AND PERCEPTION

SECOND EDITION

INTRODUCTION

1

The words (to the right) are those of the 19th-century psychologist J. Müller; they mean "one is not a psychologist who is not also a physiologist." The sentiment is more significant today than it was a century ago and will be even more true in a decade. Psychology is the science of the mind, and we are finally reaching a stage at which we can hope to relate the understanding of the mind to the physiological organ of which it is a manifestation: the brain.

The study of sensation and perception is central to psychology. The sensory systems were among the first investigated by the pioneers of this science. Through the years, perception has remained a major focus of psychology, as it is the area in which the goal of understanding how the nervous system relates to behavior is most nearly realized. In this area more than in many others, Müller's statement is undeniable.

"Nemo Psychologus Nisi Physiologus"

We have taken that statement as a guiding philosophy for this book. A person cannot understand the process of perception while ignoring the known physiology of the sensory systems that underlie the perceptual process. We are not yet in a position to provide a physiological explanation for perception, but we can deduce (from the physiology of sensation) what some of the relevant principles will be.

SENSATION AND PERCEPTION

There are two aspects to the study of our senses: sensation and perception. For our purposes, we draw the following distinction between them. *Sensation* refers to the process of detecting a stimulus (or some aspect of it) in the environment. It is the necessary collection of information about the world from which perceptions will be made. The organs of sensation are the eyes, ears, nose, tongue, skin, whiskers (in some animals), and so forth. The study of sensation is generally the study of how these organs function, often on a physiological scale.

Perception refers to the way in which we interpret the information gathered (and processed) by the senses. In a word, we sense the presence of a stimulus, but we perceive what it is. Here we enter the realm of another

1

branch of psychology: cognitive psychology. The word *cognitive* (from the Latin for "getting to know") refers to the processes by which we generate a representation of the world as we recognize it, think about it, and remember it. Perception includes the more cognitive processing by which we develop an internal model of what is "out there" in the world beyond our bodies. It is based on sensations, and it can be no more accurate than the information provided by the sensory systems.

We know the world from the energy our senses can intercept. Sound and light can travel considerable distances, and so can carry information about objects or events quite distant from our bodies. Molecules emitted by an odorant travel shorter distances, while the mechanical energy of pressure on the skin tells us about our immediate vicinity. Light (and, to a lesser extent, sound) is shaped and formed by objects it encounters; it therefore tells us more about the things around us than about the light source itself. Other forms of energy are more directly tied to their actual sources.

But the energy "out there" is of no real use to us. It must be channeled to the receptors specific to it. Light is focused on the retina of the eye to generate a useful image. Sound is channeled through the outer parts of the ear to the sensitive inner parts. Molecules are dissolved in body fluids and brought in contact with receptors in the nose or on the tongue. We usually play an active role in this process: We open our eyes, turn our heads, and aim our eyes. We turn our heads, and perhaps hold a hand cupped behind an ear. We sniff at the air, we savor our foods, we caress with our hands.

Then we can perceive. We make the most reasonable interpretations we can, given the information of the senses. *Given the information of the senses*. If the senses are fooled, we cannot help but be fooled. Have you ever seen a crime movie in which the robbers fool the security guards by placing a still picture in front of the TV camera monitoring the area? The robbers use a picture that is the exact view the camera normally scans, so the monitors display an empty room. Behind the picture, in the real room, the robbers are free to do their thing, while the guards, lacking any information that the room is occupied, are unaware of the deception.

The guards depended on the TV monitor as an extension of their senses, but your senses can be fooled directly. In Chapter 13, you will see optical illusions that appear to be quite different from what they really are. Lines that are identical can be made to seem quite different in size. Gray patches that are identical can be made to look like, well, day and night.

Optical illusions also occur in nature. Have you ever noticed that the moon looks larger at the horizon than overhead? It is not really larger; your visual system is simply applying principles that do not quite work for the moon (see Chapter 13).

Optical illusions are amusing, but similar principles are essential in the arts. A painter who wishes to create an impression of depth on a canvas, or an architect who wants a building to look taller than it is, applies the rules outlined in Chapter 13 (Figure 1–1). The mime who really seems to be carrying a huge sheet of glass is applying the principles of Chapter 11.

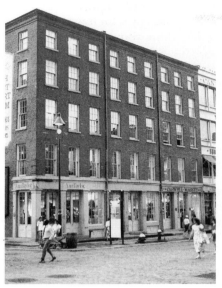 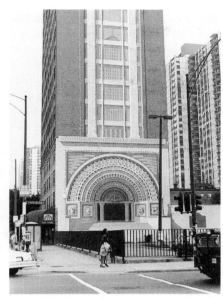

FIGURE 1-1 Two examples of how architects use perceptual principles to enhance buildings. (a) By making the windows successively smaller on higher stories, this building in New York City seems taller than it actually is. The architect exploited the depth cue of texture (see Chapter 12) (b) Here, the building presents a facade that is wholly false. Look again at the fancy doors, the imposing stairs, and arched entrance: this is a painting on a blank brick wall! (The entrance is around the side, to the left.) An artist has made use of the cues discussed in Chapter 12 to give the impression of a real, three-dimensional structure. This technique is known as *trompe l'oeil*, French for "trick of the eye."

It is not only by intent that our senses are fooled. Have you ever walked down a dark alley in a bad neighborhood at night? How easy it is to see every shadow as a threatening, armed person! A conscientious lifeguard hears the word "help" in every sudden yell. Perception is grounded in sensation, but it is far from a straightforward process.

In this book we describe sensory processes; although we do not have a complete understanding of how these systems function, with a few guesses here and there, a reasonable picture can be created. We discuss what has been learned of the cognitive processes by which perceptions are created from the sensory input; far less is known of the physiology of perception, so the principles we discuss are not as well related to the workings of the nervous system.

Students sometimes ask what these topics (particularly the more biological aspects of sensation) have to do with psychology. We reply that the science of psychology seeks to explain, understand, or even modify behavior, behavior being the response of an organism to the environment. There are stimuli in the world, and organisms or people perform actions based on their perceptions of the stimuli, with the guidance of their past experiences (memory), and perhaps some innate predilections. We cannot understand the response to the stimulus without first understanding the subject's perception of it.

There is another reason for our attention to the sensory processes: the sensory systems are parts of the nervous system that are relatively easily identified and that have relatively comprehensible purposes. If we can understand the functioning of a bit of tissue such as the retina in the eye (which is, in fact, central nervous tissue), we can hope to apply the same principles in deciphering the workings of the less well-defined, associative parts of the brain. We therefore regard our attention to the physiology of sensation as useful, not only in understanding the sensory process but also as a guide toward realizing Müller's dream of providing an understanding of behavior at the physiological level.

OVERVIEW

Our goal in this book is to present some of what is now known of how we perceive the world. We have emphasized physiological explanations for the phenomena of perception, for we believe them to be the most satisfactory ones. On the other hand, our present understanding of brain function is still rather rudimentary. We have also tried not to neglect the more cognitive aspects of the perceptual process, for which a physiological explanation lies in the future.

We have placed a heavier emphasis on vision than on audition and the other perceptual systems. We present the visual system and perception of visual stimuli in some detail to develop the principles of sensation and perception. Many of the same principles apply in other sensory systems, and we try to point out similarities between them. The emphasis is not because there are not interesting perceptual aspects to audition, touch, or smell, but because visual phenomena are more familiar, and are directly presentable on the pages of a book.

Organization

We first cover some background material in Chapters 2 and 3. These chapters introduce the principles and methodology of psychophysics (Chapter 2) and neurophysiology (Chapter 3). This material is general to the study of sensory processes, and will be drawn on in later chapters.

We discuss the visual system in Chapters 4 to 15. For the most part, we deal with the sensory and physiological aspects in the earlier chapters (4 to

9), and the more cognitive aspects in later ones (10 to 14). Chapter 15, on color vision, represents a fusion of physiological and cognitive topics.

The material on the auditory system (Chapters 16 to 19) is similarly organized. The first two chapters concentrate on sensory processing and physiology, while the last two are more concerned with cognitive aspects.

We divide the other senses into two main groups. Chapter 20 deals with the body senses: somesthesis, temperature, and pain. These are the senses that tell us about our bodies, relaying information from peripheral receptors via the spinal cord to the brain. Finally, in Chapter 21, we consider the chemical senses (taste and smell).

PSYCHOPHYSICS

2

Psychophysics is the oldest field of the science of psychology. It stems from attempts in the 19th century to measure and quantify sensation. Psychophysics and the study of sensation and perception thus stand at the very base of the family tree of psychology.

The father of psychophysics was G. T. Fechner, who coined the term *psychophysics* (*psycho* = of the mind, *physics* = tangible or measurable) and devised the classical methods of psychophysics. Fechner was a mathematician, philosopher, and scientist who hoped to derive the relationship between physical stimulus and the psychological perception of it. Modern psychophysics remains devoted to quantifying the relationship between stimulus and sensation.

Its basic methods are generally simple and straightforward, although particular experiments are often ingeniously devised to demonstrate particular points. The methods depend on the experimenter's knowledge of two things: a physical stimulus, and the response made by a subject to whom it is presented. The stimulus is chosen to be effective for a particular sensory system, and may be varied along any number of different dimensions: if it is a light, it could vary in color, size, or shape; if it is a sound, it could vary in pitch or duration. The response to the stimulus may be a verbal report[1] ("yes, I see it," "no, I saw nothing," or "these two look alike"), or a mechanical response (press *button A* when you see *stimulus 1, button B* for *stimulus 2*, and so forth). Only human subjects can make verbal responses, but either humans or animals can be taught to press buttons.

---

[1] In this chapter we speak of detecting a stimulus as "seeing" it, although psychophysics can be applied to any sensory system (and even some nonsensory systems, as in detecting "happiness," "well-being," or "value"). The use of visual-system terms is purely a convenience to avoid using the word "detectable" again and again.

CLASSICAL PSYCHOPHYSICS

Thresholds

Much early work in psychophysics was devoted to finding out how good a person (or animal) was at detecting a stimulus. This was a search for the ultimate capability of the sensory system, the minimal quantity that could be perceived. This minimum is called the *threshold* (the Latin equivalent, *limen*, is often used); threshold means just what it implies: a boundary at which one crosses from not detecting to detecting.

The concept of the threshold underlies most of classical psychophysics. If an intense light is visible and an extremely weak light is not, increasing the intensity of an invisible light eventually leads to a point at which it becomes visible; that point is the threshold.

Given the notion that there is a threshold to be measured, there are numerous ways to proceed. The most straightforward was suggested in the preceding paragraph: begin with an undetectable stimulus, and gradually increase the intensity until the subject detects it. This method, probing until the threshold is reached, is called the *method of limits*. A hypothetical method of limits experiment is shown in Table 2–1. Stimulus intensity (it could be light, sound, force of pressure against the skin, or any number of possible stimuli) is shown along the side; the subject's response to each stimulus is listed under "trial 1" ("Y" means "yes, I see it," "N" means "no, I didn't see a thing when you said I should have.") As each stimulus is presented, the subject responds negatively, although the stimulus strength is becoming progressively greater. Finally, when the sixth stimulus (S6) is

TABLE 2–1 Hypothetical Responses to Stimuli Presented in Four Ascending Trials and Percentage of Detection of Each Stimulus Based on These Results

Stimulus	Trial 1	Trial 2	Trial 3	Trial 4	Percentage Detection
S1	N	N	N	N	0
S2	N	N	N	N	0
S3	N	N	N	N	0
S4	N	N	N	N	0
S5	N	N	N	N	0
S6	Y	N	N	N	25
S7		N	Y	N	50
S8		N		Y	75
S9		Y			100
S10					100
S11					100
S12					100

Intensity (along left side, with downward arrow)

given, the subject responds "yes." There is no need to continue, for if S6 was visible, surely S7, which is stronger still, should be detected. The threshold must lie between S5 and S6.

If we repeat the experiment, however, the result is not necessarily the same. The responses to the second trial are shown in the next column of Table 2–1; this time the subject failed to detect S6, S7, and even S8. If we continue to repeat the experiment, we find that the threshold varies from trial to trial. It seems that the same stimulus the subject saw on one trial is invisible on another. Therefore, we cannot speak of a fixed threshold; we can only ask how detectable a stimulus is. Strong stimuli such as S9 and S10 are always seen; weak stimuli such as S4 are never seen. Stimuli in between are seen some percentage of the time: stimulus S8 was seen on three of four trials, or 75%; stimulus S6 was seen on only one of the four trials, or 25%. The percentage detection for each stimulus is shown in the last column of Table 2–1.

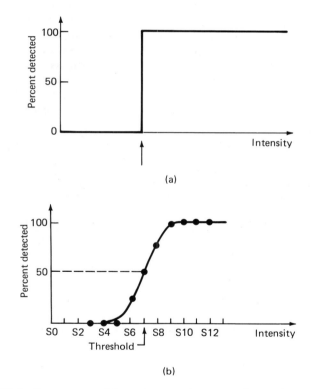

(a)

(b)

FIGURE 2-1 Percentage of detection as a function of stimulus intensities. (a) Result to be expected if there were a perfect
threshold for detection. (b) Psychometric function of the
kind generally obtained. Circles are the hypothetical data
of Table 2–1.

The ideal threshold that we were seeking was postulated to be a stimulus strength such that stimuli weaker than it would never be seen, and stimuli stronger than it would always be seen. We would then expect that a plot of percentage detection versus intensity would be represented by an abrupt change, or "step" function, as shown in Figure 2–1(a). The result of the experiment shown in Table 2–1, however, does not look like a step. The percentage detection values from the last column in Table 2–1 are plotted as a function of intensity in Figure 2–1(b). The circles can be fit with a smooth curve called an *ogive*, as shown. A curve of percentage detection versus intensity is called a *psychometric function*, and is generally an ogive.

One possible interpretation of the psychometric function is that the threshold has a slightly different value from trial to trial. This could happen either because the threshold is actually changing, or because there is a variable amount of extraneous, apparent stimulus added to the real stimulus (this is called *noise*). In any case, whatever the threshold is at a given moment, stimuli greater than threshold evoke a "yes" response, and stimuli less than it evoke a "no." Clearly, the threshold is rarely above S9 or below S4; it is usually around S7. It is usual to define the threshold stimulus as that stimulus intensity corresponding to 50% detection on the psychometric function; however, other criteria may also be used.

BOX 2–1

The previous paragraph indicates that the psychometric function represents the probability of the threshold being at each intensity or lower. That is, the psychometric function is the integral of the function describing the distribution of the threshold.[2] Suppose we assume that the distribution of the threshold is a normal-probability distribution, as shown by the bell-shaped curve in Figure 2–2(a). Integration of the normal distribution gives the cumulative-probability function shown in Figure 2–2(b). This function is similar to the ogives found for psychometric functions. We may therefore interpret the psychometric function to mean that the threshold takes on values distributed according to a normal probability distribution, with its peak at the 50% point on the psychometric function.

[2]An integral represents the sum of all the probabilities of obtaining each value up to some particular value, x. In other words, it is the area under the probability curve, from -∞ to x, or the probability of obtaining a value x or less. The integral of any probability distribution from -∞ to ∞ is 1.0—it is guaranteed to take *some* value.

So far we have treated the subject as a passive observer who does nothing but respond "yes" or "no" as stimuli are presented. There is a variant of the method of limits in which the subject is an active participant; it is called the *method of adjustment*, in which the subject has control of the stimulus intensity. When the stimulus is invisible, the subject presses a button that

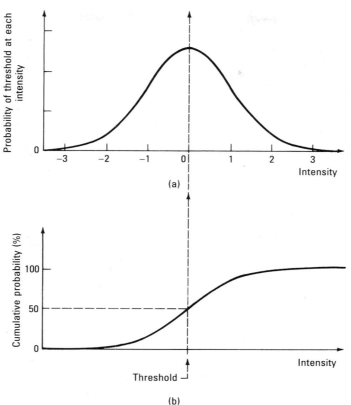

FIGURE 2-2 Interpretation of the psychometric function as a variable threshold. (a) A normal distribution representing the probability that the threshold will be at a particular intensity. (b) The psychometric function that would be obtained by integrating the curve in (a). Half the area of the curve in (a) is to the left of the vertical dashed line.

causes the succeeding stimulus to be stronger; when it is visible, pressing a different button causes the stimulus to be weaker next time. In this way, the subject "tracks" the threshold, wavering from just above to just below threshold. This is a rapid way to obtain threshold measurements, and is particularly useful when threshold is changing, such as during a period of dark adaptation (see Chapter 7).

Returning to the original hypothetical experiment, on each trial a slightly different threshold was measured. Suppose instead we begin the series with a more intense stimulus. In this case, the subject will probably say "no" to stronger stimuli. If we started with a stimulus less intense than S1, the subject would probably say "yes" at a lower intensity. There is a tendency to place the threshold according to how far down the list you think it should go, as well as whether the stimulus can actually be detected. It is good practice to start each series with a different first stimulus to avoid this effect, but the general objection still applies.

The experiments described, in which stimuli progressively increase in intensity until threshold is crossed, are called *ascending series*. Obviously, the opposite is possible: begin with clearly detectable stimuli, and gradually decrease intensity until the subject first responds, "no, I don't see it." This is called a *descending series*. The descending series suffers from the same drawback as the ascending series: the initial intensity at which the series begins can influence the point at which the subject reports threshold.

The problems associated with the method of limits are partly caused by the fact that at any point the subject knows how intense a stimulus to expect next. As the series of presentations progresses, the expected intensity changes, and the subject knows that succeeding stimuli will be either successively weaker or successively stronger. A second method of classical psychophysics is specifically designed to overcome this problem: it is called the *method of constant stimuli*. The order of presentation of the stimuli on any given trial is random, so the subject has no way of anticipating the intensity. It is not the stimuli that are constant, it is what the subject *expects* that does not change from trial to trial.

If the experiment of Table 2–1 were being run by the method of constant stimuli, we might present S6, then S2, then S1, then S8, and so forth, until each of the intensities was presented a sufficient number of times (say, 50). At each presentation of each stimulus, the subject would respond "yes" or "no," and a record would be made of the responses. Ultimately, a table such as the one in Table 2–1 would be completely filled in, and the percentage detection for each stimulus computed. Note that every stimulus must be presented on every trial; in the method of limits, the stimuli beyond threshold could be omitted.

The result of an experiment by the method of constant stimuli is a psychometric function like the one in Figure 2–1(b). From the function, the threshold can be determined.

This method overcomes some of the problems associated with the method of limits, but both suffer from vulnerability to the subjective whims of the observer. When a subject is asked to say, "yes, I see it," or "no, I don't," there is no control over the *criterion* applied in deciding whether a stimulus was actually present. One subject might refuse to say "yes" unless the stimulus was absolutely obvious, while another might be willing to claim seeing at the slightest hint. Worse, the same subject may switch criteria during the course of an experiment.

There is another classical method that removes the choice of criterion from the subject: the *method of forced choice*. The subject is presented with two or more alternatives, and must pick one even if the stimulus might not have been seen. For example, the stimulus might appear in either of two windows; after the presentation, the subject must respond by stating which window it was. Even if the subject does not know, a guess must be made. The question is not *whether*, but *which*.

Consider another hypothetical experiment using the same set of stimuli as shown in Table 2–1 and Figure 2–1(b). A stimulus light will appear in either the upper or lower window of a display, with both the stimulus intensity and location varying randomly from presentation to presentation. After each flash, the subject must respond "upper" or "lower"; depending on where it actually was, the answer is either right or wrong. The percentage correct is recorded for each stimulus level, and plotted as a psychometric function.

The results of this experiment are shown in Figure 2–3. Two features distinguish this psychometric function from that in Figure 2–1(b). First, there is 100% accuracy for stimulus values that were not detected 100% of the time in experiment 1. In effect, this method gives a lower threshold than either the method of constant stimuli or the method of limits. That is because in forced choice the subject must make a response; in the other methods the response can simply be "no" if the subject is unsure. Many of the responses can be guesses, but most subjects are surprised to learn (after the experiment) that while they thought they were just guessing they were getting many more correct than could be explained by chance.

The second difference is that the psychometric function derived from the forced choice experiment does not fall to 0% for weak stimuli; it levels off at 50%. This is readily understandable if one thinks about what the consequences of guessing will be. When the stimuli are intense, there is no question of whether to say "upper" or lower," and the score should be 100% (right side of Figure 2–3). When the stimuli are weaker, more mistakes are made. If the stimulus is actually below threshold, and invisible to the subject, a pure guess must be made. In saying "upper" or "lower" there is a 50-50 chance of being correct (the stimulus is in either one or the other). There may be runs of luck (just as there will be runs of straight heads in tossing a coin), but after enough trials the expected result is that the subject will get half right when the stimulus is not visible.

As 50% is the score expected for an invisible stimulus, it cannot be taken as the threshold. Figure 2–3 shows that the psychometric function is an ogive going from 50% to 100%. Threshold should be between the limits; the point analogous to threshold on the previous curve is at 75%.

The fact that the psychometric curve has its range limited between 50% and 100% makes it harder to measure threshold, especially as the probability of getting *exactly* 50% by guessing is small unless the number of trials is extremely large. It would be desirable to improve matters by making it difficult to do so well by guessing; this can be done by increasing the number of possible responses. In the hypothetical forced choice experiment just described, there were only two choices the subject could make; this is called a *two-alternative forced choice* paradigm, or *2AFC*. We could increase the number of alternatives to three, four, or more (3AFC, 4AFC, and so on). Con-

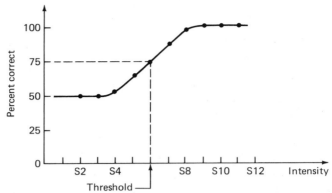

FIGURE 2-3 Psychometric function resulting from a hypothetical experiment in which the subject is required to choose which window a stimulus was in.

sider a 4AFC experiment: the subject's task is to state in which of four windows the stimulus appeared. The probability of guessing correctly when the stimulus is invisible is now one in four, or 25%. The psychometric function will thus run from 25% to 100%, and threshold will be defined as 62.5%. The more alternatives, the lower the expected score for guessing, but also the greater the chance of the subject becoming confused or missing the stimulus because it is difficult to attend to so many windows at once. As a result, the best performance is less than 100% when there are too many alternatives.

Before we leave this discussion of the classical methods used to measure thresholds, it is worth noting again that these methods can be, and have been, used to measure the sensory capabilities of animals. It is important to know that animal sensory systems are similar to humans', as sensory physiology must be done on animals. The ways these methods have been applied to animal work also serve as good examples of the use of psychophysics.

Blough (1955) used the method of adjustment to follow the change in threshold of a pigeon that had been exposed to a bright light. Pigeons were trained to peck at one key when a light appeared in a window, and another key when there was no light. Pecking the correct key a number of times resulted in a reward of food. The experiment was arranged so that pecking the key that meant "light present" caused the light to become weaker; pecking the key that meant "no light" caused it to become more intense. If the light was above threshold, the pigeon pecked the "present" key, which caused the light to become progressively dimmer until it was no longer above threshold. The pigeon would then switch keys; pecking the other ("no light") key caused the light to become brighter. When it was above threshold, the pigeon switched keys again, and the alternation continued for as long as a reward was provided. The setting of the light was always either just above or just below threshold, so threshold could be deduced from the average of several runs.

The method of constant stimuli has been applied by a number of workers to the problem of defining fishes' ability to detect colored lights (Otis, Cerf, & Thomas, 1957; Northmore & Muntz, 1974; Shefner & Levine, 1976). All of these workers used a classical conditioning procedure: the fish were administered electric shocks after the presentation of light. When it is shocked, a fish momentarily stops breathing, a wholly involuntary response. When light and shock have been paired often enough, light alone causes the involuntary gasp (this is exactly like Pavlov training dogs to salivate at the sound of a bell). Once the fish are trained, they are presented with the test stimuli. If the light evokes a gasp, the fish must have seen it (the gasp is its way of saying "yes"); if there is no gasp, it did not see the stimulus.

The 4AFC method has been used with success in many animals from pigeons to monkeys. An example is the comparison of the capabilities of human and monkey visual systems for detection of flickering of a light (DeValois, Morgan, Polson, Mead, and Hull, 1974). A monkey was trained to press the one panel in an array of four that was different from the other three. Correct selection gave the monkey a squirt of grape juice, which monkeys rather like. Once the monkey learned the task, all panels were illuminated with steady lights except the one with the intermittent test light in it; if the monkey chose that panel, it presumably could see the flicker (or guessed correctly). The procedure was repeated over and over, with different panels chosen and different rates of flicker, so that a psychometric function could be drawn and threshold deduced.

Differential Sensitivity

So far we have been considering only the problem of detection—can a subject see that a stimulus is present? The threshold for detection is the *absolute threshold* (sometimes abbreviated *RL*, for *Reiz limen*, a German/Latin concoction). But absolute threshold is only one possible kind of threshold: one could also ask whether the subject can detect a difference between two stimuli. The threshold for detection of differences is called the *difference threshold* (or *differential threshold*); it is often abbreviated *DL*, for *difference limen*, or *jnd* for *just noticeable difference*. In a sense, RL is a special case of DL—the detection of the difference from zero.

The jnd is the amount of change in a stimulus necesssary for it to be perceived as different. It is the difference between a test stimulus and a standard comparison stimulus. If we denote the intensity of the standard stimulus by I_0, and the intensity of the test stimulus by I_t, we are asking whether the subject can detect a difference of $(I_t - I_0)$ at the level I_0. It is usual to avoid having to write "$I_t - I_0$" by calling the difference "Delta I," written ΔI (Δ is the Greek letter *delta*, which is generally used in mathematics to indicate a difference). We define $\Delta I = (I_t - I_0)$. Here, ΔI is the difference between test and standard (but ΔI usually means the *threshold* difference between test and standard—that is, the jnd).

The measurement of jnd's can be made by any of the classical methods we have discussed. We could ask the subject whether a difference is visible, and by making the difference greater or smaller obtain the jnd by the method of limits. Alternatively, we could ask whether there is a noticeable difference, and present various random pairings of standard stimuli and test stimuli according to the method of constant stimuli. The forced choice method could be used by presenting the test and standard stimuli and asking which is brighter, or by presenting several (identical) standard stimuli and one test stimulus, and asking the subject to pick out the one that is different.

The result of a series of presentations is a psychometric function, like the ones in Figure 2–1(b) or Figure 2–3, except that the abscissa is ΔI instead of I. From the psychometric function a threshold value, the DL, can be deduced; this DL is the ΔI appropriate to the I_0 used. If a different I_0 had been taken, a different psychometric function would have been generated, and a different ΔI derived.

By measuring ΔI for a large number of I_0, we can develop a function that describes how the jnd changes for different levels of stimulation. If I_0 is some value of intensity of light, or sound, or weight, or pressure against the skin, increases in I_0 really would represent increases in the amount of stimulation. Variables of this type are called *prothetic continua;* they are variables in which a larger numerical value indicates a greater amount. Not all dimensions of a stimulus represent a change in amount of stimulation, however; some represent changes in the quality. It is also possible to ask how big a change is needed along a qualitative dimension; for example, how large a difference in frequency of sound is needed to produce a noticeable pitch difference, how large a difference in wavelength of light to produce a noticeable color difference? Increasing the frequency of sound makes the pitch higher, but one would not consider a higher pitched tone to be somehow "greater" than a low tone; similarly, a long wavelength light (which appears red) is not "more" of anything than a short wavelength light (which appears blue). Variables that do not imply a change in quantity are called *metathetic continua.* It is interesting and valid to ask how our frequency discrimination changes with pitch, or how well we can discriminate various similar colors, but it is not the same as asking how well we can discriminate at different levels of stimulation. The remainder of this discussion will be concerned with prothetic continua only.

The pioneering work on the relationship between ΔI and I_0 for prothetic continua was done by E. H. Weber in the 1830s. Weber found that the increment in stimulation required for a jnd was proportional to the size of the standard stimulus. That is,

$$\Delta I = kI_0$$

where k is a constant less than 1. This can be rewritten in the somewhat more familiar form

$$\frac{\Delta I}{I_0} = k$$

which simply says that the jnd is a constant fraction of the comparison stimulus.

Weber's law is a precise formulation that says the bigger the stimulus, the bigger the increment needed for change to be detectable. This should not be a surprise; stars that are invisible in the day are bright against the black night sky, $50 enriches a pauper, but far more is needed to change the net worth of a millionaire.

To understand Weber's law, it is easiest to consider an example. Weber found that the constant k (also known as the *Weber fraction*) for detection of additional weight on the finger is about 1/30. In other words, given two weights to compare, if one is exactly one pound, it will be just possible to detect a difference if the second is 1/30 pounds heavier, or about 1.033 pound. If the original weight were 2.0 lb, the DL would be approximately 0.067 lb; you could just discriminate between a 2.000-lb weight and a 2.067-lb weight. If you tried to discriminate between a 2.000-lb weight and a 2.033-lb weight (the same *difference* discriminated in the first case) you could not, for 0.033 is less than the DL for an I_0 of 2 lb. Given a 3-lb weight, the next heavier weight that could be discriminated would be about 3.100 lb; given a 6-lb weight, a 6.200-lb weight would be just noticeably different. The larger the standard weight, the larger the increment required.

BOX 2–2

The value of the Weber fraction, k, while constant over a reasonable range of stimulus strengths, is not the same for all sensory systems. In fact, the value of k in a given sensory modality can depend on how it is measured; for example, the Weber fraction for weights would be quite different if the weights were tested by placing one on each hand, rather than one after the other on the same hand. Similarly, the Weber fraction for brightness would depend on the size of the light tested, and how long the subject is allowed to look at each light.

Magnitude of Sensation

With Weber's law we move away from threshold stimulation, and can ask a rather different question: given a stimulus large enough to be clearly detectable, how large does it seem to be? Psychophysicists refer to this as the problem of *scaling*, which means measuring the psychological effect.

The first attempt to define the magnitude of sensation was done without actually making a measurement. Fechner, who devised the classical methods of psychophysics, used Weber's result to derive a theoretical relationship between stimulus magnitude and sensation. In fact, he was responsible for first stating Weber's law as a mathematical relationship, and probably is more responsible than Weber for bringing Weber's work to light (for this reason, Weber's law is sometimes referred to as the Weber-Fechner law).

Fechner did not believe it possible to measure sensation directly, but saw the jnd's of Weber's law as a potential scale for sensation. He made a bold assumption: all jnd's, being barely perceptible changes (by definition), are perceived as being equal changes in sensation. That is, the jnd's are the measure of sensation; the perceived magnitude of any stimulus is in proportion to the number of jnd's that it is above absolute threshold.

Figure 2–4 shows how the magnitude of sensation would be related to stimulus intensity according to Fechner. The Weber fraction is taken to be one-third (the approximate value for tasting differences in the saltiness of water). If we give the threshold stimulus the value 1, from threshold to 1 jnd above threshold is one-third unit on the abscissa. At that point there is a 1-jnd increase in the ordinate, representing a ''unit'' change in sensation. From that point, the next jnd is at 1.77; the change in the abscissa is just slightly larger than the first step, while the ordinate again increases by one unit. As we progress to larger I_0's the horizontal steps become longer. For example, at $I = 10$, $\Delta I = 3.33$ ($3.33 = 1/3$ of 10), which is larger than the first four steps put together. Since the vertical change is the same for each step, as the steps become wider, the climb becomes less steep. This is evident in Figure 2–4.

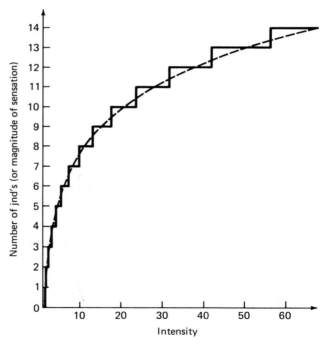

FIGURE 2-4   Fechner's derivation of how the apparent magnitude of the stimulus should relate to actual intensity, on the assumption that apparent magnitude is proportional to number of jnd's. The dashed curve is a log function.

Fechner used this argument to derive the form of the relationship between stimulus magnitude and sensation. Of course, the relationship is not a series of steps, but a smooth curve like the dashed curve drawn through the steps. The mathematical form of the curve that fits this shape is the logarithmic relationship (derived by integrating Weber's law); this is called Fechner's *log law*. It states that the magnitude of sensation (S) is proportional to the logarithm of the stimulus magnitude (I).

$$S = c \cdot \log (I)$$

Here, c is a constant of proportionality that can be directly related to the Weber fraction for the given sensory dimension.

Fechner's law says that the sensation grows as the logarithm of the stimulus. Put another way, constant *differences* in sensation are given by the same *ratios* of stimulation ($S_2 - S_1$ corresponds to $c \cdot \log I_2 - c \cdot \log I_1$, and subtraction of logarithms corresponds to division—see appendix). It is an extension of Weber's law (from which it is of course derived): the apparent difference between a 1-lb weight and a 3-lb weight is the same as the apparent difference between a 20-lb weight and a 60-lb weight.

Fechner's law should not be too surprising; we know that increments appear smaller against large backgrounds. The moon is sometimes visible in the day, but does not appear to be nearly as bright as it does at night. When we turn on a 50-100-150 three-way light, the biggest change comes when the light is turned on in a dark room; there is a noticeable increase when going from 50 to 100 watts, but practically no difference between the medium and high ranges (100 to 150 watts). The differences in light are all about the same—it is the compression of sensation with increased stimulation that makes the later increments seem smaller.

Fechner's law states that the apparent increment in sensation declines with increasing levels of stimulation (see Figure 2–4). It also means larger changes in stimulus are required for the same sensory effect at higher intensities. To go from the first to the third jnd in Figure 2–4 (a difference of 2 jnd's) requires a change in intensity from 1.33 to 2.37. This is a change of barely more than 1 intensity unit. But to go from the 10th to the 12th jnd (also a difference of 2 jnd's) requires a change in stimulation from 17.76 to 31.57, a difference of nearly 14 units. Notice, however, that the *ratios* of the changes are the same:

$$\frac{2.37 - 1.33}{1.33} = \frac{31.57 - 17.76}{17.76} = 0.78$$

In vision, the ratio of the change in light to the level of the background light is generally known as *contrast* (this particular definition is the *Weber contrast*; we shall encounter a slightly different definition of contrast in Chapter 10). What this relationship means, then, is that we obtain the same sensory effect when the contrast is the same. In essence, that is why a photograph looks the same whether it is viewed in dim light or bright: the contrast is a function of the print, not the illumination. Each bit of the photo reflects a given percentage of the incident light, so the ratio of light reflected from any two points is the same in any illumination.

What this means is that sensation grows less rapidly than the stimulus, and that large changes at high intensities are sometimes less noticeable than small changes at low intensities. The logarithm function proposed by Fechner has this "compressive" property. The curve relating sensation to stimulation in Figure 2–4 curves over and becomes less steep at high levels of stimulation. The logarithmic relationship was long believed to represent a truth, and even today some workers are attempting to find the way in which receptors "take the logarithms" of stimuli. The logarithm function is not the only curve that becomes less steep at high levels, however, and there is evidence that it may not be the correct one.

In the 1800s, J. A. F. Plateau measured the relationship of stimulus and sensation by asking artists to mix the shade of gray that lies exactly halfway between two given shades of gray, one light and one dark. He found a scale that implied ratios of sensation were related to ratios of stimulation, and proposed what is called a *power law*:

$$S = k \cdot I^n$$

where S is sensation, k is a constant, I is intensity, and n is an exponent to which the intensity is raised.

The power law was largely forgotten until the 1950s, when it was resurrected by S. S. Stevens (1956; 1957). Stevens took issue with Fechner's fundamental assumption that all jnd's are perceptually equal. Stevens said that even if 1 lb is a jnd for a 30-lb weight, and 0.1 lb is the jnd for a 3-lb weight, the observer somehow feels that the 1-lb jnd is larger than the 0.1-lb jnd.

Stevens proposed that equal physical ratios are psychologically equal; the mathematical relationship that satisfies this rule is the power law suggested by Plateau. Stevens also measured the relationship of stimulus and sensation by a method so simple it eluded investigators for 100 years: he asked the subjects how intense the stimulus appeared. This is called *direct scaling*.

As an example, the subject is presented with ten different intensities of light, and asked to assign a number to each one according to its relative brightness. This is called *magnitude estimation*, for the subject is being asked to estimate the magnitude of each stimulus. A standard light of a physical intensity we shall call "one unit,"[3] is presented to the subject, who is instructed to assign it a "brightness" rating of 1. Each of the other lights is then rated by the subject according to its relative brightness compared to the standard (several times each, so an average rating can be obtained), and the value of the rating plotted. Figure 2–5 (a) shows the result of this hypotheti-

---

[3]For our purposes, it does not matter what units are used to measure the light. In fact, strictly speaking, "intensity" is being misused throughout this chapter; technically, intensity refers to the light emitted by a point source. We shall continue to misuse the term in its colloquial sense of amount of light per unit area of a luminous source. For the correct terminology, see Chapter 4.

cal experiment. The 1-unit stimulus is rated 1, the 2-unit light is rated 1.4, the 16-unit light is rated 4. The smooth curve drawn to fit the "data" shows the property expected from Fechner's law: it becomes less steep as intensity increases. The smooth curve drawn, however, is not a logarithmic function; it is a power function: $S = I^{1/2} = \sqrt{I}$. This can be demonstrated by replotting this graph on log-log coordinates, as in Figure 2–5(b). Log-log coordinates (see appendix) mean that we are plotting the logarithm of the estimated magnitude versus the logarithm of the intensity. The logarithmic scale has the property of making ratios into differences. The logarithmic transform of intensity means we obtain constant ratio changes in intensity; the logarith-

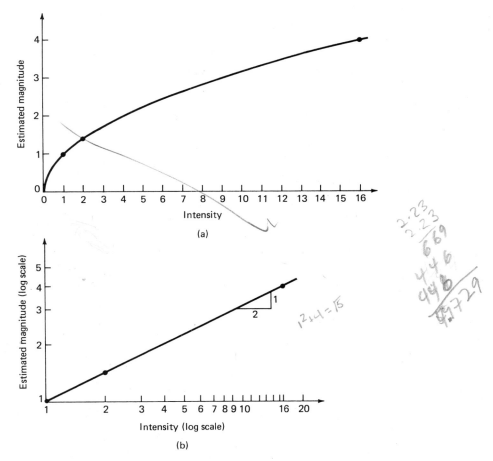

(a)

(b)

FIGURE 2–5 Hypothetical estimates of magnitude of stimulus as a function of actual intensity, assuming a power function. (a) Three "data" points plotted on linear scales. (b) The same data plotted on log-log coordinates (see appendix); they fall along a straight line with a slope of one-half.

mic transform of magnitude implies ratios of sensation. This was the defining characteristic of the power function as stated earlier, that ratios of stimulation lead to ratios of sensation.

A straight line on log-log coordinates implies a power function. This is the result Stevens obtained when he performed magnitude estimation experiments on brightness, loudness, weight, odor, and a number of other sensory stimuli. The exponents were different for different types of stimuli, but all plotted as straight lines on log-log coordinates, indicating power functions (Stevens, 1962). The slopes of the lines obtained represent the exponents of the power functions, as explained in the appendix.

There is a second method Stevens used to demonstrate power functions. It is called *magnitude production* and is just the inverse of magnitude estimation. Instead of being given a stimulus and asked to produce a number representing its intensity, the subject is given a knob controlling the intensity and asked to turn it until the stimulus intensity is some multiple of the standard intensity (this is just like what Plateau asked artists to do when he first discovered the power law). Subjects are quite consistent; the method of magnitude production gives results similar to those derived by the method of magnitude estimation.

The fact that different types of stimuli effective for different senses all gave power functions enabled Stevens to test the consistency of his data. This was done by a procedure called *cross-modal matching* (referring to two sensory modalities, or senses). The subject first is tested in two different sensory modalities so that the exponent for each can be estimated. This may be done either by magnitude estimation or magnitude production. The subject then is asked to match stimuli of one type by producing an equivalently intense stimulus of the other type. The instruction is "turn this knob until the sound you hear is as loud as the light in front of you is bright." Surprisingly, subjects can do this without becoming confused.

The data produced by the cross-modal match are intensities in one modality that match intensities in the other. They are plotted on log-log coordinates. If the power law was a correct description of the sensation/stimulation functions in each modality, the resultant plot will be a straight line whose slope is the ratio of the exponents found for each modality. This is the result Stevens obtained.

BOX 2-3

The assertion that a power law will give the result of a straight-line log-log plot in cross-modal matching is relatively easy to show. For each modality, there is a power function; let us indicate the modalities as 1 and 2, and sub-script all the variables to indicate which modality is being considered. The conditions for which a match is made occur when the sensation in modality 1 is the "same" as that in mo-

(continued)

(box continued)

dality $2: S_1 = S_2$. If we write out the power law for each, we obtain

$$S_1 = k_1 \cdot I_1{}^{n_1} = S_2 = k_2 \cdot I_2{}^{n_2}$$

or

$$k_1 \cdot I_1{}^{n_1} = k_2 \cdot I_2{}^{n_2}$$

Taking the logarithm of both sides gives

$$\log(k_1) + \log(I_1{}^{n_1}) = \log(k_2) + \log(I_2{}^{n_2})$$

or, rearranging terms and expanding the logarithms of the exponentials,

$$n_1 \cdot \log(I_1) = n_2 \cdot \log(I_2) + \log(k_2) - \log(k_1)$$

so

$$\log(I_1) = \frac{n_2}{n_1} \log(I_2) + \frac{1}{n_1} \log\left(\frac{k_2}{k_1}\right)$$

We are plotting $\log(I_1)$ versus $\log(I_2)$, so the ordinate $y = \log(I_1)$ and the abscissa $x = \log(I_2)$. Substitution gives

$$y = \left(\frac{n_2}{n_1}\right) x + \frac{1}{n_1} \log\left(\frac{k_2}{k_1}\right)$$

which is the equation of a straight line with a slope of n_2/n_1.

Ekman (1964), however, has shown that the results of cross-modal matching would be the same even if Fechner's log law were correct. Ekman's derivation is virtually the same as that shown in the preceding paragraph, but each S is defined by a logarithm:

$$S_1 = c_1 \cdot \log(I_1) = c_2 \cdot \log(I_2)$$

There is no need to take logarithms of each side; simply rearrange terms:

$$\log(I_1) = \frac{c_2}{c_1} \log(I_2)$$

As before, we substitute $x = \log(I_2)$ and $y = \log(I_1)$:

(continued)

$$y = \frac{c_2}{c_1} x$$

Again, a straight line results for the cross-modal match.

Ekman's argument is more damaging than simply demonstrating that the cross-modal match does not demonstrate a power law. It may be carried a step further: the very process of magnitude estimation (or magnitude production) may itself be considered a cross-modal match in which one modality is our perception of the number system (Attneave, 1962). There is reason to believe that we perceive numbers in a compressed fashion (Schneider, Parker, Ostrosky, Stein, & Kanow, 1974). For example, our perception of the values of money (expressed by numbers) behaves similarly to the perception of light or sound. Is a quarter a lot of money? It is a big price increase for a candy bar, but irrelevant to the price of a computer. If numbers are treated as still another sensory input, magnitude estimation is really nothing more than cross-modal matching against the sense of numerosity. By Ekman's argument, a straight-line log-log plot must result, regardless of whether the sensory stimulus is transformed according to a log law or a power law. Thus Stevens has not demonstrated that the power law is more appropriate than the log law (Rushton, 1961b).

We do not mean to imply that the idea of a power law is wrong. Various lines of evidence have implicated a power function rather than a logarithmic function (Easter, 1968a; Levine & Abramov, 1975; Schneider et al., 1974), and the argument in the previous paragraph does not *disqualify* a power function. There is still controversy over which formulation may be correct. It is even possible that both the power function and the logarithmic function are valid. Wasserman, Felsten, and Easland (1979)

(box continued)
have argued that a logarithmic function seems most appropriate when responses must be made at the instant a stimulus appears, but a power function is obtained when the subject is allowed to consider the stimulus for a longer period of time.

Richard Warren (1981) argues that the psychophysical measurements may not really relate to the intensity versus response functions of sensory systems. And perhaps the relationship is neither a power function nor a logarithmic one. After all, why must a physiological system produce a mathematically neat and concise function? The various operations and relationships could effectively produce a function similar to a logarithmic or power function. The important feature is shared by both: the relationship between stimulus and sensation is a downward curve, so larger increments are needed to have similar effects at higher stimulus levels.

Static Invariances

There is another question related to the perception of differences; that of how stimulus parameters can be changed in tandem in order that two quite different stimuli can be judged the same. In discussing the jnd, we asked for the minimal change of one parameter, such as intensity, that could be made so that the difference would be detectable. Now we ask how one parameter can be changed so that it will compensate for changes in another. If the correct compensation is made, the subject will judge that the two stimuli are the same in some way (although in most cases it is still possible to discriminate between them).

There are two classes of static invariances to consider. In the first class, the total energy is held constant, but we change the way it is delivered; the subject is asked to make judgments of intensity. In the second class, there is no attempt to equalize energy; the judgments of the subject will be that the stimuli are alike in a particular quality. In a way, these two classes parallel the distinction between prothetic and metathetic continua.

As an example of the first class of invariances, consider a circular spot of light. The total energy in that stimulus depends on three things: (1) the *intensity* of the light (technically, the *radiance*)—that is, how much light is issuing from the stimulus per unit area; (2) the *area* of the stimulus; and (3) the *duration* of the stimulus (how long it is present). The total energy delivered within the stimulus is the product of these three numbers. Let us consider them two at a time.

First, suppose that the duration is constant; all test flashes last the same amount of time. The total energy depends on the product of area and radiance. We can test a subject with spots of different areas, and ask (for each area) what radiance will result in sensations of equal "brightness." Usually, the brightness chosen is the threshold, so we ask what radiance is necessary to reach absolute threshold for each spot's diameter (Figure 2–6).

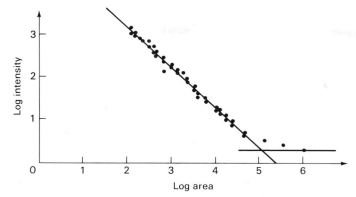

FIGURE 2-6 Log radiance needed to reach threshold as a function of log area of the test spot. The slanted line declines with a slope of − 1, indicating a trade-off between area and radiance (Ricco's law). The horizontal line indicates a failure of the relationship for large areas. Data from Graham, C. H. and N. R. Bartlett (1939). The relation of size of stimulus and intensity in the human eye. II. Intensity thresholds for red and violet light. *J. Exp. Psychol.* 24:514–587.

For small spots, the radiance required is inversely proportional to the area; this is known as *Ricco's law*. Simply put, it requires half the radiance to see a spot that is twice as large an area (1.4 times the diameter). Notice, however, that because the total energy is proportional to area times radiance, the same total energy is present in both cases. The threshold energy is the same, regardless of whether all the light is condensed into a small intense spot, or is spread out into a larger but less intense disc. We must point out that this does *not* mean the subject cannot tell the difference between a large dim spot and a small intense one, only that the two are equivalently detectable.

Ricco's law implies a trade-off between area and radiance; however, the law only applies for sufficiently small areas. When the spots become too large, additional area gives no additional advantage for detection (see Figure 2–6). Beyond this point, the radiance remains the same despite increases in area (and the total energy required increases as area increases). This means that there is a trade-off between area and radiance, but only so long as the energy falls within some limited area. This area, within which Ricco's law applies, is called *Ricco's area*, or the *summing area*. It is assumed that signals arising within that area sum together to give a signal that ultimately reaches threshold, but beyond some distance the signals no longer affect that area.

Suppose we now choose a particular stimulus size, and vary instead the duration of the stimulus. Rather than asking the threshold radiance for each of several areas, we ask the threshold radiance for each of several durations of stimulus flash. The result is analogous to Ricco's law: the threshold radiance is inversely related to the flash duration. As the total energy in the flash is the product of duration and radiance, this means that the same total energy is required to reach threshold, regardless of how it is distributed in time. An extremely brief flash of high radiance is equally as detectable as a longer flash of lower radiance. This relationship is called *Bloch's law*. Like Ricco's law, Bloch's law has an upper limit, usually about 1/10 sec (Graham, 1965). Once this critical duration has been reached, there is no further advantage to increasing the time in which the stimulus is present. This implies that the visual system sums lights over a relatively limited period of time.

The auditory system also sums energy it receives. There is no good spatial analog of Ricco's law, for the ears do not detect the size of a sound source, but there is an analog of Bloch's law (it has apparently never been given a specific name). Garner (1947) has shown that there is a trade-off between intensity and duration of threshold tones, indicating summation of signals in time.

The second class of static invariances is qualitative; that is, the invariances are not concerned with the distribution of energy in stimuli but with finding physically different stimuli that are the same in a particular qualitative way. If the quality in question is "brightness," we are simply asking what the capabilities of the system are as a function of another variable. For example, we could ask how the absolute threshold for lights varies as wavelength (color) changes, or how the absolute threshold for sound varies as the frequency (pitch) changes. In each instance, we are finding the capability of the visual or auditory system.

There are other static invariances that do not simply reflect the capability of the system. For example, the color (hue) of a light is generally associated with its wavelength, while its energy determines the *luminance* (brightness). It would seem that if we had a light of a particular wavelength, changing the energy should simply make it brighter or dimmer, but not affect the hue. This turns out not to be true. When energy is increased, the colors generally change slightly. A red light made brighter also becomes yellower; violet lights become bluer. This is called the *Bezold-Brücke hue shift*. To maintain the same hue as the energy changes, the wavelength must be changed. The Bezold-Brücke hue shift is not easy to explain (and not all color theoreticians agree on one explanation), but is a complication to be aware of when reading about color in Chapter 15.

BOX 2-4

The Bezold-Brücke hue shift can be demonstrated by placing a frosted white light bulb in front of a white wall. Look at the combination through a piece of red filter; presumably, the light from the bulb and the light from the wall are the same except that the light from the bulb is more intense. It should be apparent that the bulb appears yellow compared to the red of the wall.

An effect similar to the Bezold-Brücke hue shift is found in audition. It is generally held that he frequency of vibration of a sound wave determines the pitch of sound, while intensity (amplitude of vibration) determines loudness. If, however, a sound of a particular frequency has its intensity increased, the pitch changes slightly. A low-frequency (low-pitched hum) tone seems even lower (more basso) when the intensity increases. There is also a shift of high frequencies, such that high-frequency tones seem even higher pitched when made more intense. To maintain the same pitch when intensity increases, the frequency must be changed. More will be said of these phenomena in Chapter 18.

SIGNAL DETECTION THEORY

In modern psychophysics, the concept of the threshold has fallen into some disrepute. It is still useful for defining the capabilities of a sensory system, but the idea that there is an actual threshold or limen does not seem to be a satisfactory model for the way in which a subject determines whether there is a stimulus present. Many workers now prefer the concept of *detectability* of a stimulus, a term that can include all the decision criteria, vagaries of attention, and capabilities of the sensory system.

There is also a shortcoming to classical psychophysics: all the data are concerned with whether the subject sees a stimulus when it is actually there; there is no consideration of performance on trials in which there is no stimulus. In those cases, the subject could also be right or wrong, by correctly saying "no" when there was nothing, or by incorrectly saying a stimulus was seen that was, in fact, not there ("false alarm"). Signal detection theory, adapted from a theory developed to analyze communication systems, was intended to overcome these shortcomings (Swets, Tanner, & Birdsall, 1961).

Signal detection theory assumes that there is "noise" in the system. Noise means just what it seems to: something that interferes with "hearing" what you are intended to hear. For instance, if a radio develops a loud hum, the hum is a noise that makes it harder for you to hear the programs. The noise referred to by signal detection theory, however, is not a constant hum, it is an ever-varying level of neural activity of a type exactly like the nervous system's responses to the stimulus. There is a background level of activity in the nervous system, and sensory signals are superimposed on this activity. Noise is thus present in vision and the other senses, as well as in audition.

Noise varies at random. The activation of the sensory system during a period when a stimulus could have been (but in fact was not) present could be large, small, or in between; it is assumed that the distribution of the noise is a normal distribution, as shown by the leftmost bell-shaped curve in Figure 2–7 (marked N). The curve is centered about the *mean* (average) value of the noise, indicated $\bar{x}_N$. The variability of the noise (how much it tends to change) is given by a measure called its standard deviation, indicated by σ_N.

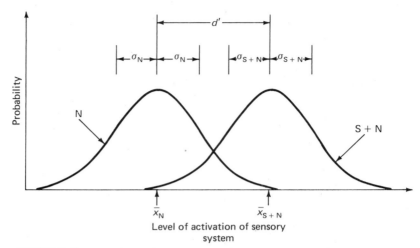

FIGURE 2–7   Hypothetical activations of a sensory system from noise in the absence of a signal (N) or a signal with the superimposed noise (S+N). The means of each distribution are indicated on the abscissa ($\bar{x}_N$ and $\bar{x}_{S+N}$), and the difference between the means at the top (d'). Standard deviations of each are shown (σ_N and σ_{S+N}).

N is the distribution of activation in the sensory channel in the absence of any stimulus. The stimulus, when it is present, simply adds some amount of activity to the noise to give the activation caused by stimulus plus noise. Activation of the sensory system when the stimulus is present will thus be given by a distribution exactly like that of the noise distribution, but shifted to a higher mean by the amount of activation from the stimulus. This is shown in Figure 2–7 as the curve marked S+N.

The observer's task in a detection experiment is to say whether the activation during a given trial was just noise, or stimulus plus noise. That is, it must be decided whether what was sensed was part of the distribution N or part of the distribution S+N. How well this can be done is determined by how far apart the two distributions are relative to their variability. If the difference is small, the two are almost completely overlapped, and any particular activation could equally well have come from either. If the difference is large (compared to the variability), there will be two quite distinct distributions; the one for N will include only small values of activation, and the one for S+N will include only large values of activation. The observer's choice is simple: if there is a large activation, choose S+N; if there is a small activation, choose N. The distance between the two distributions thus determines the *detectability*, or how well the subject can discriminate. Detectability is labelled *d'*, and is expressed in units of the standard deviation of the distributions. The larger *d'*, the more "detectable" the signal is. The problem of signal detection theory is to measure the d' for the presumed distributions of N and S+N. In a way, d' is equivalent to t in testing the statistical significance of the difference between two distributions.

Let us consider a case in which d' is moderate, as in Figure 2–8. How might a subject decide whether a given activation was from N or S+N? An ''ideal'' observer will set a *criterion;* that is, choose a particular value of activation and say: ''all values greater than this I shall call 'stimulus,' all values less I shall call 'noise'.'' Performance will depend on what criterion is chosen. For example, if it is essential to spot every stimulus that was given, one might set a lax criterion (marked *A* in Figure 2–8). Very few stimuli will be presented that will not be spotted, but at the expense of making lots of false alarms. In fact, ''stimulus present'' will be said on a large majority of the trials, whether it is there or not. This might be the way a pilot would react to blips on the radar that could be another plane with which to collide. Better to pay attention and plan to get out of the way, than to say, ''probably not, let's just see what happens.''

On the other hand, the subject might feel it more important to avoid making false alarms, and set a criterion that is quite strict (such as *B* in Figure 2–8). With a strict criterion, the subject will rarely admit to seeing something that is not there, but will similarly miss a lot of actual presentations. This might be the tactic of the person watching the early warning radar: better to be sure the blips on the screen are enemy missiles than to start a nuclear holocaust over a flight of sparrows.

The actual strategies of observers are likely to be somewhere between these extremes. Ideally, the criterion will be set so that most responses are correct. Consider the performance of a subject who sets the criterion at *C* in Figure 2–8. This subject will correctly identify the stimulus the majority of times that it is presented, for more than half of the distribution of S+N is above the criterion. The subject will correctly reject the noise a majority of the times that no signal is presented, for more than half of the N distribution lies below the criterion. There will inevitably be two kinds of errors: when the stimulus is actually presented but the activation is below the criterion (the probability of this happening is represented by the darker gray area in Figure 2–8) the subject will say nothing is seen even though the stimulus is present. This is referred to as a ''miss.'' When there is no signal but the level of activation is above the criterion level, there will be a false alarm (the probability of this is represented by the light gray area in Figure 2–8).

The effect of differences in criterion such as we have been describing can be seen by plotting for each criterion level the probability of ''hits'' (saying the stimulus was present when it in fact was—this is the white area in the lower part of Figure 2–8) versus the probability of false alarms (saying it was when it was not—the shaded area in the upper part of Figure 2–8). (Criterion must be changed in separate experimental sessions, and the same stimulus intensity always used.) This plot, shown in Figure 2–9, is called on *ROC curve* (for ''receiver operating characteristic''—remember that signal detec-

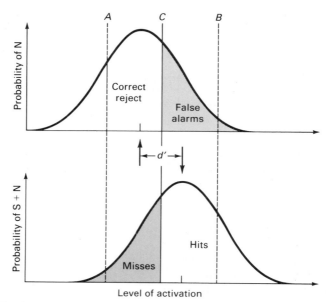

FIGURE 2-8   Noise and signal + noise distributions, with three possible decision criteria (*A, B,* and *C*) discussed in the text. The shaded areas represent the proportions of misses and false alarms to be expected if criterion *C* is used. Note that the white area representing hits extends under the light gray area, and the white area representing correct rejects extends under the dark gray area.

tion theory was originally derived from communication engineering). As the criterion changes, the probabilities of hits and false alarms both change. If the criterion is lax (at *A* in Figure 2–8), the probability of hits is high, close to unity. The probability of false alarms is also fairly high, as the subject says "yes" almost every time that the stimulus is *not* present. The subject with closed eyes who just said "yes" every time would plot a point in the upper right-hand corner, never missing a stimulus, but also making a false alarm every time there was no stimulus.

The subject with a high criterion does no better (Figure 2–8, at *B*); almost never having a false alarm, but also missing most of the stimuli. This subject plots a point near the lower left corner of the ROC curve; both the hit rate and false alarm rate are nearly zero. The subject with closed eyes who said "no" every time would never claim to see a stimulus that was not there but would also never detect a stimulus that was present.

Finally, the middle criterion shown in Figure 2–8 at *C*, would lead to the point on the ROC curve in the upper left quadrant. The percentage of stimuli correctly "hit" should be over 50%, while the percentage of noise presentations incorrectly called a stimulus (false alarms) should be under 50%.

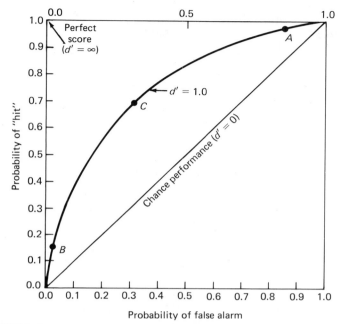

FIGURE 2–9 ROC curve expected for the noise and signal + noise curves in Figure 2–7. The points corresponding to criteria *A, B*, and *C* are indicated, as are the diagonal line corresponding to chance performance ($d' = 0$) and the point of perfect detection ($d' = \infty$).

The smooth curve in Figure 2–9 is what would be traced as the criterion changed between the extremes. The entire curve corresponds to a particular distance between the S+N and N distributions relative to their standard deviation—that is, to a particular d'. The value of d' is determined by the strength of the stimulus relative to the noise in the subject's nervous system. More about how to determine d' may be found in the appendix.

Now consider the straight line running from the lower left to upper right-hand corner (main diagonal). This line corresponds to a d' of 0, or no difference between the S+N and N distributions. Any point along the diagonal represents purely chance performance; if the observer closed his or her eyes and just said "yes" or "no" at random (so there is no difference between the S and S+N distributions), a point should be plotted on the diagonal. The position along the diagonal at which the point falls depends on the relative proportion of yesses and nos. If the response is always "yes" or always "no," a point will be plotted in the upper right corner or lower left corner, respectively. If the answer is "yes" 50% of the time, 50% of the stimuli will be hit, making a false alarm on 50% of the noise presentations (plot in the very center of the graph). Whatever is the probability of a hit will also be the probability of a false alarm.

In order (reliably) to plot to the left of the diagonal, the subject must be able to detect the stimulus to some extent. As the detectability, d', increases the curve moves up and to the left, until a stimulus that could never be confused with noise (perfectly detectable) would plot at the upper left corner. The upper left corner represents a perfect score: it indicates detection of every stimulus and correct rejection on every trial in which there was only noise.

In order to trace out more than a single point on an ROC curve (corresponding to the criterion chosen by the subject), we must make the subject change the criterion from experimental session to experimental session. Subjects can be "coerced" to change their criteria and trace out a curve by a number of means. One way to manipulate this is by changing a "payoff matrix." We have been assuming the subject is working for free, or that any payment is not going to depend on the performance. Suppose we designate payment of some amount, say 5¢, for every correctly spotted stimulus. If there is no penalty for false alarm, a clever subject can maximize the take by saying "yes" every time, or at any rate every time there is even a possibility of a stimulus. On the other hand, suppose there is also a 5¢ deduction for every false alarm; the subject who says "yes" every time will not earn anything, unless the stimulus presentations outnumber the noise presentations. In this case, the subject is well advised to say "yes" only when it is fairly certain the stimulus is actually present. The more punishing the penalty for false alarms the more care the subject must take; if there is no reward for correct answers, only a deduction for false alarms, it would be advisable to say "no" every time. Given these instructions, subjects trace out ROC curves such as theory predicts, although few subjects actually adopt as extreme criteria as might be optimal.

Signal detection theory provides a way of measuring the detectability of a stimulus, whether it can be seen, regardless of the criterion employed by the subject. It gets away from the notion of the threshold, but what it substitutes (detectability) is also a measure of the capabilities of the system. In fact, the area under the ROC curve gives the probability of a correct response in 2AFC, so signal detection measures can be related directly to classical psychophysics.

SUGGESTED READINGS

It is hard to find a book that deals exclusively with the techniques of psychophysics. We recommend a book of collected readings by W. S. Cain and L. E. Marks, called *Stimulus and Sensation* (Little, Brown and Co., Boston, 1971). In it are slightly abridged versions of articles that tell the story of psychophysics, including a good general introduction to classical psychophysics by J. C. Stevens (reprinted from the *International Encyclopedia of the Social Sciences*, D. L. Sills, editor; Vol. 13, pages 120–126, 1968). It also includes articles on static invariances, scaling and the Weber-Fechner-Stevens laws, signal detection theory, animal psychophysics, and a classical detection experiment by Hecht, Shlaer, and Pirenne (1942) that is perhaps the most elegant we have encountered.

A second account of some of the same topics may be found in W. R. Uttal's book *The Psychobiology of Sensory Coding* (Harper and Row, 1973). Chapter 6 includes signal detection theory, classical psychophysics, scaling, and a description of the Hecht, Shlaer, and Pirenne study.

GENERAL NEUROPHYSIOLOGY

3

It is impossible to talk about sensation without some knowledge of the structures responsible for receiving, integrating, and transmitting sensory information. In this chapter, we briefly describe some of the properties of the basic unit of our sensory systems: the neuron. We discuss how the neuron codes and transmits information, as well as how information is passed from one neuron to another. No pretense of thoroughness is made; the purpose of this chapter is not to create experts in the field of neurophysiology but merely to provide enough information for our discussions of sensory systems.

THE STRUCTURE OF THE NEURON

The cells of the nervous system are called neurons. Neurons come in many sizes, shapes, and configurations, depending on the function they are designed to perform. They have some structures in common with other cells in the body; these include a nucleus, a cell body, and organelles that are important for the metabolic and respiratory well-being of the cell. Neurons possess some specialized structures not found in other cells, however. One of these is the *dendrite*, shown on the left of Figure 3–1. The word dendrite is derived from the Greek word for tree, and it is obvious that the dendrites in the figure do indeed resemble the branches of a tree. The distinguishing characteristic of dendrites is their function; they are the structures that receive information from other neurons, through contacts called *synapses* (from the Greek for "coming together").

Information received in the dendrites of a neuron is processed, and the resultant signal is transmitted along another specialized neuronal structure: the *axon*. Axons are usually long thin tubes that can vary in length from several thousandths of a millimeter to more than a meter. They end in a structure called the *axon terminal* that is specialized for the transmission of information from one cell to another. Neurons may have a large number of axon terminals for information transmission to a large number of neurons.

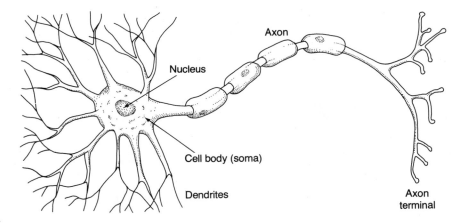

FIGURE 3-1   Sketch of a generalized neuron.

THE RESTING MEMBRANE POTENTIAL

The signals that are transmitted and processed by the nervous system are electrical in nature; in order to understand how information transmission is accomplished, we must have at least an intuitive understanding of some basic electrical concepts.

Charge, Potential Difference, Current, and Resistance

Consider the electrical circuit shown in Figure 3–2. In the left of this figure is a battery with two poles; one is labeled +, and the other is labeled − . Across the two poles is a potential difference (or voltage difference); for a normal flashlight battery, the potential difference is 1.5 volts. The difference in electrical potential between the two poles of the battery is the driving force in the circuit, causing a movement of electrons through the circuit. This flow of electrons is called electrical *current*; its magnitude depends on the magnitude of the potential difference produced by the battery, and the amount of *resistance* in the circuit. In most electric circuits, the device that is actually doing work (in this case, the light bulb) is also providing some resistance; that is, it tends to impede the free movement of electrons in the circuit.

Ions

In the electrical circuit in Figure 3–2, current is mediated by the passage of electrons within the wire. In the neuron, however, potential differences cause movement of charged particles called *ions*. An ion is an atom with either too few or too many electrons, producing a particle with either a positive or a negative charge, respectively. As an example, consider common

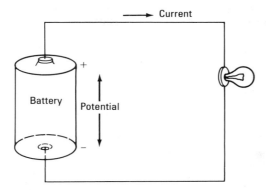

FIGURE 3-2 A simple electrical circuit.

table salt, sodium chloride (NaCl). When sodium chloride is dissolved in water, the sodium and chlorine atoms break away from each other; however, each chlorine atom takes one of the electrons formerly belonging to a sodium atom. The two atoms are said to be ionized; the chlorine has a charge of -1 (Cl^-) because it has one extra (negatively charged) electron, while the sodium now carries a charge of $+1$ (Na^+) from having lost one electron. Movement of these charged particles constitutes an electrical current just the same as does movement of electrons in a wire.

Now let us consider the axon schematically displayed in Figure 3–3. Although the axons of most neurons are extremely small (often less than 1 micron in diameter), certain invertebrates have cells with giant axons, often as large as 1 mm in diameter. Thus it proved possible as early as the 1940s to insert thin wires inside the giant axon, and measure the potential difference between the inside and outside of the cell. This potential difference was found to be approximately -70 mV (mV is millivolts, or thousandths of a volt; 70 mV = 0.07 volts) for the squid giant axon; experiments from other animals have yielded similar values. This potential difference is called the *resting membrane potential* of the neuron; it is analogous to the potential difference across the poles of a battery. Another way to describe the potential difference is to say that the membrane is *polarized*; that is, it has a negative side (inside) and a positive side (outside).

The fact that the interior of nerve cells is about 70 mV more negative than the extracellular fluid is of fundamental importance for the function of individual neurons. It is therefore worth considering how this potential difference arises. Figure 3–4 illustrates the ionic environment both inside and outside the neuron. Inside the cell (intracellular space) there is water with a relatively high concentration of potassium ions (K^+) and large negatively charged protein molecules (Pr^{--}). Outside the cell (extracellular space) there is water with a relatively high concentration of sodium (Na^+) and chloride (Cl^-) ions.

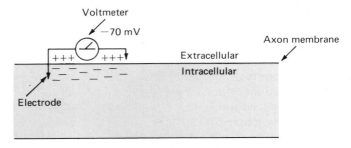

FIGURE 3-3   Measurement of the resting membrane potential across the membrane of an axon.

Suppose the positive charges and negative charges exactly balanced each other in both the extracellular and intracellular spaces, despite the fact that the charged particles were of different types. In this case, both the inside and outside of the cell would have no net charge, and the potential difference across the membrane would be zero. If no particles could cross the cell membrane, the potential difference would remain at zero forever. Consider, how-

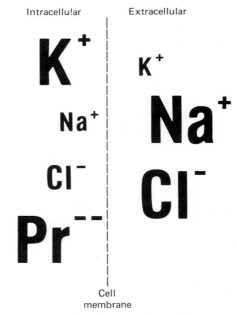

FIGURE 3-4   Ionic environments inside and outside a neuron. In the intracellular space are high concentrations of K^+ and large negative protein ions (Pr^{--}), with smaller concentrations of Na^+ and Cl^-. In the extracellular space are high concentrations of Na^+ and Cl^-, with relatively small amounts of K^+.

ever, what would happen if the cell membrane were permeable (that is, allowed passage) to potassium (K$^+$) ions and nothing else. Because there is much more potassium inside the cell, there would be a tendency for potassium ions to diffuse out of the cell into the extracellular space. The tendency for potassium ions to diffuse out of the cell would continue until there were equal concentrations of potassium inside and outside of the cell. Remember, however, that potassium is positively charged, so as it leaves the cell, it removes positive charge from inside the cell, and increases the positive charge on the outside. Thus, the inside of the cell would become negative with respect to the outside. This would tend to decrease the rate of potassium moving out of the cell, as positive particles are attracted to areas of negative charge, and repelled from areas of positive charge. Therefore, as more positive particles leave the cell, the electrical force that tends to move them back into the cell would become stronger. At some point in the process, the diffusion force tending to make potassium ions leave the cell would be identical to the electrical force pushing them back into the cell. There would still be a higher concentration of potassium inside than outside the cell, but just as many ions would be pushed into the cell because of electrical force as would be pushed outside by diffusion. At that point, there would be no net flow of potassium into or out of the cell.

The electrical potential difference that exactly counteracts the diffusion force is called the *equilibrium potential*. Its actual value depends on the relative concentrations of ions inside and outside the cell; for the concentrations of potassium measured in the squid giant axon, the equilibrium potential for potassium is equal to -75 mV. If the cell membrane were permeable to potassium and no other ions, the resting membrane potential would be exactly equal to the equilibrium potential for potassium. The cell membrane in its resting state, however, is also slightly permeable to sodium (Na$^+$) and chloride (Cl$^-$); because of this added complication, the resting potential is actually slightly less negative than the equilibrium potential for potassium.

In summary, the resting membrane potential of a neuron is about -70 mV, and it comes about for three interacting reasons: (1) the nerve cell membrane is most permeable to potassium ions; (2) the concentration of potassium ions is much higher inside the cell than outside; and (3) other ions can cross the membrane, though less easily than potassium.

ELECTROTONIC CONDUCTION

We have so far described the electrical behavior of the neuronal axon at rest; the next step is to investigate how the axon responds to small electrical stimuli. In Figure 3–5, an electrode is inserted into the axon at point 0 along its length; this electrode is connected to a source of voltage (for example, a battery) that injects a small amount of positive current into the axon at the location of the electrode. Therefore, the membrane potential at point 0 will

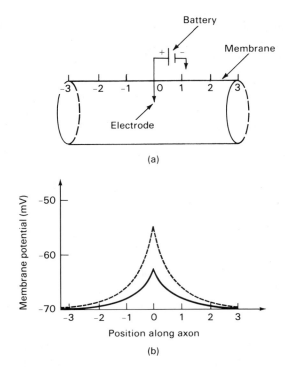

(a)

(b)

FIGURE 3-5 Spread of depolarization along the axon. (a) Stimulating electrode is placed inside the axon at the point shown. (b) Graph showing the spread of depolarization for two different strengths of stimulation.

not be equal to the resting membrane potential but will be somewhat less negative. What effect does this electrical stimulus at point 0 have at other locations along the membrane? From the solid curve in Figure 3–5(b), you can see that the effect of the stimulus is to *depolarize* (reduce the potential difference) the membrane in the region surrounding the electrode. As one measures the membrane potential at greater distances from the electrode, the amount of depolarization decreases, and finally the recorded voltage becomes indistinguishable from the normal resting potential.

Suppose the battery in Figure 3–5(a) is replaced by a stronger one, so that the amount of positive current injected into the axon is greater than before. If the stimulus is still fairly weak, its effect on membrane potential as a function of distance from the stimulus will be as shown by the dashed curve in Figure 3–5(b). The amount of depolarization in the region immediately surrounding the electrode will be greater than for the previous stimulus; this will be the case at any distance from the electrode. The potential change caused by the stimulus still decreases with distance, however, and will be indistinguishable from the resting potential at some distance not too far from the electrode tip.

This type of neuron behavior is called *electrotonic spread*, or *decremental conduction*. The potentials conducted in this way are called *slow potentials*, despite the fact that they are transmitted almost instantaneously.

BOX 3-1

To understand the way that the potential changes decrease with distance from the stimulus, think about a very leaky garden hose, as shown in Figure 3–6. Imagine that the hose is extremely long, and perforated with large, equal-sized holes all along its length. Water enters with some pressure (which is the "potential" of a fluid system) through the tap at the left end. It spurts vigorously from the holes near the tap. Farther from the tap, the pressure is less. The pressure drops because of the resistance of the hose and the water lost through the holes between the tap and the target hole. The lower pressure can be seen by the smaller geysers near the right side of the figure. Eventually, the geysers become trickles, until there is virtually no water coming from the hose very far from the tap.

How far from the tap must you look to find negligible flow? That will depend on the diameter of the hose, the size of the holes, and the pressure at the tap. A fatter hose carries water with less loss of pressure than a skinny hose; the larger the holes, the more water is lost per unit length of hose. In fact, it is the ratio of hole size (or number) to hose diameter that will determine how rapidly the pressure falls. Figure 3–6(a) shows a hose with small holes; Figure 3–6(b) shows a hose of the same diameter with larger holes. Notice how much more rapidly the geysers diminish.

The effect of pressure at the tap is slightly different. Changing the pressure changes all the geysers in the same proportion. Figure 3–6(c) shows the same hose, but with a higher pressure than in Figure 3–6(b).

A tubular piece of neuron (a dendrite or axon) is much like the leaky hose. The "pressure" is electrical potential, and the "water" is a stream of charged ions (the stimulus). The cell membrane is like the hose, channeling most of the electrical current but allowing some to leak out. The magnitude of the membrane potential at some distance from the original stimulus depends on the diameter of the neuron, the permeability of the membrane, and the size of the stimulus.

As a method of transmitting information, electrotonic conduction has some obvious problems; most importantly, the voltage change we might measure at a given point along the axon depends not only on the strength of the original stimulus, but on how far the stimulus is from the recording point. Thus, if we recorded a depolarization of, for example, 5 mV at some point on an axon, it would be impossible to determine whether such a response was caused by a weak stimulus quite near the recording point, or a strong stimulus much farther away. A second disadvantage is that no matter how strong the original stimulus might be, the characteristics of the nerve membrane are such that the membrane potential will have decayed back to resting levels within a few millimeters of the stimulus. Because neurons are often called on to transmit information over distances greater than a meter, decremental conduction clearly cannot be the only mechanism by which the neuron transmits electrical signals.

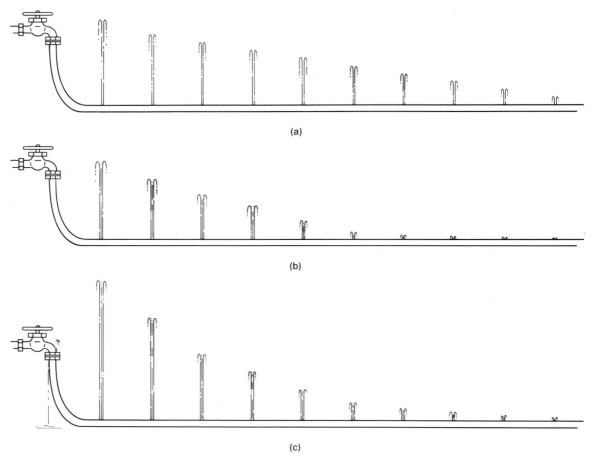

(a)

(b)

(c)

FIGURE 3-6   Analogy of the neuron as a leaky garden hose. (a) Water comes from
the tap on the left with some pressure. As water escapes through the
holes in the hose (geyser height shows how much escapes), the pressure drops and geysers to the right are smaller. (b) A hose with larger
holes loses water faster. (c) The same hose as in part (b), but with a
greater pressure from the tap. Each geyser is proportionally larger
than the one in (b).

THE ACTION POTENTIAL

The neuron must have some way of sending electrical signals across long distances without those signals decaying and becoming lost. An electrical event
known as the nerve *action potential* has been found to serve this function.

Consider the axon displayed in Figure 3–7(a). At point 1 along the axon, a stimulating electrode is inserted into the cell and the axon is stimulated with a series of brief depolarizing pulses of increasing magnitude. The membrane potential is sensed by two recording electrodes at different distances away from the stimulating electrode. The stimuli and the potential changes at the two recording sites are displayed in Figure 3–7(b). For the first two pulses, the axon behaves in the manner previously described. The depolarization caused by the stimuli are conducted electronically to the recording electrodes, with the larger stimulus producing the larger response, just as expected. For both of these stimuli, the actual potential change recorded depends not only on the

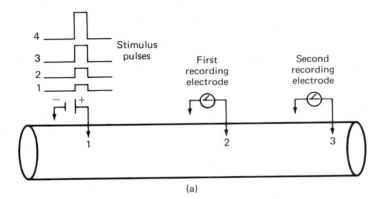

(a)

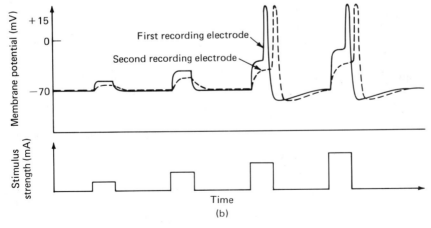

(b)

FIGURE 3–7 The results obtained when an axon is stimulated with depolarizing pulses of varying strength. (a) Shows the axon and the position of the stimulating and recording electrodes. (b) Shows a graph displaying the responses to the different pulses recorded by the two recording electrodes.

magnitudes of the stimuli but also on the distance between the stimulating and recording electrodes, as the response seen at the second recording electrode is always smaller than that observed at the first.

When the slightly larger third pulse is delivered, however, the recorded response is markedly different. In addition to a somewhat larger version of the responses to the first two pulses, the membrane undergoes a rapid and massive depolarization, so that the inside of the cell actually becomes slightly positive with respect to the outside. This response is not related to the size of the stimulus; when an even larger fourth pulse is delivered, the larger responses recorded at the two recording electrodes are not noticeably different from the responses to the third pulse. Notice also, that while the responses to the first two pulses were seen at the two recording electrodes at the same time, the larger responses to the third and fourth pulses are seen at the second electrode some time after they are observed at the first.

The responses recorded to pulses three and four are *action potentials*, or *nerve spikes*, and are the basic units of information in the nervous system. Action potentials have properties that are quite different from slow potentials transmitted by decremental conduction. One major difference is that there is a threshold associated with the generation of action potentials. From Figure 3–7, it can be seen that action potentials were only produced in response to the two strongest stimulus pulses; as a general rule, the membrane must be depolarized by at least 15 mV for an action potential to occur. Any stimulus weaker than this level will only be transmitted down the axon through decremental conduction.

Another major difference is that the size of an action potential does not vary with either distance from or the original magnitude of the stimulus. No matter where on the axon the action potential is recorded, it will always be seen as a depolarization of the membrane from -70 mV to about $+15$ mV. This is in direct contrast to decremental conduction, in which the measured potential change is related to both stimulus size and the distance between the stimulus and the recording electrode. Constant action potential size as a function of distance is obviously an important advantage over decremental conduction; it means that the signal will be the same no matter how long the axon may be. The fact that action potentials do not vary in size as a function of stimulus strength is known as the *all-or-none* principle; a stimulus will either produce an action potential, or it will not.

There is also a significant difference in the speed of conduction of signals by action potentials and by decremental conduction. Although slow potentials decay with distance, they are transmitted down the axon almost instantaneously. In contrast, action potentials travel down the axon at a finite speed that depends on the diameter of the axon. Small diameter axons conduct action potentials much more slowly than do large diameter axons; however, even the largest diameter axons conduct action potentials at speeds of only around 10 m/sec. When you think about the distance that nerve signals must travel for behaviors even as simple as a reflex, you can see that the relatively slow speed of action potentials can pose a serious problem for an organism. This problem is alleviated by a phenomenon called saltatory conduction, which is discussed later.

Action potentials are of a constant size irrespective of stimulus strength, but it is obvious that information about stimulus magnitude is available to animals. How does the nervous system code such information? Figure 3–8 provides an indication of how stimulus strength is represented in a neuron; in this figure, electrical stimuli are provided to the axon in the same way as in Figure 3–7, but they are of longer duration. All three stimuli are *suprathreshold;* that is, they are stronger than the threshold level necessary to evoke an action potential. Instead of a single action potential, the first stimulus produces a train of action potentials that lasts until the stimulus is terminated. If the stimulus is one-half of a second long, and three action potentials are produced, the stimulus results in the nerve cell firing action potentials at a rate of six action potentials per second. The second stimulus is slightly stronger than the first; you can see that the difference in the responses to the first two stimuli is that stimulus two causes action potentials to be fired at a faster rate. Instead of three nerve spikes occurring during a one-half-second stimulus, four spikes are evoked, corresponding to a rate of eight action potentials per second. The size and shape of the action potentials do not change as a function of stimulus strength, but the frequency of occurrence of action potentials does change. The response to stimulus three is a further illustration of this effect. This stimulus is stronger than either of the two preceding ones, and it produces six action potentials during a one-half-second period, corresponding to a rate of 12 spikes/sec. In this figure, you can see that the neuron codes the magnitude of an electrical stimulus by frequency of occurrence of action potentials. The stronger the stimulus, the more frequently the action potentials are generated. This is in contrast to slow potentials, which vary in magnitude as a function of the strength of the stimulus.

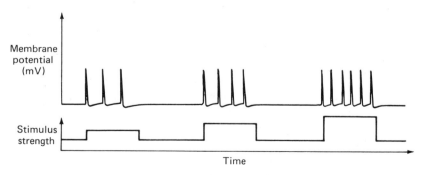

FIGURE 3–8 Graph showing the number of action potentials obtained in response to pulses of increasing strength.

BOX 3–2

We have said that the action potential is produced at a particular point on an axon when the membrane is depolarized by about 15 mV. At this level of depolarization, molecules in the membrane change their configuration to create openings, called gates, that let sodium ions (Na⁺) cross the membrane (Stevens, 1984). Na⁺ rushes into the cell, attracted by the negative potential inside, and "pushed" by the higher concentration of Na⁺ outside (Figure 3–4).

The mass movement of Na⁺ into the cell further depolarizes that area of the membrane until the inside of the membrane actually becomes somewhat more positive than the outside. The increase in **conductance** of the membrane to Na⁺ is very brief, however, returning to its resting level in less than a thousandth of a sec (msec). As soon as the membrane gates to Na⁺ close, the membrane begins to repolarize back to the resting membrane potential.

Depolarization also causes the conductance of the membrane to potassium to increase. This permeability change is much slower than that for Na⁺, and lasts several milliseconds longer. The effect of this is to increase the flow of K⁺ ions out of the cell, which tends to make the membrane potential more negative. After the sodium gates have been closed, the membrane potential becomes more negative than the resting membrane potential (Figure 3–9). This undershoot occurs because the potassium permeability is still higher than normal, so that K⁺ ions find it easier to leave the cell. During this period, the membrane potential approaches the equilibrium for potassium, which is slightly more negative than the resting level. Figure 3–9 summarizes the membrane changes that occur during an action potential.

During an action potential, some Na⁺ enters the cell and some K⁺ escapes (the same

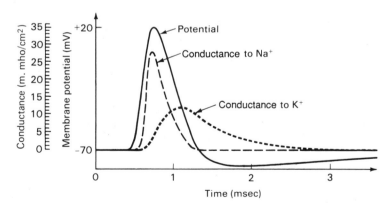

FIGURE 3-9   Graph showing the voltage changes that occur at a point along the nerve membrane during an action potential. Changes in the membrane's permeability to sodium and potassium ions are also shown. From Hodgkin, A. L., and A. F. Huxley (1952) A quantitative description of membrane current and its application to conduction and excitation in nerve. *J. Physiol.* 117:500–544. Reprinted by permission.

(continued)

(box continued)
thing happens slowly at resting potential); if this were to continue unchecked for long, the concentration of Na^+ and K^+ would eventually equilibrate and no electrical potential would remain. A "clean up" operation is needed, and it is supplied by a process called *active transport*. Within the membrane, there is a mechanism that continuously forces sodium ions out of the cell, and potassium ions in. Thus, this so-called sodium/potassium pump has the effect of maintaining the sodium and potassium concentration gradients. Pumping against the gradient is like pumping water uphill; it requires energy. The sodium/potassium pump requires energy produced by cellular respiration. If the pump is somehow disabled, the cell continues to function until the concentration gradients have dissipated.

Figure 3–10 shows an axon at an instant in time with an action potential occurring at position A along its length. At area A the membrane is depolarized from -70 mV to $+15$ mV, an 85-mV change. The charge that has flowed into the cell to cause this local depolarization does not stay restricted at area A, but will spread electrotonically, longitudinally along the membrane. This spread of potential will thus depolarize areas along the membrane adjacent to A (for example, area B). The depolarization along these adjacent areas will be greater than the threshold level necessary to initiate an action potential, so that a nerve spike will be generated at area B (Figure 3–10[b]). Similarly, the depolarization from an action potential at area B will depolarize areas adjacent to B, and the nerve spike will be generated by membrane area C (Figure 3–10[c]). In this way, the action potential will travel the entire length of the axon.

Although at any given point along an axon the depolarization caused by an action potential spreads longitudinally down the axon in both directions (for example, to both the left and the right in Figure 3–10), the nerve spike in Figure 3–10 will only travel from left to right. This is because of a phenomenon called the *refractory period* of the membrane. After an action potential has occurred along an area of the membrane (for example, area B in Figure 3–10[b]), that area is refractory; that is, it will not fire another action potential for some short period of time. Therefore, although the depolarization in Figure 3–10(b) is spreading to both areas A and C on the membrane, an action potential will only be produced at area C, because area A is still refractory.

The speed of propagation of an action potential down the axon is a function of the diameter of the axon; the larger the axon, the faster it conducts. As we have said previously, however, even the largest axons conduct action potentials at speeds less than 10 m/sec. This is too slow even to account for such behaviors as simple reflexes; therefore, there must be some mechanism by which the speed of propagation is increased. This mechanism is called

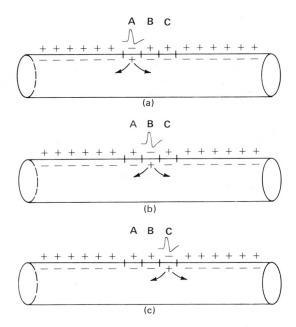

FIGURE 3-10   Propagation of the action potential. (a) Action potential is induced at area A along the membrane. (b) Depolarization from action potential at A causes spread of depolarization to area B, causing an action potential there. (c) Action potential occurring at B causes depolarization at C, causing action potential at C.

saltatory conduction, and it involves not only neurons, but another type of cell that is a member of a class of cells called *glial cells*. Glia act in many ways to provide physical and nutritive support for neurons. Some are specialized in that they consist mainly of a large area of membrane that wraps around and completely envelopes large sections of axons, as shown in Figure 3–11. The wrapping that covers the axons of most neurons is called the *myelin sheath*.

Consider what happens if an action potential is produced at point A in the cell in Figure 3–11. This action potential will propagate normally until it reaches the left-hand side of the first myelin sheath. The depolarization caused by the action potential will then be conducted *electrotonically* along the membrane. Although the amount of depolarization will decrease with distance under the myelin sheath, it will still be above the threshold level at the first node. Therefore an action potential will be produced at the left side of the node and will propagate normally until it reaches the edge of the second sheath. At that point, the sequence of events will be repeated. The entire

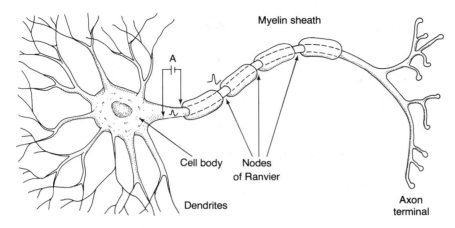

FIGURE 3-11   Axon covered by the myelin sheath. An action potential is conducted down such an axon by saltatory conduction.

process of action potential propagation at the nodes of Ranvier and decremental conduction under the myelin sheath is called saltatory conduction.

The advantage to saltatory conduction is that as most of the axon is covered by myelin, the signal is conducted down the axon mostly by decremental conduction. Because decremental conduction is virtually instantaneous, the speed of conduction of the action potential from the cell body to the axon terminal is greatly increased. It is not at all uncommon to find axons in mammalian nervous systems that conduct action potentials at speeds upward of 35 m/sec (Stone & Freeman, 1971).

RECEPTORS

So far we have been talking about the behavior of neurons in response to electrical stimulation. For a sensory system, however, the original stimulus is physical energy that is *transduced* by *receptors* that are specialized to respond to that type of energy. All receptors subserve a common function: the transformation of physical energy into electrical potential changes.

Although receptors are specialized to respond to one type of sensory input, they are able to respond to more than one kind of stimulation. For example, visual cells of the eye are specialized to respond to light; however, if you press your finger against the side of your eye (when it is closed) you get a clear visual impression. This is a result of your retinal cells responding to mechanical pressure, and it illustrates a fundamental law of sensation: no matter how a receptor is stimulated, it will produce one type of sensation. For example, whether we stimulate a visual receptor with light, pressure, or electrical current, we get only a visual response. This is because the sensory impression depends on where the sensory receptor is "wired into" the brain, just as much as it depends on the properties of the receptor itself. The concept that one will perceive a sensation of the same nature no matter how a given receptor is stimulated is called the *law of specific nerve energies*.

Properties of Receptors

Receptors have many properties in common, and we will illustrate some of these properties using a receptor called the muscle spindle as an example. Muscle spindles are stretch receptors found in skeletal muscles (see Chapter 20). When a spindle is stretched (by elongation of the muscle), it produces a *generator potential*. A generator potential is a local, *graded* potential (slow potential), whose magnitude depends on the strength of the stimulus.

A graded generator potential is common to all receptors. Katz (1950) was able to study the details of the muscle spindle generator potential by treating the spindle with a chemical that abolished all action potentials in the sensory nerve, but left the generator potential intact. He then investigated the responses to various levels of muscle stress, and obtained the results shown in Figure 3–12. For each of the five pairs of traces, the top trace records the change in length of the muscle, while the bottom trace is the generator potential. It is clear that as the muscle is stretched more and more, the generator potential also increases in magnitude.

Katz (1950) also showed that the size of the generator potential was closely related to the number of action potentials produced in the sensory nerve. Figure 3–13 shows this relationship; as the size of the generator potential increases, the number of action potentials it produces increases in a linear fashion. Therefore we can talk about generator potentials and action potentials in this sensory nerve almost interchangeably.

Receptors respond to sensory stimuli in a graded fashion, but their response is in general not a copy of the stimulus. Instead, receptors are sensitive to certain aspects of a stimulus; in particular, they give more emphasis to change than to static behavior. This is a general property of receptors; we will illustrate it here for the muscle spindle, and in later sections other receptors will be shown to function in the same way. In Figure 3–14, the muscle is being stretched over a period of 0.1 sec from one level of tension to a second, higher level. The action potentials fired in the sensory nerve in response to this stretch are shown in the top trace. You can see that the nerve is firing action potentials at a faster rate when the muscle is at the higher level of tension; however, the nerve responds with the fastest rate while muscle length is changing. This is an important observation. It shows that the rate of firing is not simply related to the amount of tension in the muscle; the muscle is stretched less at arrow 1 than at arrow 2, but firing rate is much greater at arrow 1. Instead of only responding to the steady-state level of tension, this neuron is differentially *sensitive to change*. The same principle is illustrated over a longer period of time in Figure 3–15, where a constant tension is

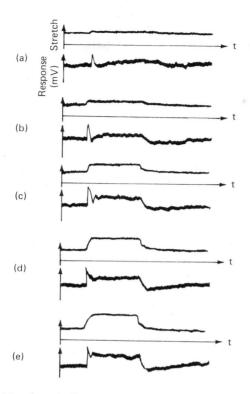

FIGURE 3-12 Muscle spindle generator potentials in response to different levels of muscle tension. The top trace of each pair shows the amount of stress put on the muscle, with the bottom trace showing the response. Amount of stress increases regularly from (a) to (e). From Katz, B. (1950) Depolarization of sensory terminals and the initiation of impulses in the muscle spindle. *J. Physiol.* 111:261–282. Reprinted by permission.

applied to the muscle over a period of 15 sec. It is clear that the period of greatest firing is immediately after the application of tension, and that firing rate decreases markedly during the period of time that the load is constant.

Having sensory receptors responding more to change than to steady-state levels has many advantages when one considers how a sensory system might be built. If one receives information about changes in steady-state values, one can figure out what those levels must be, without the necessity of constantly monitoring responses of receptors. For economy of signaling, therefore, a system that responds to change must demand the attention of the organism a smaller percentage of the time. In addition, most of the stimuli to which an organism must attend in order to assure its survival are constantly changing. Predators must be noticed when they are attacking, and animals that prey on other animals must be alert to changes in position of their potential meals. As we shall see, in many cases, higher order neurons actually respond to stimuli only during periods of change.

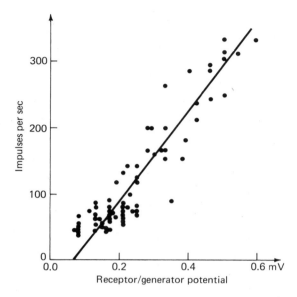

FIGURE 3–13 Relationship between muscle spindle generator potential and action potentials produced in the sensory nerve. From Katz, B. (1950). Reprinted by permission.

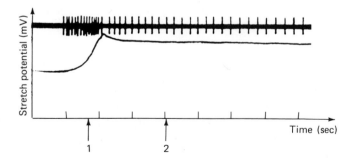

FIGURE 3–14 Response of sensory nerve coming from muscle spindle to change in muscle tension. Lower trace shows the tension placed on the muscle. From Matthews, B. H. C. (1933) Nerve endings in mammalian muscle. *J. Physiol.* 78:1–53. Reprinted by permission.

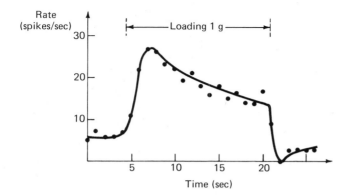

FIGURE 3-15 Response of sensory nerve from muscle spindle to a unit change in muscle tension. Firing is greatest just after change occurs. From Adrian, E. D. and T. Zotterman (1926) The impulses produced by sensory nerve endings. II. The response of a single end-organ. *J. Physiol.* 61:151–171. Reprinted by permission.

SYNAPTIC COMMUNICATION

So far we have been describing events that occur within a single neuron. Individual neurons are of little value, however—the nervous system is an enormous aggregate of neurons working together. In this section we shall see how neurons communicate with each other, and how individual neurons process the information they receive from a number of other neurons.

Neurons do not usually communicate by direct electrical links with each other; rather, they send chemical messages from cell to cell. (There are some contacts between neurons that function by electrotonic spread between the two cells, but we will not consider these further in this chapter.) These chemical messages are transmitted at synapses.

Figure 3–16 shows a single synapse as it appears in an electron microscope. This particular synapse was found in the retina of a chicken (Dowling & Boycott, 1965). Only a small section of each neuron may be seen: in the center is the cell sending the message, called the *presynaptic* neuron because it is before the synapse; below it is the receiving, or *postsynaptic*, neuron.

There is a distinct gap between the membranes of the two cells; this gap is called the *synaptic cleft*. It is across this narrow space that the chemical messengers must travel. One other specialization may be seen in Figure 3–16: the presynaptic process contains a collection of small round bodies (arrow). These are called *synaptic vesicles*, and they contain the chemical messenger, called a *transmitter*.

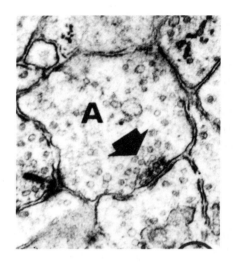

FIGURE 3-16 Electron micrograph of a synapse. Note the cluster of synaptic vesicles (arrow) in the presynaptic process and the slightly heavier postsynaptic membrane. From Dowling, J. E. and B. B. Boycott (1965) *Cold Spring Harbor Symp. Quant. Biol.* 30:393–402. Reprinted by permission of the author and the publisher.

When the presynaptic process is depolarized (by the experimenter passing depolarizing current through an electrode, by a slow potential in the neuron, or by the arrival of an action potential) vesicles tend to fuse with the cell membrane and release their transmitter into the synaptic cleft. The number of vesicles released is proportional to the depolarization. The transmitter diffuses across the cleft, and some of it reaches the postsynaptic membrane.

The transmitter that reaches the postsynaptic membrane binds to it at special structures called *receptor sites*. ("Receptors" as used here are sites, probably single molecules, in the membrane of a cell. They are not to be confused with the receptor cells that were just discussed.) The effect of the transmitter molecules being bound to the postsynaptic membrane is to change the state of polarization of the postsynaptic cell; if the postsynaptic cell depolarizes the synapse, it is called *excitatory*. If the cell becomes more strongly negative (that is, it becomes more polarized, or *hyperpolarized*) the synapse is *inhibitory*.

The action of the transmitter on the postsynaptic membrane is transient. At some synapses, the transmitter is only loosely bound to the receptors; it soon drifts away and is actively taken back into the presynaptic cell (where it can be repackaged in new vesicles for recycling). At other synapses there is a specific chemical enzyme that actively destroys the transmitter molecules. In either case, the transmitter soon vanishes from the synaptic cleft.

BOX 3–3

The way the chemical transmitter effects a change in polarization of the postsynaptic neuron is by changing the permeability of the postsynaptic membrane for certain ions. Just as depolarization increases the permeability of an axon, the combination of transmitter and receptor increases the permeability of the postsynaptic process. At some synapses, the effect is direct: the receptor itself becomes a pore through which ions can cross the membrane. At other synapses, it is indirect: the receptor acts as an enzyme to change the concentration of some other chemical that opens the pore. At some excitatory synapses, the pores allow free passage of both sodium and potassium ions. When the pore is open, sodium tends to rush into the cell, carrying a positive charge and depolarizing the cell. Some of the effect of the sodium flow is counteracted by an increased flow of positive potassium ions out of the cell, but on the whole, the effect is to depolarize.

Inhibitory synapses hyperpolarize by allowing an increased flow of chloride ions (which are negatively charged) into the cell. The pores at most inhibitory synapses specifically increase chloride conductance. At some inhibitory synapses, potassium conductance is increased instead.

The amount of transmitter released by the presynaptic cell is proportional to the depolarization of that cell, and the change in polarization of the postsynaptic process (depolarization for excitatory synapses, hyperpolarization for inhibitory) is proportional to the amount of transmitter released. The potential difference in the postsynaptic process, therefore, is an accurate reflection of the activity in the presynaptic cell. Why, then, are chemical synapses necessary at all?

One advantage is that they permit messages to pass in only one direction. Chemical transmitter is effective only on the postsynaptic membrane; lacking any direct connection, the postsynaptic cell has no way of affecting the presynaptic cell. This prevents signals from flowing backward and confounding the entire nerve network. Thus, if a particular cell that is postsynaptic to cell A is depolarized because of another set of synapses from a third cell C, cell A will not be affected by that depolarization.

Another important advantage of chemical synapses is that they allow for the existence of inhibitory synapses. An inhibitory synapse changes the sign of a signal: when the presynaptic cell depolarizes, the postsynaptic cell hyperpolarizes. We shall see shortly how important inhibitory synapses are in the processing done by the nervous system.

Most neurons receive information through both excitatory and inhibitory synapses. Whether a particular synapse is excitatory or inhibitory is built into the postsynaptic membrane. Individual postsynaptic receptors are specific to only one transmitter; when it arrives, its effect is to cause either depolarization or hyperpolarization. The same neuron may have some synapses at which a certain transmitter from other neurons causes depolarization, and other synapses at which either the same or another transmitter leads to hyperpolarization.

The computations performed by the nervous system are a balancing of excitation and inhibition. Excitation tends to raise the level of activity of a cell; the more depolarized a cell is the more rapidly it fires action potentials. Inhibition tends to depress the activity of a cell. The activity of any given neuron is the weighted sum of the excitatory inputs and inhibitory inputs it receives. Loosely speaking, excitation means "there is something there," and inhibition means "but it's not that important."

BOX 3–4

If there are slow potentials in the presynaptic neuron, the amount of depolarization or hyperpolarization in the postsynaptic process is proportional to the depolarization of the presynaptic process. Now consider a presynaptic process that is the termination of a long axon, receiving a succession of all-or-none action potentials. Each time an action potential arrives at the axon terminal it provides a powerful, albeit brief, depolarization during which a considerable number of vesicles release their transmitter all at once. The result is a sudden change in potential of the postsynaptic membrane (called a *postsynaptic potential*, or *PSP*).

This is illustrated in Figure 3–17. The top trace in the figure shows the potential in the presynaptic process as a function of time. The lower trace shows the postsynaptic potential on the same time scale. For the first part of each record, there is no activity in the presynaptic cell; during this period, both the presynaptic and postsynaptic cells are at their resting potentials. At time *A* there is an action potential in the presynaptic process. The resulting PSP appears in the lower trace after an extremely short delay. The postsynaptic membrane rapidly depolarizes in response to the flood of transmitter; the potential then declines to the resting potential as transmitter molecules break free of the receptors and are deactivated or taken back into the presynaptic process. This potential is depolarizing; this is an excitatory synapse and is called an *excitatory postsynaptic potential*, or *EPSP*. A similar sequence of events occurs at inhibitory synapses; the difference is that the potential is hyperpolarizing and is called an *inhibitory postsynaptic potential (IPSP)*.

At time *A* in Figure 3–17 we see the EPSP caused by a single action potential. Consider what would happen if a train of action potentials were to arrive in the presynaptic process. This is shown at time *B*. Before the EPSP from the first action potential has declined back to resting potential, a second infusion of transmitter arrives. This adds its effect to the transmitter still remaining from the first action potential, so an even greater depolarization is achieved. The third action potential adds its effect to the remainder of the first two, maintaining a somewhat higher level of depolarization than one action potential alone caused.

At time *C* in the figure, an even more rapid train of action potentials arrives in the axon terminal. The first EPSP has barely begun to decline when the second arrives; the third then adds to the sum of the first two. The postsynaptic process is maintained at a considerable level of depolarization. The more rapidly the action potentials arrive in the axon, the more depolarized the postsynaptic process will be. The rate at which action potentials are produced in the presynaptic neuron is proportional to the depolarization of that cell; the depolarization of the postsynaptic neuron is proportional to the rate of firing action potentials in the presynaptic cell. Change in postsynaptic potential is proportional to depolarization at the cell body of the presynaptic neuron.

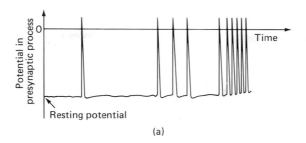

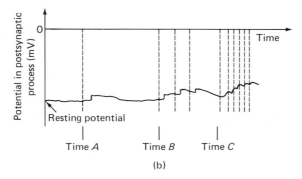

FIGURE 3-17 Transmission across a synapse. Upper trace shows the action potentials in a hypothetical presynaptic process; lower trace shows the potentials that would be recorded postsynaptically.

CHEMICAL TRANSMITTERS AND CHEMICAL TECHNIQUES

We have been speaking of the action of chemical transmitters without paying any attention to their chemical nature. A number of transmitters have been identified chemically, information that is being regarded as increasingly useful in the analysis of the nervous system. It is often found that a particular kind of neuron (one cell type, or cells with certain functions in common) all secrete the same transmitter, while other neurons in the same tissue may secrete a quite different chemical.

For most of the known transmitters, chemists can supply the transmitter in quantity, can supply chemicals that bind with its receptor site so the transmitter will have no effect (known as a *blocking agent*), or can supply chemicals that cause neurons containing that transmitter to release it without depolarizing, to prevent release or to prevent the reuptake after release. (These chemicals are the pharmacological agents we call drugs; most of the antidepressants, hallucinogens, depressants, and even psychogenic drugs work by affecting specific transmitters within the brain.)

The fact that different chemicals have an affinity for different receptors has opened rich possibilities for research. By using a chemical that specifically enhances or disables one type of neuron in brain tissue, it is possible to explore the role that cell type plays in processing information. For example, if we observe that a cell only responds to movement in a certain direction, and find that a blocker for a particular transmitter allows it to respond to movement in any direction, we know that cells normally releasing that transmitter must be preventing the responses to movements in the "wrong" directions.

It is also possible to make molecules that attach to a particular type of receptor site and mark it—that is, show which cells in the tissue receive the transmitter that normally binds to that receptor type. Alternatively, there are markers that look like the raw materials from which transmitters are built; these are taken up only by cells that make that transmitter, marking them. The mark can be a radioactive chemical, a dye that shows up in the microscope, or a chemical that glows under ultraviolet radiation. In any case, the cells marked can be seen and recognized under the microscope.

Other chemical techniques rely on the slightly different chemical "signatures" of different cell lines. Because of the different transmitters manufactured, and perhaps because of other subtle chemical differences, different cell types are recognized as different by the immune system. It is now possible to make *monoclonal antibodies* that recognize and attach to certain types of cells, either marking them or affecting their activity.

ELECTROPHYSIOLOGICAL TECHNIQUES

The electrical signals generated by individual neurons make up the code with which the nervous system communicates. Much of our understanding of how the nervous system works comes from intercepting that code, in effect "bugging" the communication channels.

There are two problems we encounter in recording the activity of neurons. The first is that neurons are quite small; even a small nerve may contain tens of thousands of individual axons. The optic nerve has about 1 million axons in it. The second problem is also one of size; the signals produced by each neuron are very small. An action potential represents an excursion of about 1/10 of a volt, but that is much larger than the signal an electrophysiologist can obtain. To record a signal, electrical contact must be made through an electrode; if the electrode is small enough to select a single cell it also will lose much of the signal. If it is larger, it cannot get as near to the cell, and therefore also loses much of the signal. The actual signals recorded are typically less than a few millivolts.

To deal with such minute signals requires considerable amplification. The principle is the same as in a boom box, where the small signal generated in the tape heads is amplified to sufficient strength to drive the loudspeakers. Modern electronics, including transistors and field effect devices, make low noise amplification relatively simple, but electrophysiology was not possible until this century, and single-cell recordings were virtually unheard of until the 1940s.

The amplified nerve signals must be displayed in a way that the experimenters can understand. If the signal consists of action potentials, it can be fed to a loudspeaker, just as the output of a stereo amplifier goes to a loudspeaker. Each time an action potential occurs, the loudspeaker produces a click. The experimenter can often get an idea of how various stimuli are modulating the rate of firing by listening to the signal.

It is also desirable to see what the signal looks like as a function of time. To draw a figure such as the graphs in this chapter, we would want a pen that moves across a sheet of paper at a constant speed, deflecting upward or downward as the voltage changes. A pen moving from left to right could trace a picture like Figure 3–17. The only kind of pen that can obtain speeds high enough to trace an action potential that is completed in a fraction of a millisecond is a "pen" consisting of a beam of electrons "writing" on a phosphor screen. An instrument that works by this principle is the *oscilloscope*, shown schematically in Figure 3–18. An electron beam is swept from left to right by a magnetic field; a second field deflects it up or down according to the voltage being recorded. Where the electron beam hits the phosphor screen the screen glows, making a visible picture of the path the beam has taken. (Television sets and video monitors also work by striking a phosphor screen with a rapidly moving beam of electrons.)

A permanent record of the voltage versus time can be obtained by photographing the oscilloscope screen, but modern technology provides far more elegant ways to preserve data. A computer can "digitize" them as they are produced; that is, the computer generates a series of numbers representing

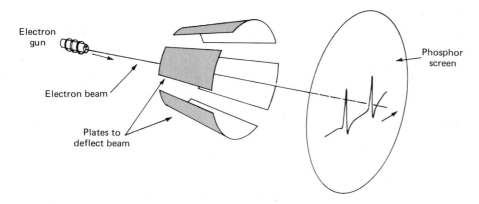

FIGURE 3–18 Schematic sketch of an oscilloscope, showing the principle of operation.

either the voltage at each point in time, or the times of occurrence of each action potential. These data may then be stored in digital form on disk; the computer can read the data back at a later time for any kind of analysis the experimenter may choose to program. Peripheral devices such as graphic terminals, plotters, and printers can be linked to the computer to present the data in their digested form, including drawing pictures of the spike train as it would have appeared on an oscilloscope (see Figure 6–1). Far more sophisticated data presentation may also be achieved with little difficulty: plots of firing rate versus time, histograms of the numbers of spikes at various times relative to the stimulus, averaged responses to several stimuli, maps of responses as a function of stimulus position, intensity, or wavelength. Often, the results of more detailed analysis can be computed while the experiment is in progress and presented while the data are being collected. This is called *on-line* processing.

Gross Potentials

There are two basic kinds of recording that can be obtained. The simplest of these to achieve (but often hardest to understand) is the *gross potential*, the sum of the activity of a large number of neurons. Often, gross potentials are recorded with flat metal electrodes that are stuck to the skin with special electrically conductive paste. Familiar examples are the EEG (brain waves) recorded from the scalp, and the EKG (electrical activity of the heart) recorded from the chest. Retinal function may be assessed by the ERG *(electroretinogram)*, a potential recorded from the front of the eye that reflects the activity of cells in the retina. Although it is not easily obtained because the inner ear is deep within the bone of the skull, there is a potential reflecting the activity of the receptors of the ear called the *cochlear microphonic*.

Gross potentials can be obtained from awake humans without causing them any pain, and are therefore useful in clinical diagnoses. Because they represent the activity of large numbers of cells, however, it is often difficult to interpret the significance to the nervous system of these potentials. Modern electrophysiology has turned increasingly to recordings from single cells, but gross potentials have provided much useful information about the functioning of the nervous system and will continue to be valuable for analyzing neural responses.

Single-Cell Recordings

The second type of electrophysiological recording is a record of the activity of a single neuron (or *unit*). With this method, an experimenter can explore the exact manner in which a particular cell responds to various stimuli. Of course, there are many possible neurons to record, and a large sample must be taken before one can say whether a particular cell is representative of the population of neurons, or if there are several functionally different types of cells in the population.

As the functional differences between neurons may be related to the different types of neurons in the same neural tissue, it is also desirable to mark the cell recorded so that it can be identified by its anatomical type. If we are recording with an electrode that is inside the cell, we can mark the cell by squirting dye into the soma from the electrode. The tissue is examined under a microscope and the marked cell located.

To record the electrical activity inside a cell, a *microelectrode* is placed in electrical contact with the cytoplasm inside the neuron. The other lead of an amplifier is in contact with the extracellular fluid, so the potential across the cell membrane is measured. An electrode that contacts the inside of the cell must be extremely delicate to enter a neuron without severely damaging it; the electrodes used for this purpose are made by heating the middle of a piece of glass tubing while pulling it (Figure 3–19). As the glass in the middle gets soft, the tube pulls out into a thin fiber. The entire tube shrinks at the middle, but the hole down the center remains. The narrowest part is a miniature tube, less than 1 micron (millionth of a meter) in diameter (too small to

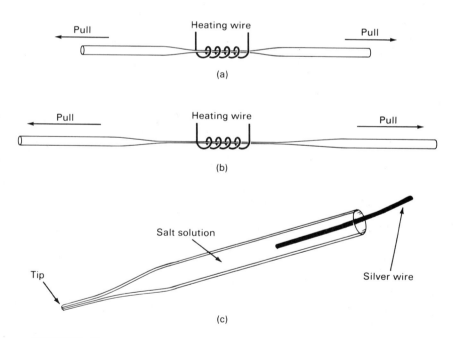

FIGURE 3–19 Anatomy of a micropipette. Glass capillary tubing is heated and pulled (a) until it draws out into a fine filament (b). The filament breaks in the center to form the tip. The pipette is filled with a salt solution, and a wire inserted in the wide end to make electrical contact (c).

be seen in an ordinary microscope because its diameter is comparable to the wavelength of light). The electrode (called a *micropipette*) is filled with a conductive salt solution, and lowered into the neural tissue. Often, the salt solution also contains a dye that can be forced out of the micropipette to mark the neuron.

Puncturing a cell with a micropipette is not quite the same as placing a plug in a socket. The electrode tip must move straight into the cell (any sideways motion or vibration would tear the membrane and kill the cell) and must stop before exiting on the far side. Once inside the cell, the electrode must remain perfectly steady, for even the slightest motion would either dislodge it or injure the cell. For these reasons, it is advanced by a *micromanipulator*, a device that allows precise and minute motions. (Often, the motion is geared down by a hydraulic link or through electrical controls. Some micromanipulators are controlled by a computer.) The micromanipulator advances the electrode, usually blindly, until the activity of a cell is recorded.

BOX 3–5

Although most recording has been done while the brain is still inside the animal (of course, with the animal completely anesthetized and unconscious, like a patient during an operation), some recording is done "in vitro"—with tissue that has been removed. It is often easier to work with a retina after it has been removed from the eye. Sometimes, thin slices of brain tissue are made, so the microelectrode can be placed directly into cells seen through a microscope. In some cases, cells (or parts of cells) are dissociated from the rest of the tissue and floated separately in a bath. This can be done by shaking the tissue gently in a bath containing an enzyme that dissolves the connections between cells. Sometimes, networks of cells are grown in a tissue culture. These methods are generally used to study the electrical properties of a single cell, usually by injecting electrical current or changing the chemical environment. It is even possible to adhere a tiny patch of the cell's membrane across the opening on the tip of the micropipette. This "patch-clamp" technique is used to study the individual ion gates in the cell membrane.

Recording from inside a cell (or *intracellularly*) is the most satisfactory way to record cells that produce slow potentials but have no action potentials. Cells that fire action potentials often are recorded without actually puncturing the cell membrane: this technique is called *extracellular* recording. In extracellular recording, a microelectrode is placed near the cell or axon being recorded, and intercepts a small portion of the electrical currents in the vicinity of the cell. The extracellular technique is simpler because electrodes do not actually have to enter the cell, but the electrical signals are much smaller.

Extracellular recordings can be made with glass micropipettes (and often are), but it is sometimes simpler to use metal microelectrodes. These are made by etching platinum or tungsten wire to a long tapered point. All but the very tip is then insulated with glass or a special varnish so that it is the only active part of the electrode. Metal microelectrodes are also advanced with a micromanipulator until the activity of a single cell is recorded.

SUGGESTED READINGS

There are many excellent books discussing the basic neurophysiology of single cells. One of the best is *From Neuron to Brain*, by S. W. Kuffler and J. G. Nicholls (Sinauer, 1976), that discusses both classical and recent neurophysiological data in a thorough and easily understood way. Another good book on this subject is *Neurobiology*, (2nd Edition) by Gordon M. Shepherd (Oxford University Press, 1988). For anybody interested in how simple neuronal systems are organized to control certain animal behaviors, a good book to start with is *Cellular Basis of Behavior,* by E. Kandel (W. H. Freeman, 1976).

There are also a number of articles that have been published in *Scientific American* that are enjoyable and explanatory. "The Nerve Impulse and the Squid," by R. D. Keynes (December 1958; offprint #58) reviews the sequence of events underlying the action potential, and the research by which it was first understood. "The Synapse," by J. C. Eccles (January 1965; offprint #1001) not only describes the mechanism of transmission at the synapse, but discusses neural processing and the ionic basis of neural function. Both of these articles have been reprinted in *Physiological Psychology*, by R. F. Thompson (W. H. Freeman, 1972). A good discussion of how receptors in various sensory systems transduce stimulus energy and generate action potentials may be found in "How Cells Receive Stimuli," by W. H. Miller, F. Ratliff, and H. K. Hartline (September 1961; offprint #99). This article was reprinted in *Perception: Mechanisms and Models*, by R. Held and W. Richards (W. H. Freeman, 1972).

The September 1979 issue of *Scientific American* is devoted entirely to topics related to the neurosciences; it contains two articles relevant to topics discussed in this chapter. "The Brain," by D. H. Hubel is a general introduction that keynotes the issue. In addition to being a general review, this article discusses some ideas about how nerve networks may function and tells some of the history of experimentation on nervous tissue. The second article is "The Neuron," by C. F. Stevens. This article reviews some of the electrical properties of neurons that we have covered here, but emphasizes how these phenomena depend on the chemical properties of the neuron itself. The entire issue has been reprinted as a book entitled *The Brain* (W. H. Freeman, 1979).

THE EYE

The preceding two chapters have provided us with the necessary tools to address the major topics of this book. We are now ready to begin our discussion of sensory systems, starting with the visual system. In this chapter, we briefly describe some of the physical properties of the basic stimulus for vision: light. We describe the general structure of the peripheral visual system, and show how the eye acts as an optical instrument.

LIGHT

Many of the attributes of vision are imposed by the nature of light. Most objects are not self-luminous, but are visible because they reflect light from other sources. The reflecting properties of most objects may be constant, but the light illuminating them is not. Nevertheless, it is the properties of the object, not the light source, that we wish to "see."

There is also a limitation of light that we make use of: It generally travels in a straight line. That means we cannot see around corners, or behind opaque objects. As we will see in Chapter 12, the occlusion of one object by another is a powerful cue to the relative distances of the objects. When light does not travel in a straight line we are fooled, as when we try to locate an object underwater.

Light can travel enormous distances, allowing us to sense a distant world. Through our visual sense, we can know about objects far beyond our reach, and thus we can construct cognitive maps of relatively large regions of the world around us. Since objects in that larger world may move (and we may move within the world), vision allows us to predict part of our future. For example, you see the low branch before you actually touch it with your advancing forehead.

Visible light is a form of energy called *electromagnetic radiation*. Qualitatively, it is similar to electromagnetic phenomena such as X-rays, radar, gamma rays, and radio waves. The continuum of electromagnetic radiation is shown in Figure 4–1; from this figure, it is clear that visible light is only a small subset of this continuum.

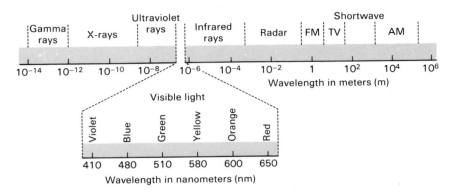

FIGURE 4–1   The electromagnetic energy spectrum; the portion of the spectrum perceived as visible light is enlarged in the lower portion of the figure.

We can think of lights (or any type of electromagnetic radiation) in two apparently different theoretical frameworks. In the first, light is considered to be composed of individual, indivisible particles called *photons*. Photons travel in a straight line at a speed that depends only on the medium through which they are passing. In a vacuum, photons travel at a speed of approximately 3×10^{10} cm/sec (or 186,000 miles/sec); in any other medium the speed is slightly less, with the reduction depending on the density of the medium. Although photons always tend to travel in a straight line, their direction of movement may be changed as they pass from one medium to another; the bending of light rays by a lens is an example of this property.

Photons are identical in their speed of movement; however, they do differ in the energy they possess. The energy of a particular photon is related to a property called *frequency*, which we will explain in the next paragraph. Frequency is related to energy in the following way: $E = h\upsilon$, where υ is the frequency and h is a scaling constant. Thus, the higher the frequency associated with a photon, the more energy it possesses.

Instead of thinking of light as being composed of many tiny particles, we can also conceive of it as a wave phenomenon. In this conception, light travels analogously to the way a wave travels when we drop a stone into a still pool. The water waves spread out from the stone at a constant speed. Figure 4–2 shows a schematic cross section of a wave. We can see that they are cyclic phenomena; there is a regular pattern of depressions and upheavals. We can define a property called *wavelength,* which is the distance from the beginning of one cycle to the beginning of the next cycle, or one peak to the next peak.

Frequency (the property of photons alluded to in the previous paragraph) can be obtained by measuring the time necessary for one complete cycle of the wave to pass a stationary point. Frequency and wavelength have an inverse relationship for wave phenomena; that is, $\lambda = c/\upsilon$, or $\upsilon = c/\lambda$,

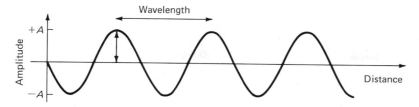

FIGURE 4-2   Cross-section of a wave.

where υ is frequency, λ is wavelength, and c is the speed of travel of the wave.

The wave and particle conceptions of light are consistent with each other because matter and energy are the same in particle physics. The existence of indivisible photons is universally accepted by contemporary physicists, and wave theory continues to be useful as a way of describing the movement of large numbers of photons. We can talk about the strength of a light using either particle theory or wave theory. When we consider light as being composed of photons, the strength of a light is related to the number of photons present; when we talk about light as being a wave phenomenon, the strength is related to the amplitude (or height, in Figure 4–2) of the wave. As wavelength and frequency are inversely related to each other, we can relate the energy of a photon to its wavelength by the following expression: $E = hc/\lambda$.

BOX 4-1

Ｈow is light measured? Consider a light source P, as is shown in Figure 4–3. There are many ways to measure the light coming from P. One choice we must make is whether to measure the energy coming from P or to count the number of photons. When the wavelength of the light is known, we can easily switch between measuring energy and counting photons, as the energy of a single photon is inversely related to its wavelength. For convenience, energy measures are most often used.

The next choice to be made is where the light should be measured. If we wished to measure all the energy coming from a light source and passing through some specified area (or falling onto a surface) in a unit of time, we would measure the *radiant flux*. We could measure the total radiant flux available from a source by enclosing the source in a transparent balloon, and measuring all the light passing through the balloon (Figure 4–3[a]). The farther the balloon surface is from the light source, the bigger it would have to be, but the total amount of light passing through the balloon would remain constant. Since the area of the skin of the balloon grows as the square of its radius, the amount of light passing through each unit area must fall as the inverse square of the radius. That is, the flux passing through a unit area "window" (a clear postage stamp fixed to the balloon) would fall as the inverse square of its distance from the source.

Alternatively, we might be interested in the amount of energy produced by a light source that reaches a surface some distance away (Figure 4–3[b]). This measure is called *(continued)*

(box continued)

the *irradiance*, and is given in units of energy per unit area. Irradiance depends on the distance between the light source and the surface, as well as the angle at which the light strikes the surface. *Radiance*, on the other hand, is a measure that depends only on the source; it is used when the light source is a surface instead of a point. Radiance is a measure of the radiant flux emerging from a surface source in a certain direction (Figure 4–3[c]).

Radiant flux, irradiance, and radiance are measures of energy and fall within a class of units called *radiometric measures*. There is another class of units that measures the effectiveness of a light for human vision; this is done by weighting different wavelengths according to how sensitive the human visual system is to those wavelengths. For example, suppose a light source could emit either 550 nm (which appears yellowish-green) or 650-nm light (which appears red). If It emitted the same energy at each wavelength, any radiometric measure would say the lights are equal. But your eye is more sensitive to 550-nm light than to 650-nm light, so you would judge that the 550-nm light is "brighter" (see Chapter 5). It would be useful to have a measuring system that weights the contributions of each wavelength according to how well we see it. Light measures analogous to those of radiometry that represent the effectiveness of the light for human vision are called *photometric units*. *Luminous flux* is analogous to radiant flux, *luminance* corresponds to radiance, and *illuminance* replaces irradiance. The weighting is determined by the average sensitivity of the human observer in normal daylight, when cones mediate vision. As you will see in Chapter 7, our relative sensitivity to wavelengths is different in very dim conditions (when only rods are active), so a somewhat different weighting must be used for dim-light vision. The qualifier *scotopic* is added for conditions in which rods mediate vision, to distinguish those units from the usual bright-light units, called *photopic* units. When no qualifier is appended, it is understood that the units are photopic.

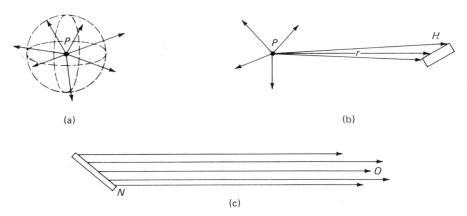

(a)

(b)

(c)

FIGURE 4–3   Different ways of measuring light. (a) Radiant flux from a source *P*. (b) Irradiance on a surface *H* a distance *r* from source *P*. (c) Radiance of an extended surface *N* in direction *O*.

Optics

Light tends to travel in a straight line; however, we can make use of optical instruments such as mirrors and lenses to alter the direction light is moving. One of the simplest optical instruments is a plane mirror, which is simply a flat polished surface. Mirrors reflect light rays according to a simple rule illustrated in Figure 4–4; light rays are reflected from a mirror at exactly the same angle that they approach the mirror. From Figure 4–4, the angle of incidence is always equal to the angle of reflection. This is a useful optical property, as it allows us to observe an image of an object at a location removed from that object.

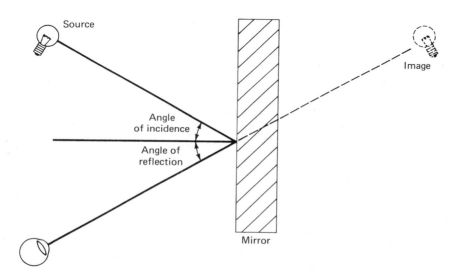

FIGURE 4–4 Light rays incident on and reflected from a plane mirror. Note that the angle at which the rays approach the mirror (angle of incidence) is equal to the angle at which they are reflected away from the mirror (angle of reflection).

Reflection is not the only way to bend light rays; *refraction* is the process of changing the path of light using lenses. A lens is an optical instrument that can produce an *image* of an object at some distance away from that object. An image is merely a reproduction of the pattern of light rays coming from an object. Because the human visual system uses a lens to produce an image on the back of the eye, it is important to understand what a lens does. Lenses can be either concave or convex; an example of a convex lens is shown in Figure 4–5. If an object is placed fairly far away from a convex lens, the lens will produce an image of the object on the side of the lens opposite to the object. This is shown in part (a) of Figure 4–5; the object is an upright arrow to the left of the lens, and the lens produces an image of that object on the right side

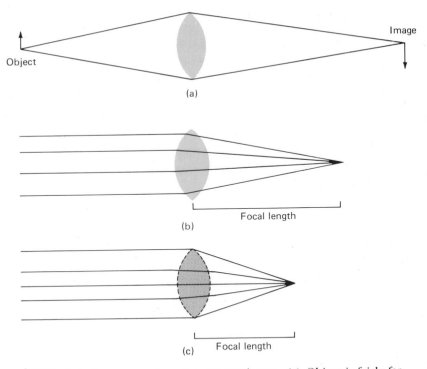

FIGURE 4-5   Images produced by convex lenses. (a) Object is fairly far from lens; inverted image is produced on opposite side from object. (b) Object is at optical infinity; image is produced at focal length of the lens. (c) Lens in (b) is replaced with a stronger lens; image is moved closer to lens.

of the lens. The strength of a lens is related to how much it can bend light rays, so that the stronger the lens, the closer the image of the object will be to the lens.

One measure of the strength of a lens is its *focal length, f*. We can determine the focal length of a lens by seeing where it will project an image of an object that is an infinite (or at least very large) distance away from the lens. Consider the light rays that emanate from a star, light years away from earth. They leave the star in all directions; however, the relatively small number that will reach the earth must travel along nearly parallel paths. Thus, in general, the farther away an object is from a lens, the more nearly parallel will be the light rays reaching the lens from that object. In Figure 4–5(b) a situation is depicted in which light rays from an object a great distance from the lens are impinging on a lens; as the object is far away, the rays are essentially parallel. In this example, let us assume that the object is a point source of light, so that the image will also be a point of light. To the left of the lens is a series of parallel light rays. To the right, the lens produces an image of the object at a distance from the lens exactly equal to the focal length. If we replace this lens with a stronger one (Figure 4–5[c]), the light rays will be bent more sharply, and the image will be formed closer to the lens. Therefore focal length is inversely related to lens strength; the shorter the focal length, the stronger the lens. Since it can be confusing for the stronger lens to be represented by a smaller number, we often use a measure related to $1/f$: the *diopter*. A lens' strength in diopters is one over the focal length in meters.

BOX 4–2

I f you happen to have a convex lens (such as a magnifying glass), you can easily demonstrate these phenomena to yourself. Go outside on a sunny day, and place the lens so that it is about 6 inches from the ground in a direct path from the sun. Move the lens up and down to find the distance where a small, bright, well-focussed spot on the ground is seen. This is the image of the sun formed by the lens. Because the sun is virtually an infinite distance away from the lens, the distance between the lens and the ground (when you have a sharp image of the sun) will be a good measure of the focal length of that lens. (Caution: never look directly at the sun through this or any other optical instrument. The sun's rays may cause permanent eye damage or blindness.)

To understand how a lens forms an image, consider Figure 4–6(a). An object (upright arrow) is illuminated by some source of light (not shown), and reflects light rays from its surface. Each point on the object is radiating rays of light in all directions; those that strike the lens are brought to focus to create the image. Two rays from the tip of the arrow are shown; one passes through the very center of the lens, and one is exactly parallel to the main axis of the lens. The ray that passes through the center of the lens is virtually unbent, because the glass faces are nearly flat and parallel to each other at this point, like a flat pane of glass. The ray parallel to the axis is like a ray from an infinitely distant object. It therefore must be bent so that it passes through the focal point of the lens (marked f). Where these two rays cross is where the image of that point is created; all other rays from that point on the object will also pass through that point on the image. Each other point on the object will project to a point on the image, so that a re-creation of the object is formed on the far side of the lens. Notice that the image is upside down; this is a general property of images made by convex lenses.

If we know the focal length of a given lens and the distance between the lens and an object, we can determine exactly where the lens will place an image of that object. If o is the distance between the lens and the object, i is the distance between the lens and the image, and f is the focal length of the lens, then

$$\frac{1}{f} = \frac{1}{i} + \frac{1}{o}$$

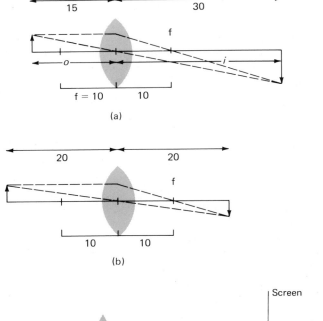

FIGURE 4-6 Demonstration of the lens equation. (a) Object 15 cm from a 10-diopter lens. (b) Object 20 cm from lens; critical rays have been drawn to show how image is created. (c) Blur circle on screen closer to lens than image.

This is the fundamental lens equation. As an example, consider the lens in Figure 4–6(a). This lens has a focal length of 10 cm, and the arrow is placed 15 cm away from the lens. From the lens equation:

$$\frac{1}{10} = \frac{1}{i} + \frac{1}{15}, \text{ or } i = 30 \text{ cm}$$

Therefore an image of the arrow should be found 30 cm from the lens.

If we change the distance between the object and the lens, the placement of the image also changes. In Figure 4–6(b), the lens is the same as in part (a), but the object has been moved farther from the lens. The effect of this is to move the image closer to the lens: from 30 cm away in part (a) to 20 cm away in part (b). The image also becomes smaller, as we would expect when the object is farther away.

BOX 4-3

Take a magnifying lens (whose focal length has been determined in the last box), and hold it parallel to a white wall in a dim room with one bright window. By varying the distance between the lens and the wall, you should be able to find a position for which a clear image of the outside scene is projected on the wall. Notice that the image is inverted.

The image exists at a certain place in space, but we are generally concerned with the way it appears when projected on a surface (such as a movie screen, the film in a camera, or the retina of the eye). When the image is exactly on the surface, it appears clear and sharp. When the image is either closer to the lens than the surface or farther away, the picture appears blurred—it is out of focus. This is because the light from each point in the object is not all at one point in the image. We have intercepted the cone of rays coming from all parts of the lens where it is still broad, and a single point on the object projects a blur circle (Figure 4–6[d]).

THE VERTEBRATE EYE

Structure

Figure 4–7 shows a cross section of a human eyeball. In most of its basic characteristics, the human eye is representative of that of other vertebrates; it is roughly spherical in shape with a diameter of about 2 cm. The eye lies in a socket of the skull, and can be moved through the action of six *extraocular muscles*, which will be described later. The outer wall of the eye is a tough, opaque covering called the *sclera*. At the front of the eye (top of the figure) the sclera protrudes and becomes clear; this portion is called the *cornea*, and is where light enters the eye. Because the front surface of the cornea is curved, it also acts as a lens and aids in bending light rays to form an image at the back of the eye. Just inside the cornea is a small compartment, the *anterior chamber*, filled with a clear fluid called *aqueous humor*. At the back of the anterior chamber is the *iris*, a smooth ring of muscle with a central opening the size of which depends on the state of contraction of the iris. This central opening is the *pupil*; the area of the pupil varies as a function of the amount of light impinging on the eye, as well as being influenced by emotional states.

Just behind the iris lies the crystalline *lens*; its purpose is to assist the cornea in producing a focussed image of the visual world onto the back of the eye. The lens of the eye is convex, similar to the lens discussed in the previous section. It is normally a clear tissue with no blood vessels in it that receives nutrition from the aqueous humor that surrounds it. (The lens sometimes becomes nearly opaque late in life; this condition is known as a *cataract*.) The lens is suspended in position by a fiber sac called the *zonule of Zinn*. This sac attaches to a set of muscles called the *ciliary muscles*. Con-

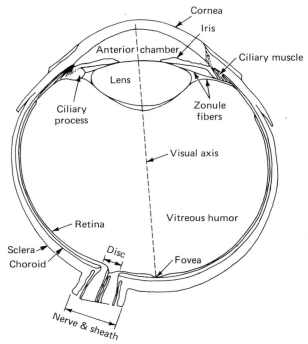

FIGURE 4-7   Schematic of the human eye. Right eye, from above. From Walls, G. L. (1967). *The Vertebrate Eye and its Adaptive Radiation*. New York: Hafner. Reprinted by permission of the Cranbrook Institute of Science.

traction of these muscles allows the eye to change its focus; details of this mechanism will be discussed in a later section.

Immediately behind the lens is the major chamber of the eye, which is filled with a clear viscous fluid called the *vitreous humor* (or "glassy fluid"). The inner wall of this chamber is lined with a thin sheet of neural tissue called the *retina*; the retina is responsible for sensing the image projected by the structures at the front of the eyeball, and encoding the information as a neural signal to transmit to the brain.

BOX 4-4

If the cornea and lens act like a convex lens forming an image on the retina, that image must be upside down. This bit of physics perplexed people in the 17th century, for the world is certainly not seen as upside down.

Descartes actually peeled a window of the sclera and choroid from a cow eye to demonstrate the image really is inverted. Why is our world not inverted? Simply because the brain is wired to "know" that cells in the lower part of

(continued)

(box continued)

the eye "see" the upper part of the world. Actually, it may not even be prewired; you may have learned that relationship when you first started to connect the patterns in your eyes with the world "out there."

But you can relearn the wiring. G. M. Stratton performed a series of experiments in the 1890s in which subjects wore eyeglasses with prisms that inverted images, making the images on the retinas right side up (see Wallach, 1987). Subjects were terribly confused at first,

but soon learned to function under these new conditions. (You have learned to function under new visual conditions, too: remember how hard it was to move your hand correctly over your face seen in a mirror the first time you tried to shave or put on makeup?) But the subjects did not just learn how to move appropriately; after a few days, they *perceived* the upside-down world as looking normal. And when they removed their prisms after nearly a week, they had to relearn normal vision.

The retina lies against a darkly colored layer of cells called the *pigment epithelium* ("epithelium" is another word for skin); the functions of this layer will be discussed in the next chapter. Between the pigment epithelium and the tough sclera is the *choroid*, which is rich in blood vessels. The blood vessels of the choroid provide nutrition and oxygen for the pigment epithelium and deep layers of the retina. The surface layers of the retina are nourished by a second network of blood vessels that lies on the surface of the retina.

BOX 4–5

It might seem that a network of blood vessels on the surface of the retina would interfere with vision, as they fall between the lens and the retina. We do not notice them in everyday vision because of an important property of the visual system: it responds only to change. The blood vessels move with the retina, and so their shadows never change.

You can see the blood vessels in your own eye by setting up a situation in which their shadows move against the retina. Take off your

glasses, if you wear them, and stare at a large uniform surface. The surface should be free of details (a blank wall is good) and not too brightly lit. Take a small flashlight or penlight, and hold it at the side of your head, aiming at your eye. Shine the light against the side of your eyeball; some light will light the retina from the side. Each time your eye (or the light) moves, you will see the branching network of the blood vessels of your eye.

Several landmarks on the back of the eye deserve mention. If we stare directly at some object in space, the position of the eye moves so that the image of that object is projected onto the central portion of the retina. This central region is called the *macula lutea*, and is easily identifiable because it is yellowish in color. Within the macula lies a small indentation, or pit, that is called the *fovea*. The fovea is a specialized region of the retina in which the capacity for fine visual discrimination is greatest; in the next chapter we discuss some of the properties of the fovea that are responsible for this fine discrimination.

    Another structure on the back of the eye that is of some importance is the *optic disc*. The optic disc is slightly on the nasal side of the retina (that is, toward the nose); it is where the axons of the retinal cells that carry visual information to the brain leave the retina and form the *optic nerve*. At the optic disc, there is a hole in the retina from which the fibers exit, so that if an object projects an image directly onto the optic disc, it will not be seen; the optic disc is therefore also called the blind spot. You can demonstrate this phenomenon for yourself by examining Figure 4–8 as described in the legend.

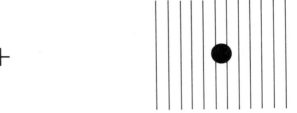

FIGURE 4–8   Find your own blind spot. Cover your left eye, and stare directly at the cross on the left of the figure. Take the book and slowly move it toward and away over a range of about 12 to 40 cm. At one particular distance, the black spot (but not the stripes) on the right of the figure should disappear; this happens when the image of the spot falls exactly on the optic disc, or blind spot.

BOX 4–6

The presence of a blind spot and its correspondence with the optic disc was known in the 1600s and taken as further evidence that the retina was *not* the photosensitive part of the eye. As far as anatomists could then determine, the retina and the optic nerve were all the same material; the retina was believed to be a broadening of the optic nerve at its head. In this view, there was no lack of "retina" at the blind spot; what was perforated was the pigment epithelium. From this, it was concluded that the pigment epithelium was the sensitive part of the eye (Priestly, 1772).

Accommodation

The function of the crystalline lens is to aid in focussing an image of the visual world onto the retina. It is not the only structure that performs this function; in fact, the cornea provides as much as 70% of the total refractive power in the human eye (Westheimer, 1975). It is because of the great focussing power of the cornea that people who have had their lenses surgically removed because of cataracts are still able to see with the help of glasses. The lens performs one function that the cornea cannot, however; it is capable of changing its refractive power to focus on objects at different distances from the eye.

Consider what happens when you look at a distant object, for example, the moon. The light rays from the moon reaching the eye are virtually parallel, as shown in Figure 4–9(a). The cornea and lens act to bend the light rays, and produce a sharp image of the moon on the retina at the fovea. From this, we can conclude that the focal length of the cornea/lens combination is about equal to the distance from the lens to the retina. Now, what happens if, instead of looking at the moon, you change your gaze and stare at a thumbtack on the wall about 1 meter away? Figure 4–9(b) shows what would be predicted given the focal length of the lens/cornea as derived from Figure 4–9(a). The image of the thumbtack will no longer be at the retina; instead, it will be projected at a distance somewhat behind the retina. This is a direct consequence of the properties of lenses we discussed earlier in this chapter; for a lens of any given focal length, as the distance between the lens and object grows shorter, the distance between the lens and the image it projects becomes longer.

If you are under the age of 45 and have normal vision, you know that your visual system somehow compensates for the problem discussed in the previous paragraph. The human eye can focus sharply either on objects that are quite far away or on objects that are practically in front of the nose. This ability depends on the fact that the lens can change its focussing power to maintain the image position at the retina. When you are looking at objects a long distance away, the lens assumes a flattened shape with a minimum amount of

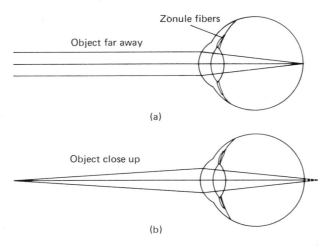

FIGURE 4-9 What happens if the lens cannot change shape? (a) Eye is appropriately focussed on far-away objects. (b) Eye is improperly focussed on close-up object.

refractive power. As the object comes closer to the eye, the lens becomes more and more rounded, increasing its refractive power (or decreasing the focal length) and so preventing the image of the object from moving behind the retina. This change in refractive power is called *accommodation*.

As an object moves closer to the eye, the lens decreases its effective focal length in order to maintain an image of the object on the retina. At a certain distance, however, the lens has become maximally curved, and a further decrease in the distance between the object and the eye will not cause change in the shape of the lens. At separations shorter than this distance, the lens will not be able to provide sufficient accommodation, and will project an image behind the retina. At the retina, then, the image of this object will be unfocussed or blurred. The closest distance for which the lens can project a focussed image of the object is called the *near point*. For very young children, the near point is about 10 cm (Brown, 1965); an object closer than this distance will not be seen clearly.

The mechanism for accommodation is illustrated in Figure 4–10. When the eye is focussing on a distant target, the zonule fibers encasing the lens and attached to the sclera are stretched tight. The stretching of the fibers flattens the lens and decreases its refractive power. This situation is shown in Figure 4–10(a). When the eye focusses on a nearby object, the ciliary muscles contract. The contraction of the ciliary muscles creates a pull in the reverse direction of the stretched zonule fibers; this results in less stretching force on the sac encompassing the lens. As the stress on the lens is decreased, the lens is free to assume its normal shape, which is quite rounded. Thus when the ciliary muscles are activated, the lens relaxes to assume the shape that produces the most refractive power (Figure 4–10[b]).

In a normal eye, the lens is flattest when distant objects are viewed, and more rounded when close-up objects are viewed. For many individuals, however, the accommodation of the lens is not sufficient to produce a focussed image for objects at all distances. As one gets older, for example, the lens becomes less elastic, and the ciliary muscles are less able to change the lens' curvature to focus on close-up objects. This decrease in accommodative ability with age is known as *presbyopia*. One consequence of presbyopia is that the near point of the eye drastically increases, making it harder to see closeup objects. It is for this reason that older people who had normal vision at a younger age usually need reading glasses.

Of course, many of us do not have normal, or *emmetropic*, eyes even when we are young. "Emmetropia" sounds like a disease, but means "correctly focussed." Refractive errors probably are largely hereditary, although there may also be some neural control over the shape of the developing eye (see Kolata, 1985). Visual deficits can also be the result of eye injury or eye surgery. For example, if the lens develops a cataract, so that light is diffused instead of focussed, the lens must be removed. The overall focussing power of the eye is therefore severely reduced, so images would be in focus far behind the retina.

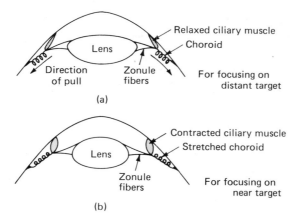

FIGURE 4-10 The mechanism of accommodation. (a) Focus on distant object; ciliary muscles are relaxed and lens ligaments are taut, causing the lens to be flattened. (b) Focus on close-up object; tension on lens ligaments is reduced by contraction of ciliary muscles, and the lens assumes its normal, rounded shape. After Crouch, J. E. and J. R. McClintic. *Human Anatomy and Physiology*. Copyright © 1971 John Wiley & Sons, Inc. Reprinted by permission.

Probably the most common visual deficit is *myopia*, or nearsightedness. When people who are myopic look at a distant object, their lenses project an image of the object at some distance in front of the retina (Figure 4-11[a]). One possible reason for this inappropriate image placement may be abnormal elongation of the eyeball; alternatively, either the lens or cornea may provide an abnormally large amount of refraction. As a distant object moves toward a myopic eye, the image of the object will move from a point in front of the retina back toward the retina, until the object comes into good focus. From that distance until the object moves closer than the near point, the eye accommodates in a normal fashion. The near point of a myopic eye is generally shorter than for a normal eye, so that myopic individuals can focus on objects closer to their eyes than can normal individuals. Note that the entire visual range has been displaced from normal. When the myopic person's lens stiffens with presbyopia, the near point moves back toward the far point, or most distant point on which the eye can sharply focus. Contrary to popular expectation, the farsightedness of old age does not cancel myopia.

Hypermetropia, or true farsightedness, is another kind of refractive error in which there is a deficit in the refracting power of the eye. When the ciliary muscles are relaxed and the lens is flattened to its maximum degree, an image of a far-away object will be projected at a point behind the retina (Figure 4-11[b]). That is, either the lens is too weak, or the eyeball is too short. When looking at a distant object, the hypermetropic eye can correct for this refractive weakness by having the ciliary muscles be constantly contracted to

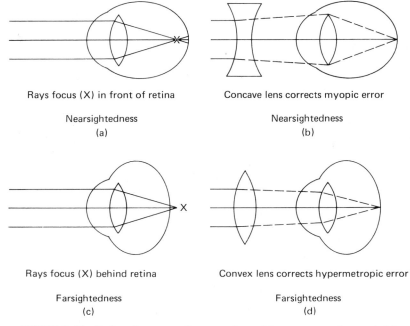

Rays focus (X) in front of retina

Nearsightedness
(a)

Concave lens corrects myopic error

Nearsightedness
(b)

Rays focus (X) behind retina

Farsightedness
(c)

Convex lens corrects hypermetropic error

Farsightedness
(d)

FIGURE 4-11   Refractive states for myopic and hypermetropic eyes. (a) Uncorrected myopia. (b) Corrected myopia. (c) Uncorrected hypermetropia. (d) Corrected hypermetropia.

some extent, increasing the refractive power of the lens. In this way, a farsighted person can bring distant objects into focus; however, that person will not be able to bring a close-up object into focus; the near point will be considerably longer than that of a normal person. When the hypermetropic person's lens stiffens with presbyopia, the near point moves back toward the far point, until even infinitely distant objects are too close for accommodation.

BOX 4-7

Both myopia and hypermetropia can be corrected through the use of lenses that cause incoming light rays to diverge for myopia, or converge for hypermetropia (Figure 4-11[c] and [d]). Another condition, *astigmatism*, results from distortion of the cornea or lens such that focus is different along different axes (that is, vertical lines might be sharp, but horizontal lines blurry). This can be compensated with a cylindrical lens. Corrective lenses can be mounted in a frame in front of the eyes (eyeglasses), placed directly on the cornea (contact lenses), or, in the case of removal of the natural lens in cataract surgery, placed inside the sac formed by the zonule fibers in the eye.

When you visit an optometrist or ophthalmologist and have your vision checked, you are usually asked to read a chart on a distant wall.

(continued)

(box continued)
This tests your *acuity*, the ability to resolve fine details. The familiar chart starting with a big "E" is called a Snellen chart; other charts require that you detect the orientation of capital E's or of the gap in an interrupted circle. Acuity can also be tested with fine grating patterns (see Chapter 10). Various lenses are placed before your eyes to determine the correction needed.

Most eyeglass prescriptions have six num-

bers, three for each eye. The two eyes are labeled O.D. (*oculus dextra*, the right eye) and O.S. (*oculus sinister*, the left eye). The "spherical" correction is the strength of the lens, in diopters. Positive spherical correction means a convex lens, for hypermetropia, while negative is a concave lens, for myopia. "Cylindrical" correction is the correction for astigmatism, and "axis" tells how to orient the axis of the cylindrical component.

Control of Pupil Size

The pupil is the aperture of the iris, and is controlled by the state of contraction of its sphincter and dilator muscles. The nervous control of these muscles is antagonistic; when one muscle is excited, the other is inhibited. Contraction of the sphincter in conjunction with relaxation of the dilator causes the pupil to constrict, while relaxation of the sphincter and contraction of the dilator causes the pupil to dilate (enlarge). The effect of light is to cause constriction of the pupil to a degree dependent on the intensity of light. As the level of ambient illumination increases, the size of the pupil decreases. Thus the pupil exerts control over the amount of light that enters the eye.

BOX 4–8

The pupil may constrict or dilate from other factors than the level of ambient light. Investigators have correlated changes in pupil size with the level of mental activity in which a subject is engaged, as well as the emotional state of the subject. A number of experiments have demonstrated that visual stimuli that have positive affective connotations will produce dilation of the pupil. Hess and Polt (1960) found that women in general increased the sizes of their pupils when presented with pictures of male nudes more than when they were shown pictures of female nudes, while the pattern was reversed for men. Similarly, Fitzgerald (1968)

reported that the pupils of infants dilated more to pictures of human faces than to geometric shapes; the infants also showed more pupil dilation to pictures of their mothers than to pictures of strangers. Hess (1965) has suggested that just as stimuli with positive affect cause the pupil to dilate, stimuli that have a negative emotional content will produce pupil constriction. Other investigators, however, have not demonstrated this relationship (Loewenfeld, 1968; Pearler & McLaughlin, 1967; Woodmansee, 1965).

Concentrated mental activity also has an effect on pupil size. Hess and Polt (1964) found
(continued)

(box continued)
that subjects' pupils dilated when they were given arithmetic problems to solve, with the amount of dilation depending on the difficulty of the problem. Other types of intellectual tasks have also been found to have the same effect (Goldwater, 1972). Kahneman and his associates (Kahneman & Beatty, 1967; Kahneman & Pearler, 1969) have attempted to determine precisely what aspect of mental activity is affecting pupil size, and have concluded that the critical variable is the amount of processing that is necessary for a subject to complete a particular task.

The size of the pupil is often thought to play a role in our ability to function in both bright and dim environments by restricting the light input under bright conditions, and allowing more light into the eye under dim illumination. In fact, however, the pupil plays only a minimal role in this regard; the pupil diameter of the human eye can vary only between 2 and 8 mm, a 16-fold change in area. Such a dynamic range is minute compared with the variations of a factor of 10^9, the range of intensities over which the human visual system operates. What the pupil does do is allow only the most optically accurate parts of the visual system to be employed, under conditions in which there is enough light for this restriction to be feasible. The edges of the human lens (or any lens, for that matter) are optically inferior to the center region; a constricted pupil restricts the passage of light to the center portion of the lens. In addition, as the pupil becomes smaller the lens becomes less important as a refractive structure. In the limit, a pinhole aperture, the visual field would be in focus even if the lens were absent. When the pupil becomes quite small, objects that were not in sharp focus when the pupil was larger look as if they are in better focus. The extent to which an object can be moved up and back in front of the lens without greatly distorting the focus is called the *depth of field*. Decreasing pupil size increases depth of field, and thus allows objects at different distances from the eye to be in sharp focus simultaneously, even without changes in the shape of the lens.

BOX 4–9

Depth of field is easy to demonstrate for yourself, if you are either nearsighted or farsighted. Make a pinhole in a piece of paper; then take off your glasses and look through the pinhole when it is placed as close as possible to your eye. The world is in reasonable focus through the hole, even though it may be quite dim. (This is one of the reasons that squinting sometimes helps.) In fact, the first cameras were merely boxes with a pinhole in one wall and a light-sensitive substance on the opposite wall. Even without a lens, an image of the world was projected onto the far wall by the pinhole.

EXTRAOCULAR MUSCLES AND EYE MOVEMENT

The eye is not stationary in the socket, but can move in two dimensions. This movement is mediated by the six *extraocular* muscles, shown in Figure 4–12. The muscles are arranged in three antagonistic pairs. Up and down movement of the eye is mediated mainly by the *superior* and *inferior rectus muscles*; contraction of one muscle in this pair is always coupled with relaxation in the other muscle. For example, to move the eye so that it is pointing upward, the superior rectus muscle must contract at the same time that the inferior rectus muscle relaxes. Similarly, sideways movement of the eye is mediated by the *lateral* and *medial* rectus muscles. The *superior* and *inferior oblique muscles* are important for producing rotational eye movements, as well as assisting the superior and inferior recti in producing vertical movements.

This is a fairly elaborate orchestration, especially since it must be coordinated with head movements that are not along the same axes. There is a relatively direct, though complex, relationship between activity in the semicircular canals of the vestibular apparatus and activation of the muscles. This pattern varies across species because the eyes may be placed either looking forward or to the sides, but the end effect is quite similar (see Simpson and Graf, 1985).

BOX 4–10

The relationship between the vestibular apparatus and eye movements may be demonstrated by a simple experiment. Have someone sit on a rotating chair (a desk chair or bar stool) with his or her eyes closed and spin the chair in one direction at a moderate speed for about 30 seconds. Stop the chair, and have the subject open his or her eyes. You will see his or her eyes move smoothly, then flick back, and move again, as if rapidly scanning a wide page of text. This pattern of movement and quick return is

called *nystagmus*, and it is just what the eyes would have to do if trying to fixate a point in the world while the body was rotating. As an aftereffect of the earlier motion, the subject feels as if he or she were rotating in the opposite direction (see Chapter 14 for visual movement aftereffects). The subject should feel like he or she is rotating the other way. This nystagmus was induced by motion, but it could also be induced by a moving visual stimulus, such as when you watch a long train move past.

Eye movements are important for several reasons. They allow the eye to follow a moving object while maintaining an image of that object at a stationary position on the retina. In addition, eye movements allow an animal swiftly to change its direction of gaze from one part of the visual field to another, perhaps in response to the introduction of some novel stimulus. These types of eye movements involve both eyes moving in the same direction, and are called *conjugate eye movements*.

Two types of conjugate eye movements can be distinguished. Eye movements that occur in response to a moving object in the visual field are called

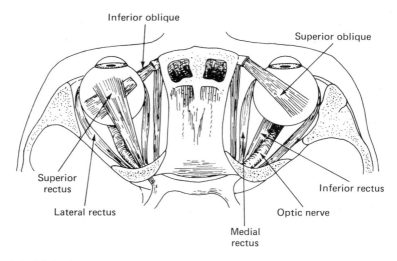

FIGURE 4–12 Extraocular muscles, as seen from above. From Walls, G. L. (1967) *The Vertebrate Eye and its Adaptive Radiation*. New York: Hafner. Reprinted by permission of the Cranbrook Institute of Science.

smooth pursuit movements. The velocity of rotation of the eye will match the movement·of the object as long as this velocity is less than about 30 degrees/ sec. Smooth pursuit movements are involuntary, in the sense that one cannot produce them in the absence of a moving object.

The other major class of conjugate eye movements are *saccadic movements*, which are sudden jumps made by the eye as it changes its point of fixation. Saccades last anywhere between 20 msec to 50 msec and can vary in size from less than 10′ of angle to as large as 20°. Saccadic movements occur continuously while scanning the visual world, as one attends to different aspects of the stimulus array. They also occur in direct response to introduction of a novel or moving stimulus into the visual field. In such cases, the saccadic movement orients the eye so that the novel stimulus projects an image onto the fovea, as opposed to the peripheral retina where the image had previously been projected.

Conjugate eye movements involve both eyes moving in the same direction; in *disjunctive eye movements*, however, the eyes move in opposite directions. When one views a close-up object, both eyes move inward, so that an image of the object can be projected onto the foveas of both eyes. This is called *convergence*; conversely, as an object moves away, the eyes *diverge*. If the images of the object are not in the equivalent places on the two retinae, a phenomenon called *diplopia*, or double vision, results. You can demonstrate this phenomenon by trying the test for stereopsis in the box on page ix. When you focus on your fingers, you see the point at the far end of the room in duplicate. The double image (or the double image of your fingers, which you see when you focus on the far point) is an example of diplopia. Disjunctive eye movements are necessary to reduce the double images into a single image.

BOX 4-11 ▬▬▬▬▬▬▬▬▬▬▬▬▬▬

The eyeballs of most vertebrates are remarkably similar, possessing many of the structures that we have described in the preceding sections. Many invertebrates, however, have visual systems that deviate greatly from the vertebrate scheme. Consider, for example, the eye of the horseshoe crab, *Limulus polyphemus*, a primitive marine animal. In contrast to vertebrate eyes that have one lens and cornea, the *Limulus* eye is a compound eye. As shown in Figure 4-13, it is composed of about 800 tiny but separate facets, or *ommatidia* (Hartline, Wagner, & Ratliff, 1956), each of which has its own lens and cornea, receptors, and optic nerve fibers that emanate from it. Each facet is oriented so that it responds to light stimuli in different areas of the visual field, with neighboring facets responding to somewhat overlapping areas. Within each ommatidium, the transparent covering of the eye acts as both a lens and a cornea to channel the light (coming from the region at which the ommatidium is pointing) to the receptor cells that lie underneath (Hartline, Wag-

ner, & MacNichol, 1952). The axons of these receptor cells leave the ommatidium and join the optic nerve that goes into the brain.

The eye of the *Limulus* is obviously quite different from those of humans and other vertebrates; however, there are some parallels that can be drawn. In place of the mosaic of receptors on which the vertebrate lens projects an image of the visual world, the *Limulus* has a mosaic of ommatidia acting as both light-gathering and light-responding units. The apparent simplicity of the *Limulus* eye is what attracted scientists to it in the first place. (H. K. Hartline and his associates have studied the properties of *Limulus* eyes in great detail; from this work, many of the basic principles that underlie human vision were first discovered. In particular, it was in *Limulus* that Hartline and his colleagues first described lateral antagonism, a main topic of Chapter 6. For his work in characterizing visual sensory processes, Hartline shared the Nobel Prize in 1967.)

SUGGESTED READINGS

George Wald's August 1950 *Scientific American* article entitled "Eye and Camera" (offprint #46) reprinted in *Perception: Mechanisms and Models*, by R. Held and W. Richards (W. H. Freeman, 1972) provides a good introduction to the comparative anatomy of animal eyes. More detailed information about light properties and the structure of the vertebrate eye can be found in Chapters 1 and 2 of *Vision and Visual Perception*, edited by C. H. Graham (John Wiley, 1965). Finally, for anyone who really wants to be immersed in eyes, *The Vertebrate Eye and its Adaptive Radiation*, by G. Walls (Hafner, 1967) is a classic description of the eyes of almost every vertebrate imaginable.

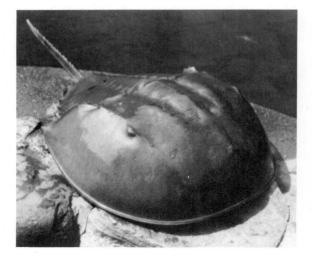
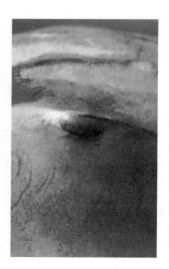

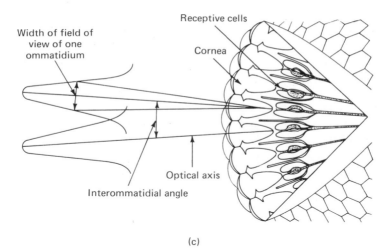

(c)

FIGURE 4–13 (a) *Limulus polyphemus*, the horseshoe crab. (b) Close-up view of the lateral eye of *Limulus*. Note the slightly darker ommatidia near the center; this "pseudopupil" is caused by the fact that the view is directly down the axes of these ommatidia. (c) Cross section of several ommatidia.

THE RETINA

5

In the previous chapter we presented the gross anatomy of the eye, and explained how it projects an upside-down image of the visual world on the sensitive neural retina. This chapter is an overview of how the retina converts an image of light and shade into a neural signal, and codes that signal for transmission to the brain. In fact, this chapter does not quite tell the whole story; the final stage of processing and encoding is performed by the retinal ganglion cells, which are the subject of the next chapter.

The coding of the signal that the retina sends to the brain is a complicated process, and has not been fully deciphered. This chapter may seem to contain an inordinate amount of detail; in fact, we have omitted many details and set forth only those that probably are most pertinent to the problem at hand. (We say probably, because until the process is better understood it will be hard to judge which aspects are really the most significant.) The concepts and principles introduced in this chapter will reappear in discussions of higher centers and other senses, and prove to be significant in understanding perception.

Pigment Epithelium

Before we begin to discuss the retina itself, we should consider the tissue with which the retina is closely allied, the pigment epithelium. As the name implies, it is a layer of cells that contain pigment, or coloring agent. Pigment epithelium is not actually neural, but is derived from the same kind of cells as the retina of the developing embryo.

Pigment absorbs light, and therefore looks dark. Light absorbed by the pigment epithelium is apparently not useful for vision, having already passed through the retina without being absorbed. If this light that failed to stimulate the retina were not absorbed by pigment epithelium, it would bounce back through the retina. It might be absorbed by the retina on the second pass, and be taken for a part of the image. On the second pass, however, it could be slightly displaced from its original position, so the image would be degraded. Some might pass through again, and strike the retina at some distant point, further confusing the image. Thus, one important function of the pigment epithelium is to prevent light from bouncing around inside the eye, an effect called *scatter*. (In this respect, pigment epithelium is the equivalent of painting the inside of a camera black.) We shall see shortly that it has another important function as well.

BOX 5-1

Not all animals have a dark-colored pigment epithelium. Animals that hunt at night have eyes designed to make the most use of a limited amount of light. The "second chance" to see sparse light on the bounce is more important than the loss of image clarity caused by scatter. Rather than having a dark layer behind the retina, these animals have a highly reflective layer called a *tapetum*. The tapetum is the reason a cat's eyes seem to glow in the dark; what is seen is the light that has entered the eye, passed through the retina, bounced off the tapetum, passed through the retina again, and out of the eye. This kind of reflection can occur in human eyes as well. It is the explanation for the effect called "red eye" in photography. If you take a flash photo of someone who is staring right at the camera, and the flash is mounted next to the camera lens, the pupils of the subject's eyes appear to be red. The light filling the pupils is light from the flash, beamed back at the camera by the lens and cornea. There is a reddish color because the pigment of pigment epithelium absorbs long wavelength light least efficiently, and also because the light passes through blood vessels on the surface of the retina. This beamed-back light is what an ophthalmologist views through the ophthalmoscope.

GENERAL ANATOMY OF THE RETINA

The retina itself is more than just a layer of light-sensitive cells; it also performs the first stages of processing the visual image. It is composed of three major layers of cell bodies, separated by two layers of synaptic connections called *plexiform layers* (Figure 5–1). The layers are named according to their position relative to the center of the eyeball; layers nearest the center of the eye are referred to as *inner*, and those nearer the pigment epithelium are called *outer*.

Starting at the layer nearest the pigment epithelium, cells in the outermost layer of cell bodies are the *receptors*. These are the cells that perform the task of absorbing light and transducing it into nervous energy. Light is absorbed by pigments in the receptors, at which time it ceases to be light, just as the sound of a voice is no longer sound when it is traveling along a telephone wire.

As the receptors are in the outermost layer of the retina (and, in fact, the light-absorbing pigment is in the outermost part of each receptor) light reaching the receptors must first have passed through all other layers of the retina (to be discussed in the following paragraphs). This might seem like an inefficient way to design an eyeball. Actually, the loss of light because of this "backward" arrangement is negligible, as the retina is extremely thin (about

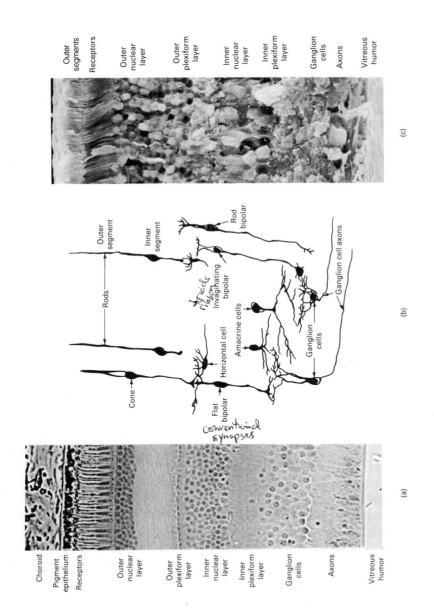

FIGURE 5-1 The retina. (b) Schematic showing the various cell types and some of their interconnections. (a) Light micrograph of a human retina with the cells shown up by a technique called phase contrast microscopy. (c) Scanning electron micrograph of a cat retina. Micrograph (a) from Boycott, B. B., and J. E. Dowling (1969) Organization of the primate retina: Light microscopy. *Philos. Trans. R. Soc. Lond.* 255:109–184. Reprinted by permission of the publisher and the author. Electron micrograph (c) courtesy of E. H. Polley, Dept. of Anatomy and Cell Biology, University of Illinois at Chicago.

0.2 mm), made of cells that are mostly water, and therefore practically invisible when immersed in the fluids of the eye. (The micrograph in Figure 5–1 was made by a special technique that makes the cells visible.) This slight disadvantage is more than compensated for by the advantages of having the receptors in close apposition to the pigment epithelium. Because the receptors are close, the spread of light that does bounce from the pigment epithelium is minimal. In addition, the pigment in the receptors must be replenished after absorbing light; the pigment epithelium apparently plays a role in this replenishment.

The cell bodies of the receptors lie in a layer called the *outer nuclear layer* ("nuclear" because the nuclei of the receptors are there). The receptors terminate in a layer of synaptic connections called the *outer plexiform* layer. It is here that the receptors are presynaptic to other cells in the retina, and possibly also postsynaptic to some of them. We will have more to say about these synapses.

The next layer of cell bodies is the *inner nuclear layer*, which actually consists of three somewhat distinct sublayers. At its outer margin are *horizontal cells*, so named because they run horizontally in the retina, interconnecting distant areas. These horizontal (or *lateral*) connections are the first stage in retinal processing of the visual image.

The bulk of the inner nuclear layer is filled with *bipolar cells*. Bipolar means "having two ends"—that is, cells that simply interconnect two points. The bipolar cells are the links between the outer and inner plexiform layers, but they also participate in the processing at both ends.

Near the inner margin of the inner nuclear layer, you can see some nuclei that are slightly larger than the bulk of those in the layer. These are the *amacrine cells* (which means "cells without axons"). The amacrine cells are the horizontal or lateral elements of the inner plexiform layer; their cell bodies are in the inner nuclear layer but they send a number of dendritelike processes into the synaptic layer, like an octopus sitting on an oyster bed. There is considerable dispute over exactly which cells should be called amacrine, how many different types of amacrine cells there are, and what their function might be. For our purposes, they are the cells that provide the lateral interconnections required for the second stage of processing of the visual image that occurs at the *inner plexiform* layer. Here, the bipolar cells are presynaptic to amacrine cells and *ganglion cells*; amacrine cells are presynaptic to other amacrine cells, to bipolar cells, and to ganglion cells.

The inner plexiform layer varies considerably in thickness and complexity among different animals. In a comparison of this layer in a number of species, Dubin (1970) found that the thickest ones were in the retinas of frogs and pigeons, while in humans they are relatively thin. Moreover, the inner plexiform layer of frogs and pigeons is considerably more complex in that bipolar cells rarely synapse directly on ganglion cells; rather, bipolar cells make synapses with amacrine cells, which synapse with other amacrine cells, which ultimately lead to ganglion cells. Human retinas show a relatively high number of bipolar cell synapses directly on ganglion cells.

The implication of this structural complexity is that the retinas of these "simpler" animals perform a more complex processing task than our retinas do. Presumably, their retinas do more processing because their brains do less. Our brains receive a more complete description of the visual world and decipher those aspects that are most important The frog's brain receives a highly processed version of the world, with the relevant information already sorted out for immediate action.

The final level of this complicated processing network is occupied by the ganglion cells. These are the only cells that communicate with the brain, so they may be considered to be the output of the retina. Ganglion cells have their dendrites in the inner plexiform layer, their cell bodies in the *ganglion cell layer* (see Figure 5–1), and send axons across the surface of the retina (to the optic disc) to join the *optic nerve*. The optic nerves (one from each eye), each contain about one million ganglion cell axons whose ultimate destinations are in the brain.

BOX 5–2 ▪▪▪▪▪▪▪▪▪▪▪▪▪▪▪▪

Although we have described a number of cell types and interconnections, we have drawn a relatively simple picture of a retina in which information tends to flow in the direction from receptors to ganglion cells, with lateral spreading at the two plexiform layers. After all, we consider the retina's main function to be telling the ganglion cells about light falling on the receptors, so the ganglion cells can convey that information to the brain. Recently, however, this straightforward picture has been disrupted by the discovery of pathways by which information can also flow in the opposite direction. In the inner plexiform layers of the retinas of fish (Ehinger, Falck, & Laties, 1969; Dowling & Ehinger, 1975), monkeys (Dowling & Ehinger, 1975), and other mammals (Boycott, Dowling, Fisher, Kolb & Laties, 1975; Dawson & Perez, 1973; Dowling & Ehinger, 1978b; Fisher,

1979), there are cells that look like amacrine cells. Unlike amacrine cells, however, these have axons that travel into the outer plexiform layer, where they are presynaptic (Dowling & Ehinger, 1978a; Dowling, 1978). These cells, which connect the two plexiform layers, have been named *interplexiform cells* (Gallego, 1971). They are *centrifugal*; that is, they conduct information from the inner layers to the outer layers.

Another centrifugal pathway arises in the brain itself. Cells in specific areas of the brains of pigeons (Dowling & Cowan, 1966) and fish (Witkovsky, 1971) send axons that run alongside the axons of ganglion cells and end in the inner plexiform layer of the retina. This pathway enables the brain to influence the processing performed by the retina. The operation of this system is not yet well understood.

RECEPTORS

Most vertebrate retinas contain two distinctly different types of receptor cells, *rods* and *cones*. They are distinguished principally by the shape of the outermost part of each cell, the *outer segment* (which is the part that actually absorbs light and generates the initial neural signal). Rods have long cylindrical ("rodlike") outer segments that are of uniform diameter for most of their lengths; cones have shorter, tapered ("conical") outer segments that are widest near the cell body and quite narrow at their outer extremities.

In human eyes, rods and cones are not uniformly distributed in the outer layer of the retina. Along the main axis of the eye, at the very center of the retina, is the fovea. The retina is thinner at the fovea because the bipolar and ganglion cells serving the receptors in the fovea are off to the sides. This sweeping out from the foveal pit may be seen in Figure 5–2. The *only* receptors in the center of the fovea are cones; there are no rods at all. The fovea is the part of the human retina that is specialized for detailed vision. When we direct our eyes to a particular object, what we are doing is turning them so that the image of that object falls on the foveas. Humans (and some other primates such as monkeys) are the only animals to have this particular specialization. Some other animals, such as cats and birds, have specialized central regions similar to a fovea, but usually there are rods as well as cones in these regions. Some cold-blooded animals have retinas that show no specialization of this type.

Because there are no rods in the human fovea, they must all be in the part of the retina outside the fovea. Figure 5–3 shows the distribution of rods and

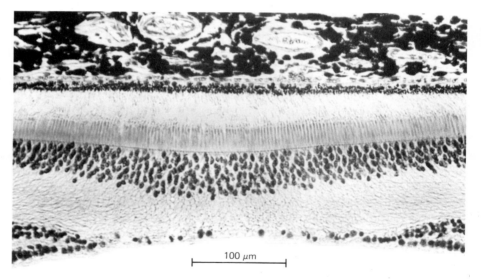

100 μm

FIGURE 5–2 Section through the fovea of a monkey retina. Cell bodies made visible by staining with haematoxylin and eosin. From Brown, K. T., K. Watanabe, and M. Murakami (1965) The early and late receptor potential of monkey cones and rods. *Cold Spring Harbor Symp. Quant. Biol.* 30:457–482. Reprinted by permission of the author and publisher.

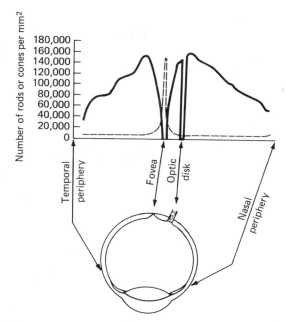

FIGURE 5-3 Distribution of rods (solid curve) and cones (dashed curve) in the human retina. Data of Østerberg (1935).

cones in the human eye; it represents the numbers of receptors encountered along the horizontal line that passes through the fovea. Cones are most numerous in the fovea, becoming more sparse as one moves either nasally or temporally. Rods are absent in the fovea, but are most dense in the region of retina to either side of it, being numerous all the way out to either the nasal or temporal edges, and outnumbering cones outside the fovea. One other point to notice in Figure 5–3: there is an interruption in both the rod and cone curves slightly nasal of the fovea. This is an area free of any receptors; it is the optic disc or blind spot, where the optic nerve exits from the eye.

There are a number of psychophysical correlates of the distribution of rods and cones. As we have said, the fovea is specialized for detailed vision, being the part of the eye in which the finest detail can be discerned; this property is called *acuity*. Acuity is best in the fovea, and considerably worse outside it. (Even though vision may be mediated by cones outside the fovea, the cones of the fovea are specialized for better acuity.) You can demonstrate the high acuity of your foveas by looking at a picture on a color television from close to the screen. Stand about arm's length from the screen. (Alternatively, you can get a similar effect by standing about 3 to 4 feet back from a windowscreen.) Concentrate on seeing the dots (or bars) of color that make up the picture, not on the picture itself. You should be able to see a small circular area in the very center of your gaze where individual dots may be clearly seen; this is the area falling on your foveas. Outside this sharp area, which will jump about as you move your eyes, the dots tend to blur together. The high acuity of your foveal vision allows you to resolve the individual dots in the areas seen by your foveas, but the rest of your retina does not have the requisite acuity.

Color vision is also best in the fovea. Outside it there are fewer cones and more rods, which seem to dilute the strength of colors (Gordon & Abramov, 1977). At the furthest periphery there are mainly rods, and little color vision at all. You can demonstrate this to yourself by having someone bring a small colored object into your field of view from behind your head. If you do not move your eyes, you may be able to see the object before you can determine its color or see its details.

Structure of Receptors

Each receptor, rod or cone, consists of two major subdivisions. The *inner segment* consists of the cell body (with the nucleus), and an axonlike process extending into the outer plexiform layer and terminating in an enlarged portion in which the synapses are made, called the *receptor terminal*.

The outer segments of rods and cones differ in shape, but appear to be similar in that each contains a tightly folded membrane that fills the segment. Electron microscope close-ups of outer segments in Figure 5–4 show this clearly; both rods and cones appear to be filled with sheets of membrane. There is a subtle difference between them, however. The membrane of the outer segments of cones is mostly one long folded sheet, like an accordion or fan, with openings to the extracellular fluid. The membranes in the outer segments of the rod consist of separate enclosed discs, like a stack of pancakes inside the membrane enclosing the outer segment (Laties & Liebman, 1970; Yoshikami, Robinson, & Hagins, 1974).

BOX 5-3

The inner and outer segments of rods and cones are connected by a fine filament located well off-center. The filament arises from a structure in the inner segment called a *centriole*, and contains nine pairs of tubular filaments. These are structures typical of *cilia*, the fine hairlike projections with which many single-celled organisms swim. The outer segment may be thought of as a highly specialized cilium, one that does not move, but instead transduces energy. The sensory portion of receptors in several other sensory systems are derived from modified cilia (Rodieck, 1973).

Function of Receptors

The outer segment of a rod or cone is the business end, the part that actually absorbs photons and begins the process of sending a neural signal to the brain. In effect, the real receptor is the outer segment. It contains molecules

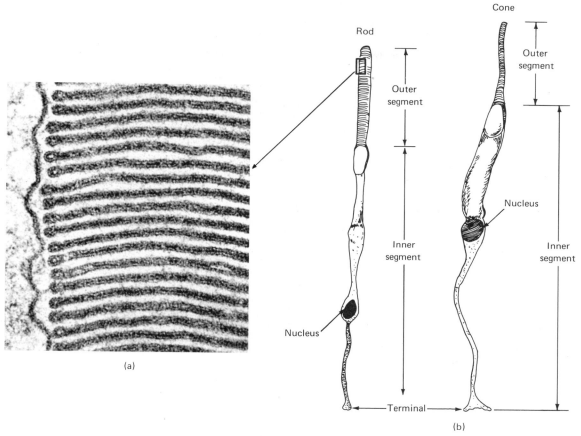

FIGURE 5-4 Structure of rods and cones. A rod is shown on the left, a cone on the right. An electron micrograph of part of the rod outer segment is shown next to it. Electron micrograph from Dowling, J. E. (1967) Figure 6 from Chapter 7, The organization of vertebrate visual receptors. In *Molecular Organization and Biological Function*. Edited by John M. Allen. Copyright © 1967 by John M. Allen. Reprinted by permission of Harper & Row, Publishers, Inc.

of pigment that absorb photons and undergo a chemical change as a result of that absorption. If light were not absorbed and its energy used to trigger this chemical change, there could be no vision.

There are two principal parts to a visual pigment molecule (more accurately, complex of molecules): the *opsin* and the *chromophore*. The opsin consists of a fairly large chain of amino acids. It is therefore a protein (although it also contains sugar and fat components). This long, stringy molecule is virtually "sewn" into the disk membrane, traversing it seven times (Bok, 1985). The chromophore is the part of the complex that is affected by light. It consists of a chemical called *retinal* that is an altered form of vitamin A (*retinol*), hence the relationship between eating vitamin A-rich foods such as carrots, and night vision. Both retinal and retinol consist of a ring of carbon atoms decorated with some side groups, and sporting a decorated tail of nine carbon atoms. When retinal is bound to opsin it is in a configuration called *11-cis*. That is, there is a bend in the tail at carbon atom number 11, as shown in Figure 5–5(b). Folded in this manner, the retinal tends to bind to the opsin, forming a single complex, the visual pigment.

When a photon is absorbed by the visual pigment, it ceases to exist as a photon and its energy is absorbed by the chromophore. When the chromophore absorbs this energy it undergoes a change called *isomerization*, which is a change in the physical configuration of the molecule of retinal. Specifically, the bend at carbon atom 11 straightens out; the retinal goes from the 11-cis isomer to the *all-trans* isomer shown in Figure 5–5(a). With its tail straightened out, the retinal no longer binds to the opsin, and rapidly breaks free. The change in form of the chromophore is the first step in the process of vision.

In order for vision to continue to be possible, there must be a continuing

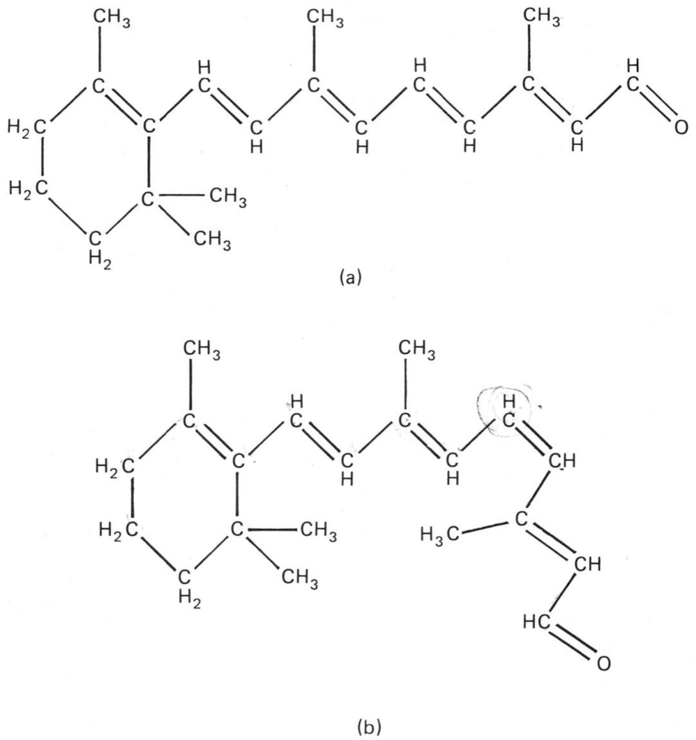

(a)

(b)

FIGURE 5–5   (a) All-trans retinal. 11-cis retinal (b).

supply of visual pigment. There are several changes the chromophore undergoes after isomerization, and a complicated set of alternative fates that could befall it. Eventually, however, it is made back into 11-cis retinal that recombines with opsin to make new pigment. Some of the all-trans retinal is converted directly back into 11-cis by an enzyme in the outer segment (called retinal isomerase); some is converted into retinol, and is recombined with opsin by a more complicated method in which the pigment epithelium plays a role (Pepperberg, Brown, Lurie, & Dowling, 1978).

BOX 5–4

There is another function of the pigment epithelium that requires it to be near the receptor outer segments. The receptors shed the folded discs from the outer segments, and these are taken up and digested by the pigment epithelium. (Why the receptors shed the tips of their outer segments is not understood, but they do. The receptors grow new discs or membrane at the innermost part of the outer segment, and the older material is pushed outward.) At first it was believed that only rods shed their discs, but we now know that cones also lose chunks of their outer segments (Young, 1978). Interestingly, the process of shedding occurs only at specific times of the day; cones shed their tips in the evening, and rods shed discs in the morning. The timing of shedding is partly controlled by lighting, and can even be influenced by the color of the light presented (Balkema and Bunt-Milam, 1982).

The absorption of a photon causes isomerization, and this leads to a change in the polarization of the receptor (see Chapter 3). It is a slightly curious property of vertebrate photoreceptors, both rods and cones, that the response to light is hyperpolarization. In most other receptors, including the photoreceptors of most invertebrates, the response to an appropriate stimulus is depolarization. Rods and cones hyperpolarize, in a sense acting as if they were excited by darkness and inhibited by light. In the dark, the membrane potential is less negative than is the case for most other neurons; during a stimulus, the receptor may hyperpolarize to levels near the normal resting potential of other cells (Tomita, 1970). This really makes no difference, as the information is the same whether the signal is excitatory or inhibitory (a photographic negative has the same information as the print made from it; it just looks strange to us).

BOX 5–5

How does the isomerization of a pigment molecule on the disk or folded membrane of an outer segment lead to hyperpolarization of the receptor? When the first edition of this book was written, we had a tentative answer to this question. We now believe that answer was wrong, although it did stimulate the research that has led to the new answer. We think this

(continued)

(box continued)

story is interesting not only for the explanation of how isomerization leads to hyperpolarization, but also as a glimpse at how science proceeds.

For an event on the disk membrane to affect the outer membrane of the receptor, some messenger must travel from disk to outer membrane. It had been observed that calcium ions are concentrated in the disks, and that adding calcium mimicked the effects of light (Yoshikami & Hagins, 1971; Brown & Pinto, 1974). The "calcium hypothesis" suggested that when rhodopsin isomerizes, it acts like an open pore in the disk and lets calcium ions out. The calcium diffuses to the outer membrane, where it blocks (or closes) pores that normally allow positive sodium ions to enter the cell in the dark and depolarize it.

There were some serious questions about the calcium hypothesis (Liebman & Pugh, 1979). Calcium may be sequestered in rod disks, but how is it segregated from the outer membrane in the folded membrane of cones? And why is there an effect of, and change in concentration of, a chemical called cyclic GMP (cGMP), a ribonucleic acid that is often a "second messenger" at synapses (Farber, Brown, & Lolley, 1978; Woodruff, Bownds, Green, Morrisey, & Shedlovsky, 1977)?

The answer came from the application of patch clamping (see Chapter 3) to the photoreceptor. Patches of outer segment membrane were recorded during exposure to various media. In both rods (Fesenko, Kolesnikov, & Lyubarsky, 1985) and cones (Haynes & Yau, 1985), a sodium gate was found that is held open by cGMP. Matthews and Watanabe (1987) showed that this cGMP-operated gate has the same properties as the sodium gate closed by light. In the dark, there is ample cGMP to hold the gates open, allowing sodium ions to enter and depolarize the cell. Isomerization of rhodopsin by light causes a decrease in the concentration of cGMP; the gates close, blocking the sodium flow, and the cell hyperpolarizes.

How does rhodopsin cause a decrease in cGMP? There is a complicated cascade similar to that in some synapses (Lamb, 1986). The "activated" (isomerized) rhodopsin breaks apart another molecule, variously called G-protein or *transducin*. Transducin molecules consist of three pieces that are bonded together. Activated rhodopsin frees one of these from the other two; the liberated piece joins another protein, *phosphodiesterase* (PDE). The PDE is thereby activated, and goes to work; its work is to break open the ring structure of cGMP, making ordinary GMP. Ordinary GMP does not open the sodium gates, so they close (until another enzyme reloops the GMP). This cascade of events allows tremendous amplification: one photon isomerizes one rhodopsin molecule, which activates hundreds of transducin molecules. The transducin activates PDE, each molecule of which breaks thousands of cGMP molecules. In this way, one photon can affect enough cGMP molecules to make a significant difference in the concentration of cGMP.

Why did calcium seem to be the culprit? There are three somewhat interlocked reasons. First, calcium can enter the cell through the sodium gates, but it is a tight squeeze. If a calcium ion gets in the gates, it occupies it and blocks the passage of many sodium ions. Thus, excess calcium "clogged" the sodium gates, and workers thought they were closed as they are by light.

Second, there is a sodium/calcium ex-

(continued)

(box continued)

change pump in the outer segment membrane (Yau and Nakatani, 1984). This pump allows sodium in, but throws calcium out (to make up for the calcium entering through the sodium gates). When the gates are blocked during light, the pump continues to expel calcium, so its concentration drops. This change in concentration made it look like it was being released as an internal transmitter.

Finally, we now think that calcium does play a part, not in the response to light, but in light adaptation (Flaming & Brown, 1979). The concentration of calcium apparently controls the rate at which the enzyme that reloops the broken cGMP can work. "Freezing" the calcium levels by preventing operation of the pump that would expel it during the light seems to prevent light adaptation in both rods and cones (Matthews, Murphy, Fain, and Lamb, 1988; Nakatani and Yau, 1988). It is even possible to ascribe differences in the rates of adap-

tation of rods and cones to their relative surface areas compared to volume (Pugh & Altman, 1988).

We may summarize as follows: In the dark, rhodopsin, transducin, and PDE are in their inactive states. There is a high concentration of cGMP, which holds the sodium gates open, letting sodium (and some calcium) enter and depolarize the cell. The sodium/calcium pump keeps the calcium level normal. Light isomerizes rhodopsin, which activates transducin, which activates PDE, which breaks up cGMP. Lacking cGMP, the gates close, and sodium cannot enter, so the cell hyperpolarizes. Calcium also cannot enter, so the pump lowers the calcium concentration in the cell. Low calcium speeds the reaction that rebuilds cGMP, so some gates reopen (causing the initial overshoot mentioned in Chapter 3), and responses to flashes added to the steady light are smaller and faster than if there were no steady light (see Chapter 7).

The hyperpolarization of a receptor is initiated in its outer segment, and spreads through the inner segment by decremental conduction. The receptor is sufficiently short that the slow potential is nearly full-sized at the terminal; there is no need to transmit the message by action potentials. In fact, all the cells of the retina (except the ganglion cells, which project all the way to the brain) are sufficiently small that action potentials are unnecessary. As will be seen when we discuss the other cells in the retina, all their responses are graded slow potentials, and all are transmitted by decremental (electrotonic) conduction.

The synapses made by receptors are similar to those made by other neurons: synaptic vesicles merge with the cell membrane and release transmitter into the synaptic cleft when the cell membrane is depolarized. Receptors are somewhat depolarized in the dark, and therefore release transmitter in the dark. Light causes hyperpolarization of the receptors, and thus decreases or stops the release of transmitter by the receptors (Toyoda, 1973; Kaneko & Shimazaki, 1975; Dacheux & Miller, 1976; Evans, Hood, & Holtzman, 1978). The information that a light is shining on a receptor is signaled by interruption of the ongoing flow of transmitter.

We may now review the sequence of events as follows: a photon of light enters the receptor, and is captured by a molecule of photopigment in the stacked or folded membranes of the outer segment. The chromophore of the photopigment isomerizes, going from the 11-cis to the all-trans form (unfolds its tail).

Through a cascade of chemical events within the outer segment (see Box 5–5), channels that allow sodium ions into the receptor are closed, and the receptor hyperpolarizes. The amount of hyperpolarization depends on the number of photons absorbed. Hyperpolarization is communicated to the terminal by decremental conduction (electrotonic spread). The terminal, which had been releasing transmitter in the dark because it was in a somewhat depolarized state, slows the release of transmitter to the horizontal and bipolar cells with which it synapses in the outer plexiform layer.

Spectral Sensitivity of Receptors

Up to this point, we have been tacitly assuming that every photon impinging on a receptor is absorbed by a molecule of photopigment in its outer segment. As we mentioned in our discussion of pigment epithelium, this is far from the case. The majority of photons pass completely through the receptor and are lost as far as vision is concerned. Let us now examine what determines whether a photon is likely to be absorbed or to pass clear through the receptor.

There are two factors that determine that probability of a photon being absorbed (we are in the world of quantum mechanics where we cannot predict anything for a given photon, only express the probability of outcomes). These two factors are the concentration of pigment (how many pigment molecules the photon is likely to encounter), and the match between the "tuning" curve of the pigment molecules and the energy (wavelength) of the photon. This can be clarified by an analogy. Photons are like bullets being fired into a clump of trees; the trees are analogous to pigment molecules. We wish to know what the probability is of a bullet shot at random (without aiming at a tree) embedding itself in a tree. Clearly, the more trees there are, the better the chance of hitting one; this is analogous to saying that the more pigment molecules there are (how concentrated), the higher the probability of photon capture. There is also a question of how well matched the bullet energies are to the type of tree. Bullet energy could refer to the muzzle velocity at which they are fired, ranging from a slow air gun to a high-powered rifle. (Of course, all photons travel at the same speed, the speed of light, but they do vary in energy, which is inversely proportional to the wavelength of the light; see Chapter 4.) If the bullets travel slowly and the trees are hard, the bullets will bounce right off. Bullets that travel rapidly will pass completely through trees that are soft or thin. When the bullet speeds are well matched to the types of trees, nearly every bullet that hits a tree will embed itself; as the speed is less well matched only certain kinds of hits will result in embedding. Photons are absorbed only if their energy is appropriate to effect an isomerization.

Rather than discuss the fate of a single photon, let us consider the fate of a large group (a visible stimulus can contain hundreds of millions of photons). If the probability of capture of each photon is 0.01 (1 in 100), we would expect one photon to be captured from a stimulus containing 100; we would expect about 10,000 captured from a stimulus containing 1,000,000. In short, the probability in this case gives us the *percentage* of photons *absorbed*. We can then characterize the relative effectiveness of a visual pigment for various wavelengths of light by presenting the percentage absorbed as a function of wavelength.

Figure 5–6 shows the percentage absorption curve for human *rhodopsin*, the pigment found in the rods. Rhodopsin (originally called visual purple because it appears purplish when extracted and dissolved in a test tube) most effectively absorbs photons when their wavelength is 505 nm; its ability to absorb photons of longer or shorter wavelength is considerably less.

Rhodopsin is the rod pigment in most mammals. (Many cold-blooded animals have a related pigment named *porphyropsin* in their rods.) The cones do not contain rhodopsin; however, they contain *cone pigment*, sometimes called *iodopsin*, which was the name given to the first cone pigment to be studied chemically (Wald, Brown, & Smith, 1955). In the normal (not colorblind) human retina there are three distinct cone pigments. Each is somewhat like rhodopsin in that it is capable of absorbing light of almost any

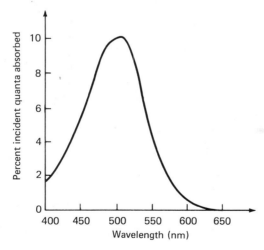

FIGURE 5–6   Percentage of incident quanta absorbed by rhodopsin as a function of wavelength. Based on nomogram presented by Ebrey and Honig (1977). New wavelength-dependent visual pigment nomograms. *Vision Res.* 17:147–151. Reprinted by permission of Pergamon Press, Ltd.

wavelength in the visible range, but the particular wavelengths to which each is most sensitive are different. Just as rhodopsin has a *peak* wavelength (505 nm), which is the light it absorbs more readily than any other, the cone pigments each have characteristic peak wavelengths. One of the human cone pigments has a peak wavelength somewhat shorter than 505 nm, the other two being longer than 505 nm. These differences are apparently caused by subtle chemical differences in the opsin parts of the photopigments.

Each cone in a human retina (or any retina that has more than one cone pigment) contains only one cone pigment (Marks, Dobelle, & MacNichol, 1964; Marks, 1965; Tomita, Kaneko, Murakami, & Pautler, 1967). There are thus three different types of cones in the human retina, distinguished from each other by the particular cone pigment each contains. In some animals, cones containing different cone pigments have also been found to be distinguishable morphologically (Scholes, 1975; Marc & Sperling, 1976). As we shall see in Chapter 15, it is because we have spectrally distinct types of cones that we can detect differences in color. As there is only one type of rod, rods alone cannot give information about the color of a stimulus.

OUTER PLEXIFORM LAYER

Let us return to the processing done in the retina. We will follow the signal initiated by the absorption of light in the receptors as it passes through the layers of the retina. We have already presented the general anatomy of the retina; here we give some details of the connections made in each of the plexiform layers, and discuss the responses of the various cell types.

The rods and the cones hyperpolarize in response to light absorbed by their individual outer segments. At the outer plexiform layer, information from these discrete receptors is passed to other cells in which messages from numerous receptors are mixed. This is the first stage of processing visual information.

BOX 5-6

As a matter of fact, the processing may have begun before the outer plexiform layer. It is convenient to think of receptors as individual point readouts of the visual image, but receptors are influenced by neighboring receptors as well. They send processes that come in close apposition to neighboring receptors (Scholes, 1975; Gold & Dowling, 1979), and apparently make electrical synapses with each other at these points. There is ample evidence from a number of different cold-blooded animals that the hyperpolarization of a given rod is caused in considerable measure by the photons captured by neighboring rods (Fain, 1975; Schwartz, 1976; Copenhagen & Owen, 1980; Attwell & Wilson, 1980). In the turtle, coupling has also been demonstrated between cones (Richter & Simon, 1974), and possibly

(continued)

(box continued)
even between cones and rods (Schwartz, 1975). In addition, receptors are apparently postsynaptic to horizontal cells, so they may be slightly depolarized by light in somewhat distant parts of the retina (Baylor, Fuortes, & O'Bryan, 1971; Lasater & Lam, 1984).

The connections made by receptors are quite specialized. Within each receptor terminal are *invaginations*, or pockets. Processes from bipolar cells and horizontal cells fit into these invaginations and form a stylized arrangement called a *triad* (Dowling & Boycott, 1966) (Figure 5–7). The central element of each triad is the dendrite of a bipolar cell; it is flanked on each side by processes from horizontal cells. The receptor is clearly a presynaptic element at the triad, as it contains synaptic vesicles and a structure called the *synaptic ribbon*, a dark double line surrounded by a halo of vesicles. (The significance of the synaptic ribbon is not known.) Horizontal cells are probably both presynaptic and postsynaptic; they contain vesicles, but are in a position that indicates receptors are presynaptic to them. Bipolar cells are apparently postsynaptic to both receptors and horizontal cells.

Although the triads are the most striking features in the outer plexiform

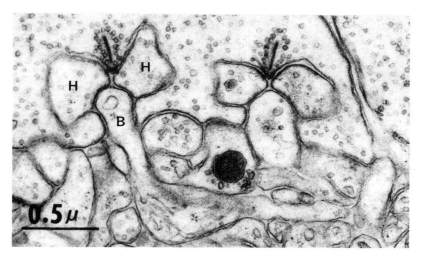

FIGURE 5–7 Triads in a monkey cone. Two triads are visible, each with a synaptic ribbon surrounded by a halo of vesicles, a bipolar cell dendrite (B), and two horizontal cell processes (H). Electron micrograph from Dowling, J. E. (1965) Foveal receptors of the monkey retina: Fine structure. *Science* 147:57–59. Reprinted by permission. Copyright 1965 by the AAAS.

layer, there are other contacts as well. Receptors are also presynaptic to bipolar cells that do not enter the invaginations. These bipolar cells, called *flat bipolars* (as opposed to the *invaginating bipolars* that provide the central elements of triads) synapse at the surface of the receptor terminals. These synapses, in which there is a single postsynaptic and single presynaptic element and no specializations such as the synaptic ribbon, are called *conventional* synapses. There are also conventional synapses between horizontal cells and bipolar cells.

We now consider the responses of the various cell types found in the outer retina by working through a simplified version of a figure first presented by Werblin and Dowling (1969) from their recordings of cells in the retina of the mud puppy (*Necturus*). The mud puppy, an aquatic salamander, is a particularly convenient animal for intracellular studies. It is an amphibian that fails to complete its metamorphosis. All the nuclei in its cells undergo mitosis and double the number of chromosomes in preparation for a metamorphosis that never happens. The *Necturus* remains water-breathing throughout its adult life, but because of unfinished metamorphosis, the nuclei contain twice the chromosomes, and hence the cell bodies are large. These large cell bodies are relatively easy to impale with microelectrodes, making it possible to record responses from the cells of the retina. Werblin and Dowling took advantage of this quirk of nature to make their recordings (as researchers continue to exploit the *Necturus* for intracellular recording). Improvements in technology have since made it possible to record cells from the outer retina of a number of other animals, including fish, toads, rabbits, cats, and monkeys. We present what is known about the cells of the retina in the framework of Werblin and Dowling's classical figure, but much of the information we give depends on more recent work in various animals.

Figure 5–8 is organized in four rows and two columns. Each row represents intracellular recordings of potential versus time for a particular neuron responding to stimulation of the retina by light. The records in the top row are from a receptor (probably a rod); those in the second row are from a horizontal cell; those in the third row are from a bipolar cell, and those in the fourth row are from an amacrine cell. Each column represents the responses to a particular stimulus. The responses in the left column are to a spot of light, about 100 microns (0.1 mm) in diameter, centered on the neuron itself. The other column shows responses to *annuli* (singular: *annulus*) of light. An annulus is a common visual stimulus; it means "ring," and is just that, a ring or circle of light. It allows stimulation of the area near a neuron without stimulating the area of retina in which the cell itself resides. The response to a large annulus is therefore caused by lateral interconnection of the cells of the retina. (In practice, however, it is impossible to produce an annulus without a small amount of light also falling in the supposedly dark central area. This is because of scatter of light within the retina. We should always bear in mind that when the theoretical stimulus is an annulus, there is actually a relatively dim illumination in the center.)

Each panel in Figure 5–8 represents the response of a neuron to a single

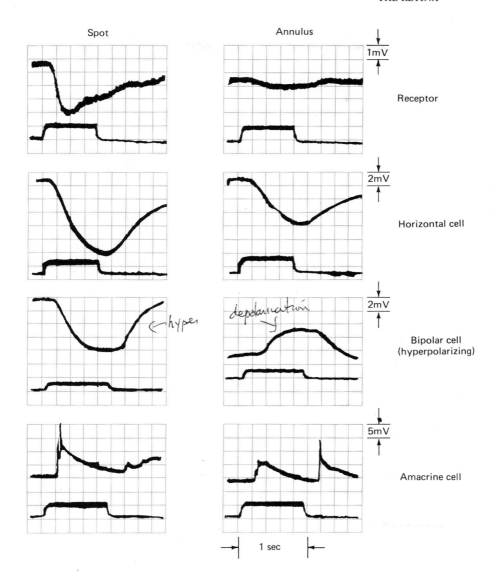

Spot   Annulus

1mV — Receptor

2mV — Horizontal cell

→hyper   depolarization

2mV — Bipolar cell (hyperpolarizing)

5mV — Amacrine cell

|← 1 sec →|

FIGURE 5-8 Responses of retinal cells in *Necturus* to flashed stimuli. Responses to spots of light are shown in the left column, responses to annuli in the right. Within each panel is the intracellular voltage as a function of time (upper trace) and a signal marker indicating the time the light was on (lower trace). The top row shows the responses of a receptor, the second row shows responses of a horizontal cell, the third row shows responses of a hyperpolarizing bipolar cell, and the bottom row shows responses of an amacrine cell. Adapted from Werblin, F. S. and J. E. Dowling (1969) Organization of the retina of mudpuppy. *J. Neurophysiol.* 32:339–355. Reprinted by permission.

presentation of a stimulus. The upper trace shows the potential measured in the cell as a function of time, photographed directly from the face of an oscilloscope. (Each trace starts at resting potential for that cell, but its position in the figure is not an indication of what that resting level was, because the position of the oscilloscope trace was arbitrarily shifted from record to record.) The lower trace in each panel is the output of a photocell that recorded the presence or absence of the stimulus light. It therefore serves as a synchronization marker, indicating exactly when the stimulus was present. Lights were on during the raised portion of this trace. The duration of the flashes was about 800 msec, or slightly less than 1 second.

The top row of the figure shows responses of a receptor; as we have already pointed out, receptors hyperpolarize when light is shone directly on them (left panel). When the light falls on neighbors (annulus, right panel) the hyperpolarization is much less; presumably this hyperpolarization is caused primarily by scattered light falling on the cell. (There may also be a contribution caused by the responses of the distant receptors; see Box 5–6.)

Horizontal Cells

The second row shows the responses of a horizontal cell. When a spot of light is shone on a horizontal cell (rather, on the position in the retina at which the electrode is located), it hyperpolarizes. This hyperpolarization is much like the responses of the receptors presynaptic to the horizontal cell, but considerably larger (note that the scale is different than in the upper row), and somewhat slower. In contrast to the receptors, however, the horizontal cell gives a robust response when the stimulus is an annulus. Horizontal cells are responsive to lights across a wide area of the retina; the area of retina in which stimulation leads to response in a cell is referred to as the *receptive field* of the cell. Horizontal cells have large receptive fields; in fact, the receptive field of a horizontal cell can be considerably larger than the lateral spread of the cell. This is presumably because horizontal cells interconnect with neighboring horizontal cells (Kaneko, 1971).

BOX 5-7

There are several varieties of horizontal cells that can be distinguished both anatomically and physiologically. One distinction is that horizontal cell dendrites do not go indiscriminately to rods and cones. In fish, there is a division between horizontal cells that contact only rods, and those that contact only cones (Stell, 1967; 1975); these two types of horizontal cells, which are segregated into separate sublayers in the inner nuclear layer, do not interconnect directly with each other (Kaneko, 1971). In animals such as the cat, some horizontal cells have a thin "axon" with a bulbous ending. The processes from the horizontal cell bodies contact only cones, while the processes from the axon terminal contact only rods

(continued)

(box continued)
(Kolb, 1974). Apparently the axon is sufficiently thin that there is no communication between the rod-specific soma and the cone-specific terminals (Nelson, Lützow, Kolb, & Gouras, 1975). (Remember that horizontal cells do not fire action potentials, so conduction along the axon is decremental in nature.)

In animals with color vision, there is a further subdivision of the horizontal cells that contact cones. The cells we have been discuss-ing, which hyperpolarize regardless of the wavelength of the light, are called *L-Type* (for luminosity). There are other horizontal cells, called *C-Type* (for color), that hyperpolarize for some wavelengths but depolarize for others. These are *spectrally opponent* responses, and presumably play a role in the processing of color information. Other spectrally opponent responses are discussed in Chapter 15, so we will gloss over this aspect of cell responses here.

Bipolar Cells

The responses of the bipolar cell shown in row 3 of Figure 5–8 demonstrate a new and important property. The response to a spot of light (left) is hyperpolarization, much like the responses of the receptors and horizontal cells. The response of this bipolar cell to the large annulus (right panel), however, is depolarization. A bipolar cell's response can be either hyperpolarizing or depolarizing, depending on the spatial configuration of the stimulus. This cell does not simply detect light, it discriminates between light falling directly on it (hyperpolarization), and light falling somewhat to the sides of it (depolarization). If a large spot of light were flashed, it would attempt both to hyperpolarize and depolarize at the same time, and there would therefore be less response.

The kind of organization observed in this bipolar cell is called *spatial antagonism;* the receptive field of this cell is *concentric* (one region inside another), and referred to as *center/surround* (the center is the middle or direct region that leads to hyperpolarization, while the surround is the distant region that leads to depolarization).

Spatial antagonism is an important concept in visual processing. The response of a bipolar cell depends on the distribution of the light within its receptive field, not simply on the total amount of light. Bipolar cells respond to the relative amount of light, or *contrast*. The hyperpolarization of a bipolar cell depends on the amount of light falling on the center of its receptive field, relative to the amount falling on the surround. There is net hyperpolarization if the light in the center exceeds that in the surround, and net depolarization if there is much more light in the surround (even though the center may also be lit). This kind of processing of spatial information is discussed in greater depth in Chapter 6.

The bipolar cell shown in Figure 5–8 is typical of one type that is found in the retina. There is also another kind of bipolar cell that is a mirror image of this one. The second type depolarizes when light is shone directly on the receptors above the cell, and hyperpolarizes when the light is in the surround part of its receptive field. To distinguish between them, this second type of bipolar cell is called "center depolarizing," while the cell shown in the figure is called "center hyperpolarizing." The two types of bipolar cells generally correspond to the two anatomical types mentioned on page 102; most of the center-depolarizing bipolars are invaginating, while most center-hyperpolarizing cone bipolars are flat (Famiglietti & Kolb, 1976; Stell, Ishida, & Lightfoot, 1977). While the division by anatomical types is not perfect (Saito, Kujiraoko, & Yonaha, 1983; Sterling, 1983), the division into mirror-image systems persists throughout the retina.

INNER PLEXIFORM LAYER

Bipolar cells represent the output of the first stages of retinal processing, in the outer plexiform layer. The signals within bipolar cells are conducted radially inward (by electrotonic conduction) to the inner plexiform layer, where the next major processing steps occur. Here, bipolar cells communicate with amacrine cells and ganglion cells.

There is another specialized kind of synapse that is found in the inner plexiform layer. It is called the *dyad*. At a dyad, a bipolar cell terminal with a synaptic ribbon is presynaptic to two amacrine cells (Figure 5–9). One of the amacrine cells, in its turn, is presynaptic to the *same* bipolar cell terminal (Dowling & Boycott, 1966; Dowling, 1968). (At some dyads, the bipolar is presynaptic to an amacrine cell and a ganglion cell.) The result of this arrangement is a *feedback* of the amacrine cell onto the bipolar cell.

Amacrine Cells

Let us consider the responses of the amacrine cells. Returning to Figure 5–8, we see that the response of an amacrine cell to a spot of light (fourth row, left) is a depolarization that appears rapidly at onset of light, but dwindles to nothing by the time the light is extinguished. This is a rather different kind of response from those of receptors, horizontal cells, and bipolar cells. In those cells, presentation of light led to a depolarization or hyperpolarization that was at least partially maintained for as long as the light was present; these are called *sustained* or *tonic* responses. The amacrine cell shown here, on the other hand, produced its response when the light level *changed*, but gave little or no response when the light was steady (regardless of whether it was steadily off or steadily on); this kind of response is called *transient* or *phasic*. The sustained response is a signal that something is present; the transient response is a signal that something has just changed. It is a general property of the visual system from this level onward that responses are at least some-

BOX 5–8

Although the amacrine cells recorded in *Necturus* all seem to be transient cells like the one shown in Figure 5–8, many of those in other animals give sustained responses (Murakami & Shimoda, 1977; Kaneko & Hashimoto, 1969; Chan & Naka, 1976; Kolb & Nelson, 1981; Weiler & Marchiafava, 1981; Nelson, 1982). Sustained amacrine cells can be further subdivided into depolarizing and hyperpolarizing types. There is a tremendous diversity of amacrine cell types in the retina (Kolb, Nelson, & Mariani, 1981). Some of the types are distinguished by their anatomy, some by their connections to other cells, some by their response type, and some by the chemical transmitter they release (see Massey & Redburn, 1987). While a few of these cell types have been implicated in specific functions (Masland & Tauchi, 1986; Vaney, 1986), we are still not clear about the roles of most of them.

what transient. Some cells maintain a level of activity throughout the duration of a stimulus, but all cells are considerably more active at the instant a

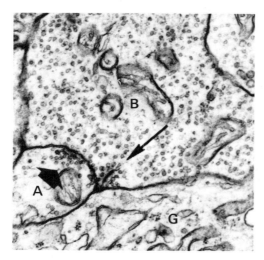

FIGURE 5–9   A dyad in a human retina. The bipolar cell (B) is presynaptic to an amacrine cell (A) and a ganglion cell (G). Where the three join, a synaptic ribbon (thin arrow) may be seen in the bipolar cell. The collection of vesicles in the amacrine cell process (fat arrow) indicates where the amacrine cell is presynaptic to the bipolar cell. Electron micrograph from Dowling, J. E., and B. B. Boycott (1965) *Cold Spring Harbor Symp. Quant. Biol.* 30:393–402. Reprinted by permission of the author and publisher.

stimulus appears (or disappears) than after it has been present or absent for a while (see Chapter 3).

The response of the amacrine cell in the figure to an annulus is similar to its response to the spot. There is a transient depolarization at onset of the light (called an ONSET response) and a second depolarization at the offset of the light (called an OFFSET response). As the stimulating light is moved farther from the cell body the relative sizes of the ONSET and OFFSET responses shift; the spot produces almost no OFFSET response, while the annulus produces a larger OFFSET response than ONSET response. This cell apparently has a concentric receptive field, but the center and surround do not antagonize each other, they simply contribute different components of the response.

We have already seen that the processing in the outer plexiform layer was largely concerned with spatial contrasts. The amacrine cells and their synapses in the inner plexiform layer process another kind of contrast: temporal contrast. Transient responses are signals of sudden changes; phasic cells respond best when there is an abrupt change in stimulation, and ignore steady stimuli.

There is another interesting aspect to the responses of the amacrine cell shown in Figure 5–8. At the leading edge of the ONSET response to the spot and the OFFSET response to the annulus, there is a spikelike depolarization in excess of the bulk of the response. This spike is not an action potential, as it is *graded* (its amplitude is different when the stimulus is stronger or weaker). It is also much slower than the action potentials observed in true spiking neurons, and there are rarely more than one or two of these "spikes" in a given response (Toyoda, Hashimoto, & Ohtsu, 1973). This spike is apparently caused by a regenerative amplification somewhat like the amplification that causes an action potential (Werblin, 1977; Eliasof, Barnes, & Werblin, 1987). This active amplification probably accounts for the rapid rise of the amacrine cell's response; notice that it reaches a peak considerably before the bipolar cells that provide its input. For example, Nelson (1982) has suggested that the function of an amacrine cell in the rod pathway (called the AII amacrine) may be responsible for the time course of the rod-driven responses.

Ganglion Cells

Finally, the cells that receive the fruits of all this processing and communicate it to the brain are the ganglion cells, located at the inner edge of the inner plexiform layer. These cells are the subject of the next chapter, so we will not discuss them here. Suffice to say that ganglion cells generally have spatially antagonistic (center versus surround) receptive fields, and may be transient in their responses (like the amacrine cell in Figure 5–8) or sustained (like a bipolar cell).

Like the hyperpolarizing and depolarizing bipolars that form a mirror-image pair, there are ganglion cells that are excited by the onset of light in their receptive field centers (ON-*center*) and ganglion cells inhibited by light in the center (OFF-*center*). The two systems continue in parallel through the retina, with a third system that combines features of both arising in the inner plexiform layer (the amacrine cell shown has what is called an ON-OFF response, and presumably receives excitatory inputs from both hyperpolarizing and depolarizing bipolars) (Marchiafava & Torre, 1978). The ON-center ganglion cells send their dendrites to the part of the inner plexiform layer that is directly above the ganglion cell layer, which seems to be the level where mostly invaginating (center depolarizing) cone bipolar cells make synapses. The OFF-center ganglion cells send dendrites through the inner plexiform layer to make synapses at its outer portion, where mostly flat (hyperpolarizing) bipolar cells terminate (Famiglietti & Kolb, 1976; Nelson & Kolb, 1983). The ON-OFF type may send a spray of dendrites through the entire plexiform layer, or have two distinct layers of branches. In any case, the ON-center ganglion cells receive direct excitation from depolarizing bipolar cells, and the OFF-center ganglion cells from hyperpolarizing bipolars (Miller & Dacheux, 1976; Naka, 1977).

However, it also seems likely that the ON-center ganglion cells receive inhibition from the hyperpolarizing bipolars, and the OFF-center ganglion cells receive inhibition from the depolarizing bipolars (Sterling, 1983; Müller, Wässle, & Voigt, 1988). Thus, their responses are actively increased when the one kind of bipolar is depolarized, but actively decreased when the other is depolarized. This "push-pull" action allows the cell to respond well to either direction of change, brightening or dimming (Levine & Shefner, 1975, 1977; Sterling, 1983).

We can summarize the responses of the various cells in the retina, and speculate on the connections between them, by referring to the schematic shown in Figure 5–10. In it, we see stylized pictures of receptors (at the top) and the other cell types leading to the ganglion cells (at the bottom). In the circle representing each cell's body is a graph showing the response of that cell to a light flashed on the receptor at the left. The cells in the column to the right are not directly illuminated by the flash; for them, the light is in the surround part of their receptive fields, as with the annular stimuli, in Figure 5–8. Synapses between cells are shown by Vs (presynaptic element) covering round spots (postsynaptic elements).

Starting at the top, the receptors hyperpolarize when the light is flashed; in effect they say, "there is light shining on me." The receptor that is illuminated hyperpolarizes far more than the one that is not. The horizontal cells say, "there is light somewhere around here," and they integrate signals from a large number of receptors and hyperpolarize when light falls anywhere in their vicinity. As the receptor is releasing transmitter in the dark and stops releasing it in the light, the transmitter released by the receptors must be excitatory to the horizontal cells.

The two bipolar cells shown are both of the hyperpolarizing, not the depolarizing, type. The one on the left hyperpolarizes in response to the

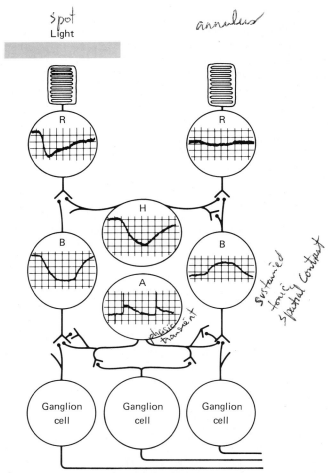

FIGURE 5–10   Summary of the connections between cells in the vertebrate retina and the responses of each cell type. From
Dowling, J. E. (1970) Organization of vertebrate retinas.
Invest. Ophthalmol. 9:655–680. Reprinted by permission of the publisher and the author.

slowed release of transmitter from the receptor on the left; the receptor
transmitter must also be excitatory for the hyperpolarizing bipolar. The bipolar on the right depolarizes. As the receptor synapsing on it was not significantly affected by the light, this response must be caused by the slowing of
transmitter release by the horizontal cell. Bipolar cells say, "there is more
(or less) light here than in nearby regions." If slowed transmitter leads to
depolarization, the transmitter must be inhibitory. It is possible, however,
that the "inhibition" actually consists of horizontal cells depolarizing the
receptors (Toyoda, 1973; Toyoda & Kujiraoka, 1982). In any case, the surround part of the bipolar receptive field seems to be caused by the activity of

horizontal cells (Naka, 1977). The importance of the surround contribution relative to that of the center may be modulated by feedback by way of the interplexiform cells (Hedden & Dowling, 1978; Djamgoz, Reynolds, Rowe, & Ruddock, 1981).

BOX 5–9 ▬▬▬▬▬▬▬▬▬▬▬▬▬

The figure does not show any depolarizing bipolar cells, but their responses would be the opposite to those of the hyperpolarizing cells shown. That is, the transmission from receptors to hyperpolarizing bipolars is "sign conserving": the bipolars mimic the depolarization or hyperpolarization, while that from receptors to depolarizing bipolars is "sign inverting": these bipolars do just the opposite. If both types of bipolar cells receive the same transmitter from the receptors, they must use it to operate different channels. We know that horizontal cells and depolarizing bipolars require chloride ions to function, but hyperpolarizing bipolars do not (Miller & Dacheux, 1976). Furthermore, the transmitter seems to close ionic channels in the depolarizing bipolars, but open channels in the hyperpolarizing type (Toyoda, 1973). All of this implies that the channels in these two types of bipolars are different. Pharmacological investigations of the synaptic chemistry have shown that the appropriate systems are present in retina (Miller & Slaughter, 1986).

The amacrine cell receives inputs from bipolar cells in a relatively large area of retina. It gives phasic responses to changes in bipolar cell outputs; it says, "something just changed." These synapses are apparently excitatory (Marchiafava & Torre, 1978). The transient nature of the amacrine cell responses is not understood, but it is probably due both to the ionic amplification that gives the graded "spike" (Werblin, 1977) and feedback at the dyad (Dowling, 1970). The feedback could be a negative regulation by which the response is "shut down" after the initial surge because of its own activity (Tachibana & Kaneko, 1988; Maguire, Lukasiewicz, & Werblin, 1989), or a positive boosting by its own bootstraps (Freed, Smith, & Sterling, 1987). Possibly, all three mechanisms operate.

Finally, the ganglion cells receive signals from the bipolar and amacrine cells in the inner plexiform layer and relay information to the brain. Werblin and Dowling (1969) hypothesized that the transient ganglion cells receive their input from the amacrine cells, while sustained ganglion cells receive input from bipolar cells. The sustained amacrine cells apparently also contribute to responses of sustained ganglion cells (Chan & Naka, 1976).

SUGGESTED READINGS

It is difficult to recommend general readings to supplement this chapter, as so much of the work is too new to have been gathered in secondary sources. Perhaps the best review of the structure and function of the retina is now somewhat out-of-date: "Organization of vertebrate retinas," by J. E. Dowling, in *Investigative Ophthalmology*, Vol. 9, pages 655–680 (1970). A good review of the chemistry of photopigments, including all the steps involved in bleaching pigment with light (which we have not discussed here) is "Molecular basis of visual excitation," by G. Wald; *Science*, 162:230–239 (1968).

A number of readable reviews may be found in a special issue of *Trends in Neurosciences* published in May 1986. Articles in that issue review topics relevant to this chapter, such as the structure of rhodopsin, the cGMP cascade, synaptic relationships between receptors and bipolar cells, neurotransmitters in the retina, the role of interplexiform cells, and the structure and function of amacrine cells. Other articles are relevant to Chapter 6. We also recommend the *Scientific American* article "The Functional Architecture of the Retina" by R. H. Masland, November 1986, for a review of the types and functions of amacrine cells. This article has been reprinted in *The Biology of the Brain: From Neurons to Networks*, edited by R. R. Llinás (W. H. Freeman, 1989).

Those who wish to tackle a serious and advanced study of the vertebrate retina cannot do better than read portions of *The Vertebrate Retina*, by R. W. Rodieck (W. H. Freeman, 1973). This work is a veritable encyclopedia of what was known of the retina as of 1973; the drawback to reading it is that it is quite detailed and complete. Visual pigment chemistry is covered in Chapters 2 and 3. The structure of the retina is discussed in Chapters 13 and 15; in addition, the book includes a translation of Ramón y Cajal's classic 1893 monograph *La Rétine des vertébrés*.

A newer book on many of the same topics is John Dowling's *The Retina*, published by Harvard University Press, Cambridge, Mass. (1987). This book covers all the topics from light transduction in receptors to ganglion cell responses, with an emphasis on those areas in which Dowling has made major contributions.

RETINAL GANGLION CELLS AND LATERAL ANTAGONISM

6

In the last chapter, we discussed the anatomical structure of the retina, and described the response properties of retinal cells. In this chapter, we focus our attention on the cells that provide the retina's output to the brain, the retinal ganglion cells. Ganglion cells receive input from bipolar and amacrine cells, and their axons leave the retina at the optic disc (blind spot) to become the optic nerve. All the processing functions subserved by the retina must therefore be observable in the responses of ganglion cells. For this reason, we will spend considerable time discussing the behavior of ganglion cells; not only is this background necessary in order to analyze the responses of visual cells in the brain, but also some of the properties of the vertebrate visual system can be explained on the basis of ganglion cell responses.

GANGLION CELL RESPONSES

Figure 6–1 shows the responses of ganglion cells to spots of white light centered on their receptive fields. These cells are in goldfish, a vertebrate whose visual system is fairly representative of vertebrates. In Figure 6–1(a), the response of one ganglion cell is displayed as a train of action potentials. Several important points should be made about this figure. The ganglion cell is a neuron that codes information by firing action potentials; in fact, it is the only cell in the retina that does not employ decremental conduction as its sole means of information transmission. It is not surprising that the ganglion cell should be different from other retinal cells in this regard, as it is the only cell in the retina that has to transmit information over long distances. Because it fires action potentials, we can record its responses extracellularly (see Chapter 3); this allows us to observe a single cell's responses with little possibility of damaging the cell.

Another property of ganglion cells that is evident from Figure 6–1(a) is that they are not silent in the absence of stimulation. Before the onset of the stimulus, the cell is firing action potentials; this is called the *maintained discharge* of the cell. Although the maintained discharge may be influenced

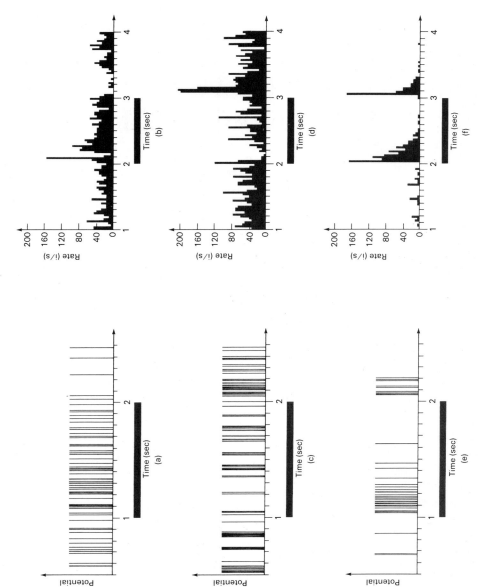

FIGURE 6–1 Responses of ganglion cells to small spots of light. The duration of the stimulus is marked by the dark bar below each response. Parts (a), (c), and (e) show the spike trains for an ON-cell, an OFF-cell, and an ON-OFF cell, respectively. (These are computer-generated plots of data from goldfish ganglion cells. See Chapter 3.) Parts (b), (d), and (f) are peri-stimulus time histograms (PSTHs) of the same responses; each PSTH is an average of 30 stimulus presentations. Spikes have been cumulated in 100 msec bins.

by the level of steady background illumination, it is present even if the eye is placed in total darkness. The origin of the maintained discharge is a matter of some contention; some investigators argue that it is caused by spontaneous activity of receptors that occurs even in the dark (Barlow & Levick, 1969; Rodieck, 1967), while others believe that it is intrinsic to the ganglion cell itself (Schellart & Spekreijse, 1973; Hughes & Maffei, 1965), and still others contend it arises somewhere between the receptors and the ganglion cells (Frishman & Levine, 1983; Levine, Saleh, & Yarnold, 1988). Whatever its origin, it serves a useful purpose that will be discussed shortly.

The cell in Figure 6–1(a) responds to the onset of light by firing a burst of action potentials; this high rate of firing decays to a plateau after the stimulus has been present a short time, although the firing rate is still somewhat higher than it was in the dark. At stimulus offset, the firing rate is temporarily reduced below the level of the maintained discharge, and gradually climbs back up to the firing rate that was observed before the stimulus. This cell therefore is responding with excitation to light onset and inhibition to light offset (an ON response), and so is an ON-center cell (ON-cell for short). As we saw in Chapter 5, there are two responses to each stimulus: the response to stimulus onset is called the onset response, while the response to stimulus offset is called the offset response. ON-cells, therefore, respond to small spots with excitatory onset responses and inhibitory offset responses.

Figure 6–1(b) shows the same response of the cell in a slightly different way. Instead of displaying the action potentials themselves, the response is shown as a *peri-stimulus time histogram* (PSTH). To obtain a PSTH, the time axis is divided into a sequence of uniform bins. For each bin, the action potentials occurring during that time are counted and plotted as a frequency histogram. In doing this, we have generated a representation of the rate of firing action potentials as a function of time. Often, the histograms from a series of identical stimulus presentations are averaged. The PSTH histogram serves as a useful means of examining the shape of a given response that is simpler than looking at the time of occurrence of every single action potential.

In (c) and (d) of Figure 6–1, the response of a second type of ganglion cell is displayed. This type of cell responds with inhibition to the onset of the spot, and with excitation to its termination (OFF response). Such a cell is called an OFF-cell; its response pattern is just the opposite of that displayed by an ON-cell. Figures 6–1(e) and (f) show how a third type of ganglion cell responds to the same stimulus. It has both an excitatory onset response and an excitatory offset response; that is, firing rate increases both at light onset and to light offset (ON-OFF response). This is an ON-OFF cell, and its function is to signal a change in light level without regard to whether the change is toward more or less light.

After inspecting the responses of the three cells in Figure 6–1, an important function of the maintained discharge should become clear. A given ganglion cell will respond to light with either excitation or inhibition, and the only way that the inhibitory component is revealed is by a reduction in the firing rate below the level of the maintained discharge. If the cell were perfectly silent in the absence of stimulation, an inhibitory response would go unnoticed, as the cell cannot fire fewer than zero spikes. Thus, inhibition at the ganglion cell level would be ignored at the next synapse in the processing hierarchy. The presence of the maintained discharge therefore provides for a baseline from which an inhibitory response can deviate.

A property common to all three types of cells is that both onset and offset of the light is signalled by all cells. The presence of both onset and offset responses is a fundamental property of sensory systems. At the ganglion cell, the onset and offset responses have been shown to be closely related to each other; if a stimulus produces a large onset response, it is likely to produce a large offset response, and vice versa. Recent evidence has shown, however, that onset and offset responses in fish are, in fact, produced by separable pathways converging onto the ganglion cell (Levine & Shefner, 1975, 1977; Levine & Zimmerman, 1988). In this sense, the onset and offset responses are manifestations of the push-pull operation of the retina mentioned in Chapter 5.

Ganglion Cell Receptive Fields

So far, we have been looking at the responses of retinal ganglion cells to spots of light falling directly on the area of retina in which the cells are located. Like other cells of the retina, however, ganglion cells are more responsive to stimulation in certain parts of the visual world than in others; the area to which a ganglion cell is sensitive is called its receptive field.

The first detailed investigation of the receptive fields of mammalian retinal ganglion cells was done by S. W. Kuffler (1953), who used small spots of light to test the responses of ganglion cells in the cat retina. He found that there were two distinct parts to the receptive fields of most ganglion cells. For cells that gave ON responses to presentation of diffuse light flashes covering much of the retina, Kuffler found that there was a specific area of the retina that also gave ON responses to small spot stimulation; he noted where in the visual field ON responses were elicited by marking that location with a plus sign (Figure 6–2). Surrounding this central region, however, was an area in which stimulation by small spots produced an OFF response. This was one of the first demonstrations of the spatial antagonism that has since been reported for various other retinal cells (see Chapter 5). Figure 6–2 illustrates the receptive field of this type of cell; the region in which small spot stimulation produced ON responses is the *center* of the ganglion cell receptive field, while the area marked with − (negative signs) that envelops the center is the *surround*. Kuffler found that most ganglion cells possessed this antagonistic center/surround organization, but that the response to light onset of the center region was excitatory in some cells and inhibitory in others. In the case where center stimulation produced an OFF response, surround stimulation produced an ON response. The center of the field seems to correspond to the spread of the dendritic field of the ganglion cell itself (Peichl & Wässle,

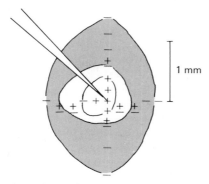

FIGURE 6-2 Mapping of the receptive field of a cat retinal ganglion cell. Center region marked + yields ON responses when stimulated with small spots; region marked − responds with OFF responses. Intermediate region marked ± gives ON-OFF responses. Microelectrode is drawn in for illustration. From Kuffler, S. W. (1953) Discharge patterns and functional organization of mammalian retina. *J. Neurophysiol.* 16:37–68. Reprinted by permission.

1983), so the surround must be due to the lateral signals carried by amacrine and horizontal cells.

PERCEPTUAL EFFECTS ACCOUNTED FOR BY CENTER/SURROUND ANTAGONISM

The center/surround organization of retinal ganglion cells provides a way for the response of the ganglion cell to stimulation of one portion of the receptive field to be modified by stimulation of a neighboring area. This relationship between neighboring areas of retina is called *lateral antagonism*[1]; it is a mechanism that allows a single ganglion cell to be selectively sensitive to contrast within its receptive field, rather than simply responding to the total amount of light directed onto the field. Consider the ganglion cell whose receptive field is shown in Figure 6–3. In (a) of the figure, an edge is positioned so that light covers the entire receptive field when the stimulus is

---

[1]Lateral antagonism is commonly known by another name, *lateral inhibition*, which you may encounter in your other reading. The word "inhibition" was applied when the process was first discovered in the eye of the horseshoe crab (see Box 4–11); in that animal, light directly on a receptor always caused an increase in firing that was decreased (inhibited) by light to the sides. In vertebrates, however, the response in the center of a field may be either an increase in firing (ON response) or a decrease in firing (OFF response). For an OFF-center cell, the light to the side *increases* the firing; it is very odd to refer to this increase as "inhibition." Nevertheless, the increase in firing is antagonistic to the response in the center (a decrease). We therefore prefer to refer to lateral *antagonism*, as a way of avoiding confusion when responses may be either ON or OFF.

presented; it produces an ON response, as shown on the right. When the edge is moved so that all of the receptive field center is stimulated but only a portion of the surround receives illumination (Figure 6–3[b]), the response evoked by stimulus onset is significantly greater than in (a). This cell is therefore more sensitive to an appropriately positioned edge than it is to a diffuse light stimulus of the same intensity covering the entire receptive field. When the edge is positioned so that only the surround of the cell is stimulated (Figure 6–3[c]), the cell responds in a different way than it did to the stimuli in (a) and (b) of the figure; it produces an OFF response.

From this we can conclude that retinal ganglion cells are sensitive to contrast within their receptive fields, rather than responding only as a function of total illumination within the field. There are numerous ways to demonstrate the visual system's preference for contrast; a number of them are shown in Figures 6–4 to 6–8. The pattern in Figure 6–4 produces a sensation called a *Mach band*, after its discoverer, Ernst Mach. The light distribution is shown under the pattern; you can see that the light uniformly and smoothly increases from left to right. But you probably see a vertical dark band (marked D) that occurs just to the left of the luminance gradient, and a vertical light band (marked B) just to the right of the gradient. *These light and dark bands are not present in the physical stimulus*; they exist in your perception of the stimulus because of the way the visual system responds to the stimulus. (Prove this by covering part of the pattern with a sheet of blank paper, as described in the figure caption.) In this and succeeding demonstrations of lateral antagonism in the visual system, we will discuss the phenomenon as if it is exclusively a property of retinal ganglion cells. It is important to note, however, that lateral antagonism exists at many levels within the visual system, and that the perceptual effects we describe here are enhanced by interactions other than those at the ganglion cell level.

To see how the responses of ganglion cells can account for your perception of Mach bands, suppose that the stimulus in Figure 6–4(a) is projected onto the retina. An image of the stimulus therefore falls onto an array of ganglion cells, each possessing its own receptive field; a sample of this array of ganglion cell receptive fields is shown at the top of the Mach band pattern. For convenience, let us suppose that all of these are ON-center cells, and consider the response of each cell, starting from left to right on the figure. The leftmost ganglion cell, like other cells near it that are not shown, is uniformly illuminated with a low level of light; it therefore fires at about its maintained discharge rate. The second cell is not being stimulated uniformly; although the center portion of the receptive field is being illuminated at the same level as its neighbors to the left, the right half of its surround is on the edge of the intensity gradient, and is therefore receiving more light. Compared to cells on the left, this cell is receiving more light in its surround and the same amount of light in its center; as the surround is inhibitory, the response of this cell should be less than the response of the first cell in the row. That is the reason you see a dark bar at this location on the pattern; the ganglion cells are signaling a smaller amount of light at this position than are the cells to the left.

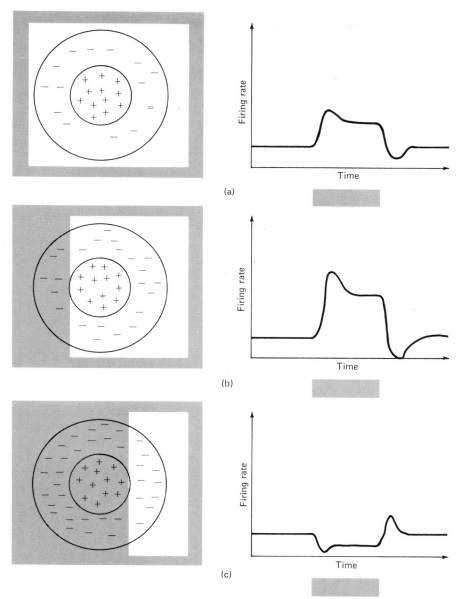

FIGURE 6-3 Responses of a hypothetical ON-center retinal ganglion cell to edge of light positioned at different places. (a) Light covers the entire receptive field; response shown on the right is an ON response. (b) Edge is moved so that entire center region is stimulated, but only part of the surround; ON response is enhanced relative to (a). (c) Surround only is stimulated; the response on the right is an OFF response.

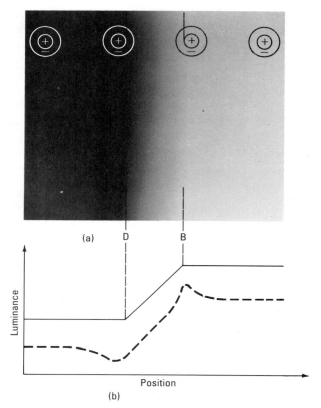

FIGURE 6-4 Mach bands. (a) Mach band pattern, with the receptive fields of four ON-center ganglion cells projected on it. (b) Luminance gradient (solid line), along with the perceptual brightness gradient it produces (dotted line).

To demonstrate that the bands are not physically present, cover the gradient part of the pattern. Take a sheet of paper and slowly move it across the figure from the left, while keeping your eye on the light Mach band. The band will vanish when the gradient is covered—just before the paper reaches it. Similarly, bringing the paper across from the right will make the dark band vanish just before the paper reaches it.

The same reasoning can be applied to the perception of the light band at the right of the luminance gradient. Start with the right-hand side of the row of ganglion cells; the first cell receives the same high illumination over its entire receptive field. Its firing is therefore only slightly higher than its maintained discharge rate. Now consider the second cell from the right; its receptive field center is illuminated at the same level as the cells to the right of it, but the left part of its surround is illuminated less than the right part because of its proximity to the gradient. The surround of this cell, therefore, will exert less of an inhibitory effect on the response of the cell than will the surrounds of cells to the right; the result of this will be a greater response from the cell. The greater responses of cells at this location along the pattern will produce the perception of a light band.

Center/surround interactions produce a brightness gradient like that shown by the dotted line in Figure 6–4(b). Even though the luminance gradient changes monotonically from dark to light as shown by the continuous line, the perceptual effect is one that tends to enhance the brightness difference between the two steady-state levels. This is, in fact, the probable purpose of lateral antagonism; it acts to emphasize borders while neglecting to some extent uniform brightness levels. If one has a clear idea where borders are, the brightness on either side of the border is known by implication, and does not have to be coded specifically by the visual system.

BOX 6-1

$\mathbf{W}$hy do we not see bands at all borders where luminance changes? Various hypotheses have been put forward. Some suggest that the effect of lateral antagonism is like taking spatial derivatives (looking for rates of change of light). When the change happens too abruptly, the changes at the one border cancel those at the other (Marr, 1982; Watt & Morgan, 1983). Another suggestion is that the sharp edge prevents the visual system from detecting the bands (Ratliff, 1984), a process called *masking* that we will discuss in Chapter 10. Another way of thinking about it is that it is simply a matter of how the brain interprets the pattern of firing. When the bands are contiguous, they are interpreted as indicating a real edge (which it normally is); when they are separated, as in the Mach pattern, the bands can be separately seen. Assumptions about how the brain might interpret patterns of firing in the sensory pathway are called "linking propositions" (Teller, 1984).

The staircase illusion shown in Figure 6–5 is another example of the visual system's tendency to emphasize borders. Although the actual physical stimulus is a series of luminance steps, the perception is that each step is brighter at its left border and darker at its right border. This has the effect of producing a brightness distribution that is shown as a dotted line in Figure 6–5(b); as with the Mach band in the previous figure, the borders between adjacent steps are perceptually more extreme than is the case for the physical stimulus. The mechanism for the enhancement of borders in the staircase illusion is identical to that described for Figure 6–4.

An illusion that demonstrates even more strongly the fact that the visual system is selectively sensitive to borders is the Craik-O'Brien illusion shown in Figure 6–6. In this figure, you should see a pattern consisting of light and dark bars. Looking at the luminance distribution taken through the figure, however, reveals that the luminance in the middle of the "light" bars is identical to the luminance in the middle of each "dark" bar. (Prove this by cover-

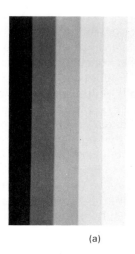

(a)

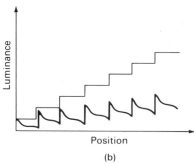

(b)

FIGURE 6-5   Series of equal luminance steps. (a) The pattern. (b) Luminance and perceptual brightness gradients.

ing the borders with pencils.) The abrupt luminance drop is enhanced by lateral antagonism and is perceived as a border. The gradual changes in luminance are not given much attention, however. The result is a perception of a brightness change at the borders, but no concomitant perception of the gradual changes on either side of the borders. (In Chapter 10 we discuss other ways of thinking about this illusion.)

The strength of this illusion can be seen by comparing Figures 6–6 and 6–7. In Figure 6–7, the bars are actually uniform in their luminances, as is shown by the luminance distribution in part (b) of the figure. The magnitude of the abrupt change at each border is identical to that in Figure 6–6; when the two figures are compared to each other, it is hard to decide which figure reflects a real luminance difference between adjacent bars. The fact that the "dark" bars in Figure 6–7 are actually darker does not seem to add additional information to the visual percept; what the visual system seems to be concentrating on is the borders, to the exclusion of information about steady-state levels.

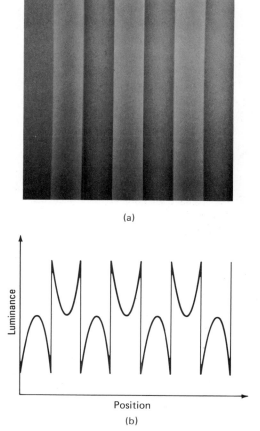

(a)

(b)

FIGURE 6-6 Craik-O'Brien illusion. (a) The luminance in the middle
of all bars is the same, even though it looks as if there are
light and dark bars. (b) The actual luminance gradient.

A final demonstration of the effects of lateral antagonism is shown in Figure 6–8. This pattern is known as the Hermann grid; it is merely a series of horizontal and vertical white bars running through a black background. By staring at the center of this grid you should get an impression of dark spots at the intersections of the white bars. These dark spots will not be present in the intersection that you actively stare at, but will occur in the periphery of your gaze. Occurrence of the dark spots is a straightforward result of lateral antagonism. Consider the responses of the two ON-center ganglion cells whose receptive fields are sketched on the figure. The cell on the right has one white bar projecting through the center of its receptive field, and through part of its surround. The cell on the left has the identical light distribution in its center, but an additional white bar is projected through its surround. This

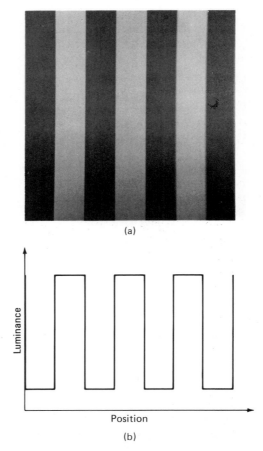

(a)

Position

(b)

FIGURE 6-7   (a) A succession of light and dark bars, mimicking the
Craik-O'Brien illusion. (b) The luminance gradient.

cell, therefore, receives more light in its surround than does its neighbor; it
will respond at a lower level because of greater antagonism by the surround.
Hence the dark spots.

BOX 6-2

Disappearance of a dark spot at the center of
the intersection of two white bars when you fix
your gaze upon it is caused by the nonhomo-
geneity of the retina. When we stare directly at
an object, an image of the object is placed on
the fovea. One way in which the retina maxi-
mizes acuity in the fovea has been discussed in
Chapter 5; the highest density of cones in the

(continued)

(box continued)

retina is found in this region. In addition, along with the high concentration of receptors in the fovea, there is also a large number of ganglion cells receiving inputs from foveal receptors. Ganglion cells in this region have much smaller receptive fields than they do elsewhere in the retina.

The fact that ganglion cell receptive fields are small in the fovea means that when you gaze at a particular intersection of white bars in the Hermann grid, the ganglion cells with the image of the intersection projected onto their receptive fields will be so small that both the center

and surround of each cell will lie within that intersection. Therefore there will be no effect of the surrounding black squares, and you will not have an impression of a dark spot. Images of intersections that are projected onto extrafoveal regions of the retina, however, will stimulate ganglion cells whose receptive fields are much bigger than those in the fovea, so that the situation sketched in Figure 6–8 will be obtained. If you look at the figure from across the room, the image of the figure will be much smaller on your retina, and a gray spot will be apparent at the intersection on which you fixate.

We have spent a considerable amount of time discussing one particular aspect of ganglion cell function: the presence of lateral antagonism. We have done so partly because this is an important function, but also because lateral antagonism provides a good example of a property general to all sensory systems; that is, sensory systems act to condense the information present in the

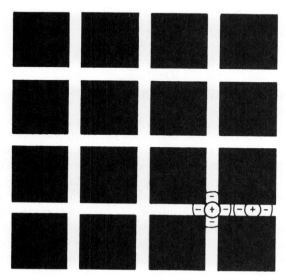

FIGURE 6–8 The Hermann grid, with two ganglion cell receptive fields projected on it.

physical world down to certain specific aspects that are essential to the organism. An animal dependent on its vision needs to know about borders; given that information, the animal can make unconscious inferences about the illumination present within a given contour. Selective attention to borders reduces the amount of information that must be taken in by the visual system, allowing the animal to concentrate on essential features.

BOX 6-3

We have been discussing the properties of lateral antagonism as it occurs in vertebrate visual systems; however, the earliest experiments on this subject were performed on the lateral eye of the horseshoe crab, *Limulus*, an animal whose visual system is vastly different from ours. As we discussed in Box 4–11, the lateral eye of the horseshoe crab is made up of about 800 tiny facets, or ommatidia, each of which has its own lens, receptors, and output fibers that leave the eye and form the optic nerve. The response recorded at these output fibers reflects, in general, the amount of light being projected onto the particular facet from which the fiber originated. Hartline and his co-workers (Hartline, 1949; Hartline, Wagner, & Ratliff, 1956; Hartline & Ratliff, 1957) found that the response to light of fibers coming from one facet could be reduced by shining light on a nearby facet. The amount that the excitation in one facet was reduced simultaneously by stimulation of another facet depended on how close the two facets were to each other, with the inhibitory effect decreasing with distance. Thus there is a lateral inhibitory network in the *Limulus* eye by which excitation in one region can affect the responses to light of a neighboring region. Functionally, this is similar to the lateral antagonism produced in the vertebrate visual system as a result of the interactions between the center and surround regions of the ganglion cell receptive field. Using quite different mechanisms, both types of visual systems employ lateral antagonism to enhance the response to borders in the visual world.

GANGLION CELLS WITH SPECIAL CODING CHARACTERISTICS

So far in this chapter, we have discussed the properties of retinal ganglion cells that derive from interactions between the center and surround of the receptive field. In some animals, however, certain ganglion cells may selectively respond to much more specific features of the visual world. The frog retina, for example, seems to extract specific features from the visual world, while ignoring more global properties. Lettvin, Maturana, McCulloch, and Pitts (1956) studied the properties of frog retinal ganglion cells and found four types of cells with distinct processing characteristics. We will describe the properties of the four cell types, as they provide an illustration of how a sensory system can be selectively sensitive to a small subset of inputs from the physical environment.

The first type of ganglion cells (Lettvin et al., 1959) were named *sus-*

tained contrast detectors. They did not respond at all to changes in overall illumination if the light was diffusely distributed throughout the receptive field of the cell. If an image of a lighted edge was passed through the receptive field, however, the cell responded vigorously. This response could be *direction-dependent*; that is, a response might be generated when the stimulus moved through the receptive field in one direction, but be absent or reduced if the edge moved in the opposite direction. Sustained contrast detectors send information to the brain about specific aspects of the visual world. Not only is this type of cell selectively sensitive to light/dark borders, but also it prefers movement of the border at certain velocities and only in certain directions. When this cell is firing, therefore, the information it is sending is considerably more specific than a mere statement of how much light is falling on its receptive field.

The second type of ganglion cells investigated by Lettvin and associates were named *net convexity detectors*. These cells provide perhaps the most dramatic illustration of feature detectors yet discovered. Net convexity detectors respond poorly to changes in illumination within the receptive field, and to light/dark edges moving through the field at any speed in any direction. They do, however, respond to the movement of a small, dark object into the receptive field. The response of the cell to such an object persists as long as the object remains in the field; if it is moved into the field and just left there, the response will persist until it is finally moved out again. Although the response is maintained to a stationary spot, the cell prefers movement within the receptive field, with jerky movements producing larger responses than smooth ones. The size of the spot is not crucial, but it must be darker than the surrounding level of illumination to evoke any response. If an array of spots (each of which is capable of producing a response if presented alone) is moved into the field of a cell, little or no response is produced. If one of the spots moves relative to the others in the array, however, the response evoked is similar to what would occur if that spot were alone in the field.

This type of cell is sensitive to a specific pattern of visual stimulation. In fact, a little reflection might lead to the conclusion that the types of patterns that activate net convexity detectors are of crucial importance to frogs: they are similar to the movements of insects in the natural habitat! Net convexity detectors have been given the somewhat romantic nickname "bug detectors"; their activation may indicate the location of a potential food source. With this type of information coming into the brain, the amount of central processing that must be performed before a response can be initiated is greatly reduced. For an animal such as the frog, with a fairly small number of different behaviors in its repertoire, this type of sophisticated peripheral processing is an efficient way of analyzing the visual world.

The other types of ganglion cells in the frog retina have somewhat less specific feature-detecting properties. *Moving edge detectors* (also called ON-OFF units) (Hartline, 1938; Barlow, 1953) are insensitive to changes in diffuse illumination, but are quite responsive to light/dark edges moving in any direction through the receptive field. This type of cell increases its firing in response to movement of either a light or a dark edge; it thus is concerned only with movement, and not with the actual amount of illumination. *Net dimming detectors* give a prolonged response to the extinction of a diffuse light stimulus; they will also respond to any moving stimulus regardless of its size, shape, or contrast, in direct proportion to the amount of dimming that the stimulus produces when passing across the receptive field of the cell.

The four types of cells just described comprise the great majority of all retinal ganglion cells found in the frog. The frog brain does not receive from the retina anything remotely similar to a photographic representation of the visual world. Rather, it receives a catalog of features whose correct detection is crucial for the animal's survival. From the sustained contrast detectors and net dimming detectors, the frog receives information about objects moving about, perhaps indicating potential predators. From the net convexity detectors comes information about potential sources of food. This type of informa-

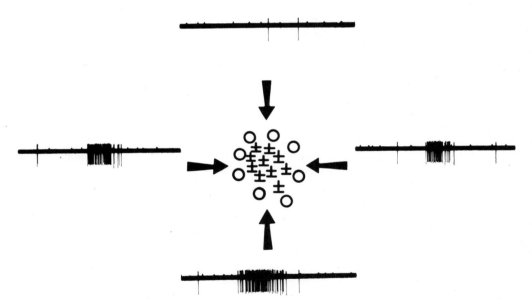

FIGURE 6-9 Responses of a directionally-sensitive ganglion cell from a rabbit. Center portion of the figure shows the receptive field of the cell, mapped with small spots. The response patterns were all generated by a moving stimulus traveling across the receptive field in the direction indicated by the arrow. Stimulus was a bar of light. From Barlow, H. B., R. M. Hill, and W. R. Levick (1964) Retinal ganglion cells responding selectively to direction and speed of image motion in the rabbit. *J. Physiol.* 173:377–407. Reprinted by permission.

tion is what is necessary for the animal to survive, but it in no way provides a general picture of the visual world.

The frog is noted for its specialized retinal feature detectors, but ganglion cells that seem to be tuned to special features in the visual world are found in all animals. Cells with concentric center/surround mechanisms seem to comprise the largest class of ganglion cells in most mammals, but significant numbers of cells are sensitive to either the orientation or direction of a moving stimulus.

Direction-selective ganglion cells give excitatory responses to both onset and offset of a flashing spot anywhere within their receptive fields, but give responses to a moving stimulus that depend on its direction of movement (Barlow & Hill, 1963). Figure 6–9 shows the receptive field organization of such a cell, along with its responses to a bar of light moving in various directions through its receptive field. This cell responds most strongly to a bar moving upward through the field; as the direction of movement varies from upward-going the response decreases and is nonexistent for stimuli moving vertically downward. The response of this cell does not depend on whether the bar is brighter or dimmer than the background.

Orientation-selective units are not concerned with the direction of movement of an asymmetrical stimulus as much as they are selective to its orientation (Levick, 1967). Figure 6–10 shows the receptive field of an orientation-selective unit, along with responses to rectangular stimuli that

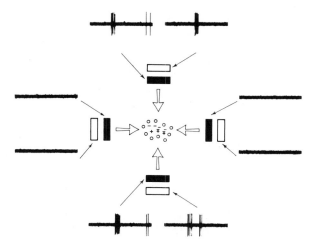

FIGURE 6-10 Responses of an orientation-selective ganglion cell from a rabbit. Center of the figure shows the receptive field of the cell; responses to light and dark bars oriented either vertically or horizontally are shown surrounding the receptive field. From Levick, W. R. (1967) Receptive fields and trigger features of ganglion cells of the rabbit's retina. *J. Physiol.* 188:285–307. Reprinted by permission.

move through the receptive field at different angles. This cell has a horizontally elongated receptive field, making it more sensitive to stimuli that are wider than they are tall. White or black bars that are moved upward or downward through the field evoke a vigorous response that is independent of direction. If the bars are rotated by 90° and passed horizontally through the field of the cell, however, no response is seen. If this cell were stimulated with stationary flashing bars of the same size, it would respond strongly to bars oriented horizontally, and make little or no response to bars oriented vertically. Thus, this cell is selectively sensitive to the shape of the stimulus, as opposed to its direction.

X-CELLS AND Y-CELLS

Most ganglion cells that have been recorded from the retinae of higher mammals (primarily cat and monkey) have concentric center/surround receptive field organizations. This does not mean, however, that they are all identical in their processing characteristics. In fact, ganglion cells with concentric receptive fields have been classified into several distinct groups on the basis of both anatomical and functional characteristics. Enroth-Cugell and Robson (1966), recording from ganglion cells in the retina of the cat, used stimuli called *sinusoidal gratings* to distinguish between what they named *X-cells* and *Y-cells*. Figure 6–11 shows an example of a sinusoidal grating (to be discussed in detail in Chapter 10); it is simply a succession of light and dark gradations. Enroth-Cugell and Robson performed an experiment in which a grating was presented to the receptive field of a ganglion cell for a short time period, and was then replaced by a diffuse light stimulus that was of the same luminance as the average of the grating. The position of the grating with respect to the receptive field of the cell was varied. Sometimes a dark bar covered the receptive field center, sometimes a light bar covered it, and sometimes parts of both portions covered the center.

The experimenters found that they could distinguish between two types of ganglion cells on the basis of their responses to the grating stimuli. Figure 6–12 shows the responses of an X-cell. When the light bar covered the center, the cell increased its firing; when the dark bar was over the center, the cell decreased its firing. By manipulating the exact placement of the grating, however, a position could be found where the presentation produced no response. At this position, the average illumination on the receptive field center and on the receptive field surround from the grating was equal to the illumination provided by the diffuse light. This type of cell, therefore, averages the amount of light falling on its receptive field, and responds accordingly.

Y-cells, on the other hand, respond quite differently when stimulated with gratings. As Figure 6–13 shows, no matter how a grating is positioned on the receptive field, a response to the onset and/or the offset of the presentation is always obtained. Y-cells, therefore, care about more than just the

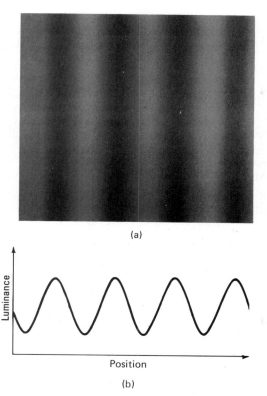

(a)

(b)

FIGURE 6-11 A sinusoidal grating. Below the figure is the luminance
distribution for the grating.

total amount of light falling on their receptive fields; the spatial configuration of the light is also important. That is, while X-cells will only respond to
the grating presentation when it produces a change in the total effective
amount of light falling on the receptive field, Y-cells will respond because
the grating represents a different spatial arrangement of the light than simple
diffuse illumination.

BOX 6–4

There is an interesting story behind Enroth-
Cugell's and Robson's discovery of X- and
Y-cells. When they began their experiments,
they had no idea there were two types of ganglion cell. Their purpose was to quantify a
model of the receptive field that they expected
(continued)

would apply to all ganglion cells. The model,
proposed by Rodieck and Stone (1965), suggested a specific mathematical description of
the way the center and the surround were sensitive to lights at different positions. Enroth-
Cugell and Robson took an unusual approach

(box continued)

to the problem: analysis by linear systems theory, for which sinusoidal gratings are the fundamental stimulus. Sinusoidal gratings had never been tried in a physiological experiment, although gratings were being used in visual psychophysics (see Chapter 10). In fact, John Robson was a pioneer in the use of sinusoidal gratings, and hoped to show (1) that they were useful for physiology, and (2) that the model could account for the quantitative details of the psychophysical findings.

The analysis technique for which gratings are suited depends on the cell combining influences from different parts of its receptive field in a linear manner. Before the analysis could be applied, therefore, this property had to be verified for the ganglion cells. The exchange of a grating for a uniform field, as described on p. 132, was Enroth-Cugell's and Robson's test for this kind of linearity. A cell would "pass" the test (prove spatially linear) if gratings positioned such that a bright bar and a dark bar that shared the field center elicited no response. As you saw, X-cells passed that test (Figure 6–12, second and fourth rows), and these were used to verify the model. Y-cells "failed" the test (Figure 6–13), and so were not suited for the study originally planned. But Enroth-Cugell and Robson realized that some cells being different could be important (in an early draft, Y-cells were called "I-cells," for "interesting"). Although a large part of their paper is devoted to the analysis of X-cells (as they had originally intended), there is also a discussion of the dichotomy they found. Their paper is one of the most widely cited in the vision literature, and most of the references are to the X-cell and Y-cell distinction.

X-cells differ from Y-cells in a number of other ways. Y-cells have larger receptive fields than X-cells (Enroth-Cugell & Robson, 1966). In general, Y-cells respond to stimuli in a fairly transient manner, showing strong response components primarily at stimulus onset and offset; X-cells, on the other hand, usually respond in a more sustained fashion (Saito, Shimahara, & Fukuda, 1970). While some researchers rely on this difference in response type as a way of classifying cells, it should be noted that all cells become more transient in brighter lights. Since Y-cells have larger receptive fields, which therefore collect more of the background light, it is possible that this difference may be due to the Y-cells being more light adapted (see Jakiela, Enroth-Cugell, & Shapley, 1976).

In addition to having larger receptive fields, Y-cells have thicker axons that conduct action potentials significantly faster than those of X-cells (Stone & Freeman, 1971). The cells are differentially sensitive to moving stimuli, with X-cells responding well to slow movements of a stimulus, and Y-cells preferring rapidly moving stimuli across a wide field. The retinal distributions of X- and Y-cells differ; the former are concentrated in the central retina, while the latter occur more or less uniformly throughout the retina (Fukuda, 1971).

At any particular location in the retina, Y-cells are physically larger, and

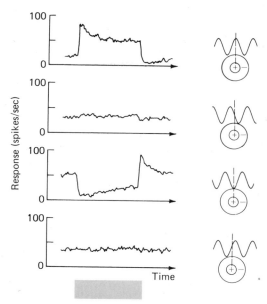

FIGURE 6-12   Responses (PSTH) of an X-cell to stimulation by a grating positioned in different ways within the receptive field. The position of the grating is shown on the right of the figure. Grating was substituted for a uniform field of the same mean luminance during the time indicated by the dark bar under the bottom PSTH. From Enroth-Cugell, C., and J. G. Robson (1966) The contrast sensitivity of retinal ganglion cells of the cat. *J. Physiol.* 187:517–552. Reprinted by permission.

the two may be differentiated by structural criteria (Cleland, Levick, & Wässle, 1975). In a heroic series of experiments, Heinz Wässle and his co-workers have been able to show that X-cells and Y-cells are anatomically distinct (Peichl & Wässle, 1981; Wässle, Peichl, & Boycott, 1981; Wässle, Boycott, & Illing, 1981). They did this by recording from many ganglion cells in a small area of retina, and noting the exact locations at which X-cells or Y-cells were found. They then stained the retina to reveal certain anatomical types, and correlated the locations of these types with the positions of the X-cells or Y-cells. They found that the Y-cells corresponded to a relatively rare, large cell called the *alpha cell*, while X-cells corresponded to a smaller cell called the *beta cell*. The relative rarity of Y-cells was a surprise, for physiologists had seen more Y-cells than any other type. This is probably because the large cell bodies and axons are more easily recorded by microelectrodes.

Consideration of the properties of X- and Y-cells, summarized in Table 6-1, has led to the hypothesis that they have radically different functions (Sherman, 1979; Rodieck, 1979). It has been proposed that Y-cells are im-

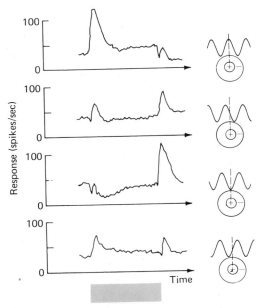

FIGURE 6-13 Responses of a Y-cell to stimulation by a grating positioned in different ways within the receptive field. Same conventions as in Figure 6–12. From Enroth-Cugell and Robson (1966). Reprinted by permission.

TABLE 6-1 A Comparison of Properties of X-, Y-, and W-Cells and Their Anatomical Correlates

	X-Cells	Y-Cells	W-Cells
Response type	brisk	brisk	sluggish
Spatial summation	linear	nonlinear	can be any
Response timing (tendency)	sustained	transient	can be any
Receptive field	center/surround	center/surround	various
Field size	small	medium	large
Anatomical type	beta	alpha	gamma
Cell body/axon size	medium	large	small
Axon conduction velocity	medium	fast	slow
Main density in retina	center	everywhere	periphery
Relative number	55%	4%	41%
Main target in brain	thalamus	thalamus and brainstem	brainstem

portant for orienting to new, potentially important stimuli, while X-cells, because of their smaller receptive fields, mainly function to provide more detailed information from stimuli after they have been attended to and fixated on the fovea. The Y-cells each cover a larger area, perhaps allowing a better analysis of direction of motion (Marr, 1982). The smaller receptive fields of X-cells allow for more fine discrimination (and perhaps identification) of a stimulus. We shall see in Chapters 8 and 9 that the X- and Y-cells are related to parallel systems that can be identified at higher levels of the visual system.

Although it is very difficult to record from ganglion cells in the human retina, psychophysical studies have been performed that suggest that there may be a similar separation of function in our own visual system. Investigators have been able to distinguish between what have been called *sustained* and *transient* mechanisms within the human visual system (Breitmeyer & Ganz, 1976; Tolhurst, 1973). The sustained system is slower in its response to stimuli, but has better acuity. The transient mechanism, on the other hand, is significantly faster in its response, but is much less sensitive to fine spatial patterns. Of course, we cannot state that the X- and Y-cell types form the basis of the sustained and transient mechanisms in human vision. Indeed, as you will see in Chapters 8 and 9, another distinction similar to that between X- and Y-cells seems to be even more important.

W-CELLS

There is also a significant third system in the retina. The W-cells are a heterogeneous group of cells with large receptive fields (but small cell bodies, making them very difficult to record) that are almost as numerous as the X-cells (Stone & Hoffmann, 1972; Stone & Fukuda, 1974). They may be either spatially linear, like X-cells, or nonlinear like Y-cells (Sur & Sherman, 1982), and include the motion-selective and other specialized cell types as well as ordinary center/surround cells (Rodieck, 1979). Anatomically, they seem to correspond to *gamma cells*, a diverse group of cells that have in common small cell bodies, large but sparse dendritic fields, and extremely thin axons (Boycott & Wässle, 1974; McGuire, Stevens, & Sterling, 1986; Stanford, 1987). Their responses are different from those of X-cells and Y-cells in that they are "sluggish," rather than "brisk" (Cleland & Levick, 1974). To understand the difference between a brisk response (X- or Y-cell) and a sluggish response (W-cell), think of how you respond to a challenge in a lively debate. That is brisk. Now think of how you respond to someone trying to wake you from a deep sleep. That is sluggish.

Another difference between W-cells and other cells is their target in the brain. W-cell axons leave the eye with other axons in the optic nerve, but few of them go to the main target—the lateral geniculate nucleus of the thalamus (see Chapter 8). Instead, they terminate on groups of cells near (or stuck inside as islands) the main target or go to the brainstem. X-cells, on the other hand, seem to go almost exclusively to the main part of the lateral geniculate nucleus. Y-cells seem to split, sending branches to both the main target and the brainstem. Properties of the W-cells are also summarized in Table 6–1.

SUGGESTED READINGS

Books that discuss properties of the retina generally include the ganglion cells. The books recommended in Chapter 5 are therefore also relevant for this chapter (*The Vertebrate Retina* by R. W. Rodieck, 1973; *The Retina* by J. E. Dowling, 1987). Topics relating to lateral interactions in the retina are nicely covered by T. N. Cornsweet (Academic Press, 1970) in his book, *Visual Perception*.

There are two (at least) *Scientific American* articles that expand on the topics covered in this chapter. C. R. Michael's "Retinal processing of visual images" (May 1969; offprint #1143), is a good treatment of ganglion cell physiology. For an authoritative treatment of Mach bands and lateral interactions, see F. Ratliff's "Contour and contrast" (June 1972; offprint #543). Michael's article is reprinted in *Perception: Mechanisms and Models* (W. H. Freeman, 1972), while Ratliff's article may be found in *Recent Progress in Perception* (W. H. Freeman, 1976).

The May 1986 issue of *Trends in Neurosciences* also includes articles on ganglion cells.

LIGHT ADAPTATION AND DARK ADAPTATION

7

In discussing the way the visual system detects and processes patterns of light, we have mentioned a number of important kinds of processing that are performed by the retina itself. We have been telling a simplified story, however, for we have not made mention of one of its most remarkable feats: *adapting* to different levels of illumination.

One might not think that there is a problem here. For any given scene, parts of the retina are stimulated by relatively intense lights, and other parts are stimulated by relatively weaker lights. What more do we need to know in order to identify objects in the visual world? In fact, that (plus information about color, movement, and so on) is all we want to be told by our retinae. The question addressed by this chapter is how they can perform this task over a wide range of luminances—the most intense lights are about 10^{13} (or 10,000,000,000,000) times more intense than the weakest lights we can detect. But, the firing rate of a neuron can range only from 0 to about 500 action potentials per second. Because of the inherent noisiness in the firing, there is only a very limited number of discriminable levels a neuron can signal; if the entire 10^{13} range were divided up, we would be unable to see subtle (and not so subtle) gradations.

A photographer faces a similar problem. The density difference between clear (unexposed) film and solid black (exposed) film is only about 100:1. With indoor film, which is very sensitive to light, you can take pictures inside a dim room by opening the diaphragm of the lens wide to let in the maximum amount of light, and setting a long exposure. In the bright sun it will be necessary to close the diaphragm to a small opening and use a fast shutter speed; otherwise the picture will be overexposed and come out solid white. If your camera does not have a wide enough range of diaphragm openings and shutter speeds, a less sensitive film must be used in sunlight.

The eyes of the photographer fiddling with the camera are functioning in the same extremes of light. True, the iris (which is like the camera's diaphragm) can close in bright light and open in dim, but the change in area is only about 16:1 (compared to at least 100:1 that most camera diaphragms can effect). Moreover, while you can change the exposure speed (time the shutter is open) on the camera, you cannot do the same with the eyes: the retina is continuously exposed to light. For the retina to work effectively at any illumination, it must be capable somehow of changing its sensitivity to light. In this chapter, we discuss some of the ways in which it can make those adjustments. Humans also have what amounts to a day retina and a night retina, with each one adjustable in sensitivity over a wide latitude.

SENSITIVITY VERSUS RESPONSE MEASURES

What do we mean by "sensitivity"? Although you probably have a pretty good feel for what it means to be "sensitive" to light, there is a specific meaning. You will need to understand the difference between sensitivity and response to understand what we mean by adaptation. The following exercise should help explain these concepts.

The curve in Figure 7–1(a) characterizes the rhodopsin of human rods; it therefore also characterizes the rods themselves. The hyperpolarization of a rod depends on the number of photons captured; the number of photons captured depends on the number delivered and their wavelengths (according to the percent absorption curve). It would seem that this curve is all we need to characterize the responses of a rod to any given light. For example, a given number of photons at 550 nm will produce just about half as much effect as the same number of photons at 500 nm, and so forth. Alternatively, we might expect that given the responses of a receptor to lights of various wavelengths, we should be able to see if the pigment in the receptor was rhodopsin (had an absorption curve like that shown in Figure 7–1[a]) or some other pigment. There is a catch: the hyperpolarization of the receptor, although it is related to the number of photons absorbed, is not linearly related. That is, the hyperpolarization due to the capture of, say, 2000 photons is *not* necessarily twice the hyperpolarization due to the capture of 1000 photons. For this reason, we must be careful about how we measure the characteristics of a visual cell when we wish to determine what visual pigment is responsible for the cell responses. There are two general methods available: response measures and sensitivity measures. Response measures are simpler (and quicker) to obtain. Sensitivity measures require more elaborate experiments, but reveal more about the intrinsic properties of the cell under study. To see why this is so, we will have to explain how the nonlinear relationship between the number of photons absorbed and amount of hyperpolarization affects response measures, and why it does not contaminate sensitivity measures.

We can characterize the relationship between numbers of photons captured and amount of hyperpolarization for a particular receptor, by presenting lights of various irradiances, all at the same wavelength, and recording the responses. When response (hyperpolarization) is plotted against the irradiance (which is proportional to the average number of photons captured), we obtain a curve called a *stimulus-response curve*, as shown in Figure 7–2.

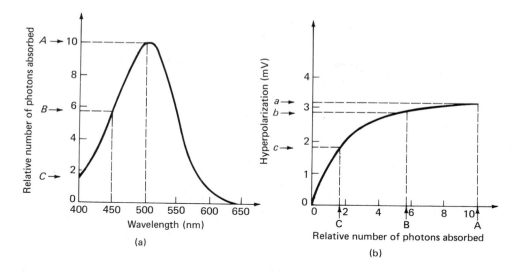

(a)

(b)

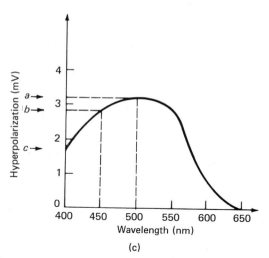

(c)

FIGURE 7-1 Demonstration that a curve of responses as a function of wavelength does not reproduce the absorption curve of the pigment in a receptor. (a) The number of photons that would be absorbed at each wavelength; this curve was shown in Figure 5–6. Three particular wavelengths are indicated, with absorptions marked *A*, *B*, and *C*. (b) The stimulus-response curve shown in Figure 7–2; the responses (*a*, *b*, *c*) that would be expected from the three absorptions (*A*, *B*, *C*) are shown. (c) The responses that would be expected at each wavelength (with *a*, *b*, and *c* indicated).

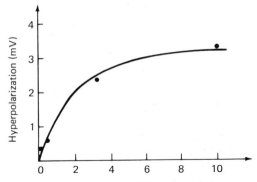

FIGURE 7-2   Stimulus-response curve from a single rod in *Necturus*.
Response is shown as a function of the relative number of
photons absorbed (actual numbers of photons about 3300
times larger). Based on Normann and Werblin (1974).
Control of retinal sensitivity. I. Light and dark adaptation
of vertebrate rods and cones. *J. Gen. Physiol.* 63:37–61.
By copyright permission of the Rockefeller University
Press.

Suppose we have impaled a receptor with a microelectrode and wish to
determine whether the pigment it contains is pure rhodopsin. We might
choose some irradiance (number of photons to include in each stimulus
flash) and record the hyperpolarization to flashes of various wavelengths. Because we are providing a constant number of photons in each flash, the percentage absorption curve can be relabeled as number of photons absorbed
(the number absorbed is the percentage times the number in each flash).
This is shown in Figure 7–1[a]. Consider three wavelengths: 500 nm, 450
nm, and 400 nm. The number of photons absorbed at each wavelength may
be read from the ordinate on the left: they are the three values labeled *A*, *B*,
and *C* (corresponding to 500, 450, and 400 nm respectively).

The receptor pigment does not absorb the same number of photons from
each of the three lights; we would therefore expect that the hyperpolariza-
tions produced by the three lights would be different. The actual hyperpo-
larizations in response to the three wavelengths depend not only on the
number of photons absorbed but also on the stimulus-response curve. As an
extreme example, notice that the stimulus-response curve shown in Figure
7–2 becomes nearly horizontal (or *saturates*) at high levels. Once the saturation has been attained, further increases in the number of photons absorbed will have no further effect on the response. If the three test lights
were presented at a sufficiently high irradiance (so that the number of photons absorbed from 400 nm of light were sufficient to reach the saturation),
they would all evoke the same response. More photons would be absorbed at
500 nm than at 400 nm, but each would evoke maximal hyperpolarization.

Of course, when we notice that all stimuli are producing the identical response we might guess what the problem is, and use a more moderate irradiance. This improves matters, but does not solve the problem completely. Let us return to the three wavelengths in Figure 7–1 and the three corresponding moderate photon absorptions A, B, and C. Figure 7–1(b) contains a stimulus-response curve, with the numbers of photons corresponding to A, B, and C indicated on the abscissa. From the ordinate, we can read the amount of hyperpolarization that each stimulus would evoke; they are labeled a, b, and c. We may now plot the hyperpolarization as a function of wavelength (Figure 7–1[c]) for the three points and all other wavelengths. The curve we obtain peaks at the right wavelength for rhodopsin, but has a distorted shape (compare Figure 7–1[c] with Figure 7–1[a]). This curve would not enable us to determine whether the pigment was pure rhodopsin, some other pigment, or a combination of pigments. The curve in Figure 7–1(c) is a *response measure*: it is not an acceptable way of looking at the spectral characteristics of the receptor.

A more satisfactory way to examine spectral characteristics is to use a *sensitivity measure*. Sensitivity means basically what you expect from intuition, although the exact definition is somewhat confusing. In sensitivity measures, you choose a specific magnitude of response; for each wavelength of light, the irradiance is adjusted until the stimulus produces exactly the requisite amount of response. Sensitivity is then defined as the inverse of the energy required to produce the criterion response, or

$$S = \frac{1}{I_{criterion}}$$

The inversion may seem strange, but it is the reason that sensitivity follows an intuitive definition. High sensitivity means a minimal stimulus is required to produce a response; low sensitivity means the light must be far stronger.

We encountered measures of this type in Chapter 2: *threshold* is simply one possible criterion that we could choose. If we measured threshold for detecting lights of different wavelengths, the *spectral sensitivity function* derived would be a function of the receptors only; it would not depend on the stimulus response curve of the subject or cell making the responses. The response is always the same (just visible, 10 mV hyperpolarization, or whatever), so each point is at the same response level on the stimulus-response curve. The shape of the curve therefore can have no effect on the outcome; the only function we measure is the absorption curve.

To measure the sensitivity of a receptor, we find the irradiance at each wavelength that gives a particular amount of hyperpolarization (say, 10 mV). As the amount of hyperpolarization is always the same, the same number of photons must have been captured from each of the stimuli. If a 400-nm light requires four times as many photons as a 460-nm light in order to give the same response (see Figure 7–1[a]), the percentage capture at 400 nm must have been one-quarter of that at 460 nm. We would say the sensitivity for 400 nm is one-quarter that for 460 nm (sensitivity is the inverse of the intensity). Table 7–1 presents a comparison of the sensitivities and percentages of absorption for five wavelengths. The percentages of absorption in the second column are read directly from Figure 7–1(a). The third column gives the number of photons that would have to be delivered to result in the absorption of one photon at each wavelength. (That is, on the average. Note that in a real experiment, the numbers of photons would be many times higher and we would not run into the absurdity of a fraction of a photon.) Verify that the products of the numbers in columns 2 and 3 are 1.0 (remember to divide the numbers given in column 2 by 100, because they are given in percentages). The last column is the sensitivity; it is 1 over the numbers in the third column. Notice that the numbers in the last column agree with those in the second (again allowing for a factor of 100 because column 2 is given in percentages).

DARK ADAPTATION

Consider the problem that you create for your eyes when you decide to go to the movies in the afternoon. You step from the bright sunlight outside the theater into the gloomy rows of seats. At first, it is hard to see anything except the aisle marker lights and the relatively bright picture on the screen. It is hard just to avoid stepping on people while trying to grope to a seat. After a while, however, it is possible to see quite well. People who were jostled on the way in can be seen so clearly that it would be fairly easy to describe them if necessary. It is as if there were much more light available in the theater.

We have described an uncontrolled psychophysical experiment that most people have performed without thinking about it. Let us consider a controlled version of the same experiment: a subject is allowed a period of time to stare at a bright surface (a controlled amount of adaptation, rather than "sun in the streets"), then is placed in total darkness. Spots of light of low luminance are shown on a screen; the subject is asked to detect them. Threshold is determined as a function of the time in darkness, as described in Chapter 2.

This experiment was performed by Hecht, Haig, and Chase (1937) using

TABLE 7–1 Sensitivities and Percentages of Absorption for Five Wavelengths

Wavelength (nm)	Percentage of Absorption	Number of Photons Required	Sensitivity
400	1.75	57.1	0.0175
450	5.65	17.7	0.0565
500	10.00	10.0	0.1000
550	5.05	19.8	0.0505
600	0.52	192.3	0.0052

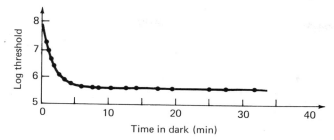

FIGURE 7–3 Threshold intensity of a small, red flash of light as a function of time in the dark after exposure to an adapting light. From Hecht, S., C. Haig, and A. M. Chase (1937). The influence of light adaptation on subsequent dark adaptation of the eye. *J. Gen. Physiol.* 20:831–850. By copyright permission of the Rockefeller University Press.

a small red spot of light on which the subject fixated. The result is shown in Figure 7–3. As the subject remained in the dark after the adapting field was extinguished, threshold dropped; the change was most rapid just after the subject was placed in the dark and tapered off to a fairly stable threshold level by 5 or 10 minutes. This stable plateau represents about 2 log units lowering of threshold, or about a factor of 100 improvement in the subject's ability to detect the red light. The improvement in sensitivity with time in the dark is what we call *dark adaptation*.

The increase in sensitivity represented by the curve in Figure 7–3 was observed when a subject was tested with a small red light presented to the fovea. It shows an improvement to a new level of sensitivity. Hecht and co-workers found a more striking result when larger test spots of violet light were used (Figure 7–4). As with the red test, there was a rapid improvement immediately after the adapting field was extinguished, gradually leveling off to a new threshold about 1 log lower than the original. About 8 min after the adapting field was extinguished, the threshold, which was apparently settling into its plateau value, suddenly plunged again. Over the next 20 min it dropped another 3 log units (1000 times), and finally settled at a value far lower than before.

What happened? Apparently, there are two distinct mechanisms; one of them acts rapidly, reaching a plateau in 5 to 10 min, while the other is much slower but apparently more potent. The plateau represents the absolute threshold of the faster system; the break in the curve at about 8 min represents the transition from the one system to the other, and the final plateau represents the absolute threshold of the slower system. You may recall these two systems from Chapter 4. The one that reached its threshold first is called the *photopic* system. When it is operating, as it does in relatively bright illumination, we are said to be in the photopic state. The slower system, which accounted for the extremely high sensitivity after about 20 min, is the *sco-*

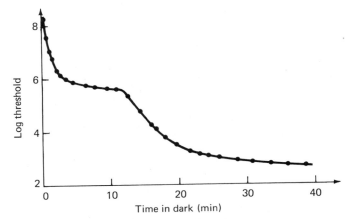

FIGURE 7-4   Threshold intensity of a large, violet flash of light as a function of time in the dark after exposure to an adapting light. From Hecht, Haig, and Chase (1937). By copyright permission of the Rockefeller University Press.

topic system; when we are dark-adapted and sensitive to dim lights, we are said to be in the scotopic state.

We can measure the spectral sensitivities of the two systems by performing the experiment of Figure 7–4 (large test stimulus) with test lights of various wavelengths. The initial plateau (before the break) represents the threshold of the photopic system some time after the adapting field was extinguished. The inverse of the threshold is the sensitivity, so we can plot the sensitivity of the photopic system as a function of wavelength (dashed curve in Figure 7–5). Similarly, the final plateau reached after a long time in the dark (absolute visual threshold) represents the threshold of the scotopic system. We can plot the sensitivity of the scotopic system on the same axes (solid curve in Figure 7–5). When we do this, we note several interesting things.

First, we notice that the scotopic system is more sensitive than the photopic for all wavelengths except for the very longest. When we are fully dark-adapted, the weakest lights we can detect (except reds) are detected by the scotopic system. Second, we notice that the shapes of the photopic and scotopic spectral sensitivity curves are different. The photopic system is most sensitive at 555 nm (green light), although the scotopic system is still more sensitive even at that wavelength. The scotopic system is most sensitive at 505 nm (blue-green). In fact, 505 nm is the light to which we are the most sensitive when dark-adapted.

The change in spectral sensitivity as we go from the photopic to the scotopic state is called the *Purkinje shift*. This is basically a shift in the peak sensitivity of the eye as a function of adaptation. Two stimuli that are equally "bright" to the photopic observer (have equal photopic luminosity) will not appear equally bright to the scotopic observer, and vice versa. An orange

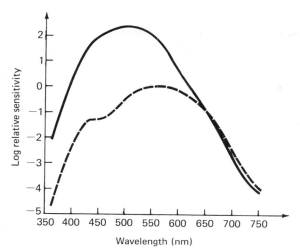

FIGURE 7-5 Relative sensitivity of the photopic (dashed) and scotopic (solid) systems as a function of wavelength. From Wald, G. (1945). Human vision and the spectrum. *Science* 101:653–658. Reprinted by permission. Copyright 1945 by the AAAS.

flower and a blue flower may seem about the same brightness (although obviously different in color) in sunlight, but in moonlight the blue flower will appear relatively light and the orange flower relatively dark. This effect was first described by J. E. Purkinje, who pointed out that in the dim light of early dawn reds look blackest of all the colors; as light increases the blues emerge first, but their brightness is overtaken by the yellows and greens in the full light of day (Purkinje, 1825).

The scotopic peak at 505 nm brings us to a third point. We saw in Chapter 5 that the peak of rhodopsin (the rod pigment) absorption curve is 505 nm. This is not a coincidence. In fact, if the scotopic spectral sensitivity curve is plotted on the same coordinates as the spectral absorption curve of rhodopsin, they may be seen to be virtually identical (Hecht, Shlaer, & Pirenne, 1942). There is a strong implication here: rods are the receptors of the scotopic system.

If the rods serve the scotopic system, it seems reasonable to surmise that the other class of receptors, the cones, serve the photopic system. (Although no cone pigment matches the photopic spectral sensitivity curve, that curve can be closely approximated by a combination of the three cone types.) Several other kinds of evidence also support the conclusion that rods serve the scotopic system and cones serve the photopic system.

1. Lights presented to the fovea stimulate only the photopic system, while lights presented outside the fovea affect the scotopic system at absolute threshold. That is why the demonstration of the adaptation of the photopic system in Figure 7–3 was performed with a light in the fovea, and the

scotopic system became evident when a larger stimulus light was used (Figure 7–4). As you may recall from Chapter 5, cones are most concentrated in the fovea, while rods are absent from the fovea but are most numerous just outside it (see Figure 5–3). The spectral sensitivity (at absolute threshold) for stimuli presented to the fovea is that of the photopic system (dashed curve in Figure 7–5); the drop in threshold following termination of a bright light does not show a break to the scotopic system when the test flashes are presented to the fovea. Only test spots presented outside the fovea, where both rods and cones are present, yield dark adaptation curves with two branches (as in Figure 7–4) having an absolute visual sensitivity after a long time in the dark that matches the sensitivity of the scotopic system (solid curve in Figure 7–5). As only the photopic system can be demonstrated in the fovea, where there are only cones, cones must be the receptors that serve the photopic system.

We may also ask what is the best place on the retina to present a test stimulus, if we wish to stimulate either the photopic or the scotopic system using the weakest possible light. The best location for a photopic stimulus (one that is detected by the photopic system) is in the fovea; the best place to present a scotopic stimulus is outside the fovea. The sensitivities of the two systems as a function of placement on the retina match the measured distributions of the cones (photopic) and rods (scotopic) respectively (see Figure 5–3).

There is a consequence of the difference in retinal location of the peak sensitivities of the scotopic and photopic systems that may be familiar: the scotopic system, which is more sensitive than the photopic (Figure 7–5), is most sensitive slightly off-axis. To detect a dim light when you are fully dark-adapted, it is best to look slightly above or below where it might be (you could look to the side, but then you might place the image on your blind spot, which is totally insensitive). This is a trick used by amateur astronomers, and taught to soldiers who stand guard duty at night.

2. Rods and cones in the back of the eye are ''aimed'' at the center of the pupil, from which the light should come (see Chapter 4). Cones in particular have inner segments that serve to channel the light to the outer segment *if* the light is coming directly down their axes (Enoch, 1963). This makes cones more sensitive to light coming from the center of the pupil than from the edges, wasting the light from the edges but giving a clearer image (the light from the edges is less well focused). Cones function in bright light and so can afford the wasted light; rods need all the light they can get, and therefore do not waste the light from the edge of the pupil. An experimenter can arrange for all the light in the stimulus to pass through a small point in the pupil, and locate that point in the center or at the edge of the pupil. If the light is effective for cones, the stimulus entering through the edge of the pupil will be less effective than that entering through the center. This is called the *Stiles-Crawford effect* (Stiles & Crawford, 1933); it is far more pronounced for photopic stimuli than for scotopic.

3. The scotopic system is served by a single type of receptor; all the rods

can do is hyperpolarize in proportion to the number of photons absorbed. There is no way for a rod to signal whether it caught one of ten available photons at 505 nm, or one of 20 available photons at 550 nm. There is thus no way for the rod to signal the color of the light—it is colorblind (see Chapter 15 for a full discussion of this). The cone system, on the other hand, has three distinct members (cones with somewhat different spectral sensitivities). With relative absorptions of a light by the three different classes of cone, the nervous system can extract information about the color of the light (see Chapter 15). You can see colors when in the photopic state but not in the scotopic state. In the dim of night, when you can see forms and shapes, you are color-blind except for some reds, to which the photopic system is more sensitive than the scotopic.

Once you are persuaded (we are certainly), that rods subserve the scotopic system and cones subserve the photopic, let us look again at what happens when you are suddenly placed in the dark and asked to detect a green light. Follow the course of dark adaptation of rods and cones on Figure 7–6. When you were in the light (adapting field) before the experiment began, both rods and cones were made less sensitive; that is, the retina was *light-adapted*. The rods, however, were far more affected by the adapting field than the cones; that is, the sensitivity of the rods became less than that of the cones. Quite possibly, the rods were made so insensitive as to be unresponsive. When the adapting field is extinguished, both rods and cones start to dark-adapt, becoming more sensitive. The cones, being more sensitive to begin with and adapting faster than the rods, determine the threshold for the first test flashes. The subject is still photopic and, as the cones are detecting the test, can also see its color.

After a few minutes, the cones have approached their ultimate sensitivity, and threshold levels off. The rods, of course, are still changing dramatically, but since their threshold is still higher than the cone threshold, the light is detected by the cones. We know that the rod curve is doing what we say it is, as studies of people who have a genetic abnormality that causes them to lack cones show dark-adaptation curves like the "rod" curve in Figure 7–6 (Rushton, 1961a).

During this photopic period, there is color vision, relatively good acuity, relatively rapid responses to flickering light, and the Stiles-Crawford effect is evident. The peak sensitivity is at about 555 nm, and maximum sensitivity is in the fovea.

At some time after 5 min in the dark, the increasing sensitivity of the rod system causes its threshold to fall below that of the cones. Because the rods are more sensitive, they are the receptors that determine threshold. Dimmer and dimmer lights can be seen, until the ultimate absolute threshold is approached by about 30 min.

This scotopic period is characterized by lack of color vision for threshold stimuli—the test flash looks colorless or pale blue (Trezona, 1970)—poorer

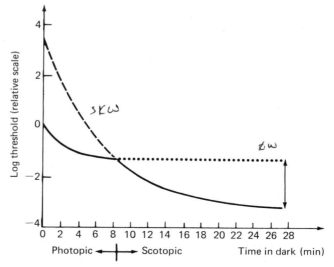

FIGURE 7–6 Theoretical course of adaptation of the cones (dotted)
and rods (dashed) as a function of time in the dark. Solid
curve shows the drop in threshold, determined by the
more sensitive system. Test light = 550 nm.

acuity, and slower responses to flickering light (a light that could be seen to
be alternately brighter and dimmer at a rapid rate in the photopic state may
now look like a steady light). The Stiles-Crawford effect is minimal, peak
sensitivity is at 505 nm, and the most sensitive part of the retina is slightly
outside the fovea. A summary of the characteristics of the photopic and scotopic systems is found in Table 7–2.

In the scotopic state, a threshold light is detected by the rods, and its color
not sensed. If the light is made stronger, however, it will soon stimulate cones
also, and color can be detected. The arrow in Figure 7–6 shows the additional
amount of light that must be added to a threshold light to make its color evident; this separation is called the *photochromatic interval*. Lights in this

TABLE 7–2 A Comparison of Properties of the Photopic and Scotopic Systems

Property	Photopic System	Scotopic System
Receptor type	Cones	Rods
Retinal location for highest sensitivity	Fovea	Outside fovea
Wavelength of peak sensitivity	555 nm	505 nm
Acuity	Good	Poor
Sensitivity	Moderate and bright lights	Dim lights
Type of vision	Color or black and white	Black and white only
Sensitivity to part of pupil light enters	Sensitive	Not sensitive

range of intensities (between absolute threshold and the photopic threshold) are visible, but uncolored. The photochromatic interval is different for different wavelengths; it depends on the relative sensitivities of the photopic and scotopic systems. Short wavelength stimuli have large photochromatic intervals, as the difference in sensitivity between the systems is large in this region of the spectrum. Lights longer than about 650 nm show no photochromatic interval; their color is seen as soon as they are detectable, as the photopic system is more sensitive than the scotopic at these long wavelengths. The photochromatic interval for lights shorter than 650 nm can be read directly from Figure 7–5; it is the space between the two curves.

BOX 7–1

Although we have been speaking of the rods and the cones as two independent systems, there is evidence that they may interact, so that the changeover from rod to cone and back again is complete. If there is an inhibitory interaction between them at the point at which one receptor type is more active than the other, it can inhibit the weaker type and so prevent it from having as much influence on the visual signal.

Evidence for an interaction between rods and cones comes from psychophysical experiments. In these the scotopic threshold is influenced differently by background lights of the same scotopic effectiveness, but that have different *photopic* effectiveness (Makous & Boothe, 1974; Frumkes & Temme, 1977; Ingling, Lewis, Loose, & Myers, 1977). That is, activity in the cones affects the rod threshold. Other evidence for rod/cone interaction comes from recordings in single horizontal cells; the range of intensities in which input from both rods and cones can be demonstrated in a horizontal cell can be changed by using anesthetic

drugs that apparently affect interactions (Whitten & Brown, 1973).

The ganglion cells of the retina have input from both rods and cones (Barlow, FitzHugh, & Kuffler, 1957; Adams & Afanador, 1971), so the interaction of the systems must be complete by that level of processing. Shefner and Levine (1977, 1981) studied rod/cone interactions by recording the activity of ganglion cells in goldfish. We stimulated with lights effective only for rods or only for cones; there was greater interaction when the two stimuli overlapped than when they were somewhat separated (although within the center of the ganglion cell receptive field). This difference implies an interaction that is distance-dependent: rods and cones that are close to each other interact more strongly than those that are somewhat separated. A similar interaction has been demonstrated in cats (Levine, Frishman, & Enroth-Cugell, 1987), and can be demonstrated psychophysically in humans (Benimoff, Schneider, & Hood, 1982; Drum, 1982; see Levine and Frishman, 1984).

LIGHT ADAPTATION

The changeover from cones to rods as the eye dark-adapts is striking, but it is actually not as remarkable as the fact that each system, rod or cone, changes its sensitivity dramatically as it remains in the dark. Similarly, each system adjusts its sensitivity according to the lighting. If we think of the system as most sensitive in complete darkness, adding a "background" light quickly reduces sensitivity. This adjustment of sensitivity is known as *light adaptation*.

In light adaptation, we speak of the change in sensitivity to lights that are superimposed on a steady background light. While the stimuli could be either brighter or dimmer than the background, we usually refer to *increment sensitivity*; that is, we are interested in how much light must be added to the background to be detected. You may recall that we already discussed this problem in Chapter 2, and concluded that Weber's Law was the typical sensory system's solution to the problem. According to Weber's Law, the size of the just noticeable increment is directly related to the luminance it is seen against; that is, the same *contrast* is just noticeable. At higher backgrounds, the system is somehow "cranked down" so that a larger increment is needed to give the same (threshold) response (Shapley & Enroth-Cugell, 1984).

What kind of change could there be in the way the retina responds to light? The solid curve in Figure 7–7(a) shows how a cell in the visual system might respond to various strengths of stimulation. For very low stimulus strengths there is no response; as the strength increases, so does the response. But there is an upper limit to the responses a cell can generate, so the cell would eventually saturate. The curve shown in Figure 7–7(a) is drawn from an equation commonly used to represent the responses of visual cells (Naka & Rushton, 1966).

A steady background light would appear along the curve at some new operating point, such as the solid circle at the middle of the curve. Increments (or decrements) of light superimposed on that background would then cause

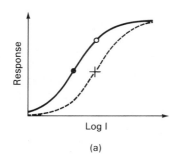
(a)

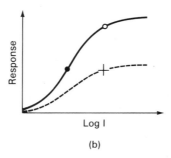
(b)

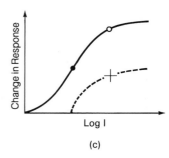
(c)

FIGURE 7–7 Responses of a hypothetical visual cell *versus* the logarithm of stimulus strength. (a) The solid curve is like that in Figure 7–2, except for the logarithmic axis. The dashed curve shows the relation in a steady strong background (open circle on solid curve) that effects a change in sensitivity. (b) The same relationship as in (a), but the dashed curve represents the relationship if the background effects a multiplicative change. (c) Responses to increments derived from the curves in part (b).

changes in response from that middle level. (Since this graph shows responses versus the log of stimulus strength, the size of the response would grow directly with the logarithm of *contrast* as long as the contrast was low enough to stay on the approximately straight central portion of the curve.)

But an even stronger background would appear at the nearly horizontal saturated part of the curve (open circle). Even very large increments would not cause any change in response (and because of the log axis, the changes would be truly enormous). How could the system compensate for the bright background?

You have perhaps found one solution to being in too bright a light: you put on dark glasses. A dark filter would reduce every light (background and increment) by the same fraction. On a log axis, a constant factor is equivalent to a constant shift (see the appendix), so the same cell (wearing dark glasses) would operate on the dashed curve shown to the right of the original solid curve. The very strong background would again be at the middle of the curve in Figure 7–7(a) (cross), and the situation would be exactly as it was for the moderate background (solid dot). If you are looking at a picture and the illumination is increased, you can get back to exactly where you had been by putting on the appropriate dark glasses. But you do not need the glasses, because your visual system light-adapts, shifting your *as if* you wore the glasses.

BOX 7–2

Notice that the dark glasses, representing a change in sensitivity, does not have the same effect as simply decreasing the *gain* of the cell. Gain refers to the multiplier between input and output. If you divided the responses represented by the solid curve in Figure 7–7(a) by some factor, the curve would shrink, as shown by the dashed curve in Figure 7–7(b). This picture illustrates the same situations for a gain-changing system. True, the sensitivity would be decreased by the background (a greater increment would be needed to give the same re-

sponse), but the high background would still saturate the responses.

If we looked at the increment responses—that is, the change in response due to flashes against the background—and ignored the steady response due to the background (as visual cells, which are somewhat transient, do), we would see a set of curves like those in Figure 7–7(c). This looks like adaptation becaues the curves shift to the right, but it is not the same as the change in sensitivity illustrated in Figure 7–7(a).

PHYSIOLOGY OF ADAPTATION

The simplest way to explain adaptation would be to assume that the loss of sensitivity in brighter lights is because there is less pigment available to capture photons. You will recall from Chapter 5 that a visual signal is initiated by a pigment molecule capturing a photon, and that the probability of a capture depends both on the number of photons and the number of available pigment molecules (among other things). Each time a molecule captures a photon it isomerizes—that is, bleaches—and is temporarily unavailable to catch more photons. A bright light bleaches a large number of molecules; that decreases the number remaining, so that there are fewer photon captures for the incoming stream of light. Hecht (1937) proposed that bleaching of pigment molecules by light caused the loss of sensitivity associated with bright backgrounds, and gradual recovery of bleached molecules (by regeneration) in the dark accounts for the increase in sensitivity we observed in Figures 7–3, 7–4, and 7–6.

Life is not that simple. Enormous changes in sensitivity occur with virtually no pigment bleaching (Granit, Holmberg, & Zewi, 1938). There is, of course, adaptation because of pigment being bleached, but there is another kind of adaptation that does not require significant bleaching. This has been termed "neural" or *field adaptation*, by Rushton (1965). Field adaptation is relatively fast, compared to that caused by the bleaching of pigment (which Rushton called *photochemical* or *bleaching adaptation*).

Where in the retina does adaptation occur? Of course, the effect of reducing the amount of pigment occurs in the receptors themselves, for that is where the pigment is. But if much adaptation occurs with minimal pigment bleaching, it might occur anywhere in the retina. Do individual receptors adapt? Cones apparently do show adaptation like that illustrated in Figure 7–7(a) (Malchow & Yazulla, 1986), but it is possible that rods (at least in retinas that also have cones to take over at higher illuminations) do not. It appears that the rods in our retinas, as judged by those in monkeys, simply shift to new operating points, like the circles on the solid curve in Figure 7–7(a) (Baylor, Nunn, & Schnapf, 1984). But rods in other animals do adapt. Recordings from single receptors have shown that at least some of the adaptive effect (over and above the part caused by loss of pigment, which is necessarily receptoral) occurs in receptors. Grabowski and Pak (1975) showed that the sensitivity of individual salamander (axolotl) rods changed far more than could be predicted by the amount of pigment bleached. Dowling and Ripps (1972), Green, Dowling, Siegel, and Ripps (1975), and Brin and Ripps (1977) studied the rods in the retina of skate, and found distinct changes in sensitivity with background lights that did not cause significant bleaching of pigment. Similar results were obtained from the frog by Hemilä (1977). A study of toad rods exactly like the study of monkey rods that showed no adaptation indicated a shift like the change to the dashed curve in Figure 7–7(a) (Lamb, McNaughton, & Yau, 1981).

While receptors adapt, there is further adaptation in the proximal retina. Like lateral antagonism, adaptation does not occur all in a single stage. One reason we can say there is adaptation after the receptors is that adaptation is not localized to individual receptors. Light in one spot also affects the sensitivity for lights in nearby regions. That is, receptors act as if they were affected by lights in a larger region, called an *adapting pool* (Rushton, 1965). These pools were first demonstrated by an ingenious psychophysical experiment in which it was found that the adaptation caused by a stroboscopic flash (too brief to allow for any eye movement) was independent of whether it was spread uniformly over an area or concentrated in fine bars alternating with dark areas (Rushton & Westheimer, 1962). Since the receptors in the dark areas were not "spared," they must have been adapted by the light in the nearby bars, even though they did not receive any of that light directly.

BOX 7–3

Adaptation that occurs in the proximal retina must nonetheless have a restricted extent; the pools cannot extend across the entire retina, as adaptation is at least somewhat local. It is reasonable to wonder whether the adaptation pools are somehow linked to the ganglion cell receptive fields.

One line of evidence indicates that the adaptation pools are indeed so related. Cleland and Enroth-Cugell (1968) and Enroth-Cugell and Shapley (1973) found that the change in sensitivity of a cat ganglion cell depended on the effective amount of light falling on the center of the field. That is, a small intense adapting field would have the same effect as a larger, less intense field if the two were equally effective in exciting the ganglion cell. It did not seem to matter how the light was distributed within the receptive field as long as it had the same effect on the center of the receptive field.

On the other hand, Easter (1968b) placed small adapting spots within the receptive fields of goldfish ganglion cells, and tested their effect on the sensitivities to test spots at various positions within the fields. He found that the effect on a test spot was determined by how near it was to the adapting spot; there were local adaptation pools within the receptive field center. Similar results have been obtained from frog by Burkhardt and Berntson (1972).

Some resolution to this apparent contradiction can be found in the work of Tong and Green (1977). They placed adapting lights within the receptive fields of rat retinal ganglion cells, and tested the effects on variously positioned test spots. As did Easter, they found a tendency for the effects to be greatest near the adapting spots; however, the greatest effect was often at a point between the adapting light and the receptive field center (Cicerone & Green, 1980). In other words, there was also a component that was associated with the receptive field center, as noted by Enroth-Cugell and Shapley. There are likely to be at least two different components of adaptation, corresponding to two different levels in the retina. The distal pools are associated with the local area around the adapting light, but there apparently is also a pool associated with the ganglion cell receptive field center. It should also be noted that these results were obtained with different animal models, and some animals may place heavier reliance on the distal pools, while others rely more on the proximal pools.

There is considerable further change in sensitivity proximal to the receptors, however. Green, Dowling, Siegel, and Ripps (1975) compared the sensitivities of the rods in skate with the *b*-wave of the electroretinogram (the electroretinogram is a massed potential that can be recorded from the retina; the *b*-wave is believed to reflect activity of cells in the inner nuclear layer). There was a distinct difference between the time courses of recovery of the rods and the *b*-wave following offset of an adapting light. This difference represents stages of adaptation in cells proximal to the receptors. Similar later stages of adaptation have been found in recordings from single cells in the retina of the mud puppy *Necturus* (Werblin, 1971; 1974).

AFTERIMAGES

There is a set of visual phenomena that are apparently related to the process of adaptation. They are called *afterimages*, literally, images seen after the stimulus is no longer present. There are two major classes: *positive* and *negative*.

Positive Afterimages

A positive afterimage is one that looks like the fading ghost of the original stimulus. Stare at a bright light and then look at a black surface; there will be a bright image of the light. This is the positive afterimage. It sometimes does not appear immediately, but "develops" after a brief delay. The afterimage gradually fades from view, although it is often possible to revive it by blinking hard, or looking briefly at a differently colored surface.

The positive afterimage is made of "light" that is not there; this "light" generated by retinal activity, has been called *dark light* (Barlow, 1964). In fact, the higher visual thresholds immediately following the offset of an adapting light can be considered as if they were caused by dark light against which the test flashes must be detected. The recovery of sensitivity with time in the dark can be equated with the gradual fading of the dark light (or afterimage), and the state of adaptation at any moment can be expressed in terms of the equivalent background light that, if present, would yield the same sensitivity.

The dark light is probably caused by continued hyperpolarization of the receptors following offset of a strong light (Baylor & Hodgkin, 1974; Kleinschmidt & Dowling, 1975; Penn & Hagins, 1972). Even the delay in onset of the afterimage may be identified with the brief dead period observed in the receptors (Baylor & Hodgkin, 1974). The reason for the continued hyperpolarization is not completely known, although it is reasonable to assume that bleached pigment molecules that have not yet regenerated continue to signal the presence of light by the fact of their isomerized state.

Afterimages do not last for the 30 min or so that is required for complete recovery of sensitivity. The reason for this is that they cannot move on the surface of the retina; they are anchored by being produced by the receptor cells in a particular area. The stimulation associated with them is therefore wholly unchanging, and as we know from Chapters 5 and 6, the cells of the retina are generally uninterested in unchanging stimuli. The afterimages move with the retina, and fade as "adaptation" occurs. A similar phenomenon occurs with actual lights that stimulate the retina without being allowed to move across it as the eye moves. These are called *stabilized images*.

Negative Afterimages

The negative afterimage is induced the same way as the positive one, except that following exposure to the original stimulus the subject looks at a light gray or white surface. The afterimage on the surface has the same form as the original stimulus, but the contrast is reversed. Areas that were bright in the original appear dark, while areas that were dim in the original appear bright (like a photographic negative). If the original stimulus was colored, the colors also are reversed, with greens appearing where there had been reds, yellows for blues, and so forth. The significance of these color reversals is discussed in Chapter 15.

To induce a negative afterimage, the luminance of the screen on which it is to be seen must be at least at the threshold for seeing a light at that level of adaptation (Gosline, MacLeod, & Rushton, 1973). That is, the lightness of the screen must be such that it is visible. That is a clue to the nature of the negative afterimage: the adaptation pools in the areas exposed to bright light have been adapted, so the cells in those areas of retina are less sensitive. The screen on which the afterimage is seen provides uniform light, but when the light falls on less sensitive areas of the retina it has less effect. It could even be below threshold, if the adaptation is strong enough and the screen is relatively dim. The areas of screen being sensed by strongly adapted areas of retina appear dim, and the other areas relatively brighter. Hence, there is a negative afterimage.

We should also note that, like the positive afterimage, the negative afterimage is stabilized on the retina. It therefore also fades more rapidly than would be expected from the time course of dark adaptation. It can be revitalized by blinking the eyes or changing the luminance of the screen on which it is seen, as these activities cause changes in the otherwise static afterimage. In fact, brightening the screen leads to a negative afterimage and dimming the screen leads to a positive afterimage. This is consistent with the idea that local areas adapted by light are less responsive; by brightening the screen, the areas adapted by light parts of the original pattern brighten less than other areas, giving a negative afterimage. Dimming the screen causes less OFF response in the adapted areas; they dim less than the surrounding regions, and we see a positive afterimage (Williams & MacLeod, 1979).

BOX 7-4

Finally, we should ask what mechanisms might lead to the field adaptation we have discussed. One intriguing possibility is that there is a "parametric feedback," in which activation of receptors serves to change the properties of the retina by some mechanism such as exhaust-

ing neurotransmitter, inactivating synapses, or accumulating some extracellular "dark adaptation substance" (Barlow, 1977). We have already seen an intracellular adapting substance, calcium, that might play a role in receptors (see Box 5–5). A possible candidate for a dark

(continued)

(box continued)

adaptation substance in the inner retina that has received considerable attention is potassium. Potassium ions (K^+) are released into the extracellular environment whenever potassium channels open, or when cells depolarize (see Chapter 3). Added to the extracellular fluid, K^+ has little or no effect on the sensitivity or responses of receptors, but has an effect on the *b*-wave of the electroretinogram that is analogous to the effect of background lights (Dowling & Ripps, 1976; Dowling, 1977; see Frishman, Sieving, & Steinberg, 1988 for a discussion of K^+ and the electroretinogram). It is therefore possible that K^+ accumulating in the extracellular environment causes a slight depolarization of retinal cells and leads to the loss of sensitivity we call light adaptation.

SUGGESTED READINGS

One of the clearest descriptions of the process of dark adaptation and the properties of the photopic and scotopic systems that we have encountered is in the book *Visual Perception*, by T. N. Cornsweet (Academic Press, New York, 1970). In particular, Chapter 7, "Cones and cone pigment," describes the differences between rods and cones, and explains the significance of the photopic and scotopic spectral sensitivity curves.

The psychophysics of dark adaptation, and the identification of the pigments of the photopic and scotopic systems are presented by W. A. H. Rushton in "Visual pigments in man" (*Scientific American*, November 1962; offprint #139). This article is reprinted in *Perception: Mechanisms and Models*, by R. Held and W. Richards (W. H. Freeman, San Francisco, 1972). A good treatment of the way individual neurons within the retina adapt to different background levels of light is presented by F. S. Werblin in "The control of sensitivity in the retina" (*Scientific American*, January 1973; offprint #1264). This article is reprinted in *Recent Progress in Perception*, by R. Held and W. Richards (W. H. Freeman, San Francisco, 1976).

A more detailed discussion of adaptation may be found in *The Retina*, by J. E. Dowling (Harvard University Press, 1987). We also recommend "Visual adaptation and retinal gain controls" by R. Shapley and C. Enroth-Cugell, in *Progress in Retinal Research*, 3:263–346. This is an excellent review of the mechanisms of adaptation in the retina, though it is quite technical and may prove difficult in places.

THE PRIMARY VISUAL AREAS
OF THE BRAIN

So far in this book we have restricted our discussion of the visual system to the processes that occur in the eye itself. Even at such a peripheral level, we have noted the existence of a number of sophisticated coding mechanisms. In this chapter, we trace the pathways of the visual system from the point at which ganglion cell axons leave the eyeball, to the cerebral cortex of the brain, and see how these higher processing centers act on the incoming signals to detect specific features of the visual world. In this chapter, we concentrate on the pathway to primary visual cortex and the responses of cells in these lower-order areas. In the next chapter, we examine how the cortical areas are organized into parallel, cooperative pathways.

THE VISUAL PATHWAY

Figure 8–1 shows three sketches of the human brain seen from different angles. Part (a) presents a side view, with the front of the brain toward the left. The area visible on the outside is a thin sheet of tissue called the *cerebral cortex*; it is only about 2 mm thick in man, but its many folds and invaginations give it an extremely large surface area of about 2000 cm² (Hubel & Wiesel, 1977). The cerebral cortex is phylogenetically the newest part of the brain; it is large and highly specialized in higher mammals, but decreases in relative size as one goes from lower mammals such as rodents to fish or amphibia. The part of the cortex that first receives the visual signal is shaded in Figures 8–1(a) and (b); it is the back part of the cortex, and is given the name *occipital cortex*. Within this region of the brain, there are a number of differentiable visual areas (creatively named *visual area I*, *visual area II*, and so on). In the cortex of the monkey (and therefore, presumably, also in man), these areas are hierarchically organized; visual area I (also called *striate cortex* or V1) receives visual information from lower centers while providing input to a number of secondary cortical regions (Van Essen, 1979). Many of the experiments to be discussed in this chapter were performed on primates because of the close similarity of their brains to those of human beings. The other major experimental animal used in research on the visual cortex has been the cat; however, as the visual cortex of the cat is organized differently from that of primates, we will note when we are talking about nonprimate data.

As are many other parts of the body, the brain is a *bilaterally symmetric* organ; that is, it is composed of two half-brains (called cerebral hemispheres) that are nearly mirror images of each other (although there are some important differences). The two halves are connected to each other by the *corpus callosum*, which is a thick band of nerve fibers (see Figure 8–1[b]). When we talk about a certain structure within the brain, therefore, we must be careful to specify to which half of the brain we are referring. For example, the visual areas mentioned in the previous paragraph exist as separate structures in each of the hemispheres.

The pathway of the visual system from the eye to the cortex is shown schematically in Figure 8–2. The axons of retinal ganglion cells leave the retina at the optic disc, and form the optic nerve. The optic nerves from both eyes run just underneath the brain (see Figure 8–1[c]) and intersect at a junction called the *optic chiasm*. At the chiasm, the nerves branch, with some of the fibers continuing through the intersection toward the half of the brain on the opposite side from the eye from which the fibers originated; this half of the brain is called the *contralateral* hemisphere. The rest of the fibers do not cross to the opposite side of the brain, but change their direction of travel at the optic chiasm and go into the same half of the brain as the eye from which they came; the half of the brain on the same side is said to be *ipsilateral* to that eye.

Which fibers cross from one side of the brain to the other at the optic chiasm is determined by where on the retina they originated. As shown in Figure 8–2, fibers coming from the side of each retina closest to the nose (*nasal retina*) will cross at the chiasm and go into the contralateral side of the brain. Fibers that originate in the area of each retina toward the temples (*temporal retina*) do not cross at the chiasm and stay on the ipsilateral side of the brain. Therefore optic nerve fibers from the temporal side of the left retina and the nasal side of the right retina both go to the left half of the brain, while fibers from the nasal side of the left retina and temporal side of the right retina go to the right half of the brain. Of course, the division is not perfect, with some cells very near the division projecting to the "wrong" side (Levick, Kirk, & Wagner, 1981). This "slop" is presumably like the "feathering" where new paint is blended to the old when a wall is patched.

BOX 8–1

The very precise route that visual fibers follow to the brain is graphically demonstrated by the visual deficits produced when different parts of this pathway are damaged by strokes, tumors, or injuries. Tests of where in the visual field a patient cannot detect stimuli can be accurate indicators of where the damage (called a *lesion*) can be found.

Not surprisingly, if one of the optic nerves is destroyed, vision from that eye is completely
(continued)

(box continued)
lost. Loss of vision affecting only one of the eyes must be near (or in) that eye. Pressure on the optic chiasm can lead to *bitemporal hemianopia*, in which each eye loses the vision on its own side (the 30° it alone sees) while the main central portion remains unaffected. (To get an idea of how much is seen by only one eye, stare at a point across the room and quickly cover your right eye with your right hand. Notice that only things to the extreme right disappear from view.) This is a result of damage to the crossing (nasal) fibers in the chiasm. It may seem rather fanciful, but ex-

actly this sort of deficit occurs when there is a tumor of the pituitary gland, which is located just beneath the chiasm. As the tumor expands, it compresses the center of the chiasm, damaging the crossing fibers.

Damage higher in the pathways (optic tract, lateral geniculate, or optic radiation) causes *homonymous hemianopia*, in which there are blanks (also called *scotomas*) in the visual field. The defects are essentially the same in both eyes, since, by this time, fibers serving the same visual area are traveling together.

This scheme of some fibers crossing to different parts of the brain may seem like a strange way to design a visual system, but a little reflection should affirm that the arrangement is indeed sensible. Human beings have eyes at the front of the head, so that the two eyes see almost the same region of the visual world. If you cover one of your eyes, there is very little change in how much of the world you see. Only about 30° at the extreme periphery is the sole province of one eye. This large overlap of the fields of view could be confusing for the visual system if it had no way of combining the analogous information from the two eyes. The partial crossing of ganglion cell axons at the optic chiasm is what allows fibers receiving information about the same point in visual space to project to the same part of the brain. In Figure 8–2, it is seen that stimulus in the right half of the visual field projects an image onto the nasal half of the right retina, and an image onto the temporal side of the left retina; these are the two half-retinas that are combined by the redistribution of fibers at the optic chiasm. Similarly, an object on the left half of the visual field will produce images on the nasal portion of the left retina and the temporal portion of the right retina. The right half of the brain receives information about the left half of the visual world, regardless of the eye from which the information comes, while the left half of the brain receives its input from the right half of the visual world.

This description of which optic nerve fibers cross from one side of the brain to the other at the optic chiasm applies only to those animals that have their eyes in the front of their heads looking forward, including humans and many predators. Eye placement in these animals is such that there is extensive duplication of visual processing by both eyes; the right eye sees almost the identical stimulus array as the left, and vice versa. Although redundant, this arrangement has one great advantage that we will discuss later; it greatly aids the perception

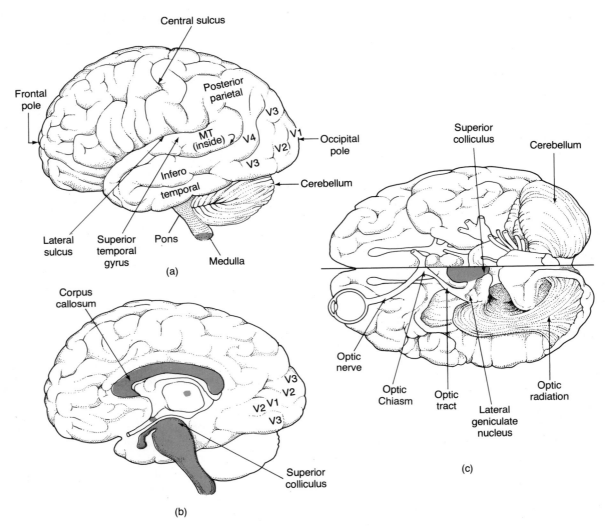

FIGURE 8-1   The human brain. (a) Side view showing the major visual areas. (b) View of the middle surface of a brain that was cut down the middle. Cut structures are shown shaded. (c) View from underneath the brain, showing the optic pathway. The left half has been dissected to reveal the structures of the visual pathway.

of visual depth or distance. Animals that are predators require a high degree of depth perception, as their existence depends on being able to judge correctly where their next potential meal is located. Hunted animals, on the other hand, are less concerned with exactly judging the position of an object in space; it is much more important for them to have as big a visual field as possible. Such animals, therefore, have their eyes placed on the sides of their heads, rather

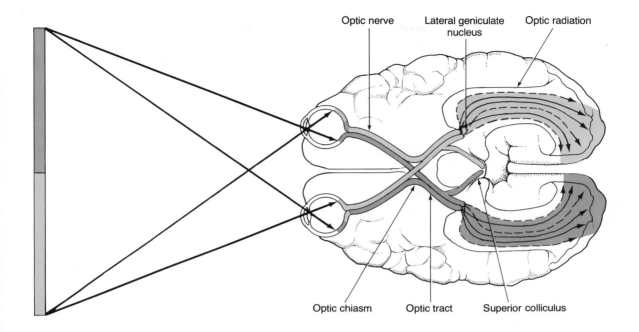

FIGURE 8-2   View of the optic pathway, showing the partial crossing of optic nerve fibers at chiasm. A visual field, shaded to the right and light to the left, is shown. Pathways are shaded in agreement with the part of the field they serve.

than at the front. This gives them a larger field of view, at the expense of a well-developed sense of visual depth. For these animals, virtually all optic nerve fibers cross to the contralateral side of the brain.

THE LATERAL GENICULATE NUCLEUS (LGN)

After the optic nerve fibers have passed through the optic chiasm, they go into the brain itself and the ones we are concerned with terminate in the *lateral geniculate nucleus* (LGN). The LGN is part of a larger section of the brain called the *thalamus*, whose major function is to act as a relay station for sensory inputs of many kinds. The ganglion cell axons make synapses onto cells in the LGN in an orderly and systematic manner. A cross section of the LGN of a monkey is shown in Figure 8–3. The structure is composed of six distinct layers. Physiological studies have shown that within any one layer there is a topographic representation of the world; that is, the visual field is mapped onto the surface of the LGN, so that ganglion cell axons synapse on LGN cells in such a way that neighboring LGN cells (within the same layer) have receptive fields that are nearby in the visual world. The central or foveal regions of the retina

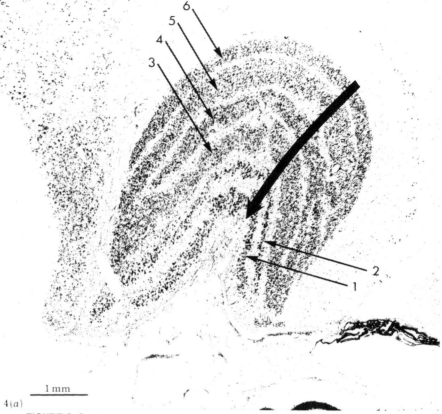

1 mm

4(a)

FIGURE 8-3   Cross section of the right lateral geniculate nucleus of an adult monkey. The preparation was stained with a chemical called cresyl violet to make cell bodies show up dark in the photograph. Arrows point to the six layers. Gray arrow represents the sample electrode track discussed in the text. From Hubel, D. H., and T. N. Wiesel (1977) Functional architecture of macaque monkey visual cortex. *Proc. R. Soc. Lond. Ser. B.* 198:1–59. Reprinted by permission.

project onto a relatively large part of the LGN, so that the topographic representation is distorted to give the central part of the retina more space than the peripheral regions. The heavy respresentation of central regions reflects the fact that this part of the retina has a higher concentration of both receptors and ganglion cells, and is specialized for high-acuity vision.

Another important feature of the lateral geniculate nucleus is that optic nerve fibers from the two eyes remain segregated at this level. Cells in layers 2, 3, and 5 of the LGN receive their inputs from the ipsilateral eye—that is, from the eye on the same side as the LGN being recorded from. Layers 1, 4, and 6 receive input from the contralateral eye. Even though the LGN receives inputs from both eyes, the information from the two eyes has not yet been combined. The topographic representations of the visual field from the two eyes are in register, but as an electrode makes a vertical penetration through the LGN (as is indicated in Figure 8–5), cells from one eye are encountered, followed by cells driven by the other eye as one passes to the next layer. Still, the receptive fields of the cells driven by different eyes are affected by stimuli in the same location in the visual field (Hubel & Wiesel, 1961; Wiesel & Hubel, 1966). The fact that cells in different layers are in register with each other provides an opportunity for interactions between layers; in fact, such binocular interactions have been reported (Sanderson, Bishop, & Darien-Smith, 1971).

There are two types of cells in the LGN: *principal* cells and *interneurons* (Burke & Sefton, 1966). The axons of interneurons remain in the LGN itself and provide a system for further processing at this level. Principal cell axons, however, leave the LGN and course upward toward the cortex in a diffuse bundle called the *optic radiation* (see Figure 8–2). In the monkey, these axons synapse on cells in visual area I of the cortex, and provide the direct source of visual information that is processed at the cortex (Van Essen, 1979). In the cat, the pattern of connections is somewhat different, with geniculate fibers contacting a number of visual areas in addition to visual area I (Wilson & Cragg, 1967; Garey & Powell, 1971).

Responses of Lateral Geniculate Neurons

In general, the responses of lateral geniculate cells closely resemble responses recorded from retinal ganglion cells. The majority of cells recorded from cat and monkey lateral geniculate have concentric center/surround receptive field mechanisms; the major difference between these and retinal ganglion cells is that the surrounds of LGN neurons are somewhat stronger than those of ganglion cells (Hubel & Wiesel, 1961). The result of this increased surround strength is to make the responses of LGN cells to diffuse illumination weaker than the responses of ganglion cells to similar stimuli. This increase in lateral antagonism over that shown by retinal ganglion cells is very slight, however (Kaplan, Marcus, & So, 1979). There is also a weak increase in the temporal tuning in the LGN (So & Shapley, 1981). Thus, the processes that we saw in retina acting to make cells more specific to particular stimuli seem to act again in the LGN. But the effect is slight, and LGN cells are barely discriminable in their responses from their retinal ganglion cell counterparts. In fact, it is most common for a cell in the LGN to receive excitatory drive from a single retinal ganglion cell (Cleland & Lee, 1985).

BOX 8–2 ━━━━━━━━━━━━━━━━━━━

The LGN is something of a puzzle. It sits in the visual pathway, taking up a chunk of valuable brain space, interposing an extra synapse, and adding noise (Levine & Troy, 1986) to the visual

(continued)

(box continued)

signal. Yet it seems to do relatively little. True, there is added lateral antagonism, and some temporal sharpening. It has been suggested that it also exaggerates the difference between the X- and Y-cells in their sensitivities to motion (Frishman, Schweitzer-Tong, & Goldstein, 1985), but this effect is so slight that it can be entirely negated by choice of stimuli (Cleland & Lee, 1985).

A possible clue is that the LGN receives a large share of its input (more than half) from parts of the brain other than the retina (Singer, 1977). These inputs come from the brainstem and from the cortex to which the LGN projects. The brainstem inputs may "turn off" the visual signal during eye movements, so we do not see the world jump when we move our eyes (Noda, 1975).

The inputs from the cortex represent a feedback, like what we saw in the retina. This feedback may affect the properties of LGN cells themselves. For example, cooling the cortex (which temporarily disables it) weakens the surrounds of LGN cells (McClurkin & Marrocco, 1984). This feedback loop may also play an important role in determining cortical cell properties (Martin, 1988a).

The receptive field properties of principal cells and interneurons appear to be similar (Dubin & Cleland, 1977). The major difference between them seems to be where their axons terminate, rather than their having different synaptic inputs.

The distinction between X- and Y-cells is also maintained at the level of the LGN; both have been found in the LGNs of cats (Cleland, Dubin, & Levick, 1971; Shapley & Hochstein, 1975) and monkeys (Dreher, Fukuda, & Rodieck, 1976; Sherman, Wilson, Kaas, & Webb, 1976). Not surprisingly, cells that have Y-like properties in the LGN receive their synaptic inputs from retinal Y-cells, with LGN X-cells receiving input from retinal X-cells (Stone & Hoffmann, 1971; Fukada & Saito, 1972; Cleland & Lee, 1985).

The Parvocellular and Magnocellular Divisions

The two eyes are segregated into separate layers in the LGN, but why are there *six* layers? There is an important further subdivision, which you can probably see in Figure 8–3. Look closely at layers 1 and 2, and you will see they are "grainier" looking than layers 3–6. That is because the cells in layers 1 and 2 are larger; the cells in layers 3–6 are smaller and more numerous. We therefore group layers 1 and 2 under the label *magnocellular* (magno for "large"), and layers 3–6 under *parvocellular* (parvo for "small").

There are differences between the properties of cells in the parvocellular and magnocellular layers. Given what we have said about the close link between the ganglion cells and LGN cells, there must also be comparable differences between the ganglion cells projecting to those layers, and that is also true (Leventhal, Rodieck, & Dreher. 1981).

A comparison of the properties of parvocellular and magnocellular cells (see Table 8–1) may lead to the idea that these cells are homologous with the X- and Y-cells in the cat. But this seems not to be the case. Kaplan and Shapley (1982) pointed out that magnocellular cells could be either X-like or Y-like in their spatial summation, but the (X-like) parvocellular cells are different from the magnocellular X-like cells. In particular, the parvocellular cells are the only ones sensitive to differences in color (see Chapter 15). Moreover, parvocellular cells are fairly insensitive to low contrasts, so only magnocellular cells can detect faint images. Figure 8–4 compares the responses of magnocellular and parvocellular cells to gratings of various contrasts. The parvocellular cells respond very poorly, giving almost no response until the contrast is at least 25%. The magnocellular cells respond well at very low contrasts (under 10%), but soon saturate; there is not much increase in response beyond 30% contrast.

Kaplan and Shapley argued that the magnocellular cells are like the familiar X- and Y-cells in the cat, and parvocellular cells are a different system. Certainly, one would expect fewer color sensitive cells in the cat, which is nearly color blind. In any case, it would appear that the magnocellular system does a considerable share of the visual task: it detects low contrast stimuli of various sizes, and is probably more sensitive to motion. The parvocellular system may be most sensitive to the finest details and to color, is not sensitive to faint patterns, but may be better at discriminating stronger contrasts (Shapley

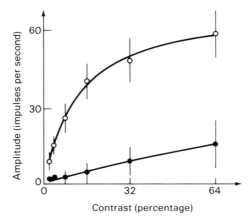

FIGURE 8-4 Comparison of the responses of parvocellular and magnocellular cells to different contrast levels. The figure shows the mean of 8 magnocellular cells (open circles) and 28 parvocellular cells (solid circles). From Kaplan, E. and R. M. Shapley. The primate retina contains two types of ganglion cells, with high and low contrast sensitivity. *Proc. Nat. Acad. Sci.* 83:2755–2757. Reprinted by permission.

& Perry, 1986). As we shall shortly see, the parvocellular and magnocellular cells project to different systems in the visual cortex. These two systems remain distinct in their further projections to higher cortical areas, although they intercommunicate at many levels. Many workers consider them the roots of parallel visual processing systems.

We have accounted for a division of the LGN into at least four layers in order to accommodate the parvocellular and magnocellular systems (with one layer per eye in each). Why then are there four parvocellular layers? The answer is not certain, but it is possible that these represent a further subdivision into the ON-center and OFF-center systems we have seen in the retina (see Chapter 6). This division is clear in at least one mammal, the ferret (Zahs & Stryker, 1988),

and seems to occur in the macaque monkey as well (Schiller & Malpeli, 1978; Michael, 1988). There are hints of a similar subdivision *within* each layer in the cat LGN (Bowling & Wieniawa-Narkiewicz, 1986), which may correspond to the magnocellular layers of the monkey (Shapley & Perry, 1986). This could explain why there are not also four magnocellular layers.

VISUAL AREA I (V1)

The principal cells of the LGN send their axons to VI (on the same side of the brain). Visual area I is composed of discrete layers as shown in Figure 8–5. This figure shows a cross section through the visual cortex of a monkey brain that has been stained to show cell bodies (Hubel & Wiesel, 1977). The cells are arranged in layers that are somewhat less discrete than those found in the retina and LGN. Axons of lateral geniculate principal neurons come into layer

TABLE 8-1 Properties of parvocellular and magnocellular cells in the Lateral Geniculate Nucleus.

	Parvo	Magno*
Retinal input	Type B (or P)	Type A (or M)
Spatial summation	linear	M_x linear, M_y nonlinear
Field size	small	M_x small, M_y large
Response timing	sustained (for pure colors)	more transient
Layers in LGN	3, 4, 5, 6	1, 2
Axon conduction velocity	slow	fast
Sensitivity to contrast	poor	good, but saturates
Sensitivity to color	many cells	none
Projection to V1 (layers)	4A. 4Cβ	4Cα

*Magnocellular cells may be further subdivided as X-like (M_x) or Y-like (M_y), but most magnocellular properties apply to both subtypes (or they have not been separately tested).

4 of the cortex exclusively. The magnocellular cell axons end near the middle of layer 4, while the parvocellular cell axons terminate above and below them, at the edges of layer 4. Cells in other layers receive their visual input from other cortical neurons rather than directly from LGN cells. It is because of the striped appearance of this part of cortex that V1 is also called striate cortex; this area can be easily distinguished from the other two visual areas in occipital cortex that lack some of the striations seen in Figure 8–5.

BOX 8–4

The layering of V1 naturally represents a segregation of function, and we are beginning to understand some of the differences among layers. As we noted, layer 4 is mainly an input layer, receiving information from the LGN. An exception, unusual for sensory cortex, is that the middle sublayer of layer 4 (called layer 4B) apparently does not receive direct LGN input, and projects to other areas of cortex forward of V1 (Tootell, Hamilton, & Switkes, 1988). Layers 2 and 3, above layer 4, project to the next higher visual area, V2. The deeper layers of V1 project to lower centers in the brain (Gilbert, 1983). Layer 5 projects to the superior colliculus (see the following box), while layer 6 provides the projection back to the LGN.

There is also a stylized interconnection among the layers. We have noted that the magnocellular input arrives near the middle of layer 4; actually, it is near the top of the lowest sublayer, called layer 4Cα. This layer projects directly above itself, to layer 4B, which we just

mentioned is the unusual part of layer 4 that projects out of V1. It also has a weak projection within V1 in layers 2 and 3, into special regions called "blobs," which we will discuss shortly. The magnocellular input also projects strongly into layer 6 (Tootell et al., 1988).

The parvocellular inputs go to the upper part of layer 4, called 4A, and to the lowest part of it, layer 4Cβ. These layers project strongly to layers 2 and 3, and from there to 5 and 6 (Gilbert, 1983).

There is considerable interchange of information among the layers, with most of the projections being radially oriented (that is, cells communicate mainly with those directly above or below them). There is also lateral intercommunication, with specific interconnections being made between cells nearby in the cortex (Eysel, Muche, & Worgotter, 1988; Gilbert & Wiesel, 1985; Komatsu, Nakajima, Toyama, & Fetz, 1988; Ts'o & Gilbert, 1988).

As in the LGN, the surface of the visual cortex is organized so that the receptive fields of cortical cells create a topographic map of the visual world. The details of this map have been determined by inserting recording electrodes systematically across the cortical surface and investigating the receptive field locations for cells in different areas of the cortex. Not surprisingly, much more cortical area is devoted to the central or foveal regions of the visual field; in fact, this magnification of foveal regions is even more extreme than that seen in the LGN (Daniel & Whitteridge, 1961; Hubel & Wiesel, 1974b). Unlike the LGN, however, the map seen on the cortex is repeated several times; the different visual areas in occipital cortex all have separate representations of the visual world mapped onto them. This multiple topographic respesentation in the several areas probably reflects the fact that each area is performing dif-

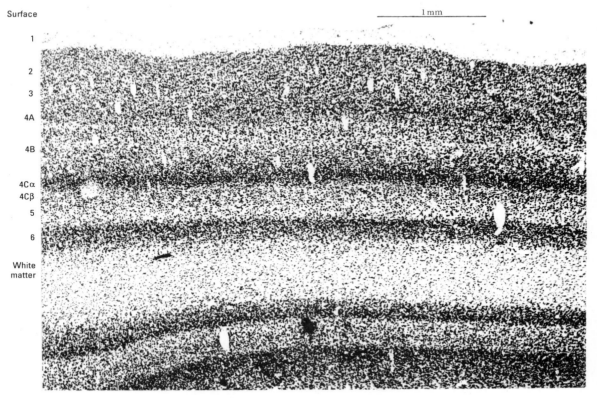

Surface
1
2
3
4A
4B
4Cα
4Cβ
5
6
White matter

1 mm

FIGURE 8–5   Cross section of a monkey striate cortex, stained with cresyl violet. The cortical layers are marked along the left of the figure. From Hubel and Wiesel (1977). Reprinted by permission.

ferent processing tasks that require knowledge of the location of a stimulus within the visual field.

BOX 8–5

The only visual pathway we discuss in this book is the *geniculostriate* pathway (from retina, to lateral geniculate, to striate cortex), but there are a number of other places in the brain that receive direct inputs from retinal ganglion cells. They include other parts of the thalamus, and parts of the hypothalamus and brainstem. The importance of these areas is shown by the fact that removal of the striate cortex in nonprimates does not lead to complete blindness (Van Essen, 1979); in humans and monkeys, its removal does cause blindness, although some very limited visual function remains (Richards, 1973; Mohler & Wurtz, 1977; Van Essen, 1979; Solomon, Pasik, & Pasik, 1981).

One area of the brainstem that has received

(continued)

(box continued)

considerable attention is the *superior colliculus* (or *tectum*), located on the rear part of the brainstem just under the cerebellum (see Figures 8–1 and 8–2). Cells in the outermost layers of the superior colliculus receive branches of ganglion cell axons, in particular from Y-cells and W-cells (Rodieck, 1979), but *not* from X-cells (Fukuda & Stone, 1974). In lower animals, cells in the superior colliculus are motion- and direction-selective (Berman & Cynader, 1972; Michael, 1972; Chalupa & Rhoades, 1977), but this does not appear to be the case in primates (Updyke, 1974; Marrocco & Li, 1977). Cells deeper in the superior colliculus also respond to inputs from other sense modalities (Bisti, Maffei, & Piccolino, 1974; Stein, Magalhães-Castro, & Kruger, 1975; Chalupa & Rhoades, 1977). Given all of this, plus the fact that the superior colliculus is located near the part of the brainstem responsible for eye movements, it is generally believed that

the superior colliculus plays an important role in orienting behavior and visual tracking of a target. In fact, cells in the monkey's tectum have been shown to be more responsive to a moving spot of light when the monkey is awake and actively following the spot with his eyes than when he is not (Wurtz & Mohler, 1976). Its removal causes a behavioral deficit in visual tracking by the cat (Norton, 1974) and the hamster (Schneider, 1969). Similarly, cells in the superior colliculus of monkeys have been found to discharge action potentials immediately before the monkey's eyes move (Wurtz & Goldberg, 1971). Superior colliculus activity seems directly related to the localization of the target of saccadic movements (Sparks & Porter, 1983). This area, therefore, seems to coordinate eye movements and visual information. It plays a role in the localization of objects in the visual world, but finegrained pattern analysis seems to be performed by the geniculostriate system (Van Essen, 1979).

Properties of Cells in Visual Cortex

While properties of LGN neurons remain similar to those exhibited by retinal ganglion cells, cells in the visual cortex have quite different response characteristics. As with the more peripheral cells, cortical cells respond to stimulation only within a restricted area of the visual field, although in general their receptive fields are larger than those of ganglion or LGN cells. Within their receptive fields, however, most cortical cells will not respond to presentations of diffuse-light stimuli, but require instead patterns of specific shapes and orientations. Responses were first recorded from single cells in the cat visual cortex by Hubel and Wiesel (1959; 1962; 1965a), who found that most cells could be placed in one of three categories that they named *simple*, *complex*, and *hypercomplex*. This classification scheme was later extended to include monkey cortical cells (Hubel & Wiesel, 1968).

Simple cells   As their name implies, simple cells have receptive fields that reflect less complex processing than the other two types. An example of a simple cell receptive field is shown in Figure 8–6. While this cell possesses antagonistic receptive field mechanisms similar to those of ganglion cell center and surround, the areas are not circularly symmetric or concentric with each other. There is a long thin area in the central portion of the field at which onset of a small spot of light will evoke a modest excitatory response (marked by the + in Figure 8–6[c]), while stimulation of either of the two antagonistic flanks that surround this central region will produce a response to offset the stimulus (marked by − in Figure 8–6[c]).

Although this simple cell may respond to the presentation of small spots of light, it is far more sensitive to the presence of a bar-shaped stimulus appropriately oriented within the receptive field. Figure 8–6(b) shows responses to bars of light whose widths were chosen to correspond to that of the central region of the receptive field. Horizontally placed bars evoke no response whatsoever from this cell, but presentation of a vertical bar the extent of which exactly corresponds to the central area of the receptive field, will result in a vigorous response. This selectivity is exactly what would be expected given the shape of the excitatory region for this cell, as the vertical bar covers the entire central area but does not intrude on the antagonistic flanks. Thus simple cells are selectively sensitive to stimuli of particular orientation and position in a way that ganglion cells and LGN cells are not. Note, however, that while

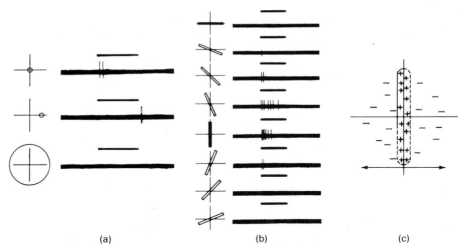

(a)   (b)   (c)

FIGURE 8–6 Responses of a simple cell in the visual cortex of the cat, and the receptive field map derived from those responses. (a) and (b) Responses to presentations of small spots and bar stimuli respectively. The bar over each response trace denotes when the stimulus was present, and the stimulus position is shown at the left of each trace. (c) Map of the receptive field, with + denoting excitatory areas and − denoting inhibitory areas. From Hubel, D. H., and T. N. Wiesel (1959) Receptive fields of single neurones in the cat's striate cortex. *J. Physiol.* 148:574–591. Reprinted by permission.

the cell in Figure 8–6 is sensitive to the orientation and width of the bar stimulus, it does not care about the length; given a bar that is long enough to cover the excitatory portion of the receptive field, additional length is not important.

Not all simple cells have receptive fields that look like the receptive field of the cell in Figure 8–6. Figure 8–7 shows receptive fields for five other simple cells; clearly there is quite a bit of variability in specific configuration. The central region of the receptive field may be either excitatory or inhibitory, and the preferred orientation can be at any angle (although in this figure all cells have the same orientation preference). In addition, as is shown in (c) and (e) of Figure 8–7, the antagonistic flanks may not be symmetric about the central region of the receptive field; in fact, the receptive field displayed in (e) simply comprises one inhibitory area and one excitatory area that are adjacent to each other. What all of these cells have in common is that their properties can be determined by mapping their receptive fields with stationary stimuli. For ex-

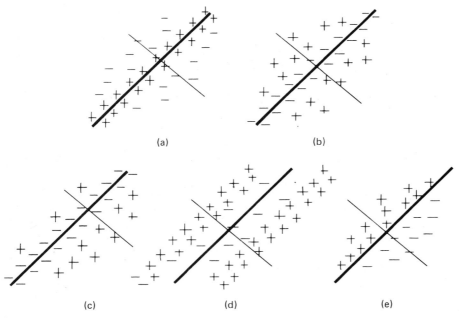

FIGURE 8–7   Receptive field maps of five different simple cells in the visual cortex of the cat. The + denotes excitatory areas, and − indicates inhibitory areas. The solid lines are parallel to the preferred stimulus orientation of each cell. From Hubel, D. H., and T. N. Wiesel (1962) Receptive fields, binocular interaction and functional architecture in the cat's visual cortex. *J. Physiol.* 160:106–154. Reprinted by permission.

ample, the cell in Figure 8–7(a) will give a response to onset of a small spot presented anywhere within the diagonal central region, and a response to off-set of a spot that is flashed in either of the antagonistic flanks. By moving such a spot throughout the receptive field of this cell, one can determine the extent of both the central region and the flanks; with this information, the orientation, placement, and width of a bar that will evoke the maximum response from this cell can be determined. As we shall see, it is a property not shared by complex cells.

Complex cells Simple cells give a vigorous response to a flashing bar of light only if the bar is of the correct size, orientation, and position within its receptive field. Complex cells share the same type of requirements for orientation and size of the stimulus, but are less restrictive as to its position. While simple cells have fairly distinct excitatory and inhibitory regions within their receptive fields, complex cells do not; in fact, complex cells usually give no responses at all when they are stimulated with small flashing spots. Figure 8–8 shows the responses of a complex cell to bar-shaped stimuli of various sizes at various positions within its receptive field. Like a simple cell, this cell is selectively sensitive to a bar stimulus of a certain width and orientation; however, the bar can be placed almost anywhere within the receptive field of the cell without affecting the magnitude of response. Thus the response of a complex cell signals the presence of a stimulus of a certain orientation, without reference to the specific position. In addition, complex cells are often selectively sensitive to movement of the stimulus in a specific direction.

BOX 8–6

The definition of complex cells is not as precise as could be hoped, and there are sometimes disagreements between groups of workers about whether the categorizations made by one group are correct. What seems to make a cell ''complex'' is that its responses are in some way independent of a stimulus feature that logically should make a difference. Thus, it should matter where a bar is placed, given that the cell does not simply add all light indiscriminately (that is, it does not respond to a wider bar, or one of the ''wrong'' orientation). It should matter whether it is a black bar on a gray field or a white bar on a gray field, but for many complex cells, the responses are the same for either contrast. On the other hand, it should

not matter (in a symmetric field) whether the bar sweeps from left to right or from right to left, but many complex cells are direction-selective. Of course, not all complex cells display all of these anomalies. It is even possible for a cell to be considered complex that does not care about stimulus orientation (DeValois, Yund, & Hepler, 1982).

Perhaps the most direct statement of what makes a cell complex is that it is spatially nonlinear. Most simple cells sum influences within their receptive fields in a linear fashion, similar to the responses of X-cells to gratings (Movshon, Thompson, & Tolhurst, 1978a). Complex cells are nonlinear in the same sense as Y-cells (Movshon, Thompson, & Tolhurst,

(continued)

(box continued)
1978b). Given this, one might consider the Y-cells as low-level complex cells. That does not mean, however, that Y-cells must be the sole inputs to complex cells, although that sug-gestion has been made (Hoffmann & Stone, 1971; DeValois, Albrecht, & Thorell, 1982). As we shall see (on page 177), the question of how these cells are "made" is complicated by the variety of subtypes of complex cells.

Hypercomplex cells   The cortical hypercomplex cells differ from simple and complex cells in that they also select for optimal length of a stimulus bar, in addition to being sensitive to its orientation and width. For example, while the optimal stimulus for a complex cell might be a bar of some particular width oriented at 45° from the vertical, a hypercomplex cell might only re-spond to such a stimulus if the bar were less than some particular length.

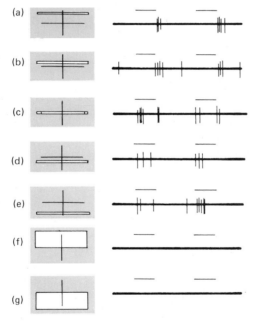

FIGURE 8-8   Responses of a complex cell in the visual cortex of the cat. Stimulus position is shown to the left of each re-sponse; the stimulus is shown by an open rectangle, with the position of the receptive field referenced by the crossed lines. The bar over the response shows when the stimulus was present. From Hubel and Wiesel (1962). Reprinted by permission.

Figure 8–9 shows the responses of a hypercomplex cell to its preferred stimulus, which is an edge moving through its receptive field in a particular direction. Unlike a complex cell, the extent of the edge in the direction perpendicular to the direction of movement is a crucial variable; if the edge is made wider than the optimal size in this direction, or is moved only slightly from its optimal position, no response is produced.

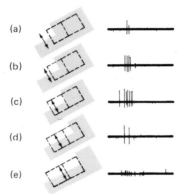

FIGURE 8-9 Responses of a hypercomplex cell in the visual cortex of the cat. Stimulus position is shown to the left of each response, with the receptive field sketched as a dashed rectangle. From Hubel and Wiesel (1965a). Receptive fields and functional architecture in two non-striate visual areas (18 and 19) of the cat. *J. Neurophysiol.* 28: 229–289. Reprinted by permission.

While Hubel and Wiesel (1965a) classified hypercomplex cells as being a third separate class of cortical neurons, more recent investigations have introduced some doubt as to whether they form a truly separable group. Dreher (1972) found that cat hypercomplex cells could be divided into subgroups according to whether the receptive field properties resembled simple or complex cells. For either subgroup, the feature that distinguished a cell as hypercomplex was its specificity for stimulus length. Thus, for example, a simple type of hypercomplex cell might have a receptive field that closely resembles that shown for the simple cell in Figure 8–6, except that, in addition to the central excitatory area and inhibitory flanks, there would also be inhibitory end zones that reduced the response of the cell if the stimulus became longer than a certain length. Similarly, a complex type of hypercomplex cell would be sensitive not only to the orientation and width of a bar-shaped stimulus but also to its length.

It is attractive to be able to consider hypercomplex cells as either simple or complex, but with an extra feature; however, more recent evidence indicates that this may not be valid. When properties of cortical cells in both cat and monkey were studied in detail, they were found to show a wide range of specificities to stimulus length, with no apparent break point that could be used to discriminate hypercomplex from non-hypercomplex cells (Schiller, Finlay, & Volman, 1976a; Gilbert, 1977). It is possible, therefore, that length specificity is a receptive field property that is shared by most cortical cells to some degree, and the classification of cells as hypercomplex is not useful.

BOX 8-7

We have discussed the properties of the major types of cortical cells; how might these properties come about? Hubel and Wiesel (1962; 1965a) hypothesized that the three types of orientation-selective cells are hierarchically organized. In their view, simple cell properties can be explained by the convergence of a number of LGN fibers with their receptive fields aligned in a straight row. That is, the LGN cells that provide the direct input to the simple cell have receptive fields whose positions (on the retina) correspond to the central region of the simple cell field (see Figure 8-10). Additional rows of LGN cells (of the opposite type) could be responsible for the antagonistic flanks. The flanks represent additional antagonism, for they superimpose on the weak flanks that would be created by the aligned surrounds of the LGN fields. The lateral antagonism begun in the outer plexiform layer of the retina was enhanced in the inner plexiform layer, enhanced again in the LGN, and is enhanced further in the cortex.

Complex cells could be formed from ranks of simple cells of the same preferred orientation. The synaptic connections would have to be such that the simple cells could only excite the complex cell, not inhibit it. Thus, if any simple cell were active the complex cell would fire, but a broader stimulus covering many of the simple cells would be ineffective because none of the simple cells would re-

spond to a stimulus that extends into its antagonistic flanks (Hubel & Wiesel, 1962).

This is an attractive hypothesis, but it is apparently not quite right. As we have noted, there are extensive intracortical connections between layers, so many cortical cells receive inputs from other cortical cells. But many cells receive only (or mainly) direct LGN input. Hoffmann and Stone (1971) showed that both simple and complex cells received direct input from the LGN, with simple cell input coming from X-cells and complex cell input coming from Y-cells. Responses of cat cortical cells tend to reinforce the notion that simple and complex cells represent parallel processing systems and not a hierarchical one. Simple cells tend to prefer more slowly moving stimuli than do complex cells, so much so that stimuli moving at velocities preferred by complex cells may be virtually ineffective for most simple cells (Movshon, 1975). For a review, see Stone, Dreher, and Leventhal (1979).

How can complex cell properties be created if not by superposition of simple cells? Spitzer and Hochstein (1985) suggested a model in which the complex cell receives inputs directly from two rows of LGN cells. These are probably X-cells (for Y-cells are too rare to account for much of the input; see Lennie, 1980). The rows of LGN cells form *subunits*, which are combined nonlinearly. The nonlinearity is called rectification: it means the cells

(continued)

(box continued)

can only signal excitation, not inhibition. In effect, the rows of LGN cells are the simple cells of the Hubel and Wiesel hierarchical model. This is exactly the kind of model proposed for Y-cells, which seem to have a large number of subunits that can only excite the cell (Cleland, Levick, & Sanderson, 1973; Hochstein & Shapley, 1976).

Different types of complex cells can be modeled by different combinations of two or more overlapping or nonoverlapping subunits, with some also receiving inputs from other cortical cells, and some receiving all their inputs from other complex cells (Spitzer & Hochstein, 1985). The fact that some complex cells respond to both dark or light bars may be because they receive inputs from both ON and OFF cells (Heggelund, 1981; Tanaka, 1985).

Another mechanism that tunes the responses of cortical cells is antagonism, in this case inhibition between cortical cells. For ex-ample, the antagonistic flanks of the simple cell shown in Figure 8–6 cause the cell to fire when a light in a flank is extinguished; this is presumably the offset response of the OFF-center LGN cells in that flank. But there is also inhibition during the presentation of the light in the flank, and this is probably due to inhibition from other simple cells in the same column (Ferster, 1988). Similarly, the orientation selectivity of cortical neurons is sharpened by inhibition from cells with similar preferred orientations (Hata, Tsumoto, Sato, Hagihara, & Tamura, 1988; Bonds, 1989). It is possible that orientation tuning is enhanced by cells with the same preferred orientation but slightly different optimum positions and by inhibition from cells with different preferred orientations (Ferster & Koch, 1987). Either of these mechanisms can be disabled by drugs that affect inhibitory transmitters in the cortex (Sillito & Versiani, 1977; Sillito, Salt, & Kemp, 1985).

Concentric cells   Orientation selectivity seemed to be the hallmark of cortical cells, a radical departure from the concentric, circular, center/surround

FIGURE 8-10   Hypothetical hierarchical scheme illustrating how receptive field properties of cells in the visual cortex could be built up from the receptive fields of more peripheral cells. In this conception, LGN cells feed into simple cells that are the inputs to complex cells. (a) LGN cells, with fields indicated to the left, combine to form the field of a simple cell (right). Three rows of LGN cells, with all cells in each row of the same type, provide the inputs. The profiles below the field maps show the relative amount of excitation or inhibition (as a function of position in the receptive field) for the cells above the profiles. Linear summation means both excitatory and inhibitory influences are transmitted, and so can cancel. (b) Simple cells with a common orientation preference in the same general region combine to form a complex cell field. Some of the simple cells have an ON middle region, some have an OFF middle region. Nonlinear summation means each simple cell can only signal that it is excited but cannot provide an inhibitory signal to cancel the excitation from other simple cells.

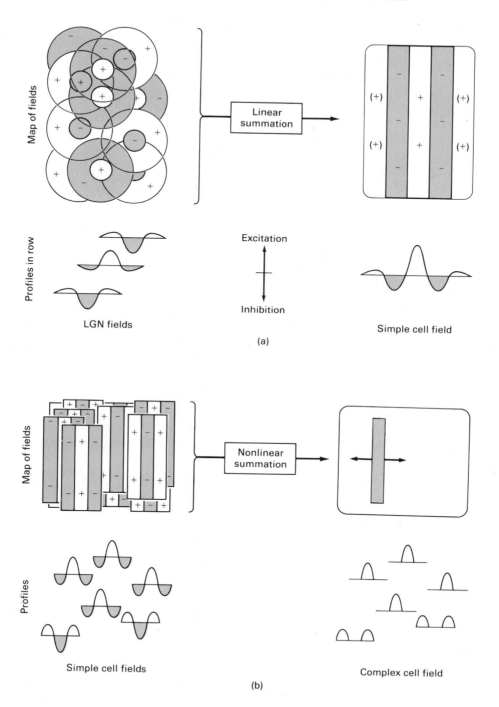

Map of fields

Profiles in row

Linear summation

Excitation

Inhibition

LGN fields

Simple cell field

(a)

Map of fields

Profiles

Nonlinear summation

Simple cell fields

Complex cell field

(b)

antagonism seen in the retina and LGN. When concentric cells were encountered in cortex, therefore, they were generally ignored in the belief that these were recordings from the ascending fibers of the LGN principal cells. However, as workers found clusters of these cells in cortex (Michael, 1981), it was gradually conceded that this was still another class of cell in cortex (Hubel & Livingstone, 1983). Many of these cells seem to be specific for the color of a stimulus (Michael, 1981).

One property that many cortical cells have in common is that they receive their visual inputs from both eyes. This is in marked contrast to LGN cells, which only respond to visual stimuli presented to one eye or the other. Cells that receive from both eyes are called *binocular* neurons; V1 is the first level in the visual system where there is an excitatory combination of inputs from the two eyes. When the receptive fields of binocular cortical neurons are examined, it is found that those from the two eyes almost always completely overlap. (A certain percentage of cells have non-identical receptive field locations; their function in the perception of depth will be discussed in Chapter 12.) This overlapping should not be surprising; if a single cell received inputs from two different areas in the visual field depending on which eye was being stimulated, it would be impossible to tell whether a response from that cell meant that a stimulus was in one location or the other.

Not only are the receptive field locations from the two eyes usually identical in a binocular cell, the particular response properties are also the same. Thus if a cortical simple cell responds best to a bar of light flashed at an angle of 30° from the horizontal when the right eye is stimulated, the optimal stimulus from the left eye will also be a bar at the same orientation. If the same optimal stimulus is presented to both eyes simultaneously, the response of the cortical cell will be greater than if just one eye were stimulated. Binocular neurons are therefore most effectively activated by stimuli presented to both eyes.

CORTICAL CELLS AND PERCEPTION

Primary visual cortex contains a rich variety of cell types. How do these cell types relate to perception of the visual world? One approach has been to ask to what parts of a complex stimulus a particular cell might respond. For example, if you were presented with an equilateral triangle, most cells in the area of cortex that "sees" the triangle would not respond. Only those cells whose receptive fields lie on the borders of the triangle will respond, and then only if their preferred orientation matches the orientation of that border. Simple cells will require exact placement of the border; hypercomplex cells will have to be appropriately near any corner.

Because the cells of the cortex respond best when specific patterns are present in their receptive fields, they are sometimes described as *feature detectors*. In this view, feature detectors are each abstracting the particular aspect of the pattern to which they are specific. In the triangle example, the features were the borders of the triangle (which had already been emphasized by the process of lateral antagonism in the retina), and the three corners. The simple and complex cells that detected the sides of the triangle were "straight line at 60°" detectors; the base was detected by "horizontal line" detectors. The corners were detected by hypercomplex cells specific for "60° corners." The significant features of the figure are abstracted by detectors; an appropriate constellation of active cells would then be the effective stimulus for a "triangle detector" higher in the processing hierarchy (probably in some other part of cortex) (see also Chapter 11).

It makes intuitive sense for the perception of a triangle to depend on recognition of the three sides and angles, but we run into problems when the feature detector model is extended. A triangle detector would be a cell that fires when a correct pattern of simple, complex, and hypercomplex cells fire; is there then an "hourglass detector" that fires when the two appropriate triangle detectors are active? Is there a "jack-o-lantern detector" sensitive to the output of certain triangle detectors and a "pumpkin detector"? Is there a cell somewhere that recognizes "mother standing at the door"? These higher order detectors would have to have "learned" their stimuli through experience; that is not a problem for a cortical cell, as we shall see in the next chapter, but how many cells are there available to become specific detectors? Each percept would have to be embodied by a constellation of cells, or the death of a single neuron (which happens all the time) would cause the loss of ability to recognize a particular thing.

There is a danger in describing cortical cells as feature detectors; it makes one forget that the same cells respond to a variety of stimuli. A cortical cell could be defined as a "55°-tilted line detector" because when the experimenter tested it with lines of various orientations, it responded best (or exclusively) if the line was oriented at 55°. Unless one has also tested for it, one cannot know that the cell would not prefer a *double* line, or a checkerboard, or a wavy line, or. . . . The nature of the detector depends on the way it was identified experimentally. (A noted neurophysiologist illustrated this point in a lecture by suggesting that if he were to pour a glass of water over a person's head, the person would probably let out a scream; he asked if that means we should define this wet individual as a "water detector.")

Lines, edges, and corners are effective stimuli for cortical cells and are the kinds of features we intuitively expect the brain to extract. An alternative interpretation of the function of cortical cells is that they are "spatial frequency analyzers," a concept we will discuss more fully in Chapter 10. The spatial frequency notion will require some development to make it clear; for now, we just want to point out that there are alternatives to the feature-detection model.

There is still another possible interpretation of these cells' responses. Cortical cells do not act alone. Not only do they have neighbors, but they also interact with the "higher" cells to which they project. We have pointed out places in which there is feedback in the visual system: the inner plexiform layer of the retina feeds to the outer layer via interplexiform cells; the cortex (layer 6) projects back to the LGN. Similarly, higher visual areas project to V1. Cooling V2 (which effectively disables it) has subtle but potentially important effects on V1 (Sandell & Schiller, 1982). It is not fair to consider responses of V1 as if they independently told the whole story.

If you think of the entire network of cells in all layers of the visual system as a whole, you can appreciate that one particular cell would not have a single, separable function. It would participate in many visual tasks, in ways that might not be well related. Indeed, there are properties of even a simple network of cells that are not "given" by the individual cells; these are called *emergent properties* (Sejnowski, Koch, & Churchland, 1988). We shall consider how perception might be an emergent property of the nervous system in Chapter 11.

SUGGESTED READINGS

For those who want to know more about responses of cells in the visual cortex, probably the best thing to do is to read some of the original work. Hubel and Wiesel have written an extensive (and very readable) review of their work on monkey (*Proc. R. Soc. Lond. Ser. B.*, 198:1–59, 1977); an earlier classic paper of theirs that also makes good reading is the 1962 paper on visual cells in cat cortex (*J. Physiol.*, 160:106–154; also reprinted in many collections including *Perceptual Processing: Stimulus Equivalence and Pattern Recognition*, ed. P. C. Dodwell (Appleton-Century-Crofts, 1971).

A readable and up-to-date version may be found in *Eye, Brain, and Vision*, by D. H. Hubel (Scientific American Library, 1988). Hubel's collaborations with Torsten Wiesel lay the groundwork for much of what we discussed in this chapter (and the next), and resulted in their sharing a Nobel Prize. His book is even more relevant to the next chapter.

ARCHITECTURE OF VISION
IN THE CORTEX

9

In Chapter 8, we learned that the information from the two retinae passes through the LGN to the primary visual cortex, V1. Cells in V1 seem to be selective for attributes of the stimulus, such as color, orientation, and direction of motion. We also saw that in addition to the X-type and Y-type, and ON-center and OFF-center cells of the retina, there is a subdivision into the parvocellular and magnocellular pathways. In this chapter, we will consider how some of these attributes are sorted out in the cortex. We will examine the anatomical arrangement in V1, and the projections into "higher" cortex. You will see that the parvocellular and magnocellular pathways form two parallel, but interdependent, pathways through the visual system.

FUNCTIONAL ARCHITECTURE OF THE VISUAL CORTEX

The visual cortex is a thin sheet of tissue on which a map of the visual world is projected. Cortical cells, however, possess many other properties beside their receptive field location, such as angle of optimal orientation and extent of binocularity. Before we can understand how the cortex performs its function of analyzing the visual world, we must understand how it organizes the visual information that its cells are designed to detect. In order to begin this process, Hubel and Wiesel (1962; 1968; 1974a; 1974b) have systematically investigated the organization of the cortex by recording from cell after cell and seeing how the properties of each cell varied with location within the cortex.

Orientation Columns

One property Hubel and Wiesel investigated was optimal orientation of a visual stimulus. Multiple electrode penetrations were made through the cortices of monkeys and cats, and the orientation specificity was determined for each cell encountered. The cells encountered in two electrode penetrations into V1 of cat cortex are shown in Figure 9–1. The solid lines show the paths of the electrode, with the short lines intersecting them representing the optimal stimulus orientation for each cell. For the electrode track on the left in the figure, all of the cells in the upper part of the penetration had horizontal optimal orientations, with orientation gradually shifting to an angle of about 45°. Clearly, this is not a random distribution; instead, cells with similar optimal orientations seem to be stacked one on another. This is in fact, a general finding; when an electrode penetration is made perpendicular to the surface of the cortex, all of the cells in that penetration tend to have the same or similar preferred stimulus orientation. The penetration shown in the right side of the figure shows what happens when the penetration is not perpendicular to the cortical surface; in this case, the electrode passes through regions of constant orientation, but there is a systematic change in preferred orientation as one proceeds down the electrode track. The penetration shown in Figure 9–2 is even more oblique; optimal orientation of the cells encountered is plotted versus electrode distance, showing a clear and systematic variation of preferred orientation as a function of distance along the cortical surface.

The data just described led Hubel and Wiesel to conclude that the cortex was organized into what they called *orientation columns*, within which all cells possessed the same optimal stimulus orientation. From Figure 9–2, it is seen that the preferred orientations of nearby columns are similar; that is, orientation changes fairly uniformly across the surface of the cortex. Over a distance of about 1.0 mm, all possible orientations are represented, so that the width of each column must be quite small.

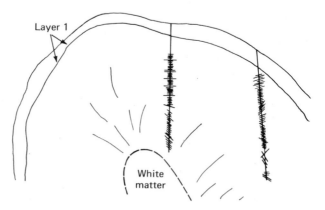

FIGURE 9–1 Cross section of cat visual cortex, showing the orientations of cells encountered during two electrode penetrations. Cells encountered during a given penetration tend to have similar preferred orientations. From Hubel and Wiesel (1962). Receptive fields, binocular interaction and functional architecture in the cat's visual cortex. *J. Physiol.* 160:106–154. Reprinted by permission.

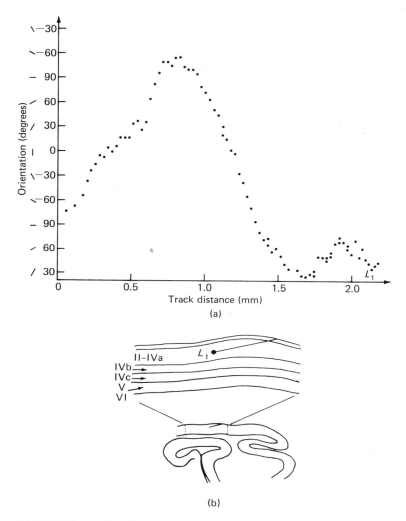

FIGURE 9-2 (a) Graph of orientation versus electrode position for an electrode penetration that was nearly horizontal to the surface of the cortex. (b) Shows the actual track of the electrode during the penetration graphed in (a). From Hubel, D. H., and T. N. Wiesel (1974). Sequence regularity and geometry of orientation columns in the monkey striate cortex. *J. Comp. Neurol.* 158:267–294. Reprinted by permission.

Ocular Dominance Columns

The preferred orientation of a visual stimulus is systematically represented along the surface of the cortex; the responses of cortical cells, however, vary along other dimensions as well. One dimension of interest is *ocular domi-*

nance, the extent to which a cell responds to stimulation delivered to one eye or both. Most cortical cells in the cat are binocular; they receive inputs from both eyes, so they will respond (at least to some extent) if one eye is closed. Some cells are monocular; they respond only when one of the eyes is stimulated and are blind if that eye is closed. However, even the binocular cells may favor one eye, so most cells can be assigned either a right- or a left-eye preference.

To examine ocular dominance, Hubel and Wiesel (1965b; 1968) went through the same procedure as when they found orientation columns; that is, multiple electrode penetrations were made through the surface of the cortex, and the ocular dominance was determined for each cell encountered. They found that if the electrode track was perpendicular to the surface of the cortex, all of the cells recorded from in a single penetration would be dominated by the same eye. Thus, the cortex is organized into ocular dominance columns, as well as orientation columns.

BOX 9–1

It is possible to show by anatomical methods the existence of both orientation and ocular dominance columns. A substance called 2-deoxyglucose (2-dg) accumulates selectively in regions where cells are actively firing action potentials (Sokoloff, 1975). Through the use of sophisticated anatomical techniques, cell groups that have high concentrations of 2-dg can be treated so that they appear to be darker on a photographic plate than do regions where 2-dg has not accumulated. Hubel, Wiesel, and Stryker (1978) injected 2-dg into the circulatory system of a monkey, after which they stimulated both eyes with a field of unidirectional stripes. After 45 min of this stimulation, the brain was anatomically prepared to show regions with high concentrations of 2-dg, so that only cortical areas that were actively responding to the striped stimulus were darkly stained. Figure 9–3(a) shows a tangential section through the visual cortex from a monkey brain treated in the above manner. One can clearly see a pattern of darkly stained regions that represent the orientation columns sensitive to the stimulus presented.

Hubel and Wiesel (1974a; 1977) used another anatomical technique to reveal the shapes of the ocular dominance columns. They injected a radioactive substance that is actively absorbed by the cell bodies of neurons into the vitreous humor of one eye. This substance was absorbed by retinal ganglion cells and transported down their axons to the lateral geniculate nucleus, where it was taken up by LGN neurons and transported to the visual cortex. When the visual cortex of an animal treated in this manner was prepared to show the presence of radioactivity, only those neurons that were functionally connected to the treated eye were stained darkly. Figure 9–3(b) shows a cross section of a monkey brain treated in this manner; the pattern of ocular dominance columns is even clearer than that shown in Figure 9–3(a) for orientation columns.

From Figure 9–3, which shows the anatomical shapes of the cortical columns, it is clear that "columns" is probably not the most appropriate term for the way orientation and binocularity are organized in the cortex. In fact,

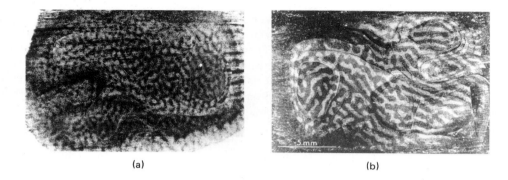

(a) (b)

FIGURE 9-3 (a) Pattern of orientation columns in monkey cortex, treated with 2-deoxyglucose. (b) Pattern of ocular dominance columns in the same region of cortex as in (a). Columns are made visible by radioactive proline injected into one eye and transported to the visual cortex. From Hubel, D. H., T. N. Wiesel, and M. P. Stryker (1978) Anatomical demonstration of oriented columns in macaque monkey. *J. Comp. Neurol.* 177:361–380. Reprinted by permission.

the cells seem to be arranged in slabs. There are clear strips of cells of similar ocular dominance or orientation specificity that wend their ways irregularly along the surface of the cortex. These strips remain about equal in width throughout their lengths. Although columns may not be the most accurate way to describe the organization of the cortex, for convenience we will continue to use that term.

The surface of the cortex has at least three types of visual information represented on it. Not only is position in the visual world determined by cortical location, the orientation and level of binocularity of a cell is also related to where it is on the cortex. At first, this may seem like a confusing way for the visual system to be set up, because as you move from one location of the cortex to another, you might be changing location of the visual field, preferred orientation, and binocularity all at the same time. If this is the case, you would think that all cortical cells having their receptive fields in a certain location would also only have one preferred stimulus orientation and one ocular dominance level. In fact, this problem does not arise, because of the arrangement of the cortex into what Hubel and Wiesel (1974a) called *hypercolumns.*

A hypercolumn is defined as a collection of either orientation or ocular dominance columns so that the collection includes all possible orientations or ocular dominance levels. Therefore an orientation hypercolumn would be a region of cortex that included orientation columns for all stimulus orientations, and an ocular dominance hypercolumn would include cells receiving exclusive input from one eye or the other, as well as binocular cells. Hubel and Wiesel (1974a; 1977) found that the sizes of both types of hypercolumns were about the same throughout the cortex; a lateral movement of about 1 mm along the surface of the cortex was sufficient to move across a complete hypercolumn. This distance corresponds well to the distance on the cortex an electrode must travel to change the receptive field locations of the cells encountered. Therefore, within a given 1mm-by-1mm chunk of cortex, all the cells recorded will have approximately the same receptive field location, and there will be a full range of preferred orientations and ocular dominance levels.

Notice that while all hypercolumns occupy about the same amount of cortical volume, the amount of visual space covered by each depends on the sizes of the receptive fields of the cells within the hypercolumn. In fact, the distance between the centers of the receptive fields represented by neighboring hypercolumns (that is, the difference in location of receptive fields of cells about 1 mm apart) is about half of the average receptive field size (Hubel & Wiesel, 1974b). We already know (Chapter 5) that acuity is best in the fovea, and becomes worse toward more peripheral parts of the retina; in other words, the receptive fields of ganglion cells (and cortical cells) serving the fovea are smallest, and those for peripheral retina are largest. If the foveal receptive fields are small, the amount of visual space covered by each hypercolumn is small, and many hypercolumns are needed to cover the relatively small visual area of the fovea. As all hypercolumns are the same size, this means a relatively large amount of cortex must be devoted to the small visual area of the fovea. This is the case; as we pointed out in Chapter 8, maps of the retinotopic projection on the cortex show a tremendous magnification of the fovea relative to the remainder of the visual field.

Blobs

The photographs in Figure 9–3 reveal two remarkable systems of columns that correspond to those inferred from single-cell recordings. Another kind of patterning was found accidentally in the visual cortex of monkey before its physiological correlate was recognized. Margaret Wong-Riley treated cortex with a stain that would reveal cytochrome oxidase, an enzyme involved in the energy system of cells. She hoped to be able to show changes in activity of areas of cortex, like those shown by 2-dg, with a stain that did not diffuse as readily and so "smear" the pattern. Her staining did show changes in energy use. But, to her surprise, the overall levels of cytochrome oxidase showed a patchy distribution, with puffs of high activity spattered in the upper layers of the V1 cortex (Wong-Riley, 1979). These puffs, now known by the elegant name *blobs*, form chains that run down the middles of the ocular dominance columns (see Figure 9–4).

It was soon found that the blobs are the lairs of the concentric cells of the cortex (Hubel & Livingstone, 1983). They contain the majority of the color-coded cells (see Chapter 15) of the parvocellular system (Martin, 1988b; Ts'o & Gilbert, 1988), in addition to a weak magnocellular input (Tootell,

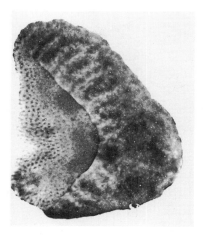

FIGURE 9-4 Cytochrome oxidase activity in the visual cortex of a squirrel monkey. V1 is at the left, V2 to the right. Blobs can be seen in V1. Thick stripes and thin stripes, separated by pale stripes, can be seen in V2. From Livingstone, M. S., and D. H. Hubel (1988) Segregation of form, color, movement, and depth: Anatomy, physiology, and perception. *Science* 240:740–749. Copyright 1988 by the AAAS. Reprinted by permission.

Hamilton, & Switkes, 1988). The areas of cortex between the blobs (called the *interblob* regions) receive parvocellular input that seems to care more about luminance than color (Tootell, Silverman, Hamilton, DeValois, & Switkes, 1988). While the cytochrome oxidase blobs are found in the upper layers (2 and 3), the functional column apparently extends through the entire cortical sheet, interrupted by the magnocellular parts of layer 4 (Ts'o & Gilbert, 1988).

We may now put all of this together into a picture of the layout of a piece of cortex (Figure 9–5). This picture is based on one first presented, and often copied, by Hubel and Wiesel (1977). Hubel and Livingstone (1983) call it the "ice cube" model. The block represents a cube of cortex about 2 mm in size; the cortical surface is at the top, the white matter underneath. The slabs parallel to the right front face (labeled "L" and "R" for the left and right eyes), are the ocular dominance columns. Their borders become vague, particularly away from layer 4; cells driven exclusively by only one eye occur only in the middles of the columns.

The slabs parallel to the left face are the orientation columns. They are thinner than the ocular dominance columns, but take about the same space to come "full circle." The preferred orientation of each column is indicated by the sloped lines on the right face.

In addition, the blobs are shown centered in the ocular dominance columns. They are shown solidly in layers 2 and 3, where the cytochrome oxi-

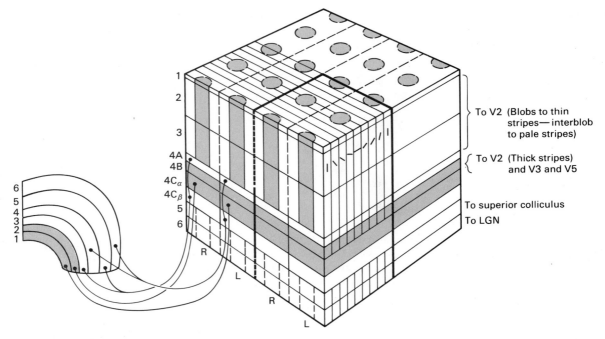

FIGURE 9-5   Model of V1 cortex, showing two hypercolumns for orientation specificity, two hypercolumns for ocular dominance, and the blobs. The
sketch of a right LGN shows the projections from each lamina to the
appropriate ocular dominance column, and the projection of the magnocellular layers to cortical layer 4Cα. The major outputs of the layers are indicated to the right (although the fibers actually exit
through the bottom of the cortex). Other inputs are not indicated. After Hubel and Wiesel (1972).

dase stain is most distinct, but are also indicated in the deeper layers where
they are functionally present. The layers are labeled at the left, and their
outputs are indicated to the right. The sketch of an LGN to the left shows
outputs of its six layers dividing among the lamina and ocular dominance
columns of the leftmost hypercolumn. Magnocellular influences are shaded
along the left face of the cube.

Notice that the ice cube represents two complete cycles of ocular dominance, and two cycles of orientation. That is, there are two hypercolumns of
each, or four complete functional units. Thus, the front quarter, outlined in
black, represents all orientations, all ocular dominances, and several blobs,
with receptive fields that are essentially in the same location. In another
quarter, there will again be a complete representation of all these aspects,
with receptive field locations shifted by about half a field width (Hubel &
Wiesel, 1974b). This cartesian regularity is appealing, but it is clearly over-
simplified. The ocular dominance columns and orientation columns do not

form regular grids (see Figure 9–3), and are not really oriented at right angles to each other (Lowel, Bischoff, Leutenecker, & Singer, 1988). The principle of the hypercolumn, however, is that a small cortical region can encode all ocular dominances and preferred orientations, plus information about color. The exact geometrical configuration of the hypercolumn is not as important.

BOX 9–2 ████████████████████

The model of cortical organization shown in Figure 9–5 is not the only possible interpretation of the data. An interesting alternative model for monkey cortex has been proposed by DeValois and DeValois (1988). They suggest that the orientation columns are not parallel slabs but are slabs that intersect at the blobs. Instead of parallel sheets, DeValois and DeValois envision a pattern like the weave in a cane chair. The columns intersect in the blobs, where there is no orientation selectivity. Blobs are centered in the ocular dominance columns, so each hypercolumn would consist of two asterisklike starbursts. Each hypercolumn represents a polar coordinate system; in each starburst (centered on a blob, responding to one eye or the other), the *angle* represents orientation. According to the DeValois', the *radius* (distance from the blob) represents spatial frequency, which we will discuss in Chapter 10. Thus, each hypercolumn (for each eye) would be read like a clock, with the "time" telling the orientation and length of the "hand" telling the spatial frequency. Many of the orientation columns in adjacent starbursts would approximately link, giving an appearance of longer slabs. However, the slabs for different orientations would run in different directions across the cortical surface. Some support for this idea may be found in the apparently "modular" organization of the cortex seen when special dyes allow one to visualize the various orientation columns in the same piece of cortex (Blasdel & Salama, 1986). Baxter and Dow (1989) found a concentric model, similar to that proposed by DeValois and DeValois, provided a good fit to orientation data from long electrode tracks like those in Figure 9–2.

How can there be two such different interpretations of the same data? Remember, the slabs are not perfectly rectangular, and we have noted that orientation and ocular dominance columns actually seem independent. Either model is an attempt to organize rather disarrayed patterns; the "ice cube" emphasizes the slablike columns, while the "starburst" emphasizes the discontinuities and interruptions (like the nonoriented blobs). What we are witnessing is a difference in the ways patterns can be organized and encoded by the perceptual systems of the scientists—the topic of Chapter 11.

DEVELOPMENT OF CORTICAL PROPERTIES AND EFFECTS OF DEPRIVATION

We now have a picture of primary visual cortex (V1), in which cells with quite specific properties are found near other cells with similar properties. Thus, a column of cells in a single vertical penetration through cortex will share a common receptive field location, preferred orientation (if any), and ocular dominance. A nearby column will have a nearby visual location, but may differ in the other properties. How did this specificity come about? Is it innate, or modified as a result of visual experience?

In an attempt to answer this question, Hubel and Wiesel have recorded from cortical cells in cats and monkeys that are either newly born or several weeks old, but deprived of any visual experience since birth (Hubel & Wiesel, 1963; Wiesel & Hubel, 1974b). In both species, they found that the properties of cells from visually naïve animals were similar to those encountered in adult animals. In the monkey, which is much more mature at birth than the cat, simple, complex, and hypercomplex cells were all found, with orientation and direction specificity that was about as sophisticated as that in the adult. Both binocular and monocular cells were seen in about equal proportions as in the adult animal. In the cat, there were more differences, with cells recorded from newborn animals being much less responsive, and often less specifically tuned to particular features (Wiesel & Hubel, 1965). Many response features seen in recording of cortical cells of mature animals were observed in cells from naïve animals, however.

Although the initial properties of cortical cells may be innate, it is possible to alter these properties by changing the visual environment of a very young animal. Ocular dominance is one property that can be changed in this way. Hubel and Wiesel (1962) classified cells according to their binocularity by creating a seven-level scale, with level 1 meaning that the cortical cell is only affected by stimulation of the contralateral eye, level 4 meaning that the cell receives equal input from both eyes, and level 7 meaning that the only input to the cell is from the ipsilateral eye. Levels 2, 3, 5, and 6 were reserved for cells that had some degree of binocularity, but were not equally sensitive to stimulation by both eyes. This seven-level scale was named the Ocular Dominance scale; with it, a cell's level of binocularity could be summarized by a single number. Hubel and Wiesel assessed the binocularity of a great many cells in cat cortex and created a histogram of the numbers of cells in each ocular dominance category. Such an ocular dominance histogram is shown in Figure 9–6; from this figure, it is seen that most cells in the cat cortex are binocular, at least to some degree. Of the relatively few monocular cells, about the same number of cells could be stimulated by the ipsilateral eye as the contralateral eye.

Wiesel and Hubel (1963) were the first to observe that if one eye of a kitten was kept closed for several months immediately after birth, more extreme changes resulted than if both eyes were kept closed. Instead of most cells responding to some extent to input from both eyes, cells from cats with one deprived eye were almost completely unresponsive to visual stimulation from that eye after it was reopened. Figure 9–7 shows ocular dominance histograms from a cat that had one eye sutured shut at birth; instead of most cells being capable of stimulation from both eyes, the majority of cells can only be activated by input from the nondeprived eye. There seems to be a critical period during which abnormal visual experiences can affect cortical proper-

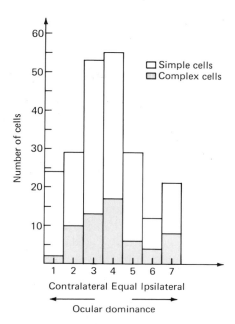

FIGURE 9-6   Ocular dominance histogram for 223 cells encountered in the visual cortex of a normal cat. From Hubel and Wiesel (1962). Reprinted by permission.

ties; if after four months of normal visual experience, cats are monocularly deprived for any length of time, no changes are seen in cortical ocular dominance (Wiesel & Hubel, 1965).

Depriving one eye of visual stimulation is not the only way to modify the binocularity of cortical neurons. If one extraocular muscle from one eye is surgically severed, that eye will not be able to participate in convergent eye movements with the other eye. The cat becomes "cross-eyed" (or "wall-eyed," depending on which muscle is severed), and the two eyes have different images of the visual field projected onto them. This should make things confusing for binocular cortical neurons. Hubel and Wiesel (1965b) performed this experiment and found that one could find approximately equal numbers of cells in the cortex driven by either eye, but that there were few binocular cells. It seems, therefore, that although binocular cells exist in cortex of newborn animals, they will lose their ability to signal binocular information if the animal's visual experience is restricted to situations in which this information is either useless or harmful.

The contention that the cortex needs appropriate binocular input in order to maintain a population of binocularly driven cells receives more support from the experiment of Blake and Hirsch (1975), who subjected kittens to a period of alternating monocular deprivation. For the first six months of each kitten's life, one eye was covered with an opaque contact lens for one

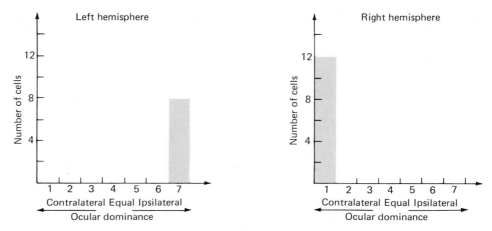

FIGURE 9-7 Ocular dominance histograms from 3-month-old kitten with its right eye closed from eight days after birth to the time of the experiment. The right eye was opened just before surgery; the histograms show that cortical cells only respond to visual input from the eye that was not closed. From Wiesel, T. N., and D. H. Hubel (1963) Single-cell responses in striate cortex of kittens deprived of vision in one eye. *J. Neurophysiol.* 26:1003–1017. Reprinted by permission of the publisher and author.

day; the other eye was covered the next day, and so on. At the end of the six months the properties of cortical neurons were investigated; it was found, as in the study discussed in the previous paragraph, that cortical cells could be driven by one eye or the other, but there were few or no binocularly activated cells.

If ocular dominance is so easily modified by abnormal visual experience, perhaps other cortical properties are equally plastic. Hirsch and Spinelli (1970) raised cats in complete darkness, except for one-hour periods each day, during which one eye was presented with a stimulus consisting of vertical lines, and the other eye was stimulated with an array of horizontal lines. After ten weeks, the response properties of cortical cells were investigated. Not surprisingly, as the cats had had no opportunity for binocular stimulation, few cortical cells could be driven by both eyes. In addition, it was found that cells driven by the eye that was presented with the horizontal lines had receptive fields that preferred horizontal stimuli, while cells that had inputs from the eye receiving vertical stimulation were differentially sensitive to vertically oriented stimuli. Cells with preferred orientations in between horizontal and vertical were not found. In a similar experiment, Blakemore and Cooper (1970) found that after rearing kittens in a visual environment that was limited either to vertical or horizontal stripes, most of the cortical cells recorded had preferred orientations that matched the early environment. Thus the orientation specificity of the visual cortex can also be altered by abnormal visual experience. These changes in physiological properties are accompanied by changes in morphology; Coleman, Flood, Whitehead, and Emerson (1981) report a change in cortical dendrite organization after rearing in a striped environment similar to that used by Blakemore and Cooper.

Experimenters have found that still other properties of the visual cortex can be modified by experience. If cats are reared under stroboscopic illumination, their visual experience consists of a succession of still images, with movement being totally absent. Cortical cells of cats reared under these conditions show an abnormally low number of cells sensitive to direction of stimulus movement (Cynader, Berman, & Hein, 1973; Cynader & Chernenko, 1976). In another experiment, kittens were raised so that their sole visual experience consisted of a stimulus array of stripes moving in one direction. Under these conditions, an unusually large percentage of cortical cells was found to be differentially sensitive to that direction of movement (Daw & Wyatt, 1976).

The general conclusion is that response properties may be genetically determined, but experience is necessary for normal development. But there are some indications that the genetic predisposition may be quite general, and the resulting organization may reflect the ways in which neural networks naturally form. In a fascinating set of experiments, Sur, Garraghty, and Roe (1988) removed the LGN from a ferret's brain and routed the incoming optic nerve fibers to the auditory part of the thalamus (having removed the auditory nerve). The visual fibers made connections in this "alien" area, and in fact formed a functioning visual system so that orientation-selective cells like those in normal visual cortex could be found in what had been auditory cortex. A similar result was obtained when hamster optic nerve was routed to somatosensory thalamus (Métin & Frost, 1989). Perhaps there is some predisposition for cortical cells to organize their inputs and their communications with their neighbors to analyze for "features," but the features must be whatever is available in the input. In this regard, it is interesting that when computers model cell networks (see Chapters 11 and 12), and the properties of intermediate cells between the defined input layer and output layer are "optimized" by the computer, these intermediate cells spontaneously develop properties reminiscent of cortical cells (Lehky & Sejnowski, 1988). Moreover, the apparent properties of these cells (bar or edge detectors) are not related to the task performed by the neural network (recognizing shape from shading).

PROJECTIONS TO HIGHER CORTICAL AREAS

In Chapter 8, we identified at least two parallel pathways in V1: the parvocellular and the magnocellular. As the information passes from V1 to higher areas there is considerable cross talk (Krubitzer & Kaas, 1989), but we shall see these two systems remaining somewhat distinct.

V1 actually contains at least three systems, for the parvocellular pathway splits into the systems of interblobs and blobs. Blobs also have some magnocellular input and input from *interlaminar* cells that lie between certain layers of the LGN. These three pathways seem to remain distinct in their projections to V2 and V3, which are the next cortical areas forward of V1 (see Figure 8–1).

The magnocellular system, except for its weak projection into the blobs, is confined to layer 4 in V1. From layer 4B it projects directly to V3 and V5 (DeYoe & Van Essen, 1988), and to the *thick stripes* of V2 (Livingstone & Hubel, 1987a). Thick stripes are part of a second cytochrome oxidase pattern found in monkey cortex (more or less clearly, depending on species). These stripes may be seen in Figure 9–4, to the right of the blobs in V1. Instead of blobs, the cytochrome oxidase stain produces a banded pattern in V2. There are two sets of dark staining stripes interleaved: thick stripes and *thin stripes*. They are separated by *pale stripes* of weaker cytochrome oxidase activity.

The projections from layers 2 and 3 of V1 (which are mainly parvocellular in origin) seem to go only to V2. The dark-staining blobs project to the thin stripes, while the pale interblobs project to the pale stripes. V2, consistent with its name, seems to be secondary to V1, with its three-stripe systems (thick, thin, and pale) corresponding to the three pathways of V1 (magnocellular, blob, and interblob, respectively). These projections are summarized in Figure 9–8. The figure has a columnar organization that emphasizes the parvocellular/magnocellular distinction. This figure emphasizes the projections "upward" to higher cortical areas, but most of these projections are reciprocal. That is, the higher areas also project back to the "lower," so most of the flow may be considered as two-way traffic (Zeki & Shipp, 1988).

V3 is "third" in that it receives a projection from the thick stripes of V2, but its main input is directly from the magnocellular system in layer 4B of V1. Since that is also the main input to the thick stripes, we may consider V3 as a part of the magnocellular pathway.

The next area forward of V3 is V4, or, more accurately, the V4 complex (Zeki, 1983a). Everything seems to converge onto V4: both the thin and the pale stripes of V2 (representing the parvocellular pathways), and V3 (representing the magnocellular). V4 is "fourth" in that it receives inputs from V3,

FIGURE 9-8 Schematic diagram of the interconnections and possible roles of areas and subareas in primate cortex. The lateral geniculate nucleus is at the bottom, with progressively higher cortical areas higher up the diagram. The parvocellular system is at the left, and the magnocellular system is at the right. Based on a summary diagram by DeYoe, E. A. and D. C. Van Essen (1988). Concurrent processing streams in monkey visual cortex. *Trends in Neursoci.* 11: 219–226. Reprinted by permission.

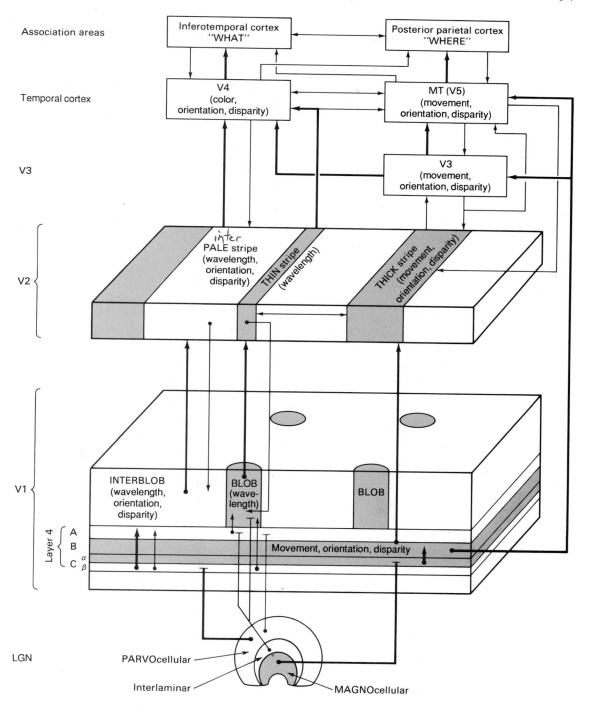

but it also receives a direct input from a special population of interlaminar cells in the LGN (Lysakowski, Standage, & Benevento, 1988). This large, heterogeneous collection of cells projects into the inferotemporal cortex near the base of the brain (see Figure 8–1).

The next visual area forward is sometimes called V5 because of its position (Zeki, 1983a), although it is at about the same logical level as V4. It is more often called the *middle temporal* region, or *MT*. It lies buried deep within a large infolding of the cortex, called the *superior temporal sulcus*. For the most part, MT receives magnocellular inputs: from V3, from the thick stripes of V2, and directly from layer 4B of V1. However, there is also some input from the thin stripes of V2, and there is an interconnection between V4 and MT. The middle temporal region projects to the posterior parietal cortex near the top of the brain (see Figure 8–1).

Functions of the Higher Cortical Areas

Some indication of possible function of the cortical areas has been placed in each of the boxes of Figure 9–8. These putative functions are based on the responses of cells in these areas and on deficits in function noticed when these areas are damaged. Thus, Figure 9–8 summarizes not only the pathways and their interconnections, but also their possible roles in vision.

A word of caution is in order. It is easy to say that an area with many cells that respond to variations in wavelength of the light is a "color-sensitive" area and forget that these same cells may also have spatial, motion, or orientation preferences. Once again, we do not wish to call an area (or a cell) a "detector" of some feature simply because that is what we tested it for.

You will also notice that most of the boxes indicate more than one function. In most cases, individual cells are sensitive along more than one dimension; in many cases, some cells in a particular area show one property, and other cells in that same area show another. It is not uncommon to find clusters of cells in a higher visual area that seem to code for one property (like color) interspersed among clusters of other cells that are insensitive to that property (Zeki, 1983a). If the pattern of cytochrome oxidase stripes had not emerged in V2, we might consider it an area with all properties represented. Perhaps some finer organization will someday be recognized within the thick stripes, or in V3, V4, or MT (see Zeki & Shipp, 1988).

We have already spoken of specializations in V1. Cells in the blobs are generally not selective for orientation or motion and are driven almost exclusively by one eye or the other. Many of them are interested in color; others may be responsive to contrast. Cells outside the blobs are orientation selective, and when they are driven by either eye, may compare the positions of the stimuli in the two eyes, a difference referred to as *binocular disparity*. Cells in layers 2 and 3 (interblob) sometimes also care about wavelength. Cells in the magnocellular layer 4B often care about direction of motion.

Since these subdivisions of V1 project fairly directly to the thin stripe, pale stripe, and thick stripe divisions of V2, it is not surprising that those areas of V2 show similar preferences (Hubel & Livingstone, 1987). V3 receives its input from layer 4B and thick stripes and so shares the preferences of those areas. This does not mean that V2 and V3 are adding nothing to the processing begun in V1. For example, some cells in V2 respond specifically to motion of a stimulus across their receptive fields (with the eyes stationary), and do not respond when the eyes sweep across a stationary stimulus (Galletti, Battaglini, & Aicardi, 1988). The motion of the stimulus across the receptive field is the same in both cases; the difference is whether the *stimulus* moved. Such discrimination has not been reported in V1. Similarly, cells in V2 (in cat) have been reported to be sensitive to motion in depth (toward or away from the animal), not simply motion across the receptive field (Cynader & Regan, 1978).

BOX 9–3

A fascinating glimpse of how processing in higher cortical areas may be more "advanced" comes from a study by von der Heydt, Peterhans, and Baumgartner (1984). They recorded from neurons in V1 and V2 of monkey, seeking cells that respond to edges. Such cells were easy to find in either area. However, the cells in V2 not only responded to edges of the correct orientation that were presented to their fields, they responded to edges of the correct orientation that were not really there (von der Heydt & Peterhans, 1989). Such nonedges, called *subjective contours*, will be discussed in Chapter 11. For now, we will just say that these "edges," which are not there but *appear* to be, can be created by the suggestion of an object overlaying a pattern. For example, in Figure 9–9(a), you may "see" a vertical white line connecting the slits in the two black rectangles. The line is not really there, but you may see it as if a thin white strip were lain across the picture.

A V2 cell receptive field is sketched between the black rectangles (dashed oval). This cell responds best to vertical lines. When the black rectangles are moved left and right (to-gether), the cell responds as if a line were being swept back and forth across its field. The response is not as strong as for a real line, but there is a response (although there is no change in the stimulus anywhere in the receptive field). And, after all, the perception of the subjective contour (the vertical white line in the area between the rectangles) is also weak.

The subjective contour depends on very subtle details of the stimulus. If you draw lines across the ends of the slits (so there is a thin white window in each of two complete black rectangles), the illusory white line vanishes (see Figure 9–9[b]). When the same cell was shown this very slightly modified stimulus, it also failed to "see" the line, and gave no responses to sideways movement of the black rectangles (Peterhans & von der Heydt, 1989).

These properties are not found in the cells of V1, and may be taken to indicate a closer agreement between the activity of the "line detectors" of V2 and the actual perception of a line. But we cannot say that this is a function of V2, for this property may depend on influences from other areas, including some "higher" than V2.

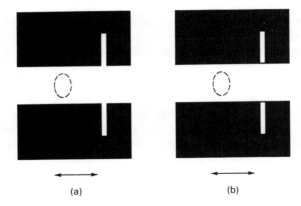

(a)   (b)

FIGURE 9-9   Subjective contours and cells in V2. The black rectangles with slits
were moved left and right, with the receptive field of the cortical cell
as shown by the dashed ellipse. (a) Open slits create impression of a
vertical white line through the gap between rectangles. A cell that responds to vertical lines responds to this stimulus. (b) Closing the slits
negates the subjective contour (the white line); the cell does not respond to this stimulus. After von der Heydt, R., E. Peterhans, and G.
Baumgartner (1984) Illusory contours and cortical neuron responses.
Science 224:1260–1262. Copyright 1984 by the AAAS. Reprinted
with permission.

Beyond V3

The next area, V4, was originally thought to be a color processing area because of a large number of color-specific cells found in it, although these
cells are found in clusters surrounded by clusters of orientation-selective
cells (Zeki, 1983a). There are at least two major systems: (1) a spatially
broad, color-selective system that probably plays a major role in the perception of color, and (2) a spatially tuned, orientation-selective system that
probably is important in pattern recognition. Of course, there must also be
some depth discrimination, since recognition of differences in distance are
key to object recognition.

A role for V4 in pattern recognition was demonstrated by Spitzer,
Desimone, and Moran (1988), who recorded from V4 of a monkey while it
matched test bars against a sample (to be rewarded with a drop of water for
correctly deciding if the test matched the sample). When the task was made
more difficult (''false'' test bars that were very similar to the sample in color
or orientation), the cells became more selective, and gave larger responses to
the ''correct'' matching stimulus. The task the monkey was engaged in had an
effect on responses within the visual system.

The main target for V4 neurons is the inferotemporal cortex. Neurons in
inferotemporal cortex may be selective for a particular shape, color, or texture anywhere within a relatively large area of visual field (Desimone,

Schein, Moran, & Ungerleider, 1985). Iwai (1985) considers this area essential for pattern perception. Inferotemporal cortex neurons, like the V4 neurons that supply their inputs, become selective for the particular stimulus parameters the animal is asked to discriminate (Fuster & Jervey, 1981). But neurons in the temporal cortex can be very selective for particular patterns. Neurons in monkey temporal cortex have even been reported to be selective for faces (Perrett, Rolls, & Caan, 1982). All of this suggests that the pathway to inferotemporal cortex may be simplistically labeled the "what" system; it is the system charged with identifying what we are seeing.

BOX 9–4

Further evidence for the inferotemporal cortex as a "what" system comes from observations on patients who have suffered damage in that area of the brain. If this area is damaged on both sides of the brain, usually because of multiple strokes (blood clots interfering with the blood supply to a part of the brain), a number of interesting clinical pictures can appear.

One such deficit is called *prosopagnosia*, the inability to recognize faces. Patients with this problem can usually recognize objects, including faces, for what they are. But they cannot distinguish among objects in the same class. They cannot say if a particular face is familiar, or distinguish one person's face from another's. The deficit is not limited to faces, but extends to any set of superficially similar objects among which distinctions must be made on the basis of relatively subtle differences. For example, a kennel owner who previously could identify each dog in the kennel will find all dogs indistinguishable. Thus, patients with this disorder have normal *generic recognition*, but have suffered the loss of *specific recognition* within a given class (Damasio, 1985). You can imagine what havoc such a problem could create in your life, even though your basic visual perception is completely normal.

Another deficit that can result from damage to visual temporal cortex is *alexia*, the inability to read. Alexia results when the visual association cortex is disconnected from the part of the left cortex that is responsible for language integration. Such patients may also be blind in the right visual field (hemianopia: see Box 8–1), but vision in the left field is completely normal—except for the inability to read. One irony is that these patients can be able to write fluently; however, they are apparently unable to read back what they have just written!

Other damage may specifically affect the color processing portions of this system. Sometimes this is associated with prosopagnosia; these patients often report that colors are "washed out" or completely absent (Damasio, 1981). This rare color deficit is known as *achromatopsia*. It is not the same as color blindness (see Chapter 15), because these patients report everything is the same color, but still can see borders formed by differences in color only. They may also see washed out blacks and whites, implicating the blob system in general (Livingstone & Hubel, 1987b).

The other major pathway is the magnocellularly driven one. Maunsell and Newsome (1987) refer to this as the "motion pathway," although it clearly has a broader function than motion detection. The main collecting station along the way is MT (V5), buried in the superior temporal sulcus.

Zeki (1974) suggested this was a movement area because it contains a high percentage of cells sensitive to movement, and because its cells are arranged in a columnar organization based on direction of movement. The preponderance of motion-selective cells has been amply confirmed (Bruce, Desimone, & Gross, 1981; Rodman & Albright, 1989). It has also been found that lesions in MT impair a monkey's ability to follow a moving target with its eyes (Dursteller & Wurtz, 1988), or even to see that a pattern is moving (Newsome & Pare, 1988). We will have more to say about the role of MT in motion detection in Chapter 14.

The major output of MT goes to the posterior parietal cortex. This area has been implicated in directing visual attention to a particular part of the visual field (Lynch, Mountcastle, Talbot, & Yin, 1977), having some neurons that respond during eye movements, and others that are responsive only during fixation. The fixation neurons are often specific for location and distance of a target, suggesting they are concerned with the position of an object in space, taking account of eye position (Sakata, Shibutani, & Kawano, 1980; Andersen, Essick, & Siegel, 1985). In fact, the neurons in this area seem to be integrating visual information with that from other senses, including *intended* hand position (Robinson, Goldberg, & Stanton, 1978). Like the cells of V4 and inferotemporal cortex, neurons in posterior parietal cortex modulate their responses in accord with the task the animal is performing (Bushnell, Goldberg, & Robinson, 1981).

The posterior parietal cortex may also play a role in pattern vision (Iwai, 1985), but it seems its main role is in locating stimuli in space. For this reason, Livingstone and Hubel (1987b) have referred to this as the "where" system, as opposed to the "what" of inferotemporal cortex. "Where" does not simply mean "where is an object?", but also "where are its parts?". That is, "where" is an essential component of integrating whole images. It may also be required by the "what" system to allow it to identify the parts of objects being recognized, or the relationships of the parts of the object.

BOX 9-5

Once again, the natural laboratory of clinical dysfunction can shed light on the normal role of a part of the brain. There is a considerable difference between the deficits caused by strokes affecting the inferotemporal cortex and those affecting posterior parietal cortex. A most spectacular disorder called *Balint's Syndrome* is due to damage in the posterior parietal cortex. Patients with this syndrome have three distinct problems:

The first prong of Balint's Syndrome is *simultagnosia*, the inability to perceive a whole structure from component parts. If you show a patient with simultagnosia a photograph of a rural scene and ask him to describe what he sees, he may pick out a tree, or a pig, or a barn. However, he seems unable to integrate these components into a unified whole. It is as if he can focus his attention on only a tiny part of the picture at any time. As a result, even if he ini-

(continued)

(box continued)

tially noted a pig in the picture, he may be unable to find it again once he has turned his attention to something else.

The second prong in Balint's Syndrome is *optic ataxia*, the inability to coordinate arm and leg movements based on visual information. A patient with optic ataxia is unable to point accurately at an object, even though she sees it clearly. She can easily point to her nose, or the spot on her skin touched by a feather, or to any other object that produces somatosensory cues. The deficit is only apparent when visual cues are isolated. While this problem most usually occurs as part of Balint's Syndrome, it is sometimes seen in isolation (Damasio & Benton, 1979).

The third prong of Balint's Syndrome is *ocular apraxia*, the inability to shift one's gaze to a new stimulus. A novel stimulus that a normal person would immediately attend to goes unnoticed, and when the patient does finally attempt to look toward the new object, the orienting eye movement is inaccurate. This problem occurs even though the patient has full eye movements and no visual-field defect evident in standard testing.

Vision and the Parvocellular and Magnocellular Systems

The roles of the parvocellular and magnocellular systems in visual perception have been examined by Margaret Livingstone and David Hubel (1987b, 1988) through a series of demonstrations. The authors were their own subjects, so we cannot be sure to what extent the effects are due to what is actually seen, and to what extent it is what the authors (or readers looking at the published figures) expected to see. Nevertheless, their ingenious approach and valuable insights will probably influence work in this area for some years to come.

Livingstone and Hubel exploited the properties of the two systems, as indicated in Table 8–1, to devise stimuli that would selectively affect only one system or the other. For example, very low contrast stimuli are below threshold for the parvocellular system, but can be seen by magnocellular cells (see Figure 8–5). Similarly, a rapidly flickering light would look steady to parvocellular cells but not to magnocellular cells. Thus, the fact that a low-contrast, counterphase grating seems to flicker even though no pattern is seen (see Chapter 6) is consistent with the magnocellular system signalling flicker, while the parvocellular system is responsible for indicating what the pattern is.

To isolate the parvocellular system, Livingstone and Hubel capitalized on the idea that magnocellular cells are "color-blind"; that is, they cannot discriminate between lights on the basis of wavelength alone. Livingstone and Hubel presented colored images that are *equiluminant*; that is, the luminance of the two colors is matched (see Chapter 4). As you will read again in Chapter 15, a color-blind person cannot discriminate between two lights that are equal in luminance, even though they may appear different in color to the rest of us.

Imagine creating an equiluminant green line on a red screen. One projector would provide a large field of red light, with a sharp shadow where the line goes. Another projector would provide a sharp green line that fits perfectly into the shadow in the red light. Now, vary the ratio of red to green light. At a high ratio, there is a bright red field with a dark line. Even a color-blind person would see that there is a dark line on a brighter field, though he could not tell the color of the field. At a low ratio, there is a bright green line on a dark field. Again, a color-blind person would easily see a light line.

Now consider what the color-blind person sees as the high ratio is gradually lowered. The bright field becomes dimmer, while the dark line gets brighter. At equiluminance, they are the same brightness; the line and field blend perfectly into a smooth field. The exact ratio needed depends on the particular person and system, but it can be found. Of course, color-normals see a green line on a red field.

The *assumption* is that at equiluminance, the magnocellular system cannot discern the stimulus, but the parvocellular system can. The blob cells, of course, signal the colors. The interblob cells may not necessarily signal color, but may be responsive to the color difference. They might respond that there is a border, even though they would indicate the appearance is the same on both sides of the border. (This is how we described achromatopsia in Box 9–4.)

Livingstone and Hubel report that at equiluminance, pictures lose their apparent depth and structure (see Figure 9–10 in Color Plate A). A picture that gives a strong impression of three-dimensionality in black and white (or at nonequiluminance) seems flat and two-dimensional at equiluminance. A pattern of moving dots that gives the distinct impression of spots on a rotating transparent sphere appears as spots dancing about at random when made equiluminant with the background. A complicated pattern (such as the silhouette of a bicycle in Figure 9–11) is difficult or impossible to recognize at equiluminance. (See Color Plate B before viewing Figure 9–11.)

Vision without the magnocellular system thus seems to lack depth and organization. In some ways, it is reminiscent of the effects of damage in the posterior parietal cortex (see Box 9–5 about Balint's Syndrome), which is a main recipient of the magnocellular pathway. Even the parvocellular function of recognizing a pattern is impaired, because the magnocellular system is needed to provide the information about depth and the relationship of the parts. We will return to the importance of the magnocellular system for the perception of depth in Chapter 12.

Perhaps it now seems like the parvocellular system is relatively unimportant (although it occupies a pretty big proportion of the visual system). The magnocellular system analyzes motion, depth, and spatial relationships; the poor parvocellular system is left with only two "minor" jobs: color

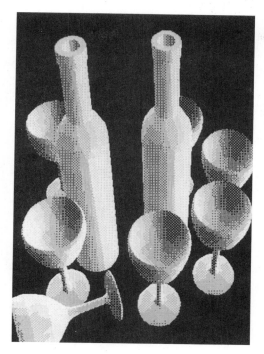

FIGURE 9-10 (Color). A picture that seems to have depth when not at equiluminance, but loses depth at equiluminance. On Color Plate A, (a) shows the equiluminant figure, (b) shows just the green portion, and (c) just the blue portion. From Livingstone, M. S. and D. H. Hubel (1988) Segregation of form, color, movement, and depth: anatomy, physiology, and perception. *Science* 240:740–749. Copyright 1988 by the AAAS. Reprinted by permission.

(which is not essential), and filling in the details. (These "details" may include the texture of surfaces, which we will return to in Chapters 10 and 11.) But vision with the magnocellular system only (say, at low contrast) is not very good, other than for seeing that "something moved." It is a vision of indistinct, shadowy shapes. Just as the parvocellular system needs information from the magnocellular system to do its tasks, the magnocellular system requires information from the parvocellular pathways. They interact at many levels, so the capabilities of both working together are far better than would be expected from what each can do working alone. This kind of complicated intertwining of systems and processes will be evident many more times as we discuss the process of perception.

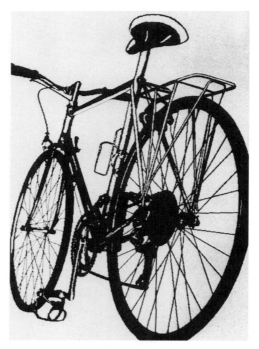

FIGURE 9-11   (Color, see Color Plate B). A picture that is hard to recognize at equiluminance. From Livingstone, M. S., and D. H. Hubel (1988) Segregation of form, color, movement, and depth: anatomy, physiology, and perception. *Science* 240:740–749. Copyright 1988 by the AAAS. Reprinted by permission.

SUGGESTED READINGS

Chapters 2 and 3 of Kuffler and Nicholls' *From Neuron to Brain* (Sinauer Press, 1976) provide an excellent discussion of the functional architecture of the visual cortex. Finally, on the subject of plasticity of cells in the visual system, Chapter 15 of R. D. Lund's *Development and Plasticity of the Brain* (Oxford University Press, 1978) provides a good review.

An excellent and readable account of how the cortex processes visual information is "Brain mechanisms of vision," by Hubel and Wiesel (*Scientifc American*, September 1979). This article reviews the types of cells found in the cortex, but emphasizes their organization into orientation and ocular dominance columns. It further speculates about how particular visual patterns might be represented within the hypercolumns of the cortex. It may also be found in *The Brain* (W. H. Freeman, 1979), that was recommended in the "Suggested Readings" for Chapter 3. It is also reprinted in *The Mind's Eye* (introduction by J. M. Wolfe) (W. H. Freeman Co., 1986).

For a more up-to-date account of the parallel processing story and the roles of higher visual centers, read "Concurrent processing streams in monkey visual cortex," by E. A. DeYoe and D. C. Van Essen, in *Trends in Neurosciences*, Volume 11 (1988), pages 219–226. A brief account that is more concerned with the roles of these areas is "Art, illusion and the visual system," by Margaret S. Livingstone (*Scientific American* 258:78–85 [January 1988]). A more technical but readable version of this has been published by Livingstone and David Hubel: "Segregation of form, color, movement, and, depth: Anatomy, physiology, and perception." *Science* 240:740–749 (1988).

Another readable account may be found in Hubel's *Eye, Brain, and Vision*, recommended for Chapter 8. A somewhat different view may be found in *Spatial Vision*, by R. L. DeValois and K. K. DeValois (Oxford University Press, 1988). This book emphasizes the cortex as a processor of spatial frequencies, the topic of our next chapter.

SPATIAL FREQUENCY REPRESENTATION

10

In thinking about or describing a visual scene, you naturally refer to areas of light and dark at particular locations in space. It is in those terms that we have described visual stimuli presented to subjects (Chapter 2), or to the receptive fields of individual neurons (Chapters 5 to 9). In this chapter, we are introducing a different, but equally descriptive, way of specifying the visual scene: spatial frequency analysis. It is another way of thinking about visual stimuli, one that has attracted considerable attention in the past couple of decades. It is a way that you have almost certainly never encountered before; because it is so different from other ways of discussing visual perception, it may seem rather confusing. Try to bear in mind, however, that this material is not harder than other material, it is just unfamiliar. There is evidence that at some level, spatial frequency analysis may be one way our nervous systems "think about" the visual scene. In any case, it is a way many researchers exploit to examine the workings of the visual system.

There are two major points to cover. First, we must explain what spatial frequency analysis is; only then can we discuss the possibility that the visual system performs this function. The first part of this chapter is therefore devoted to developing the general concepts of spatial frequency analysis. Second, we will present evidence that the visual system includes channels that amount to spatial frequency detectors. Finally, we will be able to discuss how the detectors function in perception and demonstrate perceptual effects that may be explained by assuming this kind of analysis.

THE CONCEPT OF SPATIAL FREQUENCIES

The spatial frequency representation is a *transform* of the visual image into another, mathematically equivalent, representation. As such, it is just a mathematical trick that remaps the world into a different form. There is nothing controversial here; it is a mathematical truth that the two representations are of the same thing.

The principle on which the spatial frequency notion rests was stated by the French mathematician J. B. Fourier: any function that repeats itself over and over can be synthesized as the sum of a series of sinusoids. The mathematical procedure by which functions are approximated by sums of sinusoids is called a *Fourier transform*.

What is a sinusoid? A sinusoid, of which a sine wave is an example, is a continuous waveform that oscillates in a smooth and regular fashion. As an example, consider a child on a swing; each time the child races past the lowest point, gravity slows the swing's rise. At the peak of the swing the child stops, then gradually swings faster and faster through the low point, and slows to stop on the backswing and fall again. If we plot the angle the swing ropes make with vertical as a function of time, we obtain the wave shown in Figure 10–1. This is a sine wave. It is characterized by its amplitude (A in the figure, the maximum excursion of the swing), and its *wavelength* (λ in the figure, the time between corresponding points in successive *cycles*). The wavelength is the length of a single cycle, or repetition. In general, we define the *frequency* as the inverse of wavelength. The equation of the curve in Figure 10–1 is

$$\theta = A \sin(360 \cdot f \cdot t)$$
$$\text{where } f = 1/\lambda$$

(The 360 is a "fudge factor" needed because sines are functions of angles measured in degrees. It would be inaccurate to omit the 360, but it is really irrelevant to understanding what we are talking about.)

One other parameter is needed to fully characterize a sinusoid. The two wave forms shown in Figure 10–2 have identical wavelengths and amplitudes; however, they differ in *phase*. Phase refers to the difference in timing between the two waves; in Figure 10–2, the two waves are one-quarter of a cycle apart. This is, if the curve in Figure 10–2(b) were shifted to the left by one-quarter of a cycle, it would superimpose exactly on the curve in Figure 10–2(a). As a single cycle of a sine wave is equal to a 360° change in angle, a one-quarter cycle change in phase is equal to a change of 90°. A 180° phase shift, or one-half-cycle change, would have the effect of completely inverting

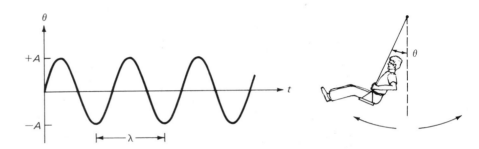

FIGURE 10-1 A sinusoid in time (sine wave). The angle from vertical made by the swing rope is plotted versus time.

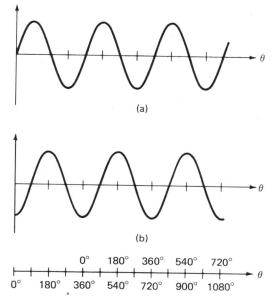

(a)

(b)

| 0° | 180° | 360° | 540° | 720° |
| 0° | 180° | 360° | 540° | 720° | 900° | 1080° | θ |

FIGURE 10-2 Two sinusoidal functions that are one-quarter-cycle out of phase.

the wave; that is, where the original wave had its peaks, the phase-shifted wave would have its valleys, and vice versa. (For more about sine waves, see the appendix.)

The sine waves in Figures 10–1 and 10–2 are functions of time, but sinusoids can also be functions of space. Ripples in a pond are waves in space; so are the ripples blown into the sand at the beach. We will be talking about sinusoids in space, but the fluctuations of interest to us are not the elevations of ripples, they are increases and decreases in the luminance of a visual pattern. In general, we refer to the frequency of spatial sinusoids in terms of the number of cycles per degree of visual angle. If we spoke of cycles per inch or mm, we would also have to specify the viewing distance; by referring all measures to visual angle, we have completely specified the size of the retinal image. We will have more to say about visual angles in Chapter 13; for now, simply consider visual angle as a measure of distance along an image.

One point should be emphasized: the spatial frequency (f in the equation of a sine) is *inversely* related to the wavelength, or "size" of the wave. A high spatial frequency (large f) is one with small wavelength; there are many cycles per degree. A low spatial frequency has a long wavelength, and there are few cycles per degree. A high-frequency pattern is therefore fine and detailed, with lots of waves in a small area. A low-frequency pattern represents long, smooth, drawn-out waves. As we will be referring to high and low spatial frequencies throughout this chapter, it is essential to get this straight.

Fourier Analysis

Now that we are clear about what a sinusoid is, let us consider the Fourier transform. First, we will simplify things by considering stimuli that vary along only one dimension. Of course, real pictures vary in two dimensions, vertical and horizontal. We could take Fourier transforms of such images, but these would have to be two-dimensional functions also, adding an extra complication to an already complicated story. If we restrict variations to one dimension, say horizontal, we can represent the entire stimulus by the single function of luminance versus horizontal displacement. This function describes how light varies as one moves across the field. As one moves vertically, the luminance is always the same as the points above or below. We have just described a vertically oriented grating, as shown in Figure 6–11. For example, two sinusoidal gratings are shown in Figure 10–3; below each is the sine function that represents the luminance at each horizontal point.

There is one other thing to notice in Figure 10–3. Because we cannot

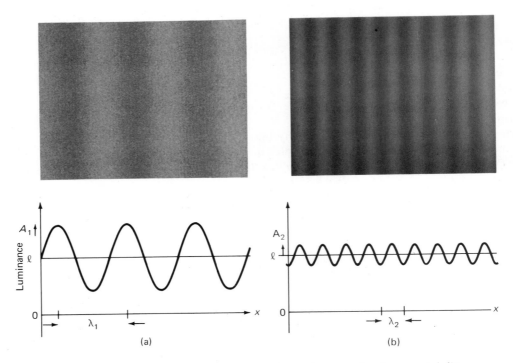

FIGURE 10-3 Two sinusoidal gratings. The relation between luminance and distance across each grating is shown below it. The grating on the left is of low spatial frequency and high amplitude; that on the right is of higher frequency and lower amplitude. Both are at the same mean luminance.

have a negative amount of light at any point, the sine wave must be shifted up so that it never goes below zero. That is, the sine wave is a *modulation* about some mean amount of light, l, where l is greater than A, the amplitude of the sine wave. Rather than talk about the amplitude, A, we generally speak of the *contrast* of the grating. We have already introduced the concept of the Weber contrast (page 19) as the relative increment of light superimposed on a mean background. For gratings, the luminance extends both above and below the mean level, and we define the *Rayleigh contrast* as the ratio of the amplitude to the mean, or

$$C = \frac{A}{l}$$

When $A = l$, the contrast is 1.0 (100%), and the dark troughs have zero light. As A becomes relatively smaller the contrast becomes less, and the ripple a less and less significant part of the illumination.

The Fourier transform represents a pattern in space by the *component* sinusoids of which it is composed. Just as the wavelength spectrum of a light tells how much energy is present at different wavelengths, so the spatial frequency *spectrum* of a given pattern tells how much contrast there is in the pattern at different spatial frequencies. The spectrum of a visual pattern is presented as a graph of contrast versus spatial frequency. For example, the gratings in Figure 10–3 consist of pure sine waves; each contains only the one frequency that is the frequency of that sine. Their spectra, shown in Figure 10–4, indicate that there is contrast at only one frequency, and all others are absent. The spectra in Figure 10–4 and the sinusoidal curves at the bottom of Figure 10–3 are two different representations of the same things. In Figure 10–3 we see the actual patterns in space; in Figure 10–4 we see their spectra. A spectrum looks very different from the actual light distribution, but it says unequivocally that the distribution of light is that shown in the corresponding halves of Figure 10–3.

Other sinusoids would also be represented by spectra in *frequency space* that are spikelike spectra; the location of the spike depends on the

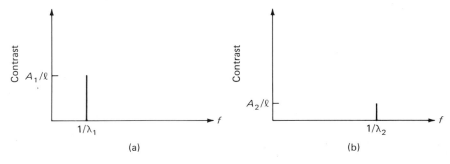

(a)   (b)

FIGURE 10-4 The frequency spectra of sinusoids shown in Figure 10-3.

frequency of the sinusoid. The height of the spike depends on the contrast of the sinusoid. A low-frequency sinusoid (coarse grating, as on the left side of Figure 10–3) is represented by a spike near the left end of the frequency axis (left panel in Figure 10–4); a higher frequency sinusoid (fine grating, as on the right in Figure 10–3) is represented by a spike to the right on the frequency axis (right panel of Figure 10–4). A high-contrast grating (left side of Figure 10–3) is represented by a taller spike than that representing a lower contrast grating (right side of the figure).

A single spike is the simplest spectrum one could imagine; only one spatial frequency is represented. For this reason, sinusoidal gratings are often the stimulus of choice when one is interested in the possibility that Fourier components play a role. Sinusoids are the most "primitive" waveforms we can use, being the only waveform that is never distorted by any linear system (Shapley & Lennie, 1985). Simple sinusoids are not what we generally see in the world about us, however; we need to demonstrate that more interesting things can also be represented by spectra in frequency space. We assert that it is possible to represent any pattern by its spectrum. As a demonstration, we shall indicate how one decomposes one particular pattern into its component frequencies. The pattern is one that is commonly used as a grating stimulus: the square wave grating (Figure 10–5). It consists of alternate light and dark bars. The pattern of light is thus described by a pattern of uniform areas—high intensity, then low, then high, then low.

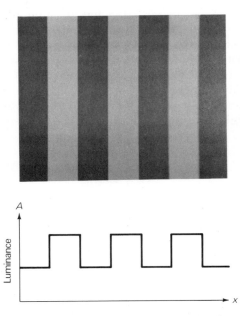

FIGURE 10–5   A square wave grating. The relationship between luminance and distance across the grating is shown below.

The four columns of Figure 10–6 are parallel representations of the building of a square wave from sines. The left column shows the actual patterns of light; the next column graphs luminance as a function of position; the right middle column shows the spectra corresponding to the patterns on the left, and the right column gives the corresponding equations.

We begin at the top in Figure 10–6, with a sine wave whose wavelength is the same as the square wave we are composing. This is called the *fundamental* component; it is both the lowest frequency present, and the largest component of the square wave. It is a sine in space, and therefore represented by a spectrum that is a single spike; its equation is given at the right.

To the fundamental sine wave, we add another sine at higher frequency but lower contrast. The particular wave needed is three times the frequency but one-third the contrast; it is drawn below the fundamental, with its spectrum and equation. The sum of these two components is shown in the third row. Notice that the higher frequency sine wave (called a *harmonic*) is negative where the fundamental reaches a peak; it therefore subtracts from the peak and flattens it. With just these two components, you can already see the form of the square wave emerging. The spectrum of the sum of the two components is simply the sum of the spectra of the individual components; that is, two spikes.

We now add another harmonic that is five times the fundamental in frequency and one-fifth of the contrast; it is shown in the fourth row. The result of adding this component to the other two is shown in the fifth row; the pattern in space is an even better approximation to a square wave, and the spectrum now has three spikes.

If we continue in this manner, adding all the odd multiples (3, 5, 7, 9, etc.) of the fundamental frequency at contrasts proportional to the inverse of their frequencies, we approach a square wave (bottom row). The spectrum has an infinite number of spikes (there are an infinite number of odd numbers), but the high-frequency components are infinitesimally small. The equation corresponding to the spectrum has an infinite number of terms (one per component), and is best represented by the summation of an infinite series. (If this notion is unfamiliar, it just means what we said in words: add all the odd multiples of the fundamental frequency, each with an amplitude inversely proportional to its frequency.)

We have been presenting the representations shown in the three rightmost columns of Figure 10–6 as being different representations of the same thing. In fact, the spectra lack a little information that is in the equations; as a result, the waveforms cannot be uniquely determined from the spectra. That extra information is the phase of each component, or the relative position of each along the left/right dimension. All that is implied by a spike on a spectrum is that there is a sinusoidal component of the given contrast at that frequency; it does not imply that this wave goes through zero at the same position as the fundamental. (The fact that all the components are sines and must pass through zero at the same points as the fundamental *is* unequivocal from the equations to the right.)

Suppose that alternate components were inverted—that is, peaked where these have valleys, and had valleys where these have peaks. This corresponds to a phase shift of 180°, as can be verified by considering the sine in Figure 10–1 shifted by one-half of a cycle. A sinusoid shifted by one-half cycle is exactly mirror image (vertically) from the original. If we take the same components as in Figure 10–6 but shift every other component 180°, the spectra will be the same as those in Figure 10–6, but the waveform and equations will be different. This can be seen in Figure 10–7. The same fundamental component is shown at top; the same harmonic is added, but with a phase shift of 180°. The result of the phase shift is that the peaks add, rather than subtract; instead of leveling the peaks of the fundamental, the harmonic builds them higher and narrower. When the full complement of harmonics has been added, the waveform shown at the bottom of the figure results. This is a *triangle wave*; it clearly looks quite different from the square wave, although its spectrum is identical. When we represent gratings, we present only their spectra, for the corresponding equations tend not to make pleasant reading. Remember, however, that the actual Fourier transform of patterns also contains information about the phase that is simply not shown in the spectra.

Let us stop and consider what we have said so far. For every pattern in space, which is representable by a function showing the luminance as a function of position, there corresponds a Fourier transform that we can graph as a spectrum of contrast versus frequency. The function of luminance versus position is a direct map of the pattern; it is the way one would generally think about what the pattern "is." The spectrum is quite different looking; however, it is a convenient way of describing the pattern mathematically.

FIGURE 10–6 How a square wave is composed of the sum of a series of sine waves. The left column shows the grating patterns; the second column shows luminance as a function of position; the right-middle column shows the corresponding frequency spectra; and the rightmost column gives the mathematical equation corresponding to the patterns. Top: A single sinusoid (the fundamental). Row 2: A sinusoid at 3 times the frequency (3rd harmonic). Row 3: The sum of rows 1 and 2. Row 4: A sinusoid at 5 times the fundamental frequency (5th harmonic). Row 5: Sum of rows 3 and 4 (fundamental plus 2 harmonics). Row 6: Result of adding all the odd multiples of the fundamental frequency (square wave).

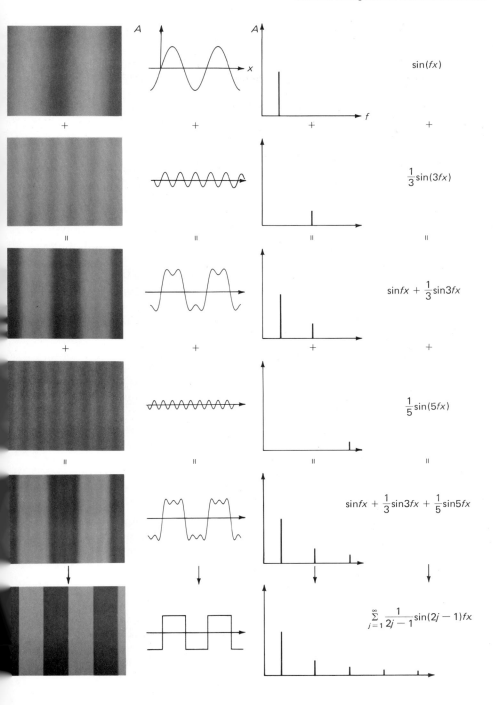

The Modulation Transfer Function

For every pattern in space there corresponds a Fourier transform; for every Fourier transform there is a corresponding pattern in space. Suppose we have an optical system (a camera or telescope) and wish to know how good an image of some pattern it can make. For most optical systems, the quality of the image that is produced depends on what spatial frequencies are present in the input signal. By looking at the quality of the images produced for input patterns that are pure sinusoidal gratings, we can predict how the optical system will perform for any arbitrary input. If the pure gratings are all of the same contrast, the performance of the optical system can be defined by the contrast of the image at each frequency. The plot of the relative image contrast versus frequency is called a *modulation transfer function* (MTF). A hypothetical example is shown in Figure 10–8(a). This is the MTF of a typical camera lens; all frequencies lower than f_0 are reproduced without a loss of contrast, but higher frequencies are progressively less well reproduced. A grating at a frequency less than f_0 would appear as strongly in the image as in the original pattern, but a high-frequency grating (closely spaced bars) will be reproduced with lower contrast; if it is sufficiently high frequency, its image would be a uniform gray field. This is typical of optical systems; low frequencies (large things) are reproduced well, but high frequencies (tiny details) are lost.

Suppose this same optical system is knocked out of focus. The highest frequencies that had been reproduced well are now lost; only the lowest frequencies survive. In general, when an image is out of focus, the highest frequencies are lost (the fine details are blurred out of existence).

The MTF of the optical system lets us predict the image that will be formed of any pattern we might present. If the pattern contains only components less than f_0 (and is in focus), it will be reproduced perfectly. If there are components greater than f_0, they will be diminished according to a factor corresponding to their frequencies. Components near f_0 will be made slightly smaller, while those well above f_0 will become vanishingly small. If we take the spectrum of the pattern, and multiply each component by the factor implied by the MTF for its frequency, we will obtain the spectrum of the image. By Fourier mathematics, the light distribution in the image may be reconstructed from that spectrum.

FIGURE 10–7 How a triangle wave is composed of a series of sine waves. Columns as in Figure 10–6. First 5 rows as in Figure 10–6, except that the harmonic is added 180° out of phase from the fundamental. Row 6: Result of adding all odd multiples of the fundamental frequency, with odd harmonics out of phase (triangle wave).

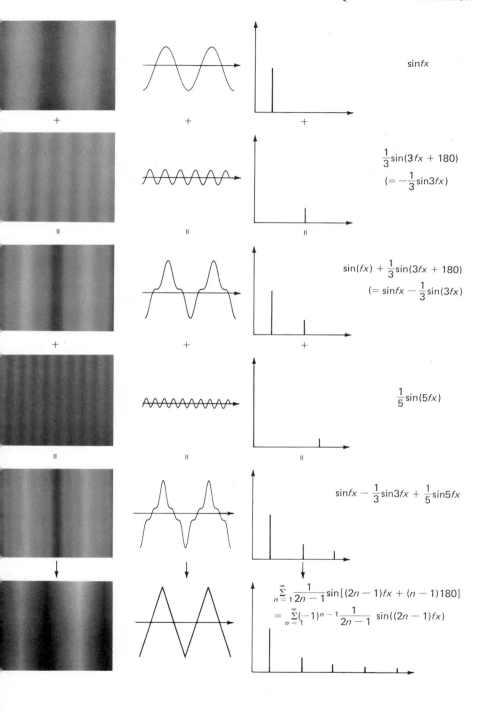

$\sin fx$

$+$

$\frac{1}{3}\sin(3fx + 180)$

$(= -\frac{1}{3}\sin 3fx)$

$\|$

$\sin(fx) + \frac{1}{3}\sin(3fx + 180)$

$(= \sin fx - \frac{1}{3}\sin(3fx)$

$+$

$\frac{1}{5}\sin(5fx)$

$\|$

$\sin fx - \frac{1}{3}\sin 3fx + \frac{1}{5}\sin 5fx$

$\sum\limits_{n=1}^{\infty} \frac{1}{2n-1}\sin[(2n-1)fx + (n-1)180]$

$= \sum\limits_{n=1}^{\infty}(-1)^{n-1}\frac{1}{2n-1}\sin((2n-1)fx)$

BOX 10-1

Wͤe have said that the spectrum of an image is simply the point-by-point product of the spectrum of the pattern and the MTF of the optical system. This simplicity is the principal mathematical advantage of transforms such as the Fourier transform. If you wished to know the output of an electronic circuit given a particular input, or the motion of a mechanical structure (bridge or tower) given a particular mechanical perturbation, or the path of a vehicle or ship with a particular steering system given a particular command, you would be faced with a difficult and complicated differential equation (differential equations are the subject following advanced calculus). On the other hand, you can take the transform of the input, simply multiply by the transfer function, and have the transform of the system output without ever having to resort to calculus or differential equations. The only problem is performing the transformations to and from frequency space, and that problem is solved by published tables of functions and their corresponding transforms.

Up to this point, we have been talking about spectra of patterns and the MTF of a physical optical system; now let us consider the human visual system as a high-class optical system. In fact, it includes a physical optical system in the traditional sense: the cornea and lens of the eye, which form an image on the retina (see Chapter 4). The tests that an optometrist or ophthalmologist makes to determine visual acuity are really just another way of characterizing the MTF of the eyes.

The visual system, however, includes more than the eye. There is no guarantee that all components imaged on the retina will be perceived (although any that are completely degraded by the cornea and lens certainly

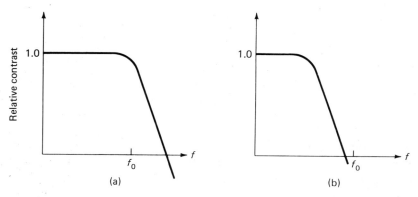

FIGURE 10-8 Hypothetical transfer functions of a physical optical system, showing relative contrast in the image as a function of spatial frequency. (a) A reasonable optical system, well focused. (b) The same system with the image out of focus.

will *not* be seen). What we wish to determine psychophysically is the MTF of the entire system: cornea, lens, retina, visual cortex, and whatever interprets patterns of firing within the cortex. The way this is done is to measure the *contrast sensitivity* for sine wave gratings at all spatial frequencies. Contrast sensitivity is defined (as are other sensitivities) as the inverse of the contrast required to attain threshold. Measuring contrast sensitivity is thus like making any other threshold measurement (see Chapter 2); the contrast is found at which the subject is just barely able to detect that the target is a grating rather than a uniform gray field. (Any of the methods discussed in Chapter 2 can be used.) If contrast threshold is measured at each frequency and the results plotted versus spatial frequency, a *contrast sensitivity function* (CSF) like the one shown in Figure 10–9 is derived. The CSF represents the underlying function (see Chapter 7 for a discussion of sensitivity *versus* response measures). The MTF and CSF are identical if the system is linear.

What does the CSF in Figure 10–9 tell us? For one thing, like the MTFs in Figure 10–8, there is drastic attenuation of very high frequencies. In fact, it is perfectly reasonable to expect this, as the cornea and lens are a physical optical system of limited capability that will transmit very high frequencies quite poorly. It is probable, however, that the exact shape of the high frequency

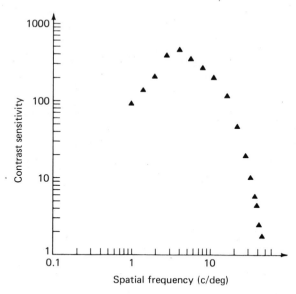

– FIGURE 10-9   The contrast sensitivity function (CSF) of a human observer; contrast sensitivity as a function of spatial frequency. From Campbell, F. W. and J. G. Robson (1968) Application of Fourier analysis to the visibility of gratings. *J. Physiol.* 197:551–566. Reprinted by permission of the Cambridge University Press.

end of the curve is also partially determined by the processing performed by the retina and cortex.

The other noteworthy feature of the CSF in Figure 10–9 is that the very low spatial frequencies are also attenuated. This is not like the characteristics of physical optical systems and is thus likely to reflect a physiological property of the visual system.

BOX 10–2

There is a particular pattern that enables you to see the shape of your own CSF. This pattern is reproduced in Figure 10–10; it is a grating in which the spatial frequency increases from bottom to top, and the contrast increases from left to right. Along any horizontal strip of the figure the frequency is the same; along any vertical line the contrast is the same. You should see a pattern in which the medium-sized "bars" in the middle are the widest—they are widest because they are visible at lower contrast (farther left on the figure). The higher frequency stripes to the top and the lower frequency stripes to the bottom are at just as high a contrast, but they cannot be seen because the human eye is less sensitive to those frequencies. Make a mark on the page to the left of the bar that appears widest, and then move to a different distance from the book. (This changes the spatial frequencies in cycles/deg; move away from the book, and all the frequencies become higher.) The peak should appear to move to a different position, indicating that it is a function of the visual system, not the way the figure was reproduced in printing.

FIGURE 10–10 Demonstration of the shape of the CSF. Grating frequency continuously increases to the top; contrast increases from left to right. Copyright G. B. Arden. Reprinted by permission.

As a matter of fact, we already know of a physiological process that attenuates low spatial frequencies: it is lateral antagonism (see Chapter 6). Remember that lateral antagonism has the effect of reducing the responses of ganglion cells when they are situated in a broad area of uniform illumination

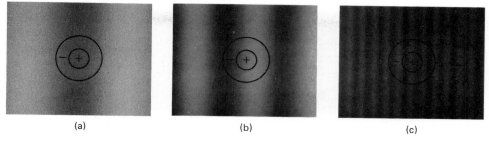

(a)   (b)   (c)

FIGURE 10-11 How lateral antagonism can account for the lower sensitivity to low spatial frequencies. (a) A ganglion cell receptive field being stimulated by a very low frequency grating; both center and surround are well lit, so inhibition cancels much of the excitation. (b) The same receptive field with a grating of optimal frequency. Center is well lit, but surround is in the dark, so there is little inhibition. (c) The same field stimulated by a very high frequency grating. Both the center and the surround are about as well lit as if the field were uniform (no grating).

(low spatial frequency). A ganglion cell with its receptive field centered on the broad plateau of a low spatial frequency grating, as shown in Figure 10-11(a), receives considerable antagonism from the well-illuminated surround of its receptive field. This is inhibition that reduces the firing of the cell from the level that it might have attained because of the illumination of its excitatory center. If the grating were of higher frequency, as shown in (b), the center could be nearly as well illuminated as in (a), but the major part of the surround would lie in the relatively darker troughs. The response in this case would be considerably greater, for there would be less antagonism.

We could go further: suppose the grating were of even higher frequency, so that several cycles could fit within the center of the receptive field (c). The center and surround would each have light areas and dark areas in about equal proportion, and the response would be expected to be less than in (a). The excitation and inhibition are balanced, as in (a), but there is less light in the center; high frequencies should therefore be attenuated also.

If lateral antagonism can be equated with the low spatial frequency attenuation noted in the MTF, we should be able to offer the MTF as an "explanation" for those visual effects attributed to lateral antagonism. We can "explain" Mach bands and similar effects by applying the MTF to the spectra of these patterns. In general, these arguments are rather complicated, but there is one that is amenable to graphic demonstration. This is the Craik-O'Brien illusion, shown in Figure 6-6. The light distribution in the Craik-O'Brien illusion is one with "glitches" in an otherwise uniform field, but the appearance is of fairly uniform steps in brightness. The pattern shown at the top left of Figure

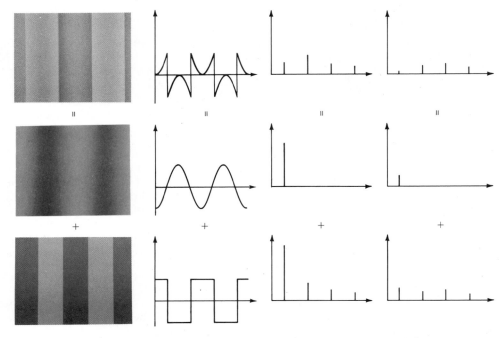

FIGURE 10–12   The Craik-O'Brien illusion explained in terms of the MTF. The left
graphs show the distribution of light in space, the middle graphs
show the spectrum corresponding to each pattern, and the right
graphs show the *effective* spectra (how effective each component
should be if it is weighted according to the CSF in Figure 10–9).
Top: The Craik-O'Brien pattern. Middle: A low frequency sinusoid.
Bottom: A step (square wave). The sum of the bottom two rows is
the Craik-O'Brien pattern in the top row.

10–12 should appear as alternate bright and dark bands, even though the actual illumination in the center of each band is the same.

The third column in Figure 10–12 shows the spectra associated with the
illusion and the two other patterns shown below it. You can better understand the spectrum for the illusion by seeing how the illusory pattern can be
broken into two components: a sine wave and a square wave. If the sine wave
in the middle row is added to the square wave at the bottom, the illusory
pattern will result (you can convince yourself of this by doing some mental
addition). The spectrum of the sine is a single spike; the spectrum of the
square wave is a series of spikes (as in Figure 10–6). The sum of these spectra
is thus the series of spikes shown at the top of the third column. Note that the
sine in the middle row is 180° out of phase with the fundamental of the
square wave; that is, it is actually *subtracted* from the square wave.

Consider what happens if each of the spectra is multiplied by the CSF in Figure 10–9. The lowest frequencies are attenuated, so the pattern the brain receives that generally means square wave (bottom) is as shown at the lower right. The sine wave, which is of low spatial frequency, is attenuated to near invisibility. The spectrum of the square-plus-sine (top) is similar to the spectrum of the square wave, so the two look alike, and the illusory pattern is seen as the more familiar square wave pattern. Put another way, the sinusoidal component (that is the only physical difference between the illusory pattern and the square wave pattern) is invisible, so the illusory pattern cannot be distinguished from a square wave. The Craik-O'Brien pattern and the square wave pattern are both members of the same "equivalence class"— patterns that are physically different but give rise to the identical neural signals (Ratliff & Sirovich, 1978). They must therefore look alike; that they both appear as square waves might be because the visual system is set up to detect edges (and therefore also square waves) by a kind of Fourier analysis (Campbell, Howell, & Johnstone, 1978).

BOX 10–3

Because the Craik-O'Brien illusion is really a square wave with its fundamental component removed, it is sometimes also called the *missing fundamental* illusion. Actually, the pattern in Figure 10–12(a) is not a missing fundamental illusion, for the sine we subtracted had the same contrast as the square wave. If you look carefully at Figure 10–6, you may notice that the fundamental component actually has a greater contrast than the resultant square wave (there is a factor of $4/\pi$ that we did not mention). Therefore, in Figure 10–12, we subtracted most, but not all, of the fundamental component of the square wave. Notice that because of this mathematical quirk, a 100% contrast square wave actually contains a fundamental component that is greater than 100% contrast!

The Craik-O'Brien illusion works well near threshold, where the low frequency fundamental may well be imperceptible. At higher contrasts, the difference between the illusory figure (Figure 10–12[a]) and the square wave (Figure 10–12[c]) is easily seen (although it may still appear that the centers of the light and dark bars are not the same luminance). Burr (1987) explored the way in which the apparent brightness of the bar centers changed at higher contrasts and concluded that two systems operate. At low contrasts (below 10%) there is a contrast-dependent system; at higher contrasts, brightness is matched. This changeover may remind you of the dual magnocellular and parvocellular systems we discussed in Chapters 8 and 9. The magnocellular system operates best at low contrasts, while the parvocellular system is ineffective at contrasts less than about 10%. It thus appears that this illusion may "fool" the magnocellular system but not the parvocellular.

THE MULTIPLE-CHANNEL HYPOTHESIS

In the foregoing discussion, we have emphasized the fact that spatial frequency analysis is no more than an alternative, equivalent description of patterns we have become used to describing in terms of light and dark. The explanations of Mach bands and the Craik-O'Brien illusions in terms of the CSF might be thought of as representing new and different explanations of these phenomena; in fact, if the shape of the CSF can be attributed to lateral antagonism, this is no more than the old explanation couched in terms of spatial frequencies. Just as spatial frequency is an equivalent description of the visual stimulus, the CSF is an equivalent description of the process of lateral antagonism.

In short, we have presented an alternative way of describing things, but have not as yet shown any evidence that it is more appropriate to use this way than the old familiar descriptions. We must now deliver on our promise to show that it is possible that the visual system considers a scene in terms of its component frequencies.

Evidence suggesting that the human visual system might perform some kind of Fourier analysis was presented by Blakemore and Campbell (1969). They measured the CSF of a subject, as previously described. Then they had the subject inspect a high-contrast sinusoidal grating. The inspection grating changed in phase by $180°$ eight times per second, so that the subject would not simply form an afterimage of the grating (see Chapter 7). Despite these phase shifts, for the minute or so that the subject was inspecting the grating, all he saw was a high-contrast pattern at a single spatial frequency. Following this exposure, the subject's CSF was again measured. The two CSFs for the same subject, one before inspecting the high-contrast grating and one after, are shown together in Figure 10–13. The CSF before exposure to the grating is shown as a solid line; it is like the CSF shown in Figure 10–9. (The only difference is that there is not as great an attenuation of low frequencies as in that other figure; this is probably because Blakemore and Campbell used a lower overall light level.) The CSF measured after exposure to the high-contrast grating is shown by the data points; it is markedly depressed for frequencies near the frequency of the inspection grating (the frequency of the inspection grating is indicated by an arrow).

A similar result was obtained when other spatial frequencies were used for the inspection grating. Whatever was used, the CSF was depressed for test gratings near that frequency, but unaffected for those much higher or much lower. Inspection of a high contrast grating has the effect of making low contrast gratings of similar frequency much harder to detect, but has little or no effect on gratings significantly different in frequency.

How might one explain such a result? Blakemore and Campbell invoked a hypothesis (first made by Campbell & Robson, 1968) that there is a large number of separate *channels* in the visual system. Each of the hypothetical channels is "tuned" to a relatively narrow range of spatial frequencies. Thus,

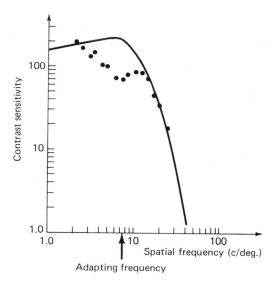

FIGURE 10-13 A CSF before (solid curve) and after (data points) adaptation to a high-contrast grating at the spatial frequency indicated by the arrow. From Blakemore, C. and F. W. Campbell (1969) On the existence of neurones in the human visual system selectively sensitive to the orientation and size of retinal images. *J. Physiol.* 203: 237–260. Reprinted by permission of the Cambridge University Press.

some channels are specific for low spatial frequencies; these channels would be activated only when there are large blobs (low frequencies) in the visual field. Other channels are specific to high frequencies and are activated only when there are fine details (high frequencies) in the visual field. Still others are specific for the frequencies in between. Detection of the presence of a grating depends on activating any channel; the one that will be activated first (and determine the threshold contrast) will be the one that is best tuned to the spatial frequency of the grating.

The overall CSF should therefore be determined by the peak sensitivities of each of the component channels, or the *envelope* of the separate channels. How a CSF is made as the sum of separate channels is shown in Figure 10–14(a). The CSF is shown as a dashed curve, with some of the channels of which it is composed shown as dotted and solid curves.

Now suppose that the subject inspects a high-contrast grating at the frequency shown by an arrow in Figure 10–14(a). The channel most stimulated by the grating is the one that peaks at that frequency; it is shown as a heavy solid curve. As each channel covers a band of frequencies, other channels that peak at nearby frequencies will also be affected by the grating; they are shown by light solid curves. Channels that peak at frequencies well above or well below the grating frequency, however, will be virtually unaffected by the grating (dotted curves).

Blakemore and Campbell assumed that a channel will adapt when it is strongly stimulated. When a channel adapts, it becomes less sensitive; that is, a higher contrast grating is needed to stimulate it. This is exactly like adaptation of retinal neurons; when they are vigorously stimulated, they become less sensitive. Adaptation depends on stimulation, so the most stimulated channel will be the most severely adapted one (dark solid curve), while less stimulated channels will be less adapted (light solid curves). Channels unaffected by the grating would not be adapted at all (dotted curves).

Adaptation means a loss of contrast sensitivity; this means an adapted channel has its sensitivity curve moved downward. Figure 10–14(b) shows the same channels after adaptation to a high-contrast grating at the frequency

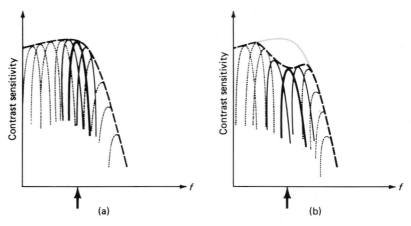

FIGURE 10-14   How the CSF could be composed of frequency-selective channels. (a) The CSF (dashed) is the envelope of a number of separate channels, each sensitive to a narrow range of spatial frequencies. A stimulus at a particular frequency (arrow) would have its greatest effect on the channel shown as a dark solid curve; it would have less effect on the channels shown by light solid curves, and virtually no effect on those shown by dotted curves. (b) The result of adapting to a high-contrast grating at the frequency shown by the arrow. The channel shown by the dark solid curve is made much less sensitive; the channels shown by light solid curves are less affected, and those shown by dotted curves are unaffected. As a result, the CSF (dashed) shows a notch in sensitivity for spatial frequencies near the adapting frequency. Modified from Blakemore and Campbell (1969). Reprinted by permission.

marked by the arrow. The channels shown by dotted curves are unaffected, and are exactly as in (a) of the figure. The channels shown by solid lines have been adapted by the grating, and are shifted downward from their former positions; the most adapted curve is the one that peaks at the frequency of the inspection grating (dark solid curve). If we now draw the envelope indicating the sensitivity of the most sensitive channel at each frequency (dashed curve), we obtain the notched CSF as observed by Blakemore and Campbell.

Channels as Fourier Analyzers

The Blakemore and Campbell experiment suggests that there are separate channels tuned to different spatial frequencies. We now leap to an assumption about the function of these channels (evidence for the assumption will be presented later): as each channel is preferentially tuned to a particular band of frequencies, we assume that activity in that channel signals how much contrast there is at that peak frequency in the visual stimulus. The visual system analyzes a scene by determining the contrast at each of the spatial frequencies: it does this by noting the activity in each of the spatial frequency channels (Graham & Nachmias, 1971).

If this assumption is true, the visual system performs a Fourier analysis of the visual scene. If we arrayed all the channels along a line in the order of the spatial frequency to which each is most sensitive, the activity in each channel (firing rate of neurons) would represent the spectrum of the visual stimulas, as extracted by the visual system. Like the spectra in Figures 10–6 and 10–7, it is a representation of the contrast at every spatial frequency.

In order for each channel to represent a particular spatial frequency, the channels must be independent; that is, activity in one channel should not affect activity in other channels. If high-frequency components could affect the responses of low-frequency-sensitive channels, one could not say that the low-frequency channels signaled the amount of low frequencies present. Independence of channels was shown by Graham and Nachmias (1971), who compared the detection of gratings made of two components. The two components they used were like the fundamental and first harmonic of a square wave; that is, a sinusoid plus another sinusoid at three times as high a frequency (see Figure 10–6, top 3 rows). The harmonic could be combined with the fundamental in phase (as shown in Figure 10–6), or 180° out of phase (as shown in Fig. 10–7). When the harmonic is in phase, it tends to flatten the peaks of the fundamental. When the harmonic is 180° out of phase it enhances the peaks of the fundamental.

Subjects could just detect that there was a grating when the fundamental was of high enough contrast to be detected. The contrast required in the fundamental was the same whether it was presented alone (no harmonic at all), or with the harmonic in either the in-phase or out-of-phase configuration. The harmonic, when it was below threshold, had no effect on the detection of the fundamental. This confirmed an earlier observation by Campbell and Robson (1968) that the threshold for seeing a square wave is determined by the threshold for its fundamental component. When only the fundamental component is above threshold, the square wave cannot be discriminated from a sine wave (see also Campbell, Howell, & Johnstone, 1978; Badcock, 1984b).

As the contrast of the harmonic component is increased, it ultimately exceeds threshold. When it does, the pattern no longer looks the same as a simple sinusoidal grating. The contrast of the harmonic at which it is seen is the same regardless of whether the harmonic is presented alone (no fundamental), or in conjunction with the fundamental (also confirming Campbell and Robson). Threshold for detecting the combination is the same when the harmonic is in phase as when it is out of phase. This demonstration of independence is actually surprising considering that the overall contrast of the pattern (difference between brightest bar and dimmest) is considerably greater in the 180° out-of-phase configuration (Figure 10–7) than in the in-phase configuration (Figure 10–6).

BOX 10–4

The equivalence of the in-phase and out-of-phase combination gratings bears further comment. It is the result to expect if phase information has been lost, as the only difference between the two patterns is their phases. At high-contrast levels, well above threshold, the two patterns do not look alike: the in-phase pattern looks like pairs of bright bars and dark bars (see Figure 10–6), while the out-of-phase pattern looks like a bright bar, medium bar, dim bar, etc. (see Figure 10–7). Near threshold, however, the phase information seems lost, and the two are equivalent.

Given that the two patterns do not look alike at high contrast, the phase information must be carried somewhere in the visual system. Where and how it is carried has been the object of considerable speculation (DeValois, 1977; Atkinson & Campbell, 1974; Stromeyer, Lange, & Ganz, 1973). Perhaps the most straightforward suggestion is that phase is encoded by the retinotopic location of the channels stimulated (Ochs, 1979). Other recent workers suggest that localization is independent of the spatial frequency channels (Burbeck, 1987), with the difference between Figure 10–6 and Figure 10–7 being coded specifically as the profile of the luminance pattern (Badcock, 1984a).

But there are problems with the simple idea that information is encoded by the activities in a large number of independent channels, each tuned to a specific spatial frequency. First, the number of channels is not as large as the early experiments had suggested. Careful psychophysical measurements have indicated that there may be relatively few channels. Williams, Wilson, and Cowan (1982) report only four size-sensitive mechanisms at each retinal location. Wilson, McFarlane, and Phillips (1983) suggest six channels. Watson and Robson (1981) believe there are ten channels, in two distinct subsets: seven operate at low temporal frequencies, while three operate only at high temporal frequencies. Whatever the actual count, there are apparently too few to provide more than a coarse Fourier analysis directly. (It should be noted, however, that a much finer Fourier analysis can be extracted from a few broad channels; see Chapter 15 for how the visual system performs an exquisite analysis of wavelength from the information in only three cone channels.)

Another objection concerns the specificity of the channels. Clearly, if there are few channels and each is very narrow in bandwidth, they cannot effectively span the frequency range. In fact, the bandwidth is limited by the mathematics of the requirement that each channel also somehow specify the position of a stimulus. In order for a channel to be narrow in its spatial frequency selectivity, it must accept input from a large spatial domain. Conversely, to be selective for a particular location, a channel must be broad in its spatial frequency bandwidth. Thus, a perfect spatial frequency channel would have an infinite spatial receptive field. As the field narrows, the spatial frequency selectivity broadens, until a point receptor (perfect spatial localization) accepts all spatial frequencies equally.

BOX 10–5

The argument in the preceding paragraph has led some to suggest that the visual system has arranged a compromise. Receptive fields must be small to allow localization, but if there is to be spatial frequency analysis the bandwidths cannot be too broad. The compromise is to have moderate-sized receptive fields that provide moderate bandwidth channels. In fact, the visual system seems to have made the compromise rather well, having receptive field sizes that jointly optimize spatial localization and spatial frequency selectivity (Daugman, 1984). The resulting channels are a close approximation to the real part of a function called a *Gabor filter*. Some workers in recent years have embraced the notion that it is this compromise, rather than a real Fourier analysis, that the visual system uses (for example, Porat & Zeevi, 1989).

Masking

Some of the most convincing evidence that the visual system actually analyzes a visual scene according to its spatial frequency components comes from an experimental paradigm called *masking*. Masking refers to using one stimulus to hide another. It is not a new technique, having been used in visual experiments for at least 30 years before the spatial frequency notion was proposed (see Chapter 11). The particular kind of masking experiments that have been invoked to support the spatial frequency idea are analogous to experiments that have long been known in audition. As shown in Chapter 17, the auditory system performs what amounts to a Fourier analysis of the temporal frequencies of sound waves in analyzing pitch. The proponents of spatial frequency analysis by the visual system often draw the analogy of the temporal frequency analysis in the ear.

There are three kinds of masking experiments that will concern us in this book: *simultaneous, backward*, and *forward masking*. In each, there is a test stimulus the presence of which the subject is requested to detect, and a masking stimulus that makes detection more difficult than it would be if the test stimulus were presented in isolation. In simultaneous masking, both the test and the mask are presented at once; if both are visual patterns, they may be printed one on top of the other on the same piece of paper. The masking pattern serves to distract the viewer from the stimulus; this is the principle of camouflage.

Backward masking occurs when the mask stimulus is presented immediately after the test stimulus; forward masking occurs when the mask precedes the test. As the timing is critical, a special piece of equipment, called a *tachistoscope* (often referred to as a t'scope), is used. The tachistoscope has the capability of presenting several different patterns, either superimposed or singly, with any timing the experimenter chooses. The timing circuitry is precise enough to allow presentations of less than a millisecond (1/1000 of a sec).

The point about masking that we wish to make here is that effective masks (those that prevent detection of the test) may lie within a *critical band* of spatial frequencies near those of the test patterns they are masking. This is consistent with the multiple channel hypothesis, for if the stimulus pattern is detected by the relative excitation of the various channels, the perception of the stimulus will be disrupted only if the mask also affects those same channels. If the mask only affected channels that peaked at a spatial frequency much different from that of the test stimulus, the channels carrying the information about the pattern would be unaffected. A mask of spatial frequency much different from the stimulus would be as ineffective as if the mask were far away from the stimulus in space; an inkspill on the desk next to the book does not interfere with reading, but an inkspill on the page could create a problem.

One demonstration of the significance of the spatial frequency content in masking was presented by Weisstein, Harris, Berbaum, Tangney, and Williams (1977). They tested the efficacy of two masking patterns: a solid black bar running across the field, and a single infinitesimal dot. The test stimuli were a bull's-eye (concentric rings at equal spacing) and a square wave grating. The spatial frequency spectrum of the bull's-eye contains mainly the odd multiples of the frequency representing the ring spacing, for all the rings are equally spaced and the edges are sharp. (The bull's-eye is a two-dimensional pattern, but a thin slice through the center of it would closely approximate a slice through a square wave grating.) Although it is not obvious, it is a mathematical fact that the spectrum of the dot contains all frequencies.

Weisstein and her associates found that a masking pattern could best forward mask a test stimulus if the mask contained the frequencies contained in the test. Although it seems rather surprising, the dot (containing all frequencies) was an excellent mask for the bull's-eye despite the greater complexity of the bull's-eye. The bar was the more effective mask for the grating because their spectra were most similar. The spatial frequency content, and not the apparent complexity, determined each pattern's effectiveness as a mask. A subsequent experiment from the same lab, however, failed to support this result at a more quantitative level (Tangney, Weisstein, & Berbaum, 1979).

The same point was made graphically using simultaneous masking by Harmon and Julesz (1973). Their stimulus, that is test and mask simultaneously, is shown in Figure 10–15. If it looks like an abstraction of gray boxes, prop up the book and look at the figure from a distance (or take off your glasses if you wear them). The picture was made by a computer process that divided a portrait into boxes and printed each box with the average intensity found in that box. This has the effect of removing high frequencies; any detail smaller than the width of a box must be averaged out. It also has the effect of adding some high frequencies, namely those that define the edges of the boxes.

Figure 10–16 illustrates graphically what the computer has done in creat-

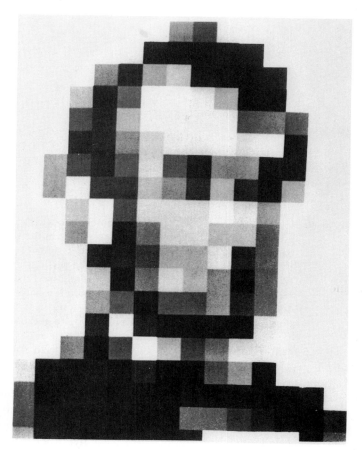

FIGURE 10–15 Computer-processed portrait. Courtesy of International Business Machines Corporation.

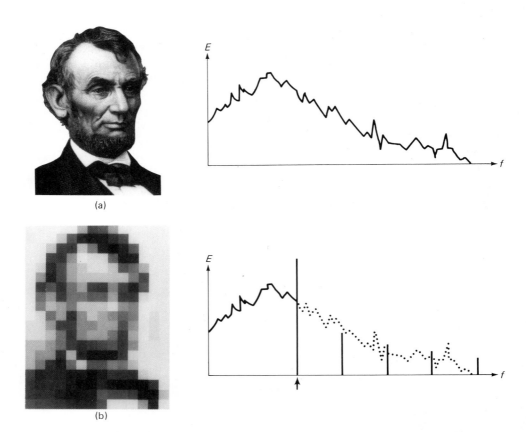

(a)

(b)

FIGURE 10-16   Various manipulations on the computer-processed photograph of Figure 10–15. Hypothetical spectra in the right-
hand column correspond to each picture. Original (top)
courtesy of Life Picture Service. Processed versions from
Harmon, L. D. and B. Julesz (1973) Masking in visual
recognition: Effects of two-dimensional filtered noise.
Science 180:1194–1197. Copyright 1973 by the AAAS.
Reprinted by permission of the publisher and authors.

ing Figure 10–15 from a portrait. Part (a) shows a hypothetical spectrum of
the original picture, with components at all frequencies. Part (b) shows the
result of the computer processing: all the picture frequencies higher than the
repeat frequency of the boxes (arrow) have been removed. (The dotted line
shows what used to be there.) In their places are the frequencies defining the
boxes; essentially, the boxes are square waves and so appear as a series of odd
multiples of the box frequency (see Figure 10–6). The hypothetical spectrum
of Figure 10–15 looks like that in (b) of Figure 10–16.

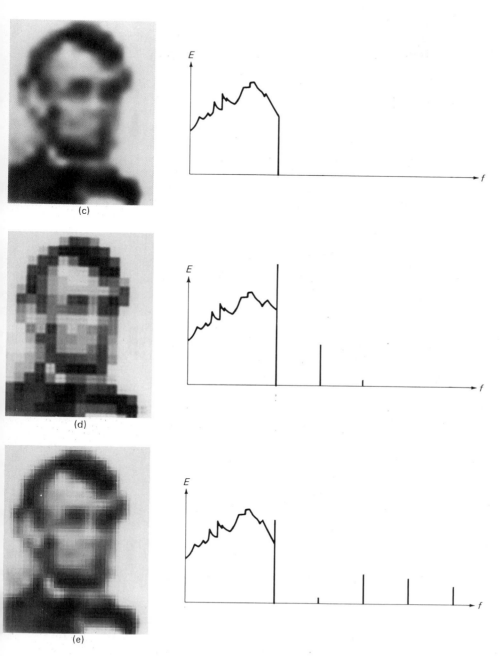

FIGURE 10–16 (Continued).

What happens when you blur the figure by moving away from it or taking off your eyeglasses? Blurring an image means removing the high frequency components (see Figure 10–8); the high-frequency components that are removed are the ones the computer introduced by making sharp boxes. The spectrum of the blurred picture is shown in Figure 10–16(c); it is nearly the same as what the spectrum of the original would be if it were blurred. There is no way to recover the lost high frequencies of the original portrait, but we can remove the additional high frequencies that made the picture information hard to see. The blurred boxed picture is about as good as a blurred original; not great, but recognizable.

The portrait is masked by the high frequencies introduced by the computer; according to the channel hypothesis, only those additional frequencies similar to the frequencies surviving in the picture should be effective in masking it. If we blurred only slightly, removing the highest frequencies but leaving the first few components of the boxes, the masking should still be quite effective. This can be seen in (d) of Figure 10–16. We cannot yet say that the slight blur that removes the very highest frequencies is less effective because those frequencies are dissimilar from the frequencies in the picture; it may simply be that we have not removed enough of the masking frequencies.

To check for the possibility that Figure 10–15 is not recognizable because there is too much masking (rather than because the masking is of a frequency similar to the picture), Harmon and Julesz prepared a picture in which the masking frequencies of (d) were removed, and the higher frequencies missing there but present in (b) were restored. This cannot be done by defocusing, but requires computer processing. The result is shown in Figure 10–16(e); the high frequencies are present, but the lowest frequencies due to the boxes are gone. The picture is about as recognizable as when all the high frequencies are removed (c). That is, the frequencies introduced by the boxing do not all mask the picture; only those within the critical band near the picture frequencies affect recognition of the photo.

BOX 10–6

There is another way of explaining the influence of the boxes in Figure 10–15. Sufficient information that this is a picture of Lincoln is carried by low spatial frequencies, which are best seen by the magnocellular system. The parvocellular system "sees" the high spatial frequencies, and, if our discussion at the end of Chapter 9 is correct, uses that high frequency information along with information from the magnocellular system to identify the stimulus. In Figure 10–15, the parvocellular and magno-cellular systems contradict each other, so the pattern cannot be found. When the high frequencies are removed, the parvocellular system has only the information from the magnocellular system to go on, but that is enough information to make the correct identification. In this regard, it is noteworthy that identification is enhanced if the picture is moved about (or the eyes move rapidly across it); motion favors the magnocellular system.

Perceptual Effects

The experiments we have been discussing provide evidence for separate channels tuned to different spatial frequencies, and further imply that the channels function as spatial frequency detectors. Now let us see what visual effects can be explained by assuming that each channel actually signals a particular spatial frequency when it is active.

Apparent size Because spatial frequency roughly correlates with the size or extent of patterns, it is natural to expect that any manipulation that distorts the pattern of which channels are most responsive would distort the apparent size of a figure. If the high-frequency channels were somehow disabled, only the low-frequency components would be sensed; low frequency corresponds to large patterns, so the pattern would appear larger than if all channels were functioning normally.

This is the premise of a demonstration prepared by Blakemore and Sutton (1969). They used adaptation to a high-contrast grating to reduce the sensitivity of channels at a particular spatial frequency; they then found that other gratings at frequencies slightly above or slightly below that of the adaptation grating appeared to be of higher or lower frequency than they actually were.

Their demonstration is shown in Figure 10–17. First, look at the two square wave gratings on the right; notice that the one on the top and the one on the bottom are of the same spatial frequency. (In fact, they are identical.) Now adapt to the two gratings on the left; fixate on the horizontal line between the two, and move your gaze back and forth along this line to avoid creating an afterimage of the two gratings. Do this for about one minute.

Then look at the dot between the identical gratings on the right. The grating on the top should appear to be of a higher frequency than the one below; that is, it should look like narrower bars spaced more closely together. Adapting to the low-frequency grating on the upper left caused the appearance of the medium-frequency grating on the upper right to shift toward higher frequencies; adapting to the high-frequency grating on the lower left caused the medium-frequency grating on the lower right to appear lower in frequency. As you see both at once, you make a direct comparison of the two appearances, and the difference is apparent.

To understand how the channel hypothesis explains this effect, consider Figure 10–18. For simplicity, we will assume that there are only three channels concerned with the detection of the gratings shown in Figure 10–17. We will also neglect the harmonics in these gratings (which are, after all, square waves). The three channels labeled 1, 2, and 3, are shown in Figure 10–18 as being equally sensitive. Suppose that the gratings on the right in Figure 10–17 are at the peak frequency for channel 2 (*t* in the figure). When these gratings are presented (before any adaptation), they evoke a large response from channel 2, and smaller responses from channels 1 and 3. Gratings of slightly higher frequency evoke less response from channels 1 and 2, but more response from channel 3; for example, a high-frequency grating at

FIGURE 10–17   Demonstration of spatial frequency adaptation. Inspection pattern on the left, test pattern on the right (see text). From Blakemore, C. and P. Sutton (1969) Size adaptation: A new aftereffect. *Science* 166:245–247. Copyright 1969 by the AAAS. Reprinted by permission of the publisher and authors.

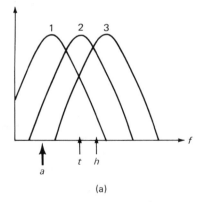

(a)

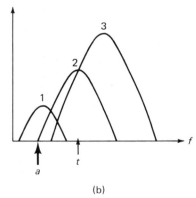

(b)

FIGURE 10–18   Explanation of the effect in Figure 10–17, showing only three channels. (a) Three equisensitive channels, with frequency of adaptation grating (large arrow), frequency of test grating (*t*), and a slightly higher frequency (*h*) indicated. (b) The same three channels after exposure to the adaptation grating has depressed the sensitivity of channels 1 and 2. Test and adaptation grating frequencies are indicated by arrows.

h would evoke equal responses from channels 2 and 3, and a much smaller response from channel 1.

Now suppose this system is adapted by a low-frequency grating, as in the top part of Figure 10–17. The adapting frequency is marked *a* in Figure 10–18; the adapting grating has a large effect on channel 1, a moderate effect on channel 2, and virtually no effect on channel 3. Channel 1 will therefore adapt the most, channel 2 somewhat less, and channel 3 practically not at all, as shown by the sensitivities in Figure 10–18(b). The responses evoked by the test grating (at frequency *t*) in channels 2 and 3 will therefore be approximately equal, with a much smaller response in channel 1. This is essentially the response pattern that would be evoked by a grating at the higher frequency *h* before adaptation; if the system has no way of compensating for the adaptation of the channels, it has to assume that the stimulus evoking these responses is of frequency *h*. That is, adaptation to the lower frequency grating causes the test grating to be perceived as higher frequency than it actually is. It is easy to see that if the adapting grating had been at a higher frequency than *t*, channels 2 and 3 would be most affected and the test would appear to be of lower frequency. This was the case for the bottom half of Figure 10–17.

BOX 10–7

The Blakemore and Sutton demonstration is closely related to another phenomenon called a *figural aftereffect* (FAE). The most famous example of this is the one studied by Köhler and Wallach (1944), reproduced in Figure 10–19. First, notice that the four white squares in the lower part of the figure are equally spaced about the fixation cross in the center of (b). Next fixate on the cross in (a) of the figure for about a minute. Then stare at the fixation cross in (b); the two squares on the left side of the figure should appear further apart than the two on the right.

Early attempts to explain aftereffects such as this one postulated electrical fields on the cortex (subsequently shown not to exist), or relied on eye movements (since shown to be irrelevant). Ganz (1966) proposed an explanation based on lateral antagonism, but his explanation is not wholly satisfactory. We can follow the lead given the explanation of the Blakemore and Sutton effect, however, and explain other figural aftereffects in terms of the multiple channel theory. In this case, the black square in (a) is smaller than the space between the boxes; it therefore adapts higher frequency channels and makes the space between the two boxes on the left appear to be of lower frequency (larger) than it is.

Orientation We have been considering patterns that varied along one dimension only; the gratings we have discussed were always oriented the same way. A bit of thought should convince you that a two-dimensional pattern must have two dimensions of frequency components, and that there must be separate sets of spatial frequency analyzers corresponding to different orien-

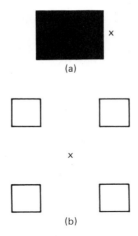

(a)

(b)

FIGURE 10-19 A figural aftereffect of size. Adapting to the pattern at the top causes an apparent shift in size of the test pattern, below. From Köhler, W. and J. Wallach (1944) Figural after-effect, an investigation of visual processes. *Proc. Am. Philos. Soc.* 88:269–357. Reprinted by permission.

tations. In fact, this is the case. Adaptation to a vertical grating (bars that run up and down) has virtually no effect on the detection of a grating of the same frequency that is oriented horizontally (bars running across) (Blakemore & Campbell, 1969). Vertical and horizontal frequencies are detected by their own sets of channels.

As with the selectivity of the channels for spatial frequency, selectivity for orientation is not perfect. Adaptation to a grating that is tilted slightly from vertical will affect the detection of a vertical grating of the same frequency, although not quite as much as it would had the adaptation grating also been vertical. The greater the angle between a test grating and an adapting (or masking) grating, the less effective the adaptation (or masking) will be.

Figural aftereffects based on adaptation to specific orientations may easily be explained by the multiple channel hypothesis. If you adapt to a grating that is tilted slightly to the right of vertical, a subsequently viewed vertical line will appear to be tilted to the left (for example, Gibson, 1937). The explanation could be made using Figure 10–18, only this time the abscissa would be labeled "angle of inclination," and all these channels would be tuned to the same frequencies. (In effect, then, there is a third dimension of the channel picture: preferred orientation of the channels.) If channel 1 is most sensitive to an orientation to the right of vertical, channel 2 is most sensitive to vertical, and channel 3 is sensitive to the left of vertical, adaptation would affect channels 1 and 2, causing the vertical test (t) to appear to be tilted left of vertical.

BOX 10-8

The fact that the channels are tuned to spatial frequency and orientation, allows us to make a further test of the Fourier analysis idea. Consider a checkerboard pattern, as shown in Figure 10–20. Although it seems that the components of a checkerboard are vertical and horizontal, like the edges of the boxes of which it is made, the principal Fourier components are oriented

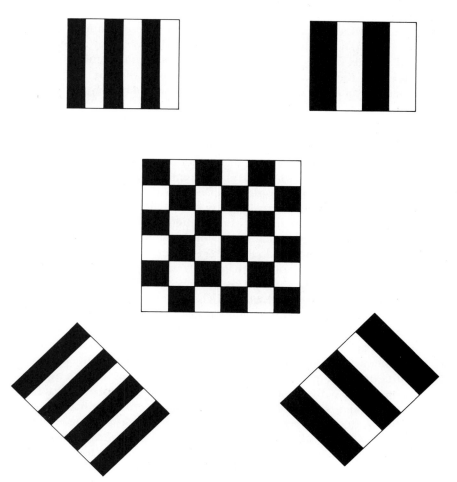

FIGURE 10-20   A checkerboard pattern, and four gratings whose detection might be affected by adaptation to it. Top gratings are vertical; bottom are oriented at 45°. Gratings on the right have a wavelength corresponding to the size of the checkerboard pattern; those on the left have a wavelength 1.4 times as large as the edge of each square.

(continued)

(box continued)
diagonally (Kelly, 1976). You can verify this by defocusing the checkerboard; when only the lowest frequency components are seen, it appears as a sort of plaid at 45° to vertical. Moreover, the fundamental frequency is not determined by the edge-to-edge size of each pair of squares, as might be expected; it is determined by the length of the diagonals of the squares. This spacing is smaller than the edge-to-edge size of each pair of squares by a factor of $\sqrt{2}$.

According to Fourier analysis, adapting to a checkerboard should have the greatest effect on a grating oriented at 45° to the edges of the board, at a spatial frequency whose wavelength is $\sqrt{2}$ larger than the size of the squares. This prediction was tested (Green, Corwin, & Zemon, 1976), and found to be correct. The grating most affected by adapting to a checkerboard such as that in Figure 10–20 would be the one on the lower left in the figure. A similar result was obtained by May and Matteson (1976).

Motion and color   Direction of motion is also selected by channels in the visual system. Among vertically oriented channels, there are some that prefer leftward motion, and some that prefer rightward motion. ("Stationary" gratings, where there is approximately equal motion in both directions because of eye movements, would affect both directions equally.) Adaptation to a rightward moving vertical grating of a particular frequency will affect detection of any vertical grating of the same frequency, but will have the greatest effect on another vertical grating of the same frequency that is moving to the right at a similar speed (Pantle & Sekuler, 1969; Pantle, 1970).

Another aspect of the channels is that they may be color selective (Bradley, Switkes, & DeValois, 1988). Inspection of an orange and black vertical grating and a blue and black horizontal grating causes a black and white vertical grating to appear bluish green and a black and white horizontal grating to appear slightly orange (McCollough, 1965). If you adapt to a red vertical grating and a green horizontal grating by alternately viewing one and then the other and then inspect a pattern made of black and white gratings of the same frequency (Figure 10–21 and Color Plate G on inside cover), the vertical black and white areas appear greenish, and the horizontal areas appear reddish. Rotate the book 90°, and the colors reverse. The reason that a red stimulus produces a green afterimage and vice versa is explained in Chapter 15.

An interesting and disturbing finding is that the McCollough effect is very long-lasting. If you looked at the color plate for a long time (more than a minute or two) in bright lighting, you will see the colors in Figure 10–21 for a long time. The effect lasts hours, days, and sometimes even weeks! This, of course, is very odd for a sensory effect. It suggests that these aspects are not part of the primary sensory process, but occur much higher in the brain. Murch (1976) has suggested that the McCollough effect is actually a form of classical conditioning. Consistent with this, the McCollough effect has been reported to vary with the amount of sleep a person has had, just as other learning tasks do (Lund & MacKay, 1983). For these reasons, it is possible that color is not an attribute of the spatial frequency channels after all.

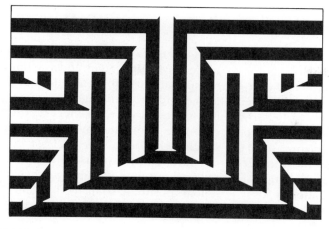

FIGURE 10–21 The McCollough effect. First adapt to the red-and-black and green-and-black gratings on Color Plate G on the inside cover; then inspect this figure.

BOX 10–9

An interesting controversy has developed around an effect similar to the McCollough effect shown in Figure 10–21 and Color Plate G on the inside cover of the book. Riggs (1973) had subjects adapt to a red and black pattern of convex upward curves, and a green and black pattern of convex downward curves (Color Plate D). Inspection of a black and white pattern (Figure 10–22) led to the perception of greenish convex upward curves and reddish convex downward curves.

That result would be consistent with what

Test

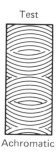

Achromatic

FIGURE 10–22 Color aftereffects based on curvature. (See Color Plate D on the inside cover.) Adapt to the 2 patterns on Color Plate D (printed in red and black and in green and black); the downward-facing curves should now look greenish, and the upward-facing curves should now look reddish. After Riggs, L. A. (1973) Curvature as a feature of pattern vision. *Science* 181:1070–1072. Copyright 1973 by the AAAS. Reprinted by permission of the publisher and author.

(continued)

we have been saying, except that the color seemed to persist through the middle of the figure (that is, the central vertical slice), where the adapting and test curves are all nearly horizontal. Orientation would seem not to be the explanation; Riggs postulated curvature-sensitive channels. He pointed out that the number of types of channels has grown out of hand, and suggested a rethinking of the channel hypothesis.

Others have objected to the results reported by Riggs. Sigel and Nachmias (1975) found that the color really did not persist well in the middle of the figure. Stromeyer (1974) has suggested ways the effect reported by Riggs could be explained by invoking orientation-specific channels. Nevertheless, we must wonder how many aspects of the stimulus each channel is tuned to, and whether it is reasonable to postulate so many different channels.

PHYSIOLOGICAL BASIS OF THE CHANNELS

It is now time to ask what these hypothetical channels might be. What would be the shape of a receptive field that is suited to detecting spatial frequencies? The expected receptive field profile is not a sine wave, as you might expect. A sinusoidal profile, with an infinite number of excitatory hills and inhibitory valleys, would be good for detecting an infinite sinusoidal grating—it would actually be too good. The channels are not exquisitely selective; they accept a fairly wide band of frequencies. According to the mathematics of Fourier transforms, a not-quite-so-selective channel would have a profile in pattern space that looks like the one shown in Figure 10–23. There would be a large central area, flanked by an antagonistic surround, then a much less potent facilitatory region, and so on. Of course, the "sign" (excitatory or inhibitory) is arbitrary, so the same picture upside down would serve just as well.

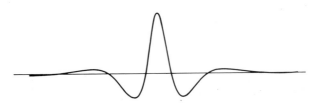

FIGURE 10–23   Receptive field profile corresponding to a channel like those postulated. From Stromeyer, C. F. and S. Klein (1974) Spatial frequency channels in human vision as asymmetric (edge) mechanisms. *Vision Res.* 14: 1409–1420. Reprinted by permission of Pergammon Press, Ltd.

If we neglect the less potent areas outside the first inhibitory surround, this is a cross section of an ON-center ganglion cell receptive field. There is the excitatory center, and the inhibitory surround. If different ganglion cells have different sized receptive fields, they will be differentially selective for spatial frequencies.

The ganglion cell receptive fields lack some important attributes, however. They are circularly symmetric; they would not be orientation-selective, as the channels are. They also seem not to have the extra excitatory and inhibitory regions beyond the surround.

When we think of all the properties of the channels (tuning for frequency, orientation, direction of motion), we naturally begin to suspect the cortex of having the cells corresponding to the channels. Albrecht, DeValois, and Thorell (1980) have reported that both the simple and complex cells of the monkey cortex are considerably more selective for spatial frequencies than they are for the widths of bars. Cortical cells also would seem to be implicated by the fact (not previously mentioned) that adaptation by a grating presented to one eye affects detection of a grating presented to the other eye.

Simple cells of the cortex have most of the requisite properties; they are orientation-selective, can be motion-selective, and can have a profile such as the one in Figure 10–23. (In the cortex, the central region is long and thin, and the antagonistic regions are the "flanks;" see Figure 8–10.) In fact, there are reports that simple cortical cells might have the additional excitatory and inhibitory regions suggested in Figure 10–23 (Maffei & Fiorentini, 1976; Schiller, Finlay, & Volman, 1976a). A model of cortical simple cells as Gabor filters has been presented by Jones and Palmer (1987). Maffei and Fiorentini (1973) report a progressive narrowing of the spatial frequency selectivity as one progresses from retina to lateral geniculate to cortical simple cells.

The complex cells of the cortex do not have receptive fields like the one in Figure 10–23, as their fields cannot be mapped in the traditional way. They certainly do, however, have all the other properties such as orientation and motion selectivity. Selectivity of complex cells to gratings of various frequencies has been measured (Glezer, Cooperman, Ivanov, & Tsherbach, 1976; Schiller, Finlay, & Volman, 1976b), and found to be appropriate for a role as frequency channels. Spatially periodic areas of excitability have been reported (Pollen & Ronner, 1975; Pollen, Andrews, & Feldon, 1978).

A number of researchers have shown that cortical cells have the requisite properties to perform spatial frequency analysis. DeValois, Albrecht, and Thorell (1982) found cells with narrow bandwidths, appropriate for a multiple channel system (see also Robson, Tolhurst, Freeman, & Ohzawa, 1988). Moreover, they found a correlation between spatial frequency tuning and orientation tuning such as would be expected for two-dimensional spatial filters. The spatial frequency tuning is apparently sharpened by a frequency-specific inhibition between cortical cells, as one would expect if spatial frequency were a feature that is being analyzed (DeValois & Tootell, 1983;

Greenlee & Magnussen, 1988). Single cells were also found to be "fooled" by the missing fundamental illusion (similar to Figure 10–12) (Albrecht & DeValois, 1981).

The question of how phase (spatial position) might be encoded is also a concern. Simple cells can encode phase (Pollen & Ronner, 1981), but most of the cortical projection to higher areas is from complex cells. Complex cells apparently do not encode phase, for they do not care where in their field a stimulus may lie (Lee, Elepfandt, & Virsu, 1981; Pollen & Ronner, 1982). However, they do apparently encode the *relative* phase of components of a compound grating, and relative phase is what is needed to distinguish Figure 10–6 from Figure 10–7 (Pollen, Gaska, & Jacobson, 1988).

If spatial frequency is what visual cortex is analyzing, one would expect some structural organization (like the orientation columns or color blobs) that corresponds to spatial frequency. Maffei and Fiorentini (1977) report that selectivity for different spatial frequencies is specific to layers of the cortex. Thus, in the ice cube of Figure 9–5, different spatial frequency channels would be represented in separate horizontal layers. However, given the functions of the layers, it is more likely that the apparent spatial frequency layering is simply due to the different cell types in the different layers. A spatial frequency column system, comparable to the orientation columns but apparently at right angles to them, has been suggested (Berardi, Bisti, Cattaneo, Fiorentini, & Maffei, 1982; DeValois & DeValois, 1988; Tolhurst & Thompson, 1982; Tootell, Silverman, & DeValois, 1981) but is apparently very weakly organized (Shapley & Lennie, 1985). An alternative concentrically organized spatial frequency column system has also been proposed for monkey (see Box 9–2).

SUMMARY

The basic premise of this chapter is that the visual stimulus might at some level be analyzed in terms of the spatial frequency components into which it may be decomposed; in this respect, the visual system performs a Fourier analysis of the stimulus. Rather than a representation of the luminance at each point in space, there is a representation of the contrast at each spatial frequency. This is realized by a series of frequency-selective channels, perhaps cortical neurons. The firing of a given cortical neuron would be interpreted to indicate the presence of contrast at a particular frequency, in the appropriate orientation, moving in the right direction at the appropriate speed, and possibly of the correct color.

BOX 10–10

Does spatial frequency analysis play a role in the way we perceive the world? We have seen that Fourier analysis provides a tool for the study of the visual system, but that does not mean that our perceptions are based on that formulation. There are investigators who maintain that the only reason we find evidence for spatial frequency analysis is that we are testing with stimuli intended to reveal these particular aspects. In that view, the visual system processes spatial frequency information concomitant to processing other, more relevant features. For example, Ullman (1986) suggests that there are receptive fields of various sizes in order to provide for multiscale computations. In his view, the receptive fields (such as those in Figure 10–23) serve to locate edges. In a complex scene, a mixture of different sized edge detectors is far more efficient at finding all the edges than is a collection of identical detectors.

On the other hand, it is difficult to dismiss the apparently elaborate channel system that seems so suited for spatial frequency analysis. It has been suggested (Graham, 1979) that the channels are vital for the mechanism by which we perceive textures, the general roughness or graininess of objects. In this view, the actual identification of objects is based on features coarser than those detected by the spatial fre-quency channels (see Chapter 11); the channels are suited for abstracting secondary characteristics of the object, such as texture. This is like the view presented in Chapter 9, in which the coarse magnocellular system located parts of an object, while the finer grained parvocellular system "filled-in" the details that are often essential for identification of the object.

In this regard, it is noteworthy that psychophysics has shown one or only a few transient (possibly magnocellular) channels, and several sustained (perhaps parvocellular) channels (see page 230). The parvocellular system might perform a Fourier analysis to represent textures, which are recognized independently of the particular placement of details. For example, you recognize a lawn without any reference to the particular placement of the blades of grass; you may not even "see" any of the individual blades.

The more extreme view is that an approximation to Fourier analysis is an integral part of visual perception (Carl & Hall, 1972). According to this view, the spatial frequency components extracted by the visual system form a "pattern" in the frequency domain that is compared to the spatial frequency component patterns stored in memory in order to classify the stimuli presented.

Fourier analysis is no more than another way of representing a pattern in space; it is mathematically equivalent to the more familiar point-by-point description. Perhaps it is surprising that the visual system could operate with a description that we find bizarre, but we do not normally have access to the inner workings of our brains. All we know of the processing is the output, the perception that is generated as the final step. How the nervous system gets from input to perception is hidden from our view; it is, in fact, the topic of this entire book.

SUGGESTED READINGS

Few secondary or general sources have a treatment of the spatial frequency idea; this reflects in part the relative newness of work in the area, and in part the conceptual difficulty the material poses. One exception is the clear exposition in *Sight and Mind*, by L. Kaufman (Oxford, 1974); Chapter 13 develops the concepts of the MTF and the channel hypothesis from a viewpoint somewhat different than the one taken here. A simpler treatment of the way components add to generate complex patterns and of the significance of the MTF may be found in *Visual Perception*, by T. N. Cornsweet (Academic Press, 1970), Chapter 12 (this treatment does not include the channel hypothesis.) For those interested in the mathematical basis of Fourier analysis, we recommend the rigorous but clear and well-illustrated book *The Fast Fourier Transform*, by E. O. Brigham (Prentice-Hall, 1974), Chapters 1–5.

Further illustrations of gratings and the CSF can be found in a *Scientific American* article entitled "Contrast and spatial frequency," by F. Campbell and L. Maffei (November 1974; offprint #1308). Another *Scientific American* article, "The recognition of faces," by L. Harmon (November 1973; offprint #555) includes discussion of computer "boxed" pictures such as the portrait in Figure 10–15. Both of these articles have been reprinted in the collection *Recent Progress in Perception*, edited by R. Held and W. Richards (W. H. Freeman, 1976).

FORM PERCEPTION

11

In the past several chapters we described physiological evidence for the visual system acting to extract useful information from the retinal image while it neglects aspects that are less informative. We have noted that the cells of the retina are sensitive to changes (temporal as well as spatial), but that they disregard long unchanging stimuli. Whether we express the tuning as a spatial frequency filtering that emphasizes higher spatial frequencies, or as a lateral antagonistic network that emphasizes steep gradients, we are saying the same thing: the cells of the retina are more excited by the presence of a border than of a uniform light. We have also seen that the cortex contains cells that seem to be specific for particular features in the array of information presented by the ganglion cells of the retina. We can express the relevant features as lines of particular orientations or as spatial frequencies; either way, cortical cells act to extract information of significance for analysis of the visual scene. Different cortical areas seem also to concentrate on somewhat different aspects of the visual stimulus.

In this chapter, we consider how the features detected by cortical neurons might be used in the generation of a percept. The physiological data we have already discussed take us only a short way into the process; from this point onward we can only guess what physiological correlates there might be for the observed facts of perception. We will consider cognitive descriptions of perception, consider how engineers have devised ways for computers to "perceive," and compare the predictions made by these approaches to observed perceptual phenomena.

First, let us consider what is meant by perception. Perception is the development of an internal representation of the outside world based on the information presented by the senses. This representation is a complete functional description of our environment. It enables us to categorize the objects and images we see; the categories into which stimuli are placed by subjects are often the only data we can have to measure aspects of a subject's perceptions. We should bear in mind, however, that categorization is not the same thing as perception: a sieve categorizes ore particles according to their sizes, but one would never accuse a sieve of perceiving (MacKay, 1967).

If perception is the formation of an internal representation of the world,

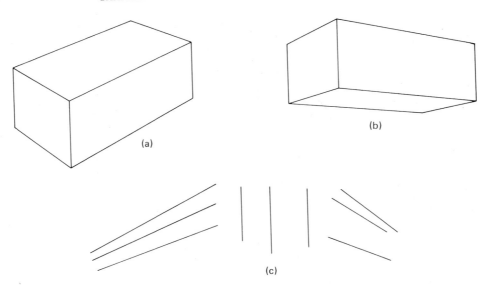

FIGURE 11-1   Visual stimuli. (a) A visual pattern. (b) A pattern that can be seen to be another view of the object in part (a). (c) The component lines of which the pattern in (a) is composed.

information from which the percept is formed are the "features" reported by lower order processors in the sensory system. These features provide a way of summarizing the scene without requiring a point-by-point description. Sutherland (1973) has pointed out that a description could be at a number of different levels. For example, consider the pattern in Figure 11-1(a). When you look at the figure, there is a pattern of light and darkness projected on your retinae; those receptors onto which the image of a black line is projected are in relative darkness, compared to those receiving a projection of an image of white paper. Until the next saccade moves the image, we could describe the figure by listing which cones are in light and which are in darkness.

Your retinae do not pass a point-by-point representation of the image to your brain, however; we have already seen that only ganglion cells with their receptive fields near one of the lines will be firing at rates significantly different from their maintained discharges. Cortical cells are specifically tuned to lines of appropriate length and orientation; we might therefore describe the figure as a collection of nine lines, each at a particular orientation, meeting at seven points to form angles. This is one kind of analysis the cortex appears to be doing.

We may now speculate that cells in some other part of the cortex, sensing particular patterns of excitation of the visual cortical cells, could signal certain plane figures that are formed from the lines. (We mentioned the possibility of these higher order detectors in the discussion of feature detectors in

Chapter 8.) At this level, we could describe Figure 11–1(a) as a collection of three quadrilaterals, each sharing two edges with the other two.

Rather than any of the above descriptions, you are most likely to describe Figure 11–1(a) as a cuboid, a rectangular solid box with three sides visible. That is the percept you probably first experienced when you looked at the figure. It is also the only level of description that would enable you to realize immediately that the object in Figure 11–1(a) and the object in Figure 11–1(b) are one and the same, viewed from different perspectives. This point was emphasized by a school of psychology that arose around the turn of the century, called *gestalt*. In the gestalt view, the whole figure is imbued with a property as a unit that is not evident when one analyzes it as a collection of features. The solidity of the cuboid is not simply an extension of the nine lines of which it is constructed. The same nine lines, rearranged as in Figure 11–1(c) give an impression that is nothing at all like the figure in Figure 11–1(a); the properties of the latter depend on the picture in its entirety.

PATTERN RECOGNITION

A perceptual system capable of determining the three-dimensional nature of Figure 11–1 is obviously performing some complex processing tasks. Before we begin our discussion of these perceptions, let us consider how a perceptual system might analyze the two-dimensional properties of a stimulus. In particular, how might it go about recognizing that Figure 11–1(a) can be described as three quadrilaterals? We accept the notion that cells in the visual cortex can specifically recognize lines, and question how we recognize three lines as a triangle, or another three lines as the letter *H*. This is the problem of pattern recognition.

The simplest form of recognition might be the task performed by a sieve; an object is "recognized" only when it possesses certain size and shape characteristics that match the properties of the sieve. In a similar way, one might compare a stimulus to a set of possible alternative patterns and reply "this one" when the stimulus matches one of the patterns. This scheme is called *template matching* (Selfridge & Neisser, 1960); it is the way the bank's computer "reads" the stylized letters and numbers printed along the bottoms of checks. The premise of template matching is that each stimulus pattern is matched to templates (or patterns) that are internal to the recognizer. One has to assume that the templates can be shifted in orientation or position to be the same as the image, and changed in relative size to effect a match. These assumptions would allow an *H* to be recognized as an "H," no matter whether the image looks like **H** or *H*, and no matter where in the visual field it may be. They do not answer the questions of how the shifting of position or changing of size is accomplished, or of how the mechanism decides it has done all it can and still failed to match a particular template.

There is evidence for template-matching activity in human perception. Subjects asked to recognize that two pictures are different views of the same object (as the two views in Figure 11–1[a] and [b]) take an amount of time to make their decision that depends on how much of a "mental rotation" of the stimulus must be made for the two views to match (Shepard & Metzler, 1971). This mental rotation can even be shown to have a neural correlate in the motor cortex of monkeys (Georgopoulos, Lurito, Petrides, Schwartz, & Massey, 1989). When a subject is shown a pattern that can be interpreted in either of two ways (an ambiguous figure, discussed later in this chapter) after being shown a pattern that is unambiguously one interpretation or the other, the interpretation of the ambiguous version will depend on which unambiguous interpretation was shown. If each of the unambiguous versions is presented to separate areas on the retina, the interpretation given to the ambiguous pattern will tend to agree with the unambiguous version that was shown to the same area of the retina as the ambiguous pattern (Wallach & Austin, 1954). This implies some kind of position preference for the template. Finally, we may note that when a subject is shown a novel pattern (a shape he or she has never seen before) he or she tends to classify it as similar to some known shape except for some set of noted deviations. That is essentially how we see patterns in the clouds: a cloud may look like a dog with two tails, or a face with no nose.

There are, however, a number of serious problems with the template theory. The main problem is that figures that are easily recognized as being of the same class may be quite different physically. A pattern can be drawn with clean black lines on white paper, or it can be done in smudgy pencil; it could even be white chalk on a blackboard. Nevertheless, all three are immediately perceived as the same. We might assume that the feature detectors have somehow cleaned up the smudgy image and treated white on black as equivalent to black on white, but how does the template tolerate wide deviances in details of the figure? Even more disturbing, a character may be recognized as one thing, even though it more nearly matches the ideal template of another. For example, most people would identify the character on the left in Figure 11–2 as a distorted "A," but it is more similar to the template for an "R." Two people's handwritten "H"'s are probably quite different, but we can still read other people's handwriting (well, usually). You have no hesitancy in recognizing a drawing of a face as a representation of the same thing you immediately recognize on the heads of your friends, but think how different these representations are. You can immediately recognize a sketch, or a caricature cartoon, not only as a human face, but as the particular human who is being represented. It is hard to imagine how templates could achieve these results.

The major alternative to a template matching scheme is a "feature-extracting" model. We have already seen that cortical cells seem to be specific to certain features of the visual scene, such as lines, angles, and slopes. It is from such features that the visual system may first construct what David Marr

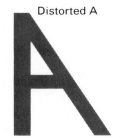 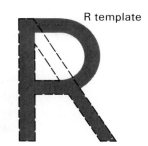 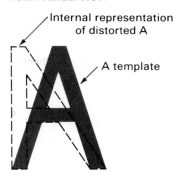

Distorted A   R template   Internal representation of distorted A

A template

FIGURE 11-2 Distorted "A" on the left more nearly matches the template for "R" (center) than for "A" (right). From *Visual Information Processing*. By Kathryn T. Spoehr and Stephen W. Lehmkuhle. Copyright © 1982 by W. H. Freeman and Company. Reprinted with permission.

(1976) has termed a "primal sketch." These would be the "primitives" from which the percept is constructed (although, as Ullman (1986) reminds us, the primitives could just as well be spatial frequencies or Gabor-like components; see Chapter 10). Indeed, the receptive fields we have been discussing in Chapters 6 and 8 are well suited for extracting edge information.

We also know that features such as edges, curves, and lines are the parts of a visual scene that convey the most information about the scene. Attneave (1954) pointed out that there is considerable *redundancy* in a visual scene. Consider a picture such as Figure 11-3 that is made up of a square matrix of picture elements, each of which could be black, white, or gray. Blocks of the same tone tend to cluster together; a block that is surrounded by white blocks will almost certainly also be white, so it is not necessary to specify that particular block. Attneave suggested that if we play a "guessing game" in which you attempt to guess the color of each block successively, the only places you will make mistakes are where there is an as yet undiscovered contour, or where a contour suddenly changes direction. In short, the contours and their limits (corners) contain the information that must be guessed; filling in the solid areas is a foregone conclusion. In fact, it is the same foregone conclusion that the retina assumes the cortex will make when it sends messages only about boundaries. This incorrect assumption can provide a basis for perceiving the Craik-O'Brien pattern as uniform stripes separated by sharp borders (see Figure 6-6; a more complete description of the Craik-O'Brien illusion in terms of its spatial frequency components may be found in the discussion of Figure 10-12).

Artificial Intelligence

Assuming that features such as lines, edges, and corners are the raw materials of which the percept will be built, how might the higher centers proceed to recognize patterns? When the question is phrased in that way, it is natural to

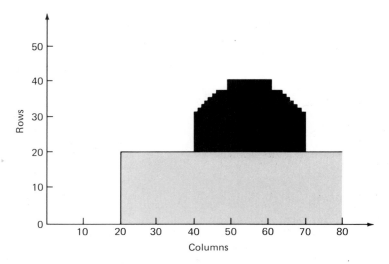

FIGURE 11-3 Figure to demonstrate the importance of redundancy. A subject asked to guess the color of each box will generally only make errors where there is a change in an established pattern. From Attneave, F. (1954) Some informational aspects of visual perception. *Psychol. Rev.* 61:183–193.

ask the related question: how could one build a machine to recognize patterns? Models of perception that start with the feature-extraction notion tend to look like pattern recognition schemes designed for computers (Uhr, 1973), and theories in this area of perception are drawn heavily from the field of artificial intelligence. This is a two-way street: as the psychologist learns from the computer expert what kinds of models will and will not work for specific recognition tasks, the artificial-perception machine designers learn from the psychologist how the most successful pattern recognizers (humans) operate. (For a further discussion, see Barlow, Narasimhan, & Rosenfeld, 1972.)

The artificial intelligence models share many features. Nearly all are the same in that there is a hierarchical structure; that is, the outputs of the computations made at one level go to a higher level structure that performs the next level of processing. We have already seen the lowest levels of a hierarchical structure: ganglion cells extract information about changes in luminance from the array of cones; cortical cells extract information about lines of various orientation from the array of ganglion cells; and presumably the higher level detectors extract information about specific patterns from the array of cortical neurons. At each level the information about the visual scene is represented in progressively more abstract form.

A closer look at one particular artificial intelligence model may help to clarify the way models of this sort operate. The model is called "Pandemonium'' (Selfridge, 1959), and is not only the most cited, it is sufficiently general that many other models are considered special cases of Pandemonium.

Pandemonium assumes a hierarchical organization; at each level is a population of demons, imaginary creatures who scurry about performing their assigned tasks. The demons in each level (does this perhaps bring to mind Dante's *Inferno*?) are individuals, but they have in common a similar level of complexity. Demons at each level receive their information from the inferior demons below them, and in their turn serve the superior demons at the next level above. Communication is by shouting: each demon yells about how well the information he received fits the mold of what he is programmed to seek, and the demons at the higher level extract their information by listening to what particular lower level demons shout to them. Hence the name pandemonium, in reference to the general confusion generated by all the shouting demons. (In fact, the name is extremely apt; it is not a coincidence that the word ''demon'' is embedded in pandemonium. The word is derived from the name of the principal city of Hell in *Paradise Lost*.)

Figure 11–4 shows a pandemonium at work. The demons at the lowest level are the *image demons*. Each reports whether there is light at a particular place in the visual field; they are probably cells in the retina or lateral geniculate nucleus. *Feature demons* listen to all the image demons, but each is hoping to find different groupings of image demons that are shouting loudest. There are ''vertical line'' feature demons, ''left curve'' feature demons, ''right angle'' feature demons, and so forth. Each feature demon shouts out when he can find evidence in the shouts of the image demons for the feature he represents; the better the evidence, the louder he shouts. (Feature demons are reminiscent of cortical neurons.)

The feature demons shout in hope of being noticed by their supervisors, the *cognitive demons*. The model simply extrapolates what has come before: each cognitive demon seeks evidence from the shouts of the feature demons that will support a claim that what he is programmed to recognize is present. The better the evidence, the louder he shouts in hopes of attracting the attention of the omnipotent *decision demon*, who ultimately decides what pattern was, in fact, present.

At each processing level there are demons (detectors) who recognize specific patterns of activity in the demons at the next lower level. The demons at any level are acting in *parallel*; they all look at the same input information at the same time. The concept of parallel processing is a key feature of the Pandemonium model. In fact, Selfridge and Neisser (1960) use the term Pandemonium to refer to *any* parallel processing model. Parallel processing stands in sharp distinction to the *serial* processing often supposed to be present in template matching.

The Pandemonium model also is a serial model, because each level depends on the shouting of the demons at the next lower level. The levels are thus serially arranged, while the demons within each level act in parallel. We shall now consider how both the purely serial and purely parallel processor

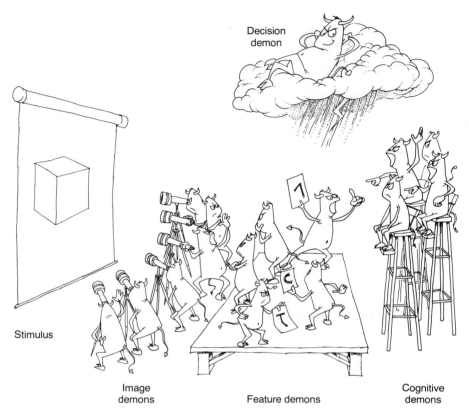

FIGURE 11-4 The Pandemonium pattern recognizer of Selfridge (1959).

might work; of course, one could easily imagine models in which some operations are performed serially, and some are in parallel.

As an example of a serial processing template-match, consider a computer that is programmed to recognize various encoded numbers. In its memory bank is a list of the codes, and a corresponding list of the numbers each represents. A code is given to the machine to identify; it is compared with each of the codes in the memorized list until it is found to match one of them. At this point the search ends, and the number corresponding to the match is reported. How long it takes to recognize the input code depends on how far down the list the search has to go before the match; the *average* search time depends on how long a list must be searched. (Of course, searches can be sped by making some preliminary tests that classify the codes, so that only a portion of the list actually need be searched.)

One advantage to parallel processing is speed. A parallel processor would have a small special computer for each possible code. The input code would go to all the computers at the same time; the answer would be typed out by the one computer that found the code that matched the pattern in its single memory location. Assuming all the computers to be equally efficient, the search time would not vary from input code to input code. The search time would also remain extremely short regardless of how many possible codes there were, but the cost of the system (one computer per code) would increase for long lists.

Perhaps of even greater importance for a perceptual system, parallel processors are less prone to make mistakes. A wrong decision at an early stage would lead a serial processor down the wrong path. For example, if one of the first tests of the character in Figure 11–2 was for vertical line on the left (which would be found), the later tests would be among "B," "D," "E," "F," and so on. "A" would no longer be under consideration, and so could never be found. A parallel processor would simultaneously seek all the possible features, and so the vertical left line would sound only one false note in a chorus otherwise proclaiming an "A."

We have now blurred the distinction between template matching and feature extracting. Templates can be compared in parallel (in fact, the bank machine that reads the numbers on checks does make its comparisons in parallel). What then are "feature detectors" but parallel templates for particular patterns in the input array? The feature demons form an array (not in physical space, but in a transformed "feature" space), and cognitive demons are templates that match particular patterns in feature space. We may think of the feature-extracting model as a more elaborate kind of template matching, with the added sophistication of parallel processing and hierarchical structure.

The advantage to hierarchical structure is that the information presented to the templates is processed into a form that can be readily examined. Moreover, the processed information retains only those aspects of the stimulus array that are relevant for pattern recognition. We need not hypothesize a large number of "equivalent formulation" templates, because the essence has been extracted for presentation to the template. The feature-extraction models, therefore, can overcome many of the objections to ordinary template-matching models (see page 251), even though they are essentially a kind of template matching at each level.

BOX 11–1

Recent artificial intelligence theory has embraced a formulation that is superficially similar to the Pandemonium model. It is called *parallel distributed processing*, or PDP. In PDP, a neural network is hypothesized to con-
(continued)

sist of layers of cells. Cells in the lowest layer receive a pattern of input from the environment (these are the receptors). They communicate with cells in the second layer, with each cell in the lowest layer sending its message to

(box continued)

each cell of the second layer. Cells in the second layer communicate with the cells of the third layer, and so forth.

So far, PDP sounds just like Pandemonium. An important difference is that all cells in a layer do not "hear" all cells in the next lower layer equally well. The linkages from various cells have various strengths, or weightings, so that a particular cell may receive most of its information from a small subset of the lower level cells and feel only a small influence from other lower level cells.

An important theoretical difference between PDP and Pandemonium is that the cells in PDP do not have the personalities of demons. We do not identify cells in one layer as "image demons," and those in another as "cognitive demons." We do not identify a cell as a "vertical line detector," or an "H detector." Activity in a cell is just that: activity. It is not a shout of "I see a horizontal bar." Thus, the same cell may participate in perception of innumerable different stimuli.

What makes the PDP networks "perceive" is that they are modifiable. A pattern of inputs leads to a pattern of outputs, depending on the array of connections among the cells of the various levels. An algorithm that adjusts those connections can adjust the output to a "desired" pattern. The strengths are adjusted "adaptively," until the pattern is learned. Of particular relevance for a perceptual system, which must perceive myriad different patterns, is that learning a new pattern does not eradicate any earlier learning. That is, there are enough connections, with so many possible ways to get from a particular input pattern to a particular output pattern, that many different codings can coexist in a PDP network. A PDP network can learn to process speech, or to read (Bien, 1988). Other PDP networks can deduce the shape of objects from patterns of shading (Lehky & Sejnowski, 1988).

All the models we have been discussing have been hierarchical; that is, information received at the lowest levels is processed by higher levels that pass it to still higher levels. We have made no provision for feedback from higher levels affecting the way the lower levels process information. You may recall, however, that the inner plexiform layer of the retina sent information back to the outer plexiform layer (Chapter 5), that the visual cortex projected back down to the LGN (Chapter 8), and that higher cortical areas sent information to lower areas (Chapter 9). It should not be surprising, then, that processing is not a one-way street.

One way in which a higher level may be affecting lower levels will be discussed later in this chapter, under the heading "Perceptual Set." This refers to effects of context, in which what is perceived depends on what is expected. It is due to these higher influences on perception that you may clearly "see" a threatening person lurking in the shadows of a dark alley; if you stay around to investigate, the "person" turns out to be a smudge on the wall or a cat on a garbage can.

Less dramatic influences of higher centers in guiding the performance of lower levels are referred to as *top-down* processing. Since accurate perception is ultimately guided by the stimulus presented, it is sometimes hard to see evidence of top-down processing. One of the best examples (although it was not presented as top-down processing) is an experiment done by Johnston and McClelland (1974). They presented brief (tachistoscopic) arrays of four letters, and asked subjects to determine whether a particular target letter had been presented. In one condition, subjects were asked to fixate the center position and read the word; in the other condition, they were told which position the target would be in (if presented), and to watch only that position. Surprisingly, subjects did better reading the whole word than monitoring the critical position. That is, it was easier to read an entire four letter word and deduce whether it contained the target letter anywhere within it than to find the target letter in a forewarned position. One would think we recognized the letters in order to read the words, but in this experiment the words were read to identify the component letters. A similar result was obtained for finding lines imbedded in coherent or incoherent figures (Weisstein & Harris, 1974; Wong & Weisstein, 1982).

DEVELOPMENT OF FIGURE AND GROUND

Let us accept the notion that there is a hierarchical feature-extracting system responsible for pattern recognition. Given what we know of physiology, it is not too hard to imagine how the feature demons might work. What can we say about the cognitive demons? Cognitive demons organize features into patterns, and it is these patterns we perceive.

Organization of Features

The question of how features are organized into whole "figures" was actively researched by the gestalt psychologists in the beginning of the 20th-century. They observed that when features were organized into a figure, the figure existed as an entity that was greater than the sum of its individual features. This was pointed out early in our discussion, when we noted that the objects in Figures 11–1(a) and (b) consist of more than three quadrilaterals, or the nine lines Figure 11–1(c). Figures 11–5 through 11–17 will further demonstrate this point.

The gestalt psychologists derived a compendium of the rules by which features (they did not generally use that term) are organized into a coherent whole. These are presumably the rules by which the cognitive demons decide which features comprise a particular figure that they might identify. The principles of organization are relatively obvious once they have been stated, so we will not spend too much time discussing them. For a more elegant discussion, see Wertheimer (1923; abridged and translated into English by his son: Wertheimer, 1958). See also Hochberg (1971a) and Kaufman (1974).

● ●   ● ●   ● ●   ● ●   ●

FIGURE 11-5   Grouping by proximity.

Two of the gestalt principles are concerned simply with the grouping of features; that is, which features will be seen as being part of the same subpattern. The first of these is the *principle of proximity*. Proximity means nearness; things that are close to each other seem to go together. The dots in Figure 11–5 are immediately perceived as four pairs and a single, rather than three triplets. We tend to group nearby items together; however, this is not a simple collation by proximity of the images upon the retina. When we view a person standing in front of a car, the images of the person and the car may be contiguous, yet we do not see person-and-car as a unit.

BOX 11-2

Kaufman (1974) provides an elegant demonstration of the importance of perceived proximity rather than retinal proximity. It is shown in Figure 11–6. In both halves of this figure, the dots are closer to their neighbors to the sides than to the ones above or below; as a result, we tend to organize each figure into horizontal rows of dots. If the figure is viewed as a stereogram, however (see instructions on page viii), we see three *columns* of dots, each column at a different distance than the others. The differences in distance (depth) are greater than the distances in height, so we organize the figure into columns. The apparent spatial proximity rules apply, rather than those of retinal proximity (Rock & Brosgole, 1964).

Another demonstration given by Kaufman (1974) shows the complexity of organization by proximity, although it is not too difficult to explain. The pattern of dots on the left in Figure 11–7 are equally spaced in the horizontal and vertical directions; as a result, the pattern can be seen either as columns or as rows of dots. The percept may spontaneously switch from the one to the other, or both may be seen simultaneously in different areas of the figure. The pattern on the right, however, is spaced so that a clear organization into vertical columns is evident. If you look at the pattern on the right for a minute or two, and then examine the ambiguous array on the left; it will no longer seem ambiguous. There should be a clear tendency for the pattern on the left to be organized into *rows*.

This aftereffect, in which staring at one

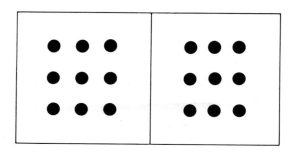

FIGURE 11-6   From *Sight and Mind: An Introduction to Visual Perception* by Lloyd Kaufman. Copyright © 1974 by Oxford University Press, Inc. Reprinted by permission.

(continued)

(box continued)
pattern induces an opposite effect on an in-

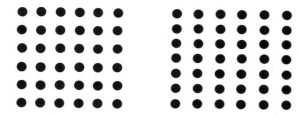

FIGURE 11-7 From *Sight and Mind: An Introduction to Visual Perception* by Lloyd Kaufman. Copyright © 1974 by Oxford University Press, Inc. Reprinted by permission.

spection pattern, is reminiscent of aftereffects discussed in Chapter 10. A group of similar aftereffects was presented in Figure 10-17 (in which inspection of fine gratings made medium ones look coarser), and Color Plate (C) (in which inspection of a red grating made a black and white grating appear green). We can postulate that the reason the pattern on the right in Figure 11-7 appears as vertical columns is that the dots are better at stimulating cortical neurons tuned to vertical lines (or spatial frequencies) than any other orientation. The pattern on the left is ambiguous because it is equally effective for vertical and horizontal detectors. Staring at the figure on the right adapts the vertical detectors (which it stimulates most), so when your gaze is returned to the figure on the left, horizontal detectors are the most responsive.

The *principle of similarity* states that we group like things together. Some examples are given in Figure 11-8. In (a) we see diagonal groups (even though all the elements are equally spaced) because we tend to group solid circles together with other solid circles, and open circles with other open circles. In (b) we see that there is more involved than the amount of stimulation of cortical cells of particular orientations, as the X's group together and the O's group together even though neither is darker than the other. Some complex processing of the shapes must take place before the grouping. This is evident in (c), where there is an obvious boundary between the vertical/horizontal elements and the diagonally oriented ones (Beck, 1972).

The relative importance of proximity versus similarity may be gauged by putting them into conflict (Hochberg & Silverstein, 1956). For example, in Figure 11-9(a), the principle of proximity would dictate that columns be visible, while the principle of similarity would predict the appearance of rows. Chances are, you can see Figure 11-9(a) either as rows of X's between rows of O's *or* as columns of "things." Unlike the ambiguous case shown in Figure 11-7, you probably cannot see both at once. We seem to be capable of choosing whether to see the individual elements in the array, and thus group by similarity, or ignore their identities and group by proximity. By adjusting the spacing between columns, we can favor one principle over the other so that

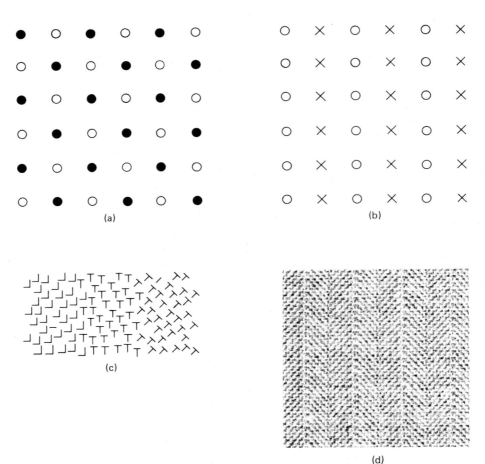

FIGURE 11-8   Grouping by similarity. (a) Dots of similar darkness are grouped. (b) Columns are seen because circles group with circles and "X"s with "X"s. (c) The pattern divides into two segments distinguished by orientation (even though the "T"s in the middle segment are really the same figure as in the right segment, but for a rotation of 45°). (d) A herringbone pattern. All the elements (and spatial frequency components) are diagonal, but vertical stripes are seen. Part (c) from Beck, J. (1966) Effect of orientation and of shape similarity on perceptual grouping. *Percept. Psychophysics* 1:300–302. Reprinted by permission of Psychonomic Society, Inc. and the author. Part (d) from Marr, D. (1982) *Vision*. New York: Freeman.

subjects almost never group the "wrong" way; thus we can devise a metric relating proximity and similarity in this situation.

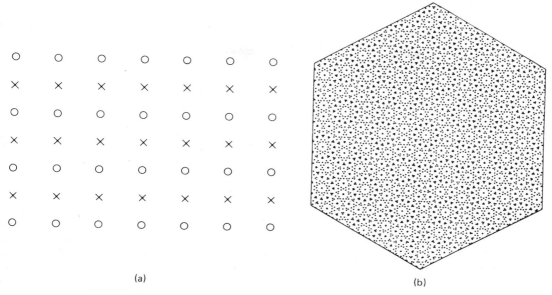

(a)   (b)

FIGURE 11-9   (a) Competition between grouping by proximity (columns) and grouping by similarity (rows). (b) Demonstration of active grouping when multiple possibilities are available. (b) from Marr, D. (1982).

BOX 11-3 ▬▬▬▬▬▬▬▬▬▬

Recognition of the boundaries in Figure 11-8(c) is often cited as an example of texture discrimination. Julesz (1981) refers to a texture discrimination system that is *preattentive*; that is, it is effortless and instantaneous. This system recognizes the units of the pattern, called textons. Textons are discriminated by first-order statistical properties, not simply orientation (Bergen & Adelson, 1988) or spatial frequency (Julesz & Krose, 1988).

A preattentive process would presumably be performed by parallel, rather than by serial search. In fact, Sagi and Julesz (1985) report that recognizing *where* aberrant textons are imbedded in a pattern is indeed a parallel process. On the other hand, recognizing *what* the aberrant elements actually are is a serial process

in which attention is focused on each element in turn. This is an example of how different aspects of the same visual image can be processed in different ways, presumably by separate systems. Notice that *where* and *what* have also been attributed to the magnocellular and parvocellular systems, respectively (see Chapter 9).

If textures are handled by a separate system from that which identifies patterns, you might expect a separate physiological correlate of that system. A class of complex cells in visual cortex, localized in two bands in layers 3 and 5, seem to be the texture-sensitive cells (Edelstyn & Hammond, 1988). These cells respond well to patterns of random dots, and are not particularly sensitive to direction of motion of the patterns.

As you look at Figure 11–9(a) (or the left side of Figure 11–7), you may notice the grouping switching between the possibilities. That is because there is ambiguity, and you can control which "version" you wish to perceive. We will return to this phenomenon later in this chapter. An even more striking example of the active grouping process may be seen in Figure 11–9(b). Marr (1982) describes this figure as one that "seethes with activity as the rival organizations seem to compete with one another" (page 50).

The remaining gestalt principles are slightly more abstract; they suggest that features are grouped according to *prägnanz*, which we generally translate as "good form." We tend to see things as belonging together if they will combine to form a "good" figure; the better the figure, the more strongly they tend to group.

What makes a figure "good"? One aspect is *continuity*, the appearance of a single entity. For example, the dots in Figure 11–10(a) are seen as two curves that cross at the center, as indicated by the dots of two heavinesses in Figure 11–10(b) (where we make use of grouping by similarity to be sure the groups we wish to demonstrate are the ones that are seen). These two continuous curves have more prägnanz than simple grouping by proximity (as indicated in Figure 11–10[c]). A similar effect can be seen in Figure 11–11, the grouping in (b) is more readily seen than that in (c).

Another aspect closely related to continuity is *common fate*, which applies to patterns that are changing in time. Common fate means that items that are moving in the same direction at the same speed are grouped together. Thus slowly moving high clouds are seen as distinct from the more rapidly moving low clouds. Another example is the way we group marching columns formed by a band at football halftime. Columns of

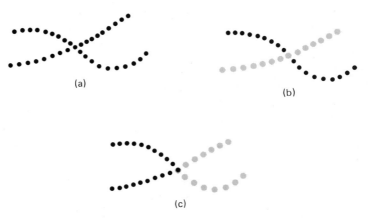

(a)

(b)

(c)

FIGURE 11–10 An example of continuity. (a) A pattern seen as two curves. (b) The two curves into which most people divide the pattern in (a). (c) Alternative pairs of curves that are generally not seen in (a).

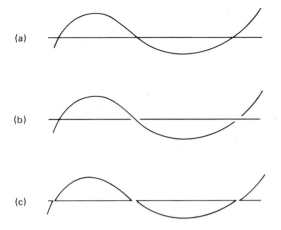

(a)

(b)

(c)

FIGURE 11-11   An example of continuity. (a) A pattern seen as a curve superimposed on a line. (b) The two components usually seen in (a). (c) An alternative grouping of the pattern in (a).

marchers traveling in the same direction are grouped together, and separated from those marching the other way (to whom they might actually be physically closer).

Still another principle of prägnanz related to continuity is *closure*, the tendency to see figures as unitary, enclosed wholes. We not only prefer figures that are enclosed, we may even perform the enclosing ourselves in our mind's eye. Figure 11–12 is an example of this; we have no difficulty in seeing the figure as a circle, even though it fails to meet the simplest definition of a circle as a "plane, closed figure." In fact, at a quick enough glance (or in a tachistoscopic presentation) an observer might not even notice the small gap in the circumference.

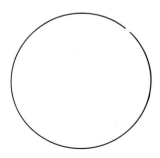

FIGURE 11-12   An almost-circle.

Another contributor to prägnanz is *symmetry*, which is when the right half of the figure is a mirror image of the left half. In geometry, symmetry could be about any axis, not just the vertical midline, but we seem to be considerably better at detecting this form of symmetry than any other (Barlow & Reeves, 1979). Adults' preferences for left-right symmetry are probably related to the fact that small children seem nearly unaware of left-right inversions (for example, in writing the alphabet) although they rarely confuse top and bottom (Rock, 1974). A symmetric form may be more readily perceived than an asymmetric one; for example, the symmetric array of open circles embedded in a background of dots (Figure 11–13[a]) is more readily perceived as a form than the asymmetric array (Figure 11–13[b]). (The form is only visible in any case because of grouping by similarity.)

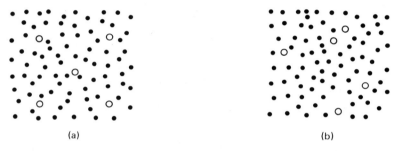

(a)   (b)

FIGURE 11-13   Demonstration of the goodness of symmetry. (a) A symmetric pattern of five circles in a field of dots. (b) An asymmetric pattern of five circles in a field of dots.

Good forms are easier to see (as the form in Figure 11–13[a]) than less good forms (Figure 11–13[b]); they are also harder to decompose into other shapes. As an example, it is harder to see a circle as a forward C butted against a backward C than it is to see the figure in Figure 11–14(a) as the combination of the two patterns in Figure 11–14(b).

BOX 11-4

It is possible to consider the gestalt principles from the standpoint of the spatial frequency concepts presented in Chapter 10 (see Ginsburg, 1975). At least some of the principles may be restated in terms of the spatial frequency spectra of the patterns.

Perhaps the most direct example is closure. The near circle in Figure 11–12 has a spatial frequency spectrum that differs from the spectrum of a whole circle only in the very highest spatial frequencies. If both the circle and the near circle were filtered to remove the highest spatial frequencies (that is, slightly defocused), they would look the same. Closure

(continued)

(box continued)

may be interpreted as a tendency to pay the most attention to the medium spatial frequency components (which are also the largest components). In fact, this particular figure has been used for some time as a test of high frequency capabilities, or *acuity*. It is called a *landolt C*. As discussed in Chapter 4, a person whose eyes are being tested is shown small landolt Cs with their gaps oriented differently, and must say where the gap is (12:00 o'clock, 6:00 o'clock, 9:00 o'clock, and so forth). Acuity, or ability to see fine details (high spatial frequencies), is defined by how narrow a gap can be located accurately.

Proponents of the spatial frequency hypothesis have been quick to point out that the grouping demonstrations may be "explained" by their spatial frequency components (Ginsburg, 1975). Clearly, there is a strong verti-

cally oriented component in Figure 11–7 (right side), and a diagonal component in Figure 11–8(a). These low-frequency components might easily be used to group elements.

The patterns in Figure 11–8(b) and (c) would depend on high spatial frequencies, for it is the details of the elements that are important. Nevertheless, it is notable that there are strong diagonal components in only one of the regions in Figure 11–8(c).

Others argue that spatial frequency is not an essential ingredient. Marr (1982) points out that a herringbone pattern (Figure 11–8[d]) has absolutely no energy in the vertical Fourier component, yet is seen as vertical stripes. Similarly, if the dots in Figure 11–7 (right) are replaced with dark and light "ripples" on a medium-gray background, the grouping persists even though there are no low-frequency components (Jáñez, 1984).

The foregoing should give a fair intuitive sense of what is meant by prägnanz, but it would be preferable to be able to define it in a more precise way. Two lines of investigation into the quantification of prägnanz are particularly worthy of mention; one of these is to equate it with simplicity; a good figure is less complex than a poor figure. Complexity can be defined as a weighted sum of a number of attributes such as curvature, angularity, num-

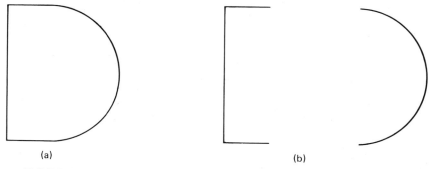

(a)   (b)

FIGURE 11–14 Decomposition of a figure into two good forms. (a) The figure. (b) The two components.

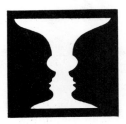

FIGURE 11-15   A pattern in which figure and ground may exchange roles. The pattern may be seen either as 2 silhouetted faces or as a white vase.

BOX 11-5

Just as the figure appears to be in front of the ground, the ground seems to extend behind the figure. How compelling this appearance is was demonstrated by Weisstein (1970). She had subjects inspect the picture shown in Figure 11–16, a drawing of a cube standing in front of a regular grating. Within 50 msec after presentation of this pattern, the subjects were shown a sinusoidal grating of the same spatial frequency as the ground. The grating fell on the area of retina corresponding to the blank white top surface of the cube (Figure 11–16[b]). Subjects were asked to rate the apparent contrast of the test grating;

contrast was decreased after inspection of the cube pattern, just as it would be following adaptation to a similar frequency grating (see Chapter 10). The grating in the background lowered the contrast of the test, implying that the subjects adapted as if the frequency channels somehow knew the grating extended behind the cube. (It should be noted that this effect could also be explained if one merely assumed the spatial frequency channels that are being adapted cover a large area of visual space, as suggested by Weisstein, Harris, Berbaum, Tangney, and Williams, 1977.)

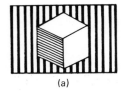
(a)

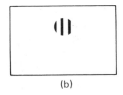
(b)

FIGURE 11-16   Stimuli used to demonstrate masking ''in back of'' an object. (a) Adaptation stimulus. (b) Test pattern to be detected after adaptation. From Weisstein, N. (1970) Neural symbolic activity: A psychophysical measure. *Science* 168:1489–1491. Copyright 1970 by the AAAS. Reprinted by permission of the publisher and author.

ber of sides, and most important, the ratio of the perimeter squared to the area (P^2/A) (Attneave, 1957; Stenson, 1966). Alternatively, complexity may be related to the number of features (lines, angles, areas) that need be sampled in order to apprehend the entire figure (Vitz & Todd, 1971).

The other way to look at prägnanz also equates it with simplicity, but of a different kind. In this view, simplicity means low information content, with information defined in the strict mathematical sense used in communication theory. Information is measured by how many "bits" are needed to specify a figure. If a figure is a member of a class that could only contain two figures, a single bit is needed (one two-choice question must be answered); if there are four members of the set, then two bits are needed (two questions: one to divide the four into two groups, and one to decide which of the two remaining is "it"). Eight figures in a class requires three bits and so on. Using this reasoning, the more predictable the figure, the less information (in terms of number of bits) the figure contains. Very predictable figures are, in general, said to have good form. This way of looking at figural goodness was suggested independently by Hochberg and McAlister (1953) and Attneave (1954). Attneave found that the visibility of figures partially obscured by extraneous details was inversely related to their information content. He also found that

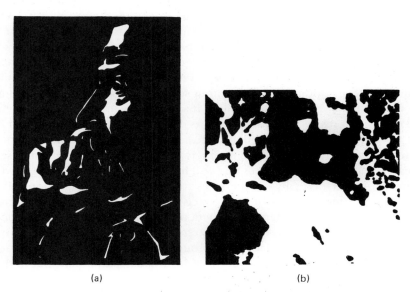

(a)   (b)

FIGURE 11-17 Two figures that are initially difficult to recognize. Part (a) from Mooney, C. M. and G. A. Ferguson (1951) A new test of closure. *Can. J. Psychol.* 5:129–133. Reprinted by permission of the author. Part (b) from Porter, P. B. (1954) Another picture puzzle. *Am. J. Psychol.* 67:550–551. Copyright © 1954 by the Board of Trustees of the University of Illinois. Reprinted by permission.

figures that seemed complicated but were symmetric, and therefore contained no more information than apparently simpler figures, were as visible as the seemingly simpler ones. (In fact, they were slightly *more* visible, indicating that information content is not the whole story.)

Figure and Ground

We have been discussing the principles by which the cognitive demons organize features into figures. What then? When features are organized into a figure, do their properties somehow change?

The answer is yes; the figure becomes a distinct entity with properties that set it apart from the remainder of the scene. The figure becomes real and apparently solid (the gestaltists said it had "dingstoff"—"thingness"). The rest of the scene, referred to as the *ground*, seems less substantial, and appears to recede behind the figure.

The distinction between figure and ground is dramatically illustrated by Figure 11–15. This is an ambiguous pattern; it can be seen in either of two ways. On the one hand it can be seen as two silhouetted faces staring at each other, nearly nose-to-nose. On the other hand, it can be seen as a white vase or goblet, in front of a black wall. Once you have seen it each way, you can easily switch from the one to the other. The thing to notice, however, is that when you see the two faces they appear to be substantial, they stand in front of the white background (of no particular depth or substance), and the borders between the black and white areas "belong" to the black faces. When the vase is the figure, the reverse is true: the white vase seems to be in front of a nondescript black background, and the contour seems to belong to the white figure.

Once a figure has become evident, it seems to be imbued with a strength and reality that resists dissolution into its elements. For example, look at Figure 11–17. It probably seems that there are two random groupings of meaningless shapes. In fact, these are photographs, at extremely high contrast, of faces. Sketches of these pictures that will help you find the faces are shown in Figure 11–18. Once you see the faces, the pictures no longer look like a smattering of meaningless blobs. Notice that they acquire a three-dimensional depth that was certainly not evident when they were seen as blobs.

The faces in Figure 11–17 demonstrate another point: despite the apparent emphasis the retina places on contours, a perceived figure need not be neatly bounded by a complete outline. Closure may play a part, but in these cases, there is less contour present than absent. Similarly, four dots appropriately placed are immediately seen as forming the corners of a square, even though none of the contours of the square is present.

It is sometimes possible to suggest contours where there are none, and still form a figure. The suggested contours are generally called *subjective contours* (Schumann, 1904). An example of a triangle formed by subjective contours is shown in Figure 11–19; the three vertices are suggested as superimposed on the three black circles, but the sides themselves are not drawn. Despite the lack of actual sides, the triangle appears as a quite distinct figure.

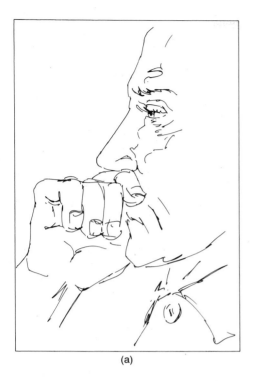

(a)

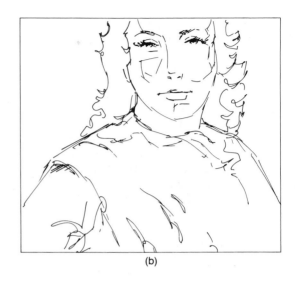

(b)

FIGURE 11-18 Sketches that will help you see the faces in Figure 11–17.

It has the properties we have already mentioned figures tend to have: it appears to have substance, it appears to be in front of the ground, and the subjective contour "belongs" to the triangle rather than to the eclipsed circles. The triangle also has one other feature commonly associated with the figure:

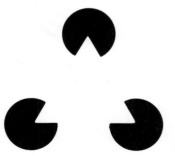

FIGURE 11-19 A triangle generated by subjective contours. After Coren (1972) Subjective contours and apparent depth. *Psych. Rev.* 79:359–367. Copyright © 1972 by the American Psychological Association. Adapted by permission.

it appears lighter than the ground. This is an anomalous brightness, as the triangle consists of the same white paper as the rest of the page; it somehow seems that there is a change in lightness at the subjective contour, even though the contour is not actually present.

BOX 11-6

Subjective contours, like the triangle in Figure 11–19, are usually explained as the visual system's means of "explaining" an apparent occlusion of one set of objects (the black circles) by an overlying object (the white triangle). That determined, the triangle appears lighter (compared to the circles), and so appears whiter than the surrounding paper. Notice the top-down flow of information: the occlusion generates the boundary (an edge, which should have been a primitive) and the edge generates the lightness gradient (which should be how we find edges).

Subjective contours do not require luminance gradients. Figure 11–20(a) shows a curved edge created by a change of the spatial phase in the striped pattern. This can even give rise to a second-order effect, as shown in Figure 11–20(b). Four "pac-men" are generated by phase changes (the shift in position of the stripes) like the curve in part (a). The pac-men in turn generate a square that stands in front of the striped background.

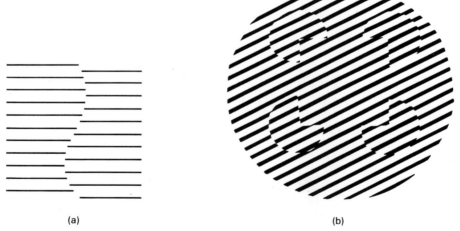

(a)   (b)

FIGURE 11–20   Phase-induced subjective contours. (a) A curved edge is seen where the phase of the lines changes. (b) The corners of a subjective square are generated by "pac-men" that are themselves generated by a phase change (from Petry & McShane, 1988). Part (a) from Gaetano Kanizsa, *Organization in Vision: Essays on Gestalt Perception* (Praeger Publishers, New York, 1979), p. 204. Copyright © 1979 by Gaetano Kanizsa. Reprinted with permission.

(continued)

(box continued)

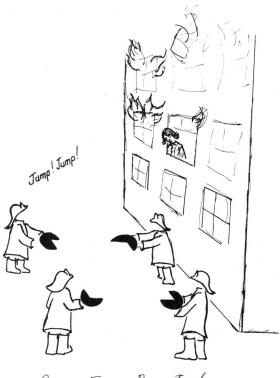

Jump! Jump!

GESTALT FIREMEN PLAY A JOKE!

Demonstration that humor is subjective (and illusory). By Meyer, G.E. (drawn by S. Petry) (1987) *Perception* 16:412.

A confirmation of the occlusion hypothesis can be found by deliberately making the occluder lie in front of or behind the occluded pattern (Braddick, 1988). The stereogram in Figure 11–21(a) is set up so that the horizontal strips appear in front of the face; that in Figure 11–21(b) is set up as if the face were "painted" on the strips. Notice that the same strips of face appear quite different in the two stereograms.

We have already seen that subjective contours can be "detected" by cortical cells (page 199). Which systems are responsible? Livingstone and Hubel (1987b) report that subjective contours are not seen at equiluminance, and take this as evidence that the magnocellular system is responsible for this effect (see page 208). Others find that subjective contours *are* present at equiluminance (Ejima & Takahashi, 1988). However, there are at least two aspects to subjective contours: the sharpness of the edge and the brightness of the surface. These aspects can be dissociated. Sharpness of the contour is enhanced under conditions that favor the parvocellular system; on the other hand, the brightness of the illusory shape is enhanced when the magnocellular system should be most active (Petry & Siegel, 1989).

The solidity of figures formed of subjective contours may be demonstrated by showing that they are nearly as effective as real contours in generating illusions. This is shown in Figure 11–22. In (a) of the figure is a familiar illusion, the *Poggendorf* figure. The usual way presenting it is to have a rectangle eclipse a straight line; the interposition of the rectangle makes the two visible segments of the line appear to be misaligned. There are nearly as many theories about why this occurs as there are psychologists who have devoted attention to it; many postulate either an interaction of the interrupted line with the contour of the rectangle, or an overestimation of the acute angles formed between the

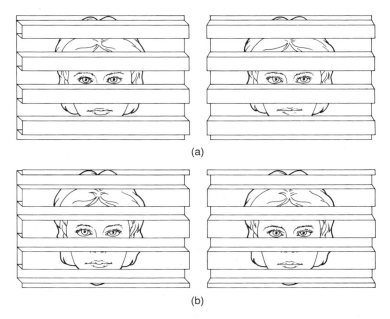

FIGURE 11-21   The same strips of a picture give different results when made to appear behind occluding strips (a) or pasted on the strips (b). View these stereograms as indicated in the box on page x. From Braddick, O. (1988) Contours revealed by concealment. *Nature* 33:803–804. Based on work by Nakayama, later published in *Perception* 18:55–68 (1989). Reprinted by permission of the author.

line segments and the contour. Confirm their alignment by placing a straight-edge along the lines, or by sighting along them from the edge of the page.

Figure 11–22(b) shows the same line segments as in (a), without the rectangle. In this case there should be no difficulty seeing the line segment to the right aligns with the one on the left. Part (c) repeats the same line segments, eclipsed by a rectangle formed by subjective contours. Most people find that there is an illusory effect caused by the subjective rectangle; most likely, the continuation of the line to the left appears to fall below the segment to the right. The Poggendorf illusion can be quite strong, but you apparently learn to overcome it and not be fooled. Some people seem never to get this illusion and very young children are most readily fooled (Leibowitz & Gwozdecki, 1967).

Another indication of the importance of the figure as a whole is the demonstration that it can have properties independent of its parts. This is most dramatically demonstrated when the same shape takes on a new identity because of a change in orientation. The two shapes in Figure 11–23 are identical but for a rotation by $45°$. The one on the left is a square; on the right it is a diamond. Turn the book $45°$ and cover the frame around the figure; the diamond is really the square turned on end. Until this intellectual discovery is

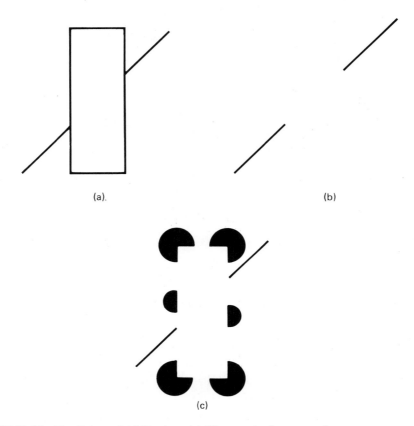

(a).   (b)

(c)

FIGURE 11-22   The Poggendorf illusion. (a) The standard pattern; the
presence of the rectangle makes it difficult to see which
of the diagonal lines on the right aligns with the diagonal
line on the left. (b) The same diagonal lines as in (a),
without the rectangle. Alignment is easy to determine.
(c) The illusion with a rectangle generated by subjective
contours. Most people find alignment hard to determine.

made, however, the diamond and the square are perceived as different figures. For example, an obvious attribute of the square is that the four corners

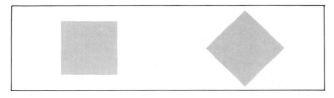

FIGURE 11-23   A square and a diamond. The diamond is the same as
the square except that it has been rotated 45°.

are right angles, but this is not as obvious in the diamond. Even the apparent sizes of the figures are affected, the diamond seeming larger than the square.

BOX 11-7

Whether an equilateral quadrilateral will be seen as a diamond or a square depends on its orientation; this implies a frame of reference against which orientation is measured. In Figure 11–23, the figure to the left appears to be a square because it is oriented the same way as the book (which you are presumably holding right side up); we have further enhanced your perception of vertical being toward the top of the page by drawing a rectangular frame around the entire figure. In this case, there is no conflict between actual vertical (the pull of gravity), retinal vertical (the direction on your retinae from cheeks to forehead), and apparent vertical (the frame around the picture).

We can now disrupt any one of these cues to the vertical and see whether the percept goes with it or with the others. For example, tilting the book and your head 45° to the side while looking at Figure 11–23 should have no effect on your perception of the square and the diamond; gravity is not a very important cue to the vertical. The visual frame is the most important cue in this case: turning the book 45° but leaving your head erect is not likely to change the square into a diamond. (It might have some effect on the diamond in that you *can* see it as a square; remember, however, that you have rotated only a part of the visual frame: the room around the book remains vertical.) Changing the visual frame, on the other hand, has a potent effect. Figure 11–24 shows a pattern of diamonds. The diamonds in the line along the top of the figure are seen as diamonds, but the cluster in the lower right create a 45° frame of reference, so the figures can easily be seen as squares (Attneave, 1971). Notice that the same figures in the upper right can be seen either as diamonds or as squares, depending on which other figures they are grouped with.

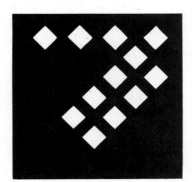

FIGURE 11-24   A pattern of diamonds that can be seen either as diamonds or squares. From Attneave, F. (1971) Multistability in perception. In *Recent Progress in Perception*, by R. Held and W. Richards. Copyright © 1976 by Scientific American, Inc. Reprinted with permission by W. H. Freeman and Company.

(continued)

(box continued)

Rock (1974) pointed out that the visual frame of reference is dominant only in the case of simple figures such as squares and diamonds. More complex figures, such as letters or faces, depend more strongly on retinal orientation than the visual frame of reference. This is why when you read lying on your side in bed, you must turn the book sideways also. Rock demonstrated his point with a series of "invertible" faces, faces that look like one person when viewed right side up but appear to be a different character when viewed upside down (180° rotation). Look at the face in Figure 11–25(a); now turn the book upside down and look at it again to see the alternative face. Turning the book over changes both the retinal and the visual frame of reference for vertical. You could change the visual frame by turning the book over, but maintain the retinal orientation by also turning yourself over. The easiest way to do this is to hold the book upside down behind your legs and bend over to view it from between your knees (we don't recommend trying this demonstration in a public place). You will see only the face that you saw in the normal right side up orientation of the book.

This not only applies to faces, but to other complex stimuli like writing. The logo in Figure 11–25(b) was designed by space scientists working on an interplanetary probe that would fly past Saturn, then go to Uranus.

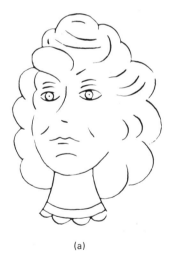

(a)

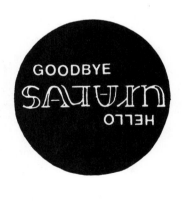

(b)

FIGURE 11–25 Invertible figures. (a) When the book is turned upside down, a different face is seen. (b) The word "Saturn" becomes "Uranus" when turned upside-down. (a) From "The perception of disoriented figures," by Irvin Rock. Copyright © 1974 by Scientific American, Inc. All rights reserved. (b) Copyright Chicago Sun Times.

Masking

We have already discussed visual masking, in Chapter 10, as a method of demonstrating that test patterns of a particular spatial frequency are most affected by other patterns of similar frequency. Visual masking is a far older idea than the spatial frequency channel hypothesis; the original masking experiments were performed in the hope of elucidating the way in which figures are perceived. Both simultaneous masking and backward masking have been exploited toward this end.

Simultaneous masking, in which the test pattern and the mask are present at the same time, is a form of camouflage. If the test is enough like the mask, it will be effectively hidden. One way in which the test and mask must be similar is in terms of their spatial frequency spectra; this was demonstrated by Figure 10–16, in which Lincoln's portrait is hidden best when the mask (boxes) have energy in spatial frequencies near those of the portrait. Other aspects of the mask also play a role, and these are often predicted by the principles of organization we have discussed. If the mask is as likely to be grouped with the features as the features are with each other, incorrect groupings will be made and the figure will be obscured. For example, in Figure 11–26 the same figure, a printed numeral 4, is hidden in all three parts of the figure. The camouflage is best in (a), where the masking elements are just like the figure elements, and approach them in ways that promote closure, continuation, and general prägnanz. In (b) the camouflage is not as good, despite the similarity of the mask elements to the figure, because closure and continuation are not implied. In (c), the mask elements are somewhat different, and continuation works against confusing the figure with the mask. Similar principles may be invoked to explain the camouflage in Figure 11–27; the person is hard to see because he fits the "s" of the writing by continuation.

BOX 11–8

For simultaneous masking to be effective, the mask and target must share certain properties, including location. If the mask and target appear to be at different distances from the observer, there will be less masking (Lehmkuhle & Fox, 1980; Schneider, Moraglia, & Jepson, 1989). This can be arranged with stereoscopic images. For example, the letter hidden in the stereogram of Figure 11–28 is difficult to find in either frame alone. But when the frames are fused, the letter stands out clearly from the masking lines.

Backward masking was used by Werner (1935) to demonstrate the importance of contour in the perception of figures. He used a tachistoscope to present two figures to the same part of the visual field: the first figure was a solid square, the second was a heavy open square that fit around the first square (see Figure 11–29). A gray interval of 150 msec intervened between

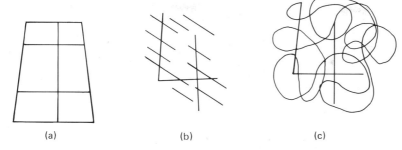

(a)   (b)   (c)

FIGURE 11–26   Camouflage (simultaneous masking) of the numeral 4. (a) The 4 is well masked. (b) and (c) The 4 is poorly masked.

the two presentations. The open square masked the smaller solid one; Werner hypothesized that the contour defining the solid square had had insufficient time to be established by the time the outer square appeared and canceled it. As the "dark inward" contour was lost, the entire dark area was not perceived. This is reminiscent of the "filling in" of areas bounded by a contour that is responsible for the Craik-O'Brien illusion (Figure 6–6).

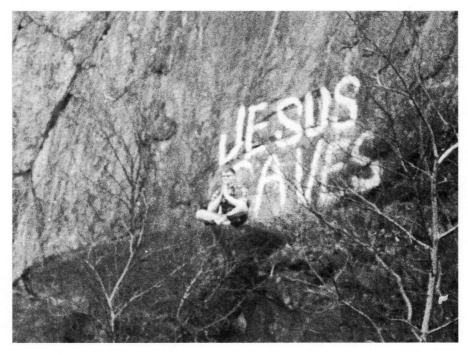

FIGURE 11–27   Camouflage on a mountainside. A person is seated cross-legged before the first S in SAVES.

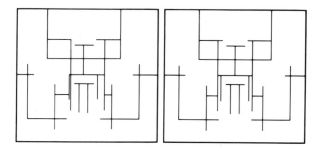

FIGURE 11-28   Stereogram in which depth information "unmasks" the hidden letter. View according to instructions in the box on page x.

(a)   (b)

FIGURE 11-29   Backward masking. (a) A square the subject is asked to detect. (b) Mask, that prevents detection of (a) if presented shortly after it. After Werner, H. (1935) Studies on contour. *Am. J. Psychol.* 47:40–64. Reprinted by permission.

BOX 11-9

A special name has been given to backward masking in which the test figure and the mask fall on different areas of retina: it is called *metacontrast*. The contour loss postulated by Werner is not the only interpretation of why this occurs. Weisstein (1968) has suggested that metacontrast may be explained as a form of lateral antagonism, if we assume that the antagonistic effect (from the mask) develops more slowly than the excitatory effect (from the test). It is likely, however, that metacontrast is more complex than simple retinal interaction; for example, Bernstein, Fisicaro, and Fox (1976) have suggested that the mechanism of metacontrast may be different for short delays between mask and test than the mechanism for long delays. They also suggest that information about the test and the mask are extracted separately before the two interact.

PERCEPTUAL HYPOTHESES

Up to this point, we have been discussing pattern recognition as if the categorization of stimuli were the principal goal of a perceptual system. Except for an occasional reference to our ability to influence perception by conscious effort, we have treated the human visual system as if it were no more than a fancy and versatile version of the machine that reads the code numbers on bank checks. It is now time to try to deal with those properties that set it apart from a sieve that sorts ore by size.

Synthesizer Models

An alternative to a model in which a stimulus is sorted and channeled to the appropriate cognitive demon is one in which an internal representation consonant with the stimulus is constructed by an active synthetic process (Neisser, 1967). In this kind of model, perception is viewed as an active process in which the perceiver makes and tests hypotheses about what physical things in the outside world could give rise to the pattern of stimulation reported by his or her retinae. Here we are drawing a distinction between two kinds of stimuli: the *distal stimulus*, which is the real set of objects "out there" in the world, and the *proximal stimulus*, which is the pattern of stimulation on the retinae. This same distinction will prove important in our discussions of distance perception and constancies, which comprise the next two chapters.

The act of perception, then, is to make a best guess about what distal stimulus is likely to correspond to the proximal stimulus being sensed. This subconscious guess is termed the *perceptual hypothesis*. The active synthesis theories postulate that an internal cognitive model is built, and views of how the model should appear are compared with the proximal stimulus. If the comparison proves valid, the hypothesis is accepted and we "see" the model we have constructed; if it is at variance with the facts (proximal stimulus), the hypothesis is rejected or modified. Probably the best example of an analysis-by-synthesis perception model is the motor theory of speech perception (Liberman, 1957), which we shall consider in Chapter 19. The construction of models of the three-dimensional world (Marr, 1982) will be considered in Chapter 12. In each case, the hypotheses about what is being seen guides the way the sensory information is used to make the models. In this sense, these schemes include top-down processing.

Although the synthesis of an internal model is quite different from the decision making of a decision demon, it is not necessary to assume that perception is either synthetic or feature extracting (or template matching). MacKay (1967) pointed out that both a parallel set of feature extractors (he refers to these as "filters") and a synthesizer have their own distinct advantages. The parallel filters have the advantage of speed (see page 256), while the synthesizer has the advantage of generality. The synthesizer would take a long time to build a model from "scratch," but it presumably could eventually construct one for nearly any input. The parallel filters are fast, but an inordinate number of them would be needed to cover all possible inputs (and in designing a system, it would be impossible to be sure all possible future contingencies have been covered). MacKay suggests that the perceptual system is designed to capitalize on the advantages of each: a set of parallel filters extracts features from the proximal stimulus, and it is this highly digested representation of the stimulus that is presented to the synthesizer.

Cognitive Learning

There is another aspect of human (and probably most animal) perceptual systems of which we have not made a point, but undoubtedly is essential. If we assume the existence of cognitive demons, we must ask how there could be a demon that recognizes the letter H—it is absurd to believe that English-speaking people are born with the alphabet built into their cognitive systems. When we speak of a perceptual hypothesis, whether we refer to it as a guess about the real world, or as an active synthesis of a model of the world, we must ask how the rules for making these guesses were derived. At some point, we must postulate that at least some of perception is learned.

A theory of form recognition based entirely on learning was proposed by Hebb (1949). It is called the "cell-assembly theory," and it postulates that for each proximal stimulus some particular group of cells is excited. When these groupings recur, the synaptic attachments among them are strengthened; cell assemblies in the associated cortex would link assemblies corresponding to particular interpretation of the world (derived from various senses). Assemblies of this sort might correspond to cognitive demons, or they might correspond to sets of rules that guide the perceptual hypothesis mechanism (see Box 11–1).

Our current understanding of how learning (of any kind) occurs in the brain is still far too incomplete to justify a more specific description than the notion of a "cell assembly." Synapses might be strengthened, new ones may form, or chemical changes might occur in neurons; the important point is that some kind of learning may be required to "teach" the brain how to perceive. This does not mean that all of perception is learned; we have already seen in Chapter 9 that cells of the visual cortex have many of their adult properties in the neonate. Aberrant visual experience seems only to modify or negate these "inborn" properties (a kind of "learning" in the cortex). Remember, however, that the cells we were discussing in Chapter 9 probably correspond to the most elemental feature detectors, not to the cognitive demons or hypothesis makers higher in the processing hierarchy.

BOX 11–10

Some evidence of the importance of early experience in "teaching" perceptual systems how to perform their tasks comes from cases in which humans who were blind from birth have had their sight restored later in life. Usually, the blinding was because of a cataract, and the restored sight a result of successful removal of the cataract.

Cataract operations were performed successfully in the 1770s; when sight was re-

(continued)

(box continued)

stored, patients went through a period of "learning to see." One patient was "far from making any judgment about distances" and "could form no judgment about . . . shape." This young gentleman having often forgot which was the cat, and which the dog, he was ashamed to ask; but catching the cat (which he knew by feeling) he was observed to look at her steadfastly, and then setting her down said, 'So Puss, I shall know you another time' (Priestly, 1772, p. 722).

More modern accounts of restored sight bear out these earlier accounts. Gregory (1978; Gregory & Wallace, 1963) reported on the restored sight of a man who had a corneal transplant. Although the patient did not "sud-

denly see" when the bandages were removed, he was capable of considerable visual perception after a few days. He was not really required to learn to perceive, however, for he had already learned to map the world using his other senses. What he was required to do was to learn how the visual stimuli he was receiving corresponded to the familiar tactile and auditory stimuli accompanying them. He performed best at perceiving things he knew from his other senses, but had considerable difficulty with purely visual phenomena (such as judging height from a window). He did show evidence of visual learning, in that his drawings of the world gradually came to include features he did not know by touch, such as writing.

Perceptual Set

If there is cognitive learning, perception is to some extent a function of what has been learned. There are two factors at work here: one is the overall question of what demons have been developed, what hypotheses encouraged; the other is the question of which of the many available sets of demons or types of hypotheses to try first in the current situation.

The first factor supposes a difference in perception among people of differing perceptual backgrounds, more generally a *cultural* difference. Anyone accustomed to the English alphabet will immediately perceive two poles with a crossbar at midheight as an H, but that description would probably not occur to a Japanese. We immediately recognize a distant airplane as a large, distant object, but a transplanted prehistoric person might see it as an odd, slow-flying bird—even going so far as to "see" the wings flapping.

These cultural differences have been invoked to explain differences in the susceptibility of certain groups of people to illusions that seem to depend on misinterpretation of line figures (these illusions will be discussed in Chapter 13). Segall, Campbell, and Herskovits (1963) found differences between European and African people, and attributed them to the Europeans' familiarity with a "carpentered environment." That is, Europeans are accustomed to straight walls, roads, and so on, and easily form impressions of depth from the implications of linear perspective (see Chapter 12). People from undeveloped cultures are not familiar with linear perspective, and therefore are not fooled by the illusions; they simply do not make the same perceptual hypotheses when shown a pattern of nonparallel straight lines. This interpretation has come under some criticisms; for example, Jahoda (1966) verified the findings for European and people from undeveloped countries, but found no difference between the people from undeveloped countries who lived in carpentered and those who lived in uncarpentered environments. This does not mean that perceptual experience plays no role, only that this particular cultural difference may not account for the differential results with these illusions.

The second factor, _set_, depends on the more immediate experience of the perceiver. This may best be demonstrated by perception of what have been called *ambiguous figures*. Ambiguous figures are patterns that can be perceived in either of two ways; often, the perception switches back and forth between the interpretations once each has been seen. Such a pattern is shown in Figure 11–30, called the "my wife and my mother-in-law" drawing (Boring, 1930). This pattern can be seen as either an old woman with her chin down on her breast, or a young woman with her head turned nearly away looking over her shoulder. With slight modifications, the figure can be made much less ambiguous, much more likely to be seen as the "wife" (Figure 11–31[a]) or as the "mother-in-law" (Figure 11–31[b]). Leeper (1935) used similar unambiguous drawings to create a set for subjects who were shown the ambiguous version. Subjects shown the "wife" first saw the young woman when shown the ambiguous version, while those shown the "mother-in-law" saw the old woman.

This might be considered a demonstration of the persistence of a figure, however, rather than of the influence of set. Quite possibly when you first saw Figure 11–30 you saw only the younger or only the older woman and could not find the other until you used Figure 11–31 as a guide. Once you saw it both ways, however, you probably had little trouble in seeing either configuration. This similar to the demonstrations in Figure 11–17; once you saw the faces in that figure, they appeared spontaneously whenever you looked at it. Similarly, the person in Figure 11–27 may have gone unnoticed when you looked at the picture, but once you saw him he stood out vividly.

Perhaps a better demonstration of set is the way you interpret particular patterns according to context. For example, you have no difficulty in seeing that Figure 11–32 shows the word "title" written twice: once in capital letters, once in lower case. You also have no difficulty in recognizing that the straight vertical line that is the second letter in the uppercase version is an "I," while the identical straight vertical line that is the fourth letter in the lowercase version is an "L." You perceive the same single stroke differently depending on whether you are in a capital or lowercase mode.

Context effects can be even more complex than a change of mode. You have no difficulty with Is and Ls in mixed upper and lowercase writing. You also can immediately perceive an ambiguous letter in one form or another depending on context. For example, the second letters in each of the two

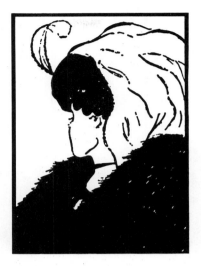

FIGURE 11-30   "My wife and my mother-in-law." An ambiguous figure
from Boring, E. G. (1930) A new ambiguous figure.
Am. J. Psychol. 42:444–445. Reprinted by permission.

"words" in Figure 11–33 are physically identical, but you read the figure as
"the cat."

Another example of the way context guides your hypothesis making is
shown in Figure 11–34. When you first glanced at this picture, you probably
saw a gesticulating Japanese character. Closer inspection reveals that the
head and hand are made up of miniature figures. Once you notice them, they
are hard to avoid seeing—but when you first looked at the picture, the lines
seemed only to represent the larger face and hand. Interpreting the lines as
part of the larger figure rather than the unexpected component figures is another indication of top-down processing affecting the way you handle sensory information.

Illusions Dependent on Perceptual Hypotheses

There are numerous visual illusions and effects that help demonstrate the
role of perceptual hypothesis making. In this section, we will deal only with
those concerning formation of figures. In Chapter 13 we will encounter a
larger group of illusions explicable by faulty perceptual hypotheses about
depth and distance.

Ambiguous figures, such as the wife/mother-in-law in Figure 11–30, can
be interpreted in either of two ways, because either of two perceptual
hypotheses can be accepted. The observer may begin with the hypothesis
that the loop to the left is a face; which means the triangular projection on
the far left is a nose, the black band below is a necklace, and so on. As each

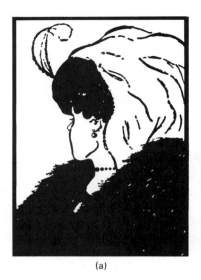
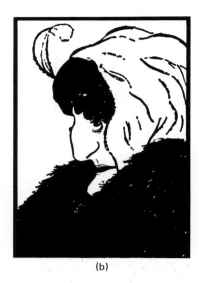

(a)   (b)

FIGURE 11-31   Unambiguous versions of Figure 11-30. (a) The young
woman. (b) The old woman.

part falls into place, no hypothesis need be rejected, and the young lady is
seen. Alternatively, if the first hypothesis was that the loop to the left is a
nose, then the triangle is a wart on it and the band is a mouth. No hypothesis
need be rejected, and the old lady is seen. There are no details drawn completely enough to cause the rejection of any particular hypothesis. In the
unambiguous versions shown Figure 11-31, certain details are drawn too
well to satisfy the "wrong" hypothesis: the necklace/mouth is too distinctly
a necklace in Figure 11-31(a) to satisfy the "mouth" hypothesis, and too
clearly a mouth in Figure 11-31(b) to satisfy the "necklace" hypothesis.

We have also seen another ambiguous figure, in which the figure and
ground could exchange roles (these are generally referred to as *reversible*
figures). This was Figure 11-15, which could be seen either as a white vase
or two silhouetted faces. Either hypothesis can be taken as "true," so either
figure may appear. Since both hypotheses cannot be true at the same time, it
is nearly impossible to see both the vase and the faces simultaneously.
Whichever we see as the figure at a given time takes on the attributes of a

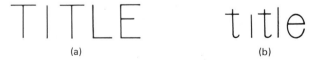

(a)   (b)

FIGURE 11-32   Effect of context on perception. A straight vertical line
can be seen as either an I (in TITLE) or as an 1 (in
title).

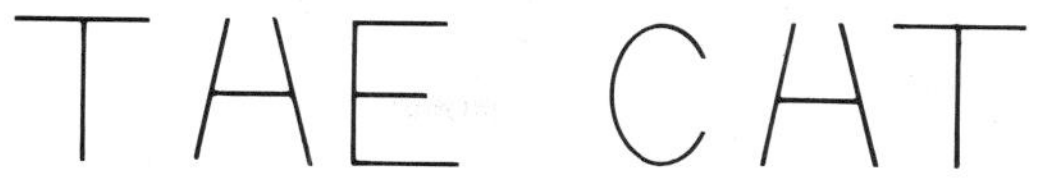

THE CAT

FIGURE 11-33   Effect of context on perception.

figure. There is also a demonstration of the active nature of our perceptual processes in both the wife/mother-in-law figure and the vase/faces: we can see either pattern in whichever configuration we wish by an act of willing it to be so.

One of the most famous reversible figures is shown in Figure 11-35(a); it is the Necker cube. As all the edges of the cube are shown (like a cube made of wires), it is possible to see the Necker cube in either the configuration shown in (b) or (c). Once both have been seen, the cube seems to oscillate between them.

If you build a cube out of toothpicks or wires, and view it (with one eye)

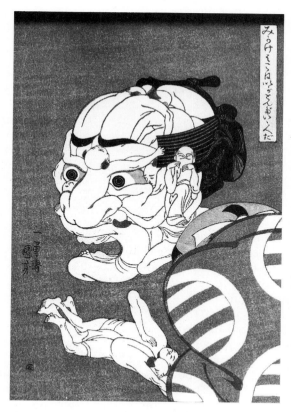

FIGURE 11-34   Japanese woodcut of a man by Hiroshige (early 1800s). Notice that the head and hand are made of tiny figures.

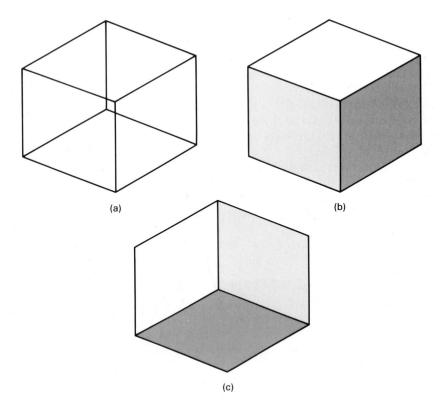

(a)

(b)

(c)

FIGURE 11-35   Necker's cube. (a) An isometric drawing of a cube made of sticks; it may be seen in either of two configurations. (b) and (c) Unambiguous cubes illustrating the two possible configurations of the Necker cube in (a).

from an angle that makes it look like a Necker cube, you may be able to see the same apparent reversals as in the drawing. There will be, however, a remarkable effect. The real cube is not symmetrical like the drawing; the nearest edges project a larger image on your retina than the edges farther away. This is a natural result of linear perspective (see next chapter), and causes no concern. When the figure reverses, however, those edges that appear closest are actually farther away, and therefore project smaller images. Distant edges projecting larger retinal images is not consonant with our experience and tends to invalidate the perceptual hypothesis that they are farther (making the real cube harder to reverse than the drawing in Figure 11–35[a]). To restore consistency, a second hypothesis, that the farther edges are also physically larger, must be made. This is what happens: when the cube reverses, it also appears to distort into a noncubic hexahedron. This distortion can be seen in the drawing of Figure 11–36(a), which is an accurate perspective view of a Necker cube. When it appears to be in the position of the cube in

Figure 11–35(c), for which the perspective is correct, it is a cube; when it reverses, it distorts. Similarly, the perspective drawing of a fanfold paper in Figure 11–36(b) distorts when it is reversed, so the corner marked with a dot seems closest (which requires considerable effort). This demonstration can also be done with a real folded sheet of paper viewed with one eye.

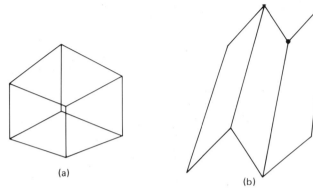

(a)   (b)

FIGURE 11-36   (a) Necker cube drawn in correct perspective for the configuration of Figure 11–35(c). When it is perceived in the configuration of Figure 11–35(b), the cube appears distorted. (b) Another reversible figure drawn in correct perspective. It appears distorted when the corner marked with a dot is seen as closer to the observer than the adjacent corners.

This brings up a point about perceptual hypotheses: we tend to make the simplest hypothesis consistent with the proximal stimulus. We can consciously invoke a less simple hypothesis that requires further hypotheses to maintain internal consistency, but we generally choose the simpler solution. This is demonstrated by the patterns in Figure 11–37. Both of these patterns are views of Necker cubes: (a) is a familiar view, (b) is from a perspective that makes the forward corner and rearward corner superimpose. It is possible to see (a) as a plane figure consisting of 12 lines (which it is), but the tendency to organize it into a cube is nearly overpowering. A cube is a simple hypothesis that explains the location of the 12 lines. The figure in (b), however, is more easily seen as a plane figure than as a cube. It is possible to see it as a cube, but slightly easier to see it as a hexagon with the three diagonals drawn in. The simpler hypothesis prevails.

Artists exploit the tendency to view the simplest alternative. We shall see that perceptual hypotheses about depth, coupled with the learned facts about perspective, allow two-dimensional canvases to appear to have depth, and theatrical stage sets to simulate a real scene. Other demonstrations are even more deliberately misleading. Figure 11–38(a) shows what appears to

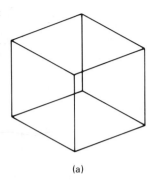 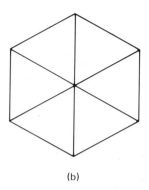

(a)   (b)

FIGURE 11-37 Demonstration of the efficacy of the simplest perceptual
hypothesis. (a) A Necker cube; this is generally seen as
a 3-dimensional cube. (b) A Necker cube viewed along
a major diagonal; this figure is more often perceived as
a plane hexagon with the diagonals drawn.

be a chair of sticks; in Figure 11–38(b) we see the same "chair" viewed from
a slightly different perspective. Sticks that appeared to be adjoining other
sticks because of their apparent proximity prove to be a considerable distance away. The simplest hypothesis is that these sticks really do touch
(Gogel, 1970), and there really is a chair; no cues are given to dispel this
idea. Even after seeing the real situation, it is nearly impossible not to see the
chair when viewing from the correct position.

There is an excellent natural example similar to this phenomenon: the
stars all appear as if they were affixed to a dome forming the sky. The stars
that form the Big Dipper look like a single unit (grouped by proximity, forming a good figure) even though they are all at incredibly different distances
from us. Even with the intellectual knowledge that the stars are not equidistant it is difficult not to see them as a group, for there are no cues to disrupt
that simplest of hypotheses.

Another kind of misleading object was devised by Adelbert Ames, the
designer of the "chair" in Figure 11–38. Ames' trapezoidal window is
shown in Figure 11–39. It is just what its name implies: a window of trapezoidal (rather than rectangular) shape. As we are accustomed to rectangular
windows, we make the hypothesis that this is a rectangular window that casts
a trapezoidal image because it is being viewed from an angle: the large side
seems closer to us. If a trapezoidal window cut from cardboard is mounted
on a spindle, as shown in the figure, it can be made to rotate uniformly in one
direction. When the taller edge passes closer to the observer there is no difficulty; but when the taller edge, which appears closer, passes *behind* the
spindle the observer thinks it is again passing in front. The window seems to
oscillate in its motion, with the taller edge waving from side to side in front
of the spindle. The hypothesis of a waving window is easier to accept than
the actual situation of a trapezoidal window rotating in a complete circle.

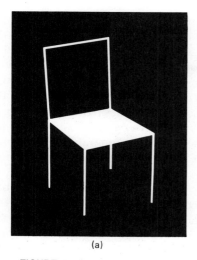 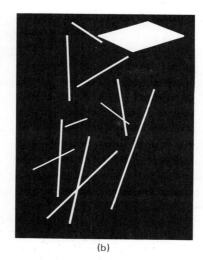

(a)   (b)

FIGURE 11-38 Ames' chair. (a) When viewed from the correct point, the chair is seen. (b) When viewed from another position, the chair becomes a collection of sticks in space. From W. H. Ittelson (1968) *The Ames Demonstrations in Perception.* New York: Macmillan Publishing Company, Reprinted by permission of the author.

If some other object such as a pencil is affixed to the window so that it projects through the frame, a strange effect is created. There is no difficulty in seeing that the pencil is normal and following a circular orbit, which is both the actual case and the simplest hypothesis. It is impossible, however, for the

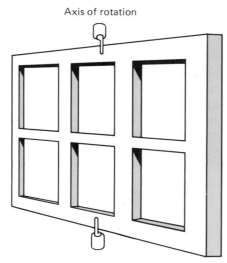

Axis of rotation

FIGURE 11-39 The Ames trapezoidal window.

pencil to travel in a circular path while the window oscillates, without the pencil somehow moving independently of, and passing clear through, the window frame. An additional hypothesis must be made to rectify the conflict between the circling pencil and oscillating window. Different observers make somewhat different hypotheses; most report the window oscillating and the pencil bending around as if made of rubber, then cutting through the frame at the extreme of each cycle. (Of course, any cues that the tall edge of the window is actually not nearer than the short edge tend to destroy the illusion. For this reason, the window is best viewed with only one eye, preferably from some distance. A movie of the rotating window is generally more effective than the actual apparatus.)

Finally, there are patterns that are not exactly illusory, but can disturb us because there is no way to make a complete set of perceptual hypotheses that will be internally consistent. These are the *impossible figures*, drawings that cannot be physically realized. Four examples (of many) are shown in Figure 11–40. The triangle on the left looks as though it might be built of three wooden slats (like a pool ball rack), except that the perspective is different for different corners. Any given corner is a perfectly valid joint, but as one follows from corner to corner the third simply will not mate. There is no reasonable hypothesis that is consistent with the proximal image, because the total pattern violates spatial closure (Draper, 1978).

The drawing in Figure 11–40(b) is an even more extreme example. The left half of the figure is a perspective drawing of a U-shaped rectangular block; the right half is a drawing of three round rods. A reasonable hypothesis can be made about either half of the figure, but the two are completely inconsistent. The significance of the six horizontal lines change halfway across: the third line down, for example, is the rear underside of a square beam on the left, but becomes the *top* edge of the second rod to the right. (Obvious as the impossibility may seem, one of us spent more than 10 minutes painstakingly pointing out these inconsistencies to his 6-year-old son, and in the end the child was still not convinced that they couldn't build one of these in the shop if they tried hard enough!)

The examples in Figure 11–40(c) and (d) are more subtle. In part (c), the perspective on the left and the right sides disagree. In part (d), there are no changes in the meanings of particular lines, and no apparent inconsistencies—until we realize that if we start at any place and start climbing steps we will go completely around the structure, always climbing, and be back at the starting point. The trick here is that the perspective is wrong; the whole structure is designed on a spiral in the opposite direction (Gombrich, 1961). (Bell Laboratories has produced a 2-minute Film entitled "A Pair of Paradoxes," based on this figure. In it, a ball is seen bouncing up the stairs; each bounce is accented by a tone that seems one step higher than the previous, although it also does not actually get any higher.)

All the figures in Figure 11–40 share the property that the visual system has no difficulty "understanding" each part of the picture, but that the parts

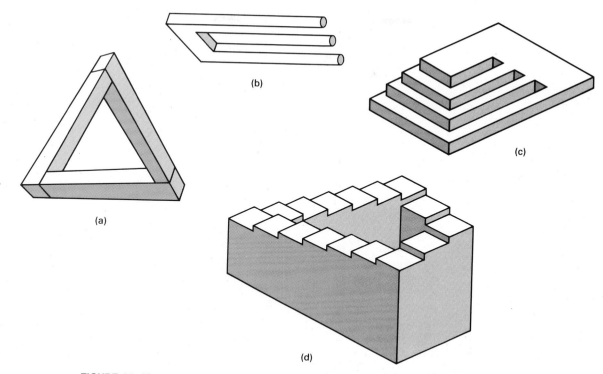

FIGURE 11–40 Some impossible figures. (a) Impossible triangle. (b) Structure in which two arms become three prongs. (c) "Ziggurat," a more subtle violation of structure. (d) Perpetual staircase. Parts (a) and (d) from Penrose, L. S. and R. Penrose (1958) Impossible objects: A special type of visual illusion. *Br. J. Psychol.* 49:31–33. Reprinted by permission of the British Psychological Society. Part (c) from Draper, S. W. (1978) The Penrose triangle and a family of related figures. *Perception* 7:283–296. Reprinted by permission of Pion, Ltd., London.

are inconsistent with each other. Apparently, local processing can invoke perceptual hypotheses that apply to local regions. Minsky and Papert (1969), pioneers of the artificial intelligence approach to vision, referred to this ability to isolate portions as the "context problem." However, it is clear that some larger process must integrate these local hypotheses into a unified percept. This larger process is missing in Balint's syndrome (see Box θ=θ).95

Impossible figures have been used in works of art, most notably in the drawings of M. C. Escher. An elaborate version of the perpetual staircase (Figure 11–40[d]) forms the basis of his *Ascending and Descending*, in which the details and buttresses of the building camouflage the distortions of the stairs. Failures of spatial closure like those in Figure 11–40(a) are featured in *Belvedere. Waterfall*, shown in Figure 11–41(a), is another use of the impossible triangle. This perfectly reasonable waterfall turns a wheel, then flows downhill along its course to arrive again at the top of the falls. The sketch of the watercourse in Figure 11–41(b) shows how the picture is actually a double impossible triangle. Notice how the craft and elaboration hides the source of the deception.

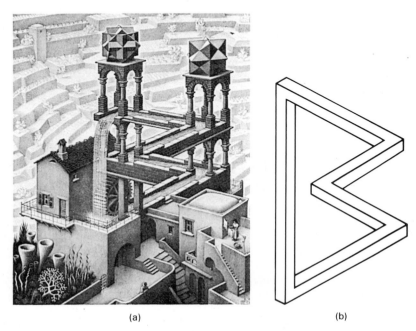

(a)   (b)

FIGURE 11–41   (a) An impossible scene: *Waterfall* by Maurits C. Escher. © 1990 M. C. Escher Heirs/Cordon Art-Baarn-Holland. Reprinted by permission. (b) The shape of the watercourse in (a), revealing how it is essentially like Figure 11–40(a). After Draper, S. W. (1978). Reprinted by permission of Pion, Ltd., London.

SUGGESTED READINGS

Several books have treatments of form perception that are readable and comprehensive; they differ considerably, however, in their points of view. A modern view of the more traditional topics may be found in *Sight and Mind*, by Lloyd Kaufman (Oxford University Press, 1974). A comprehensive view of the traditional topics is given in Julian Hochberg's ''Perception. I. Color and shape,'' which is Chapter 12 of *Experimental Psychology*, by J. W. Kling and L. A. Riggs (Holt, Rinehart, and Winston, 1971). A cognitively oriented presentation that includes some of the work in artificial intelligence is given by Ulrich Neisser in his book *Cognitive Psychology* (Appleton-Century-Crofts, 1967).

A number of *Scientific American* articles bear on specific topics covered in this chapter; in most cases, the titles reveal the contents. O. G. Selfridge and U. Neisser present "Pattern recognition by machine" (August 1960; offprint #510). "Visual illusions," by R. L. Gregory (November 1968; offprint #517) also includes illusions covered in Chapter 12. "Texture and visual perception," by B. Julesz (February 1965; offprint #318) has some material pertinent to the next two chapters, but also includes a modern view of organization by similarity, and of the concept of symmetry. How an infant first begins to perceive shape and form is the subject of "The origin of form perception," by R. L. Fantz (May 1961; offprint #459). All of these articles are reprinted in the collection *Perception: Mechanisms and Models*, edited by R. Held and W. Richards (W. H. Freeman, 1972). An article that deals with ambiguous figures and the figure ground/relationship is called "Multistability in perception," by F. Attneave (December 1971; offprint #540); a similar theme is explored by M. L. Teuber in "Sources of ambiguity in the prints of Maurits C. Escher" (July 1974; offprint #560). "The perception of disoriented figures," by I. Rock (January 1974; offprint #557) stresses the importance of the frame of reference in perception. These three articles, plus the Julesz article mentioned above, are reprinted in *Recent Progress in Perception*, edited by R. Held and W. Richards (W. H. Freeman, 1976). The articles by Attneave, Gregory, Julesz, and Rock also appear in *Image, Object, and Illusion*, by R. Held (W. H. Freeman, 1974). A classic discussion of "Subjective contours" was presented by G. Kanizsa (April 1976). A newer treatment of ambiguous figures may be found in "The interpretation of visual illusions," by D. D. Hoffman (December, 1983). Both of these are reprinted in *The Mind's Eye*, (introduction by J. M. Wolfe), (W. H. Freeman Co., 1986).

A beautifully illustrated book that covers many of the topics in this and the next four chapters is *Perception*, by Irvin Rock (Scientific American Books, 1984). In addition to explaining the principles of perception, Rock provides examples of how these principles are used in art and apply to everyday scenes. Another book that might be of interest is *Art and Illusion*, by E. H. Gombrich (Princeton University Press, 1961). Basically an art book, there is an emphasis on the use of illusory, impossible, and ambiguous figures in works of art. This book is also relevant to Chapter 13.

The application of artificial intelligence to cognitive processing is a new and exciting area, but it is hard to find appropriate readings. Two articles appearing in *Science* in 1988 merit attention for giving specific examples of how neural networks might perform cognitive functions. The first is by P. S. Churchland and T. J. Sejnowski, "Perspectives on cognitive neuroscience" in volume 242, pages 741–745. The second is by T. J. Sejnowski, C. Koch, and P. S. Churchland, "Computational neuroscience" in volume 241, pages 1299–1306. *Science* is written at a technical level, but these articles are generally accessible. For those who are serious about understanding how cognition could be based on neural interactions, we recommend *Neural Darwinism: The Theory of Neuronal Group Selection*, by G. M. Edelman (Basic Books, Inc., 1987). Edelman discusses ways in which synapses might change as a network ''learns'' to recognize objects, and he proposes a way in which neurons might coalesce into functional groups. He presents a model for a cognitive system in which functional groups interact at various levels—strikingly like the various brain regions discussed in Chapter 9. However, we hesitate to recommend this book to any but the most serious student, as it is conceptually difficult and written in a way that seems almost deliberately opaque.

DEPTH PERCEPTION

12

All the information we have regarding the visual world comes from stimulation of our two retinae. The retina, although it is curved into a hemisphere in the back of the eyeball, is equivalent to a flat, two-dimensional layer of tissue. How does stimulation of a two-dimensional retinal surface get translated by the brain into perceptions of depth? Such perceptions are an integral part of our world; when reaching for a glass of water on a table, you have a clear idea of exactly what position in space that glass is occupying. The activities of hitting tennis balls, shooting baskets, and just walking around on a city street all require vast amounts of information about spatial relationships between us and the physical world, as well as among various objects within the physical world.

We can divide the cues available for depth perception into several fairly distinct classes. *Monocular cues* are those that require the use of only one eye. Some monocular cues may be available from a stationary inspection of the visual scene; these are the types that are most often employed by artists and are therefore called *pictorial cues*. Others are only present when either the observer or the objects in the visual scene are in motion; these are called *kinetic cues*. A final source of monocular information regarding depth can be obtained from the state of accommodation of the lens when it focuses on a given object.

Another class of depth cue is available because our brains receive two views of the visual world, one from each eye. These are *binocular cues*, derived from the fact that the two retinal images are slightly different from each other. In addition, information regarding the state of contraction of the extraocular muscles of the two eyes may be used by the brain to determine the point in space at which the two eyes are pointing.

In this chapter, we discuss in some detail all of these cues, and try to determine which ones are the most important for our perception of depth. In addition, we discuss what is known about the physiological mechanisms that underly the processing of some of these depth cues.

MONOCULAR DEPTH CUES

Pictorial Cues

Size   As an object moves toward or away from an observer, the size of the retinal image produced by that object will vary in inverse proportion to the distance. For example, an object placed 5 meters away from the observer will cast an image on the retina that is exactly double what the image size would be if the same object were moved so that it were 10 meters away. Thus, the size of the retinal image can act as a cue for determining how far away the object actually is. (As we shall see in Chapter 13, perception of distance can also affect apparent size.)

There are two different ways in which this cue might be applied to the perception of depth or distance. If you are looking at two similar or identical objects whose distances from you are different, they will cast images whose sizes are also different. When making judgments regarding the relative positions of the two objects, the *relative sizes* of the images may be considered. To make this judgment, the observer does not have to know anything about the actual sizes of the objects; it is necessary only to assume that they are really identical. Under these conditions, many investigators have shown that relative size can be an effective cue. Ittelson and Kilpatrick (1951) presented subjects with two balloons at the same distance from the subjects; the sizes of the balloons could be controlled by bellows. When the balloons were viewed monocularly under dim illumination (to eliminate other depth cues), the relative distances assigned to them by the subjects depended on the relative sizes. When the two balloons were of equal size they were viewed as being the same distance away, but when they were different in size, the larger one was always thought to be closer to the subject. A demonstration of the effectiveness of relative retinal image size as a cue for distance is given in Figure 12–1. (If this figure is not compelling, it is because the cue of relative size is acting in opposition to the other depth cues that are present; for example, under the conditions you are viewing the figure, it is clear that all the triangles are actually lying in the plane of the book. For this figure to give a convincing feeling of distance, one would have to view it under

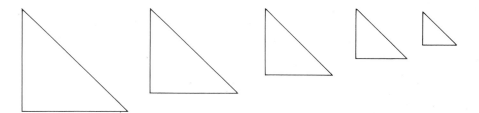

FIGURE 12–1   A demonstration of the effects of size on perceived distance.

conditions in which it was not so clear that the stimuli were on the same piece of paper.)

Although relative size can clearly play a role in the perception of depth, there are other size cues that are also effective. *Familiar size* applies when the actual size of an object is well known to the viewer. For example, everyone knows the approximate size of an automobile, but the size of its retinal image will vary with distance from the viewer. If familiar size is an effective cue for distance, the absolute retinal image size of the car should tell the viewer approximately how far away the car actually is. The importance of familiar size as a cue for depth seems to depend partially on what other cues are available. Under rich stimulus conditions, Fillenbaum, Schiffman, and Butcher (1965) found that familiar size was not used in distance judgments; however, subjects did use the cue in experimental situations where other cues were not available (Schiffman, 1967). In another study, Epstein and Baratz (1964) found that when extremely familiar objects such as coins were used as stimuli, their sizes did affect how far away subjects judged them to be. For objects that subjects were less familiar with, changing the size had no effect on distance judgments.

Interposition If two opaque objects are in the same line of sight, one will occlude the other. This is *interposition*, and its effectiveness can be seen easily in Figure 12-2. Although all of the geometric forms in the figure lie in the plane of the paper, the circle is seen as lying behind the rectangle, which itself seems to be behind the triangle. The relative depths of the three objects can be deduced from the facts that the circle is blocked by both the rectangle and the triangle, while the rectangle blocks the circle but is blocked by the triangle. The above interpretation is not the only one that could be given to the figure; the forms in Figure 12-2 could conceivably be the ones shown in Figure 12-3, in which case they could all be lying in the same plane. One reason that we get the illusion of depth from Figure 12-2 instead of seeing the forms as shown in Figure 12-3, was discussed in Chapter 11. If there is a choice between perceiving something as a complicated form or as a simpler form, we generally perceive the simplest shape possible—that is, we tend to maximize figural goodness. Perceiving the forms in Figure 12-2 as a triangle,

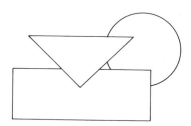

FIGURE 12-2 Interposition as a cue for distance.

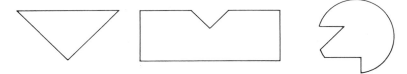

FIGURE 12-3   An alternative way of perceiving the forms
in Figure 12-2.

rectangle, and circle is simpler than having to conceptualize the rather complex shapes in Figure 12-3. Thus, in this case the perception of depth allows us to code the ensemble of lines and curves in Figure 12-2 more easily than if they were all thought of as being coplanar.

Lighting and Shadow   Objects that have depth associated with them usually cast shadows; these shadows can be used to give the impression of a three-dimensional form on a two-dimensional surface. Consider the photograph of a crater shown in Figure 12-4. There is a clear impression of the depth of the crater, at least partially because part of it is in shadow. To see the importance of the shadow gradients on perception, turn the book upside down and look at the photo again. The shadow gradients are now reversed; because of this, there should be the strong impression of a hill. A more abstract demonstration of this same phenomenon is shown in Figure 12-5.

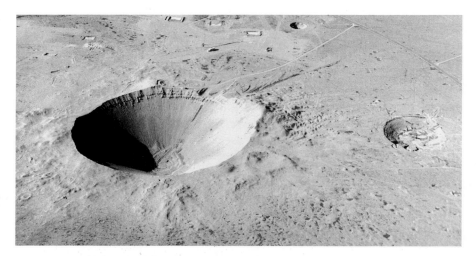

FIGURE 12-4   Lighting and shadow as a cue for depth. Turn the book
upside down and the crater turns into a hill. Photo courtesy of the U.S. Dept. of Energy.

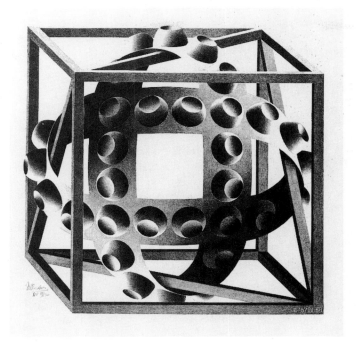

FIGURE 12-5   Drawing by M. C. Escher using light and shadow as a depth cue. © 1990 M. C. Escher Heirs / Cordon Art - Baarn - Holland. Reprinted by permission.

BOX 12-1

Workers in artificial intelligence have found that this apparently simple and straightforward process can be quite difficult to implement in machine vision. A considerable amount of effort has been devoted to the problem of deducing the shape of an object from the shades of gray in a two-dimensional photograph. It is relatively "easy" to determine the appearance of objects to be expected given their surface properties and the lighting conditions; extraordinarily lifelike representations can be generated as computer graphics requiring only a few *hours* of computation (Greenberg, 1989). The reverse problem, determining the object given the image, does not even have a unique solution. Quite complicated algorithms have been devised, but these require assumptions about the nature of surfaces and the lighting conditions in order to reach their solutions (Brown, 1984). Our visual systems solve the same problems instantly. Newer approaches in which model neural networks "learn" to recognize the shapes seem to be more successful than strictly mathematical approaches (Lehky & Sejnowski, 1988; Sejnowski, Koch, & Churchland, 1988).

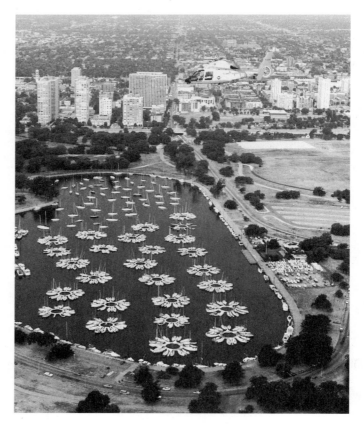

FIGURE 12-6   Scene demonstrating depth due to clarity and elevation. Copyrighted, Chicago Tribune Company, all rights reserved. Used with permission.

Clarity and elevation   Look at the aerial scene in Figure 12–6. The helicopter is obviously closer than the buildings. Of course, interposition plays a role here, but a large part of the appearance of depth is due to the relative *clarity* of the helicopter. Particles of dust and moisture in the atmosphere interrupt and scatter the light; the longer the light path from object to observer, the less clear the image. (In this sense, clarity is not simply loss of focus, but loss of *contrast*.) Clarity can thus serve as a cue for distance; however, since the amount that atmospheric particles disrupt light transmission depends on location and weather conditions, this cue is not normally critical for depth perception.

Figure 12–6 also illustrates the cue of *elevation*, the location within the picture frame. As we look from nearer objects to farther, the farther objects are generally higher in the visual field. Except for the helicopters, this is true in Figure 12–6. The closest objects (in the harbor) are at the bottom of the

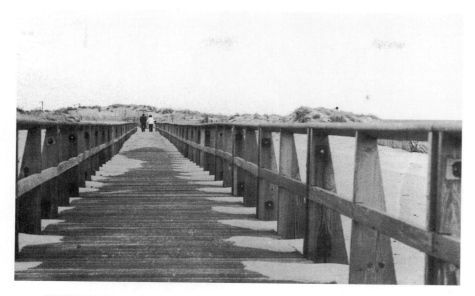

FIGURE 12-7 An example of linear perspective.

picture; midrange objects (the tall buildings near the waterfront) are higher; the farthest objects (the smaller buildings inland) are at the very top of the frame. For a particular scene, therefore, objects placed higher in the scene will tend to be perceived as being farther away.

Perspective Imagine standing in the middle of a boardwalk, gazing down the walk as it recedes toward the horizon; the view will be something similar to that shown in Figure 12–7. The railings along the walkway remain parallel as they extend away from you, and you perceive them as such; however, the retinal image of the railings is far from parallel. The images of the portion of the near railings are quite far apart on the retina, just as they are well separated from each other in the figure. Gaze farther down the walkway, and their images on the retinae become closer together, tending toward a single point at the horizon. This is exactly what happens in Figure 12–7. This phenomenon is termed *linear perspective*; it is a ubiquitous component of our retinal images, and imparts a strong depth component to line drawings and photographs.

Linear perspective is a necessary consequence of projecting a three-dimensional world onto a two-dimensional surface (that is, the retina, a photographic negative, or a piece of drawing paper). For any object that extends in depth toward and away from the observer, the near portions of the object will be imaged larger on the retina than the more distant portions. Another example of linear perspective is shown in Figure 12–8; in this photograph of the inside of a cathedral, the pews and arches near the camera take up much

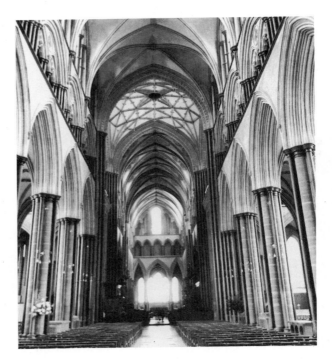

FIGURE 12-8   A second example of linear perspective.

more of the picture than the areas farther away. Just as the railings in Figure 12-7 seemed to converge at the horizon, the line of pews converges with distance down the aisles of the cathedral, as do the ceiling supports at the top of the figure.

Texture   Another depth cue is derived from the fact that there is depth-dependent distortion in a two-dimensional representation of a three-dimensional world. It is called *detail perspective*, or *texture gradients* (Gibson, 1950). Imagine again standing on the boardwalk depicted in Figure 12-7; besides the fact that the railings appear to converge as they recede from the observer, the spacing between adjacent posts decreases with distance from the observer. The reason for this is the same as for the railings converging; although the distance between the posts is always the same in the physical world, the posts more distant from the observer will project closer together on the retina than those that are close to the observer. In the case of the photograph in Figure 12-7, the camera's film is taking the place of the observer's retina, so we get the same impression of depth by looking at the photograph. This is an example of a texture gradient combining with linear perspective to produce an impression of depth.

A graphic demonstration of texture in the absence of any linear perspective cues is given in Figure 12-9. The halves of the figure differ only in the

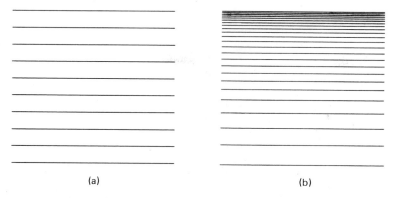

(a)   (b)

FIGURE 12-9   A pure example of texture as a depth cue. Parts (a) and
(b) are similar except for the texture gradient in (b),
which gives it a strong depth component.

placement of the horizontal lines, but we get a strong depth impression in
(b) and not in (a). This impression comes from the fact that the lines in (b)
form a texture gradient, while in (a) they are equally spaced. In this example, the only cue providing depth information is the texture change; it is
strong enough to produce a depth impression in the absence of other cues.

If you prop the book up and step back from it, you may notice that the
apparent depth in Figure 12–9(b) seems less compelling. This is true even
though you can still see the lines plainly. What is different when you step
back is that the image is smaller; that is, everything is shifted to higher spatial
frequencies. Perhaps appearance of depth depends on a system that is most
sensitive to lower spatial frequencies—the magnocellular system (see Chapter 9). If that is so, depth should not be evident when the pattern is made
effective only for the parvocellular system. Another way to achieve this is to
produce the picture in Figure 12–9(b) of equiluminant red lines on a green
background. If the red and green are equiluminant, the color-blind magnocellular system cannot see the lines, even though the parvocellular system
allows the viewer to see that they are present. When this is done, viewers
report seeing lines, but with no apparent depth (Livingstone & Hubel,
1987b). This is an indication that the magnocellular system is required for
the appearance of depth from pictorial cues (see also Figure 9–10).

BOX 12-2 ▄▄▄▄▄▄▄▄▄▄▄▄▄▄

The pictorial cues were employed to make a
statement about the nature of artistic representation in the painting *Les Promenades
d'Euclide* by René Magritte (Figure 12–10). A
(continued)

view of the world extending in great depth is
seen through a window, as if it were a pictorial
projection on the window. In front of the window is an artist's canvas with a pictorial repre-

(box continued)

sentation painted on it so that it appears we are actually seeing the world through the canvas. (Of course, this entire scene is itself painted on a canvas, seen through the eye of the camera that photographed the painting.) All the pictorial cues we have discussed can be seen in this painting: distant buildings are smaller than nearby buildings; the nearby objects (such as the pointed tower just left of center) are interposed between the viewer and more distant objects; there are shadows cast by buildings and the tower; the distant horizon is higher than the buildings and is less distinct; the sides of the street (right of center) converge as the street recedes toward the horizon (linear perspective); and the textures in the street become finer the farther down the road we look.

Of interest is the fact that the pointed tower and the street are formed by identical triangles having their apices coincident with the horizon. Whether we take the converging lines to imply linear perspective (as in the street), or an erect conical object (the tower), depends on context, texture, and shadowing. Thus, the convergent point of the tower is perceived as much closer than the point at which the road disappears over the horizon, and the triangle forming the street seems larger than the one forming the tower. We shall have more to say in Chapter 13 about how the perceived distance of objects affects their perceived sizes.

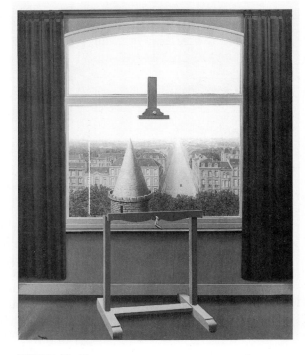

FIGURE 12–10   *Les Promenades d'Euclide* by René Magritte. Notice the pictorial cues are all used to generate a feeling of depth in the picture-within-the-picture. Notice also that the tower and road are formed by identical triangles but are perceived differently because of context, shading, and texture gradients. The Minneapolis Institute of Arts. Reprinted by permission.

Accommodation

When we shift visual attention from a nearby object to one that is far away, the lens adjusts its shape to maintain a sharp image of the particular object to which we are attending. This process is called accommodation; it was discussed in Chapter 4. When we view an object that is far away, the ciliary muscles are relaxed and the lens is pulled into its flattened position. For close-up objects, the ciliary muscles contract and the lens relaxes into its maximally curved shape. The fact that the level of activity of the ciliary muscles is correlated with the distance of the object to be viewed means that the brain could use information about this activity to make decisions about the distance of the object. Such information could be available from sensory receptors monitoring the level of activity of the ciliary muscles, or it could come directly from the centers in the brain responsible for sending the signals that actually control the muscles.

There is considerable doubt as to whether information regarding the state of accommodation of the lens provides a usable distance cue. Hochberg (1971b) reviewed the literature on this question and concluded that there is little reason to believe that the state of accommodation is an important cue for the perception of distance.

Kinetic Cues

Except for accommodation (which we have said is not an important cue for perceived depth), all the cues we have discussed involve a stationary subject looking with one eye at a stationary visual scene. In this section, we will keep the subject one-eyed, but ask what kind of depth cues are available when either subject or stimulus is moving in space.

When a person moves within the physical world, objects that are stationary in space nevertheless have images on the retina that continuously change position. The relative movement of objects at different distances from the observer is called *motion parallax*. Motion parallax occurs in many situations—for example, while looking out the window of a moving car or train. If the eyes are fixated on the horizon in such a situation, then all objects closer than the horizon will move in the opposite direction from the vehicle. If we attend to an object a moderate distance away, however, all components of the visual world situated behind that object will appear to move with us, while everything in front of that object will move in the opposite direction (Figure 12–11).

BOX 12–3

Y ou need not move about the world to cause motion parallax. Your eyes are farther forward in your head than the axis about which your head pivots on your neck. When you turn your head from side to side (as you normally do to look around yourself), you also move your eyes from side to side. To see the motion parallax induced by turning your head, "just say no." *(continued)*

Close one eye and hold the index finger from each hand out in front of you, so that one finger is quite near your eye, and the other is about 18 inches away. Keeping your fingers steady, turn your head from side to side while fixating on the far finger. Under these conditions, as you turn your head in one direction, the image of the near finger should move in the opposite direction. Now perform the same experiment while fixating on your near finger; the image of your far finger should move in the same direction as your head. Finally, if you fixate on something behind your far finger (for example, the wall), the images of both fingers will move in the direction opposite to your head movement, but the image of the close-up finger will appear to move much faster than the other.

Motion parallax clearly is a potential source of information about the relative distances of objects in space. Many studies have been performed to try to isolate this cue from other sources of distance information, to see just how effective it really is. As far as your retina is concerned, moving objects in space can exactly mimic movement of the observer, thus many of these studies kept the subject still and manipulated the external environment. In one such study, Gibson, Gibson, Smith, and Flock (1959) used an instrument called a point-source shadow projector to simulate motion parallax cues in the absence of other depth information. The shadow projector simply consisted of a light source that lit a projection screen viewed by the subject on the other side of the screen from the light. Between the light and the screen could be placed one or more transparent plastic sheets erratically covered with splattered paint or talcum powder; images of these irregular patterns could then be projected onto the screen and so seen by the observer. Figure 12–12 shows a schematic of the shadow projector.

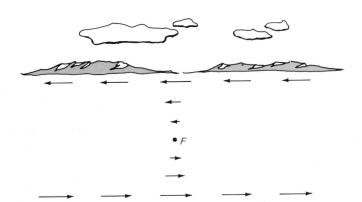

FIGURE 12-11   Motion parallax as a cue for depth. If a subject fixates on point *F* and is moving to the left, all objects more distant than *F* will move with the subject, while objects in front of *F* will move in the opposite direction. From Gibson, J. J. *The Perception of the Visual World.* Copyright © 1950 by Houghton Mifflin Company. Used with permission.

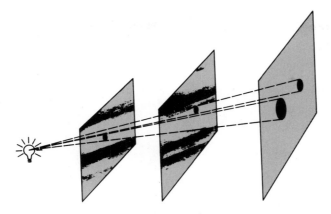

FIGURE 12-12 A schematic of the kind of shadow projector used by
Gibson, Gibson, Smith, and Flock (1959).

Gibson *et al.* placed two splattered plastic sheets parallel to the projection
screen but at different distances from the light source. The sheets were then
moved across the field at the identical velocity; because of motion parallax,
the sheet that was nearer to the light source cast an image onto the screen that
moved faster than the image of the sheet that was farther away from the light.
Thus the observer saw a moving textured field with some elements moving
faster than others, just as if the sheets were being viewed directly while the
observer was moving and the sheets were remaining stationary. Under these
conditions, subjects reported an impression of depth; however, they could not
always determine which sheet was beyond the other. Notice that they could
recognize the two sheets because of common fate (see Chapter 11).

The experimenters then removed one of the plastic sheets and tilted the
remaining one so that its bottom was nearer to the light source than the top,
producing a continuous size gradient on the projection screen; the paint
spots at the bottom of the screen were larger than at the top. When the sheet
was moved parallel to the projection screen in the same way as discussed in
the last paragraph, a gradient of motion parallax was produced, with the bottom paint spots moving faster across the screen than the spots at the top of the
screen. Under these conditions, subjects not only reported a perception of
depth created by the moving screen, but were able reliably to report the
direction that the sheet was tilted. Thus, when an entire gradient of motion
parallax is present, subjects are able to make more accurate discriminations
of depth than when objects move at one of only two velocities.

Motion parallax is a cue that is derived from the observer's movements.
In the shadow projector experiments, stimulus motion simply mimicked effects that in the real world would have been produced by movements on the
part of the subject. There is, however, a related class of motion cues that
depends on movement in the physical world. Wallach and his colleagues
(Wallach & O'Connell, 1953; Wallach, O'Connell, & Neisser, 1953) used

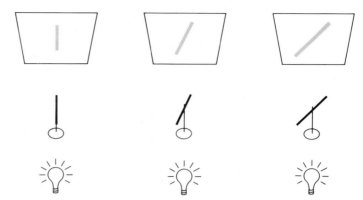

FIGURE 12-13   Demonstration of the kinetic depth effect (KDE). A rotating bar casts a shadow that changes in both orientation and length, producing a 3-dimensional impression.

the same shadow projector technique described above, except that between the light source and the projection screen was a rotating object oriented in different directions. For example, a straight rod would be positioned so that the top of the rod was tilted toward the projection screen and the bottom was toward the light source (Figure 12–13). It was then rotated in the horizontal dimension about a point at the center of the rod. When the rod was positioned so that it cast a vertical shadow on the viewing screen, the length of its shadow was smaller than when it was rotated one-quarter of a cycle in either direction. The different shadows produced by the different positions of the rod are shown in Figure 12–13; as the rod rotates, the shadow changes both in orientation and in length.

When a rod was rotated in the manner described above, subjects viewing the continuously changing shadow received the clear impression of a rod rotating in three dimensions; that is, they perceived the shadow as three-dimensional much in the way that they would have perceived the image of the rod itself. Thus, even though the shadow was in two dimensions, it was able to produce an impression of depth. Wallach and his coworkers called this the *kinetic depth effect* (KDE).

A related effect may be obtained from a field of about 50 dots that each move sinusoidally to and fro at the same frequency. This is the pattern that would arise if opaque dots were placed at random on a transparent, rotating sphere, and you were looking at the shadow of the dotted sphere. If the sphere were stationary, you would see a circular field of random dots. When the dots move, the sphere "jumps out" as a three-dimensional shape.

However, if the dots are made equiluminant with the background (for example, green dots on a red background, such that the two colors are equally effective for the magnocellular system), there is no apparent depth. Instead of a rotating field, you would see a circular field of dots that are apparently moving about at random (Livingstone & Hubel, 1987b). As we noted for depth from texture, it appears that the magnocellular system is needed to perceive depth.

BINOCULAR DEPTH CUES

The collection of cues for depth that have been discussed so far in this chapter allow human beings a fairly accurate perception of the three-dimensional world. These are all monocular cues; if you have ever had to wear a patch over one eye for any length of time, you know that these cues are adequate for most perceptual needs. People with only one eye can drive cars, catch baseballs, and perform many other tasks requiring an exact impression of the depth associated with the physical world. By comparing your perceptual experiences under monocular and binocular conditions, however, you should get the clear impression that depth perception is greatly enhanced by the use of two eyes. In this section, we will discuss some of the depth cues that depend on binocular vision.

Convergence

We have mentioned earlier in this chapter the accommodative changes in the lens that accompany changes in stimulus position for objects quite close to the eye. Associated with lens accommodation are eye movements called disjunctive eye movements, which are discussed in Chapter 4. Disjunctive eye movements occur as a stimulus moves either toward or away from the subject. In the example shown in Figure 12–14, a subject is staring at an object located at point A in space. The eyes are therefore positioned so that an image of the object is projected to both foveas; as point A is located directly in front of the two eyes, the eyes have been rotated so that their angles of gaze are not parallel, but converge at point A. If the stimulus is now moved from point A to point B as shown in Figure 12–14(b), two physiological changes should occur. As discussed earlier, lens accommodation should take place, with the lens assuming a more rounded shape to provide the extra refractive power to maintain focus of the stimulus on the retina. In addition, a disjunctive eye movement should occur, with both eyes turning inward to maintain the stimulus' projection onto both foveas. This is an example of *convergence*: the two eyes turn inward to prevent the occurrence of double images. If we now reversed the sequence and moved the stimulus from point B back to point A, the two eyes would rotate away from each other; that is, they *diverge*.

The amount of convergence between the two eyes is a potential source of depth information. In fact, unlike most other cues for depth, the angle at which the eyes converge to produce an image of the stimulus at corresponding points on the retinae provides a measure of the absolute distance be-

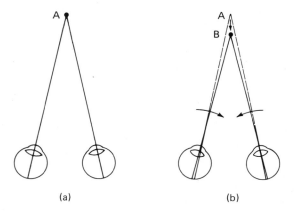

FIGURE 12-14 An example of convergence.

tween the observer and the stimulus. From a knowledge of simple trigonometry, as well as information about the distance between the two eyes and the angle of convergence, the absolute distance between the observer's head and the point at which the lines of sight of the two eyes intersect can be calculated (Figure 12–15). We would not expect our visual systems to perform a trigonometric calculation, but it is reasonable to expect that we would learn the significance of the convergence signal.

Although accommodation and convergence are closely related phenomena, evidence supporting the contention that people use convergence cues to make decisions about depth is much stronger than the evidence regarding accommodation. Heinemann, Tulving, and Nachmias (1959) presented luminous discs to subjects *dichoptically*; that is, separate discs were presented to the two eyes so that each eye only saw one disc. By simply changing the

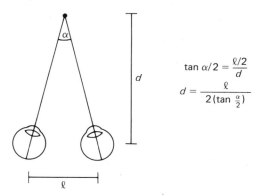

$$\tan \alpha/2 = \frac{\ell/2}{d}$$

$$d = \frac{\ell}{2\left(\tan \frac{\alpha}{2}\right)}$$

FIGURE 12-15 Demonstration of how amount of ocular convergence can provide information about the absolute distance between observer and point of fixation.

lateral position of the discs, they could manipulate the amount of ocular convergence that was necessary to maintain the image of the discs on corresponding points of the retinae. When the stimuli were arranged so that convergence was increased, subjects reported the discs as being smaller than when the eyes were caused to diverge, even though the physical size of the retinal images remained constant in both cases. Large amounts of convergence accompany the viewing of a nearby object, while the eyes diverge when one views distant stimuli; as the retinal image size was constant in both cases, it makes sense that the stimuli were perceived as being smaller when the convergence cues indicated the object was nearby. Thus apparent size changes of the stimuli provide support for the idea that convergence is used as a depth cue (see Chapter 13). Other experiments on this subject have yielded similar results (Leibowitz, 1971; Komoda & Ono, 1974).

In these studies, there were no changes in accommodative state as the stimuli to the two eyes were moved. Other experiments investigating the importance of convergence as a cue for depth have employed conditions in which accommodative and convergence information was in conflict; that is, the amount of lens accommodation necessary to place the stimulus in sharp focus was inconsistent with the convergence necessary to keep images of the stimulus located on the corresponding areas of the retina. Under these conditions, experimenters found that depth judgments were made solely on the basis of the convergence information rather than considering the state of accommodation of the lens (Ritter, 1977; Gogel & Sturm, 1972). From these experiments, it seems probable that ocular convergence information is far more important for depth perception than information arising from state of accommodation.

Binocular Disparity

In the previous section, we discussed the fact that the two eyes converge or diverge in order to place images of the stimulus being attended to on corresponding locations of the retinae. In general, however, the two eyes receive slightly different views of the world by virtue of their different locations on the head. Because of this difference, corresponding areas of the two retinae will not always receive exactly the same visual image. This phenomenon is known as *binocular disparity*, or *binocular parallax*; it provides an important cue for binocular depth perception.

As an example of binocular disparity, consider Figure 12–16. In this figure, two eyes are shown fixated on a nearby square stimulus. Because this is the stimulus being attended to, images of the square are projected to corresponding locations on the foveas of the two retinae. The images of the closer stimulus in the figure, the circle, cannot be projected onto the retinae without some disparity. From the perspective of the right eye, the two stimuli are quite close together, while from the left eye, they will look as though they are considerably farther apart. The fact that the views from the two eyes look

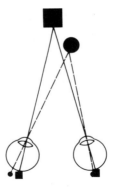

FIGURE 12-16 Binocular disparity. The square and circle are imaged quite close together on the right retina, but are imaged considerably farther apart on the left retina. If observer fixates on the square, there must be a disparity in the retinal locations of the image of the circle.

different tells the visual system that the stimuli are at different distances from the observer.

Notice that what is important is that the two views look different, not which object appears "displaced." If we directed our gaze at the circular stimulus, then the square would have been projected on two different locations in the two retinae. Whatever object we fixate on, other objects at the same distance will appear at corresponding points on the two retinae, while objects at different distances will not.

The direction and magnitude of binocular disparity provides information about which of two objects is closer to the observer, as well as how far apart the objects might be. To see how the direction of the disparity gives information about relative distance, consider the stimulus configuration portrayed in Figure 12–17. In this case, two stimuli are arranged so that one is directly behind the other. If the observer fixates on the close-up stimulus (the disc), the more distant square will appear as if it is to the left of the disc when viewed by the left eye, but will seem to be located to the right of the disc when viewed monocularly by the right eye. This is an example of *uncrossed disparity*; it occurs any time one fixates on the nearer of two stimuli. You can demonstrate uncrossed disparity for yourself; hold your finger out in front of you so that it is directly in line with the light switch on the far wall. If you fixate on your finger, and alternatively close one eye and then the other, the light switch should appear to be to the left of your finger when viewed through your left eye, and should seem to be to the right of your finger when looked at by your right eye.

Alternatively, if you keep your finger in front of you and now fixate on the switch, the position of your finger should change as a function of what eye you use to look at it. When viewed with your left eye, your finger should

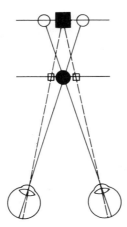

FIGURE 12-17 Crossed versus uncrossed disparity. If observer fixates on the circle, the disparity of the position of the square on the retinae is of the uncrossed variety. If observer fixates on the square, there is crossed disparity of the images of the circle.

appear to be to the right of the wall switch, while it should move to the left of the switch as you open your right eye and close your left. This is a case of *crossed disparity*, and is a signal to the visual system that the object being fixated upon is in back of the other object. In Figure 12–17, crossed disparity occurs when the observer fixates on the square and looks at the relative position of the disc under monocular conditions.

From this, it should be clear that stimuli in front of and behind an object to which an observer is attending will be seen by the two eyes with some amount of binocular disparity. What about objects that are the same distance from the observer as the object being fixated? Figure 12–18 shows two eyes that are converged so that point *F* in the figure is imaged on the foveas of both eyes. In such a situation, there is a whole population of other points in the visual field that will also be imaged on corresponding points of the two retinae. The middle curve in the figure shows one dimension of this surface, which is called the *horopter*. For a given fixation distance, all points on the horopter will have images that fall on corresponding points of the two retinae, in the same way that the single point being fixated on falls on the identical retinal area of the two eyes (that is, the fovea). All of the points on the horopter will be perceived as being at the same distance from the observer as the fixation point F. All points not on the horopter for this particular fixation distance will stimulate disparate retinal points.

If the stimulus is placed outside the region bounded by the two dashed curves, the visual system will not be able to combine the two images of the stimulus into one single percept, and a double image of that stimulus will result. This is an example of *diplopia*, or double vision. The dashed curves

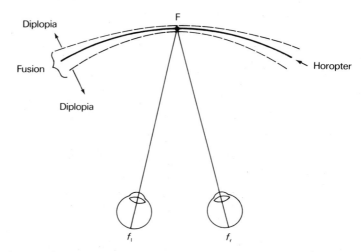

FIGURE 12-18   The horopter. If observer fixates on the point *F*, the middle solid curve represents the surface of points where images on the retinae will be projected at corresponding locations. This is the horopter. For locations off the horopter but within the bounds of the two dashed curves, there will be some amount of retinal disparity, and subject will report seeing the object in depth. Outside of these bounds, double images will result.

delimit the region in which the visual system can combine images; this region is called *Panum's fusion area*. A stimulus that is anywhere in Panum's area will be seen as a single object at a different depth from the fixation distance. As it is still seen as a single object even though it stimulates disparate regions of the two retinae, the visual system is said to *fuse* the two images.

Within certain limits, objects that stimulate disparate retinal regions in the two eyes result in an impression of depth. This fact was realized many years ago; in 1838, the English physicist Charles Wheatstone invented a device called a *stereoscope* that took advantage of binocular disparity cues to produce pictures that appeared in three-dimensional depth. The stereoscope took two pictures of the same visual scene that were slightly different in perspective (that is, one picture was taken from the position of the right eye, and a second picture was taken from the position of the left eye), and projected one picture to each eye. When the pictures (called *stereograms*) were appropriately positioned in space, the viewer received the impression of a single scene that had a distinct depth component. The modern analog to Wheatstone's stereoscope is the stereo slide viewer that allows the observer to view dichoptically (one picture to each eye) photographic slides of the same scene that have been taken by a stereo camera. A stereo camera is just a camera that has two lenses and two film compartments, separated by about the same distance that separates our two eyes. The shutter opens simultaneously for the two components of the camera, so that the same scene is photographed from the different perspectives. Viewing the photographic stereograms in the viewer results in a striking impression that the scene is three-dimensional, rather than a flat picture (see Figure i–2).

BOX 12–4 ▬▬▬▬▬▬▬▬▬

A small percentage of people do not get an impression of depth when they look through a stereo viewer. These people are called *stereoblind* (see Figure i–1). In general, stereoblind people perform more poorly than those with normal vision at any type of task that requires an accurate perception of depth. There are a number of causes of stereoblindness; the most common one seems to be some sort of disruption of normal binocular experience in childhood. For example, if a person grows up through early childhood with a cataract in one eye, or if one eye is very nearsighted and the other is normal, stereoblindness may result. Such monocular deprivation in childhood is quite similar to the deprivation experiments Wiesel and Hubel (1963) performed on kittens. When one eye was deprived in these experiments, the kittens grew up with a lack of binocular cells in their visual cortex (see Chapter 9).

The pictures viewed with Wheatstone's stereoscope or with modern stereo viewers are usually of familiar scenes having strong contours associated with them. That is, the stimulus presented to each eye is both well defined in shape and readily identifiable. In a series of studies on binocular perception, Julesz (1964; 1971; 1974) asked whether these factors were necessary for binocular disparity to produce a sensation of depth. He had subjects dichoptically view a pair of stimuli that he called *random dot stereograms*, an example of which is shown in Figure 12–19.

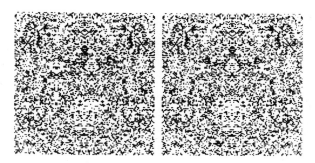

FIGURE 12–19 Random dot stereograms. View this figure using the method described on page x. When seen stereoscopically, a square floating in space should be evident.

The patterns in Figure 12–19 were generated by computer to be a random array of black and white dots. The computer began at the upper left corner of the right-hand frame; for each position in the top row, it selected a random number to decide whether to make that point (pixel) black or white. It then moved to the next position to the right, and did the same, until it reached the middle of the row. From the middle onward, it read the preceding sequence backwards to fill in to the right edge. This made the row mirror symmetric, which allows the stereogram to be viewed by either the direct or the mirror method (see page x). (Note that random dot stereograms usually do not have this mirror symmetry.) It then filled in the second row from the top, then the third, until the entire right panel was filled. Each half of the panel is completely random. You can see the mirror symmetry about the vertical midline because symmetric figures are "good" (see Chapter 11), and therefore stand out.

The left panel is a duplicate of the right panel, except that a square region in the center has been displaced to the right. If you follow the line of mirror symmetry in the left panel, you can see that it jogs 2 mm to the right about 1/3 of the way down; it returns to the central position about 2/3 of the way down. To create this panel, the computer simply reproduced the outer portion of the panel on the right. It moved each dot in the central portion 2 mm to the right. The rightmost 2 mm of the central portion, which would have overlapped the unchanged right side of the panel, was omitted. Similarly, the gap that was created when the leftmost part of the middle portion was moved right (away from the unchanged left portion) was filled with a new sequence of random dots.

The end result is that each panel is an array of random dots. Were it not for the mirror symmetry imposed in the right panel (and copied into the left), they would each be completely random and formless. However, the outer parts of the two are identical, and the central portions are also the same except for the rightward shift. When the patterns are viewed dichoptically, the shifted area will not be imaged on the exact corresponding locations of the two retinae; that is, there will be some amount of binocular disparity. If this disparity produces an impression of depth in the absence of any pictorial or kinetic depth cues, it would be a demonstration of the strength and importance of binocular cues in the perception of depth.

If the stereogram in Figure 12–19 is viewed using the method described on page x, a surprising thing happens. After about five seconds, there should be the strong sensation of a square floating in front of the rest of the pattern. Those who cannot see this will just have to take our word for it.

The appearance of the random dot stereogram is not surprising if there are disparity detectors that interpret disparity as depth. But it is surprising that disparity can be determined when there is no structure in the images in the two eyes. How do the detectors determine which dots go with which? Clearly, in this case they cannot base it on corresponding points in independently recognized figures (Julesz, 1974). Similarly, it cannot simply be an alignment of contrasts, for images of opposite contrast can also fuse to form a three-dimensional image (see Figure 12–20).

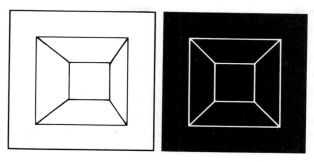

FIGURE 12–20 Stereo pair that gives an impression of depth despite having opposite contrasts in the two frames. View according to the instructions on page x. After Helmholtz (1925).

Another feature that does not seem to aid in the matching process is color (Livingstone & Hubel, 1987b). In addition, equiluminant random dot stereograms do not produce a perception of depth (Lu & Fender, 1972). As was the case in depth from texture and depth from motion, it appears that depth from stereopsis depends on the participation of the magnocellular system.

BOX 12-5

When an observer's two eyes are presented with similar views of the same scene with a small amount of binocular disparity, the observer sees a single unified scene that includes a strong depth component. What happens when the disparity between the scenes presented to the eyes is increased, either by changing the position of the scenes or by actually presenting the eyes with totally different stimuli? Under these conditions, a condition called *binocular rivalry* results. Suppose, for example, the two patterns of lines oriented in different directions shown in Figure 12–21 are presented dichoptically to a subject. There is no way that these two patterns can be integrated to produce a unified percept; what happens is that the subject usually reports seeing a horizontal pattern for a period of a few seconds, and then spontaneously changes to seeing the vertical pattern. In fact, it is likely that part of the field will be seen as vertical lines and part as horizontal, giving a "patchy" appearance that shifts with time. In other words, you see each region monocularly with the one eye, and then with the other, but the information from the two eyes does not fuse to form a single binocular percept. When the subject reports seeing the stimulus presented to the right eye, we say that eye is *dominant*, while the left eye is being *suppressed*.

Under conditions of binocular rivalry discussed in the last paragraph, where the two

(continued)

(box continued)

eyes are presented with equally compelling stimuli, subjects report frequent fluctuations in which eye is dominant and which is suppressed. In addition, they find it difficult or impossible to control which eye they are attending to at any particular moment. If one eye is presented with a well-defined stimulus and the other with a blank field, however, the eye that is seeing the stimulus will almost always be dominant (see Fahle, 1982). You can verify this for yourself by covering one eye with your hand; instead of alternating between seeing the world with one eye and seeing darkness with the other, you only see the world. Therefore, the uncovered eye has become the dominant eye in this situation.

Binocular rivalry results in the suppression of information coming from one eye under conditions in which the two eyes receive very disparate inputs. We have shown, however, that there is almost always some disparity in the image of the world projected onto the retinae. How does the visual system unite the two slightly different pictures of the visual world? One possibility is that we somehow fuse images that are slightly disparate into one percept that has a depth component associated with it. If this is the case, then we should not have a dominant and suppressed eye when looking binocularly at a visual scene; instead, information from both eyes should be processed simultaneously. Blake and Camisa (1978) were able to demonstrate that, in fact, when a subject dichoptically viewed patterns that were either identical or only slightly different from each other, both eyes were equally sensitive in detecting the presence of a small flash that could be presented to either eye. When the subject viewed a patterned scene with one eye and a blank field with the other, the eye with the blank field presented to it was always less sensitive to the test flash than the eye receiving patterned stimulation. From this study, Blake and Camisa concluded that when the two eyes viewed the same or similar scenes, the visual system used information from both eyes equally to create a single fused percept. Under conditions of binocular rivalry, however, information from the suppressed eye was actively ignored.

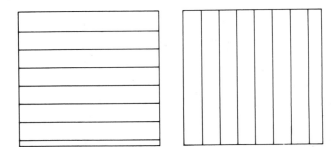

FIGURE 12-21 Two competing patterns that would cause binocular rivalry when viewed dichoptically. View this figure using the method described on page x.

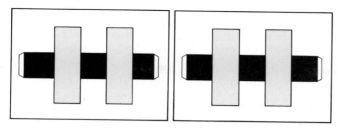

FIGURE 12-22   A stereo pair in which the depth of the middle segment is given entirely by monocular cues. View according to the instructions on page x. From *Vision*. By David Marr. Copyright © 1982 by W. H. Freeman and Company. Reprinted with permission.

Of course, the monocular and binocular cues are ultimately combined into a single percept. A good example of this integration may be seen in Figure 12–22. In this stereo pair, the two vertical bars appear to be in front of the horizontal bar both because of the monocular cue of interposition, and because of their relative disparity. But there is no stereoscopic cue to the depth of the middle segment of the horizontal bar; its image is identical in both frames. It appears at the same depth as the end segments because of the monocular information that it is to be interpreted as a continuation of the two end segments (Marr, 1982).

The combined information from monocular and binocular cues tells us the relative distances of objects from ourselves. However, this is not how we perceive the world. If it were, all the distances would shift every time we move, and relative positions of objects would be difficult to comprehend. David Marr, in an influential monograph (1982) published shortly after his death, referred to this viewer-centered representation as the "2 1/2-D sketch." It is not the flat, two-dimensional representation of edges captured by the "primal sketch," but neither is it a real three-dimensional model of the world. That representation must be derived from the 2 1/2-D sketch.

Physiological Studies on Binocular Depth Perception

In looking for a physiological substrate that might mediate binocular depth perception, one is naturally drawn to the visual cortex, as that is the first part of the visual system to possess binocularly responsive cells. Most of the binocular cortical cells discussed in Chapter 9 had receptive fields from the two eyes that corresponded quite closely with each other. That is, there was little or no disparity in the positions of the receptive fields of the eyes. Such cells would be effectively stimulated by objects at the fixation distance, but to perceive objects either in front of or behind the fixation point, one would expect to find binocular cells that had receptive fields with disparate retinal receptive field positions.

Binocular cortical cells with disparate receptive field locations have been found in the brains of a variety of animals, including cats (Barlow, Blakemore, & Pettigrew, 1967; Nelson, Kato, & Bishop, 1977), monkeys (Hubel & Wiesel, 1970), and owls (Pettigrew & Konishi, 1976). In the monkey, Hubel and Wiesel found that the binocular cells encountered from V1 all had receptive fields that showed no binocular disparity, but that cells in V2 often responded best to dichoptically presented stimuli that were slightly displaced in some way. These cells often did not respond at all to monocular stimulation, and responded best to a very small range of disparities. Some cells respond to zero disparities (locations on the horopter), some to disparities representing positions in front of the horopter, and others to positions behind the horopter (Clarke, Donaldson, & Whitteridge, 1976; Poggio & Talbot, 1981). That such cells may actually signal stimuli at specific depths in an awake, behaving animal was shown by Poggio and Fischer (1977). These investigators trained a monkey to fixate on a small spot a certain distance away, and presented stimuli that could either be in front of or in back of the fixation spot. While the animal was performing the fixation task, the experimenters simultaneously recorded from single cells in the visual cortex. They found some cells that only responded to stimuli in front of the fixation distance, and others that only responded to stimuli that were farther away than the fixation spot. At the level of the visual cortex, therefore, cells can be found that are selectively sensitive to stimuli that have specific distance relationships to the point of fixation. Cells with other properties appropriate for depth detection have also been reported. For example, Poggio, Motter, Squatrito, and Trotter (1985) found cells that responded to the disparity in a random dot stereogram. Other cells respond to motion in depth (Cynader & Regan, 1982).

To what systems do these cells belong? We have pointed out several instances in this chapter in which equiluminant stimuli failed to produce a depth effect, implicating the magnocellular system. As we said in Chapter 9, the magnocellular system responds well to depth, and leads ultimately to a "where" locating system. Indeed, the cells tuned to specific disparities near the horopter, or to detecting crossings of the horopter, seem to be found in the magnocellular pathways: the thick stripes of V2, and in V3 (Poggio, Gonzalez, & Krause, 1988).

Of course, the parvocellular system (at least the interblob) also responds well to depth, as it must if it is to determine "what" the objects are. It is not clear whether the parvocellular depth capabilities are dependent on those of the magnocellular system or represent a parallel determination of distance. In this regard, it is noteworthy that a coarse and a fine depth system have been identified (Norcia, Sutter, & Tyler, 1985).

The experiments previously discussed indicate that there are binocular cells in the cortex that have the capability of participating in the perception of visual depth. The question still remains, however, of whether the presence of these binocular cells is necessary for binocular depth perception to occur. To investigate this problem, Blake and Hirsch (1975) took advantage of the fact that if kittens are raised with alternating monocular visual stimulation (so that each eye receives stimulation, but never both simultaneously), their cortex contains abnormally few binocularly responsive cells (see Chapter 9). Blake and Hirsch tested such cats for their depth perception abilities, and found that they were inferior to normally raised cats in this regard. On other behavioral tests of visual performance, such as visual acuity, the monocularly reared cats performed normally, suggesting that the deficit was specifically in their abilities to perceive depth.

Psychophysical experiments performed on human subjects also support the contention that binocular cortical cells are necessary for binocular depth perception to exist. Blake and Cormack (1979) attacked the problem in the reverse way from Blake and Hirsch's experiment. They found a human population that was stereoblind, and tried to determine whether these people had binocular cells in their visual cortices. The experimenters reasoned that if stereoblind observers had only monocularly responsive cells, they should be superior to normal subjects in tasks that required deciding to which of the two eyes a given visual stimulus was presented. They found that this was, in fact, the case; normal observers often had great difficulty in determining which eye a given stimulus was presented to, but stereoblind observers performed this sort of task with facility. It therefore seems quite likely that the binocular disparity cells discovered by Hubel and Wiesel and others do mediate the binocular perception of depth.

SUGGESTED READINGS

The chapter on visual space perception in C. H. Graham's *Vision and Visual Perception* (Wiley, 1965) provides a detailed and fairly complete treatment of the topic of depth perception. Even more complete are the two chapters on depth and binocular stereopsis in L. Kaufman's *Sight and Mind* (Oxford Press, 1974). Finally, J. J. Gibson presents the topics of depth and distance perceptions quite elegantly in *The Perception of the Visual World* (Houghton Mifflin, 1950); the book is somewhat dated, but still quite useful.

Bela Julesz has written an excellent review of his work on binocular depth perception that appeared in *American Scientist* (1974, 62:32–43). In addition, Julesz has written two articles for *Scientific American* on this topic: "Texture and visual perception" (February 1965), and "Experiments in the visual perception of texture" (April 1975; offprint #563). The former article has been reprinted in *Perception: Mechanisms and Models*, edited by R. Held and W. Richards (W. H. Freeman, 1972), while the latter article can be found in *Recent Progress in Perception*, edited by R. Held and W. Richards (W. H. Freeman, 1976). Also in the 1976 collection is "The neurophysiology of binocular vision," by J. Pettigrew (*Scientific American*, August 1972; offprint #1255); another relevant *Scientific American* article that has not been reprinted elsewhere is "The resources of binocular perception," by J. Ross (1976, 234:80–87; offprint #569).

The process of determining depth from shadows and grays, such as in Figures 12–4 and 12–5, is considered in "Perceiving shape from shading," by V. S. Ramachandran (August, 1988); this article is reprinted in *The Perceptual World*, edited by Irvin Rock (W. H. Freeman, 1990).

PERCEPTUAL CONSTANCIES

13

We have discussed some ideas about how you can see and recognize an object (Chapter 11) and how you can locate it (Chapter 12). Now we will consider how you perceive certain attributes of the object—its size, shape, and color. Despite the fact that a given object can be viewed from different angles or distances in a variety of different lighting conditions, an observer will usually be able to correctly identify the physical characteristics of the object. The physical sizes, shapes, and colors do not change in these different viewing conditions. Similarly, the apparent sizes, shapes, and colors tend not to change; they remain constant, and we refer to the *constancy* of these properties.

This is really *the* fundamental problem for a perceptual system: how to create a logical and stable internal representation of the world (which is, of course, logical and stable) from the distorted and changing representations delivered to our sensory receptors. This is the heart of the problem identified by Ragnar Granit, a Nobel laureate for his early work in visual physiology, in his inquiries into the functioning of the brain:

> [W]e must not underestimate what the interpreting brain itself adds to make the seen world more intelligible than does a pure peripheral input, dependent though the cortex is on information from feature detectors. The purposive brain requires a considerable degree of invariance, size constancy, a fixed verticality, approximately invariant surface colors, some constancy of velocity and direction of movement and, above all, a steady world; in short, a large number of what one is fully entitled to call "reliable illusions." They are all constant errors with respect to the informational content of the primary sensory message. A world in which, for instance, my hands all the time varied in size with the retinal image would be intolerable! And so the brain does what no computer can imitate: in growing and developing, it creates the world it needs. Granit (1977; page 128).

As an example, consider an all-too-familiar object: this book. It has certain physical properties, such as size (7³/₈ x 9¹/₄ inches), a shape (rectangular solid), and a color (black cover). As it is carried about, it can be seen from various angles (straight on, tilted, edge on, and so forth) but it always appears as a rectangular solid. You see it from various distances (right next to you on the table, over there on the desk where you ''forgot'' it) but it does not appear to grow and shrink in size when viewed from different positions. You see it in bright sunlight on your way home (with lots of light reflecting from its cover to your eye) and in the dim light of the cafeteria (with little light reflected from the cover), yet the cover always appears black. In this chapter, in addition to examining the way in which we perceive the size, shape, and color of objects, we will also see a number of visual illusions that result from inappropriate judgments of these attributes.

LIGHTNESS CONSTANCY

The first constancy we will discuss is *lightness constancy*. The more general term for this is *color constancy*, for we are dealing with the ability of the observer to assign a judgment of color to an object despite changes in the illumination. However, we will be talking about the whiteness or blackness of uncolored (''gray'') objects, and ''color'' brings to mind changes of hue; we therefore use the more narrow term *lightness*.

Actually, it is not lightness at all that we are dealing with, for objects generally do not radiate their own light. They reflect light from some source such as the sun or an electrical fixture. What we are really talking about is the *reflectance* of an object, which is the percentage of the light incident on it that is reflected from it. That light that is not reflected is absorbed by the object; what percentage of light is absorbed and what percentage reflected depends on the pigmentation and texture of the surface. An object that is highly pigmented will be an excellent absorber and will appear black. A reflective object, on the other hand, will absorb very little light and reflect nearly all the light incident upon it; such an object will appear white. The blackness or whiteness of an object depends on its reflectance (another term for this is *albedo*); black objects have reflectances of only a few percent and white objects have reflectances near 90%. It is really a property of the object that is being judged; we therefore prefer to use the term lightness rather than *brightness*, a term that is commonly used to mean the same thing. (Another term that is occasionally used is *whiteness*.) Regardless of the name it is given, it should be borne in mind that we are asking subjects to rate target objects as white, black, or shades of gray, and not to say how much light appears to emanate from them. We will use the term *brightness* when subjects are asked to judge the total amount of light emanating from (or reflected by) a scene or object (see Arend & Goldstein, 1987).

Optical measuring devices (including our eyes) cannot measure reflectances directly; all that a photodetector (or a rod or cone) can do is respond to the light it is receiving. To measure reflectance, a physicist would measure the light incident upon an object as well as measuring the light coming from it; the ratio of these two measurements is reflectance. As our eyes only receive information regarding the reflected light and not the incident light, we are apparently unable to detect reflectance directly. What we respond to is the light reflected from an object, which is the product of the incident illumination and the reflectance.

Consider a sheet of white paper. It has a high reflectance, perhaps as much as 90%. Imagine looking at the sheet of paper in a room lit by a single light bulb; the paper reflects 90% of the light incident upon it, but 90% of a small number is still a small number. Now consider a black cat, whose furry coat absorbs most of the light incident upon it; the reflectance may be as low as 5%. When the cat walks in the sunlight, only 5% of the incident light reflects off the fur—but 5% of a very large number is still a lot of light. There may be thousands of times more light reaching your eye from the cat fur in sun than from the paper indoors, yet the cat looks black and the paper white. How do you make these determinations?

Suppose the same black cat steps in front of the car headlights some dark night on a clear open road. If the light bathes the cat but there are no other objects also in light, the cat will look ghostly white. We cannot detect that a small percentage of the light is being reflected because there is no way to estimate how much light is incident upon the cat. That is also why the moon appears self-luminous in the sky. It is reflecting sunlight, but observers on the nighttime earth cannot see that source of illumination.

This was the basis of an experiment performed by Gelb in 1929. He had observers look into a dimly lit room in which there was a black disc. A projector, hidden from the observers' view, cast a bright beam of light on the disc so that it was well lit, but no other visible object in the room received any of the extra light. The disc appeared white; in fact, with a bright enough light from the projector, it appeared self-luminous (see Henneman, 1935). When Gelb placed a small rectangle of white paper in the beam just in front of the disc, however, the disc immediately appeared black and the paper white. It was as if the white paper, revealing the true nature of the illumination, dispelled the question of how much light was incident, and lightness could be correctly judged. When the paper was removed, the black disc again appeared white, indicating it was not the observers' conscious (or intellectual) knowledge of the situation that was critical.

The converse demonstration can also be performed. Kardos (1934) set up a field of objects lit by a single source, with a white disc for the observer to judge. A solid object (out of the observer's view) cast a shadow only on the white disc, which then appeared black. Removing the screens that hid the true situation so that the observer was intellectually aware of the shadow did not reverse the illusion. The cues for lightness constancy must reside in the scene being observed, not in the intellectual knowledge of the observer.

BOX 13-1

Shadows present an interesting situation. If two identical objects are seen against the same surface but a shadow falls across only one of them, they still appear the same color and lightness. Nonetheless, it is clear that the one in shadow has less light coming from it; the judgment of lightness seems to be one of reflectance rather than of light reflected.

When a shadow falls across a relatively uniform surface, we can generally recognize it for what it is: a shadow. We can clearly see that the shadowed area is "darker," yet we do not think of the surface as being different in the area of the shadow. (Sometimes we are fooled by an odd fold in the surface and mistake a shadow for a stain; in that case the shadowed area does appear to be different from the rest of the sur-

face. Conversely, we may sometimes mistake a stain for a shadow.) As an example, take a sheet of white paper and cast a shadow on it. The shadow should be relatively crisp and distinct; a reasonable arrangement is shown in Figure 13-1. Here, a wooden ruler casts a clear shadow if the only light in the room is a single bulb at some distance; it is best if the bulb has no lampshade. (We could use the sun as a source, but the shadow will move slowly as the earth rotates on its axis.)

The shadow cast by the ruler is relatively distinct, but there should be no trouble recognizing it as a shadow. This recognition is caused in part by the fact that the shadow's edge is slightly blurred. The shadow cast by an object lit by a finite light source has two parts:

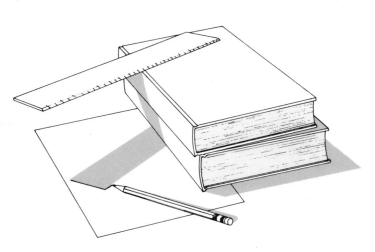

FIGURE 13-1 A shadow cast on paper.

(continued)

(box continued)

the *umbra*, or darkest part, is where the surface on which the shadow falls is fully shielded from the light source. The *penumbra*, or outer shadow is the part near the edge where the source is only partially eclipsed, so the light is partly diminished. This slight blurring of the shadow's edge serves to indicate the fact that the dark area is a shadow and not a different surface.

If we now remove the blurred edge and replace it with a firm outline, the shadow changes its nature (Wallach, 1963). To do this, take a dark pencil or black felt-tip pen and carefully outline the shadow, as shown in the figure. (This is why the sun makes a poor light source: we do not want the shadow to move away from its outline.) The outline into which the shadow exactly fits makes it look like a different surface than the rest of the paper; when it is outlined, it also appears darker than it did as a simple shadow. Our perceptions of lightness depend on the apparent illumination of the surface being judged.

Simultaneous Contrast

That judgments of lightness depend on the perceived illumination of objects raised the question of how the incident illumination can be estimated. Wallach (1948) suggested that what we are doing is simply comparing the amount of light reflected by the object in question with the amount of light reflected from adjacent regions in the visual field. Thus an object of moderate reflectance should look lighter in front of a black background than it would in front of a white background. This is called *simultaneous contrast*.

The idea of simultaneous contrast is often considered an alternative to the theory of *adaptation level* (Helson, 1948; 1964). Adaptation level refers to the mean luminance of a field; the visual system is presumed to respond to changes above and below the average level of luminance (and average color as well). In the experiments we will be discussing, the only things in the visual field other than the test objects being judged are uniform surrounding fields; the average luminance of the scene is therefore really just the luminance of these surrounding fields. In the real world, the objects we observe are surrounded by complicated arrays of other objects of various shades and sizes. These would determine the adaptation level; from the point of view of simultaneous contrast, some average of those objects nearest (or bordering) the test object would be taken as the surrounding luminance. The difference between the simultaneous contrast and the adaptation level theories would therefore reside in how large an area surrounding the test object would determine the surrounding (or adaptation level) luminance. It would also depend on whether the surround was taken to be that area adjacent to the test object in the proximal stimulus, or those things perceived to be near the test object (in distance as well as position). It should also be noted that the adaptation level depends in part on the recent history of illumination, as well as on the current scene.

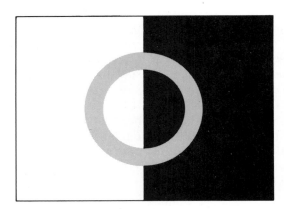

FIGURE 13-2 Simultaneous contrast; when a pencil is placed across the border between black and white, the halves of the ring appear different.

Simultaneous contrast is demonstrated in Figure 13–2. Careful inspection should show that the shaded ring is uniform; if we now create a border between the part of the ring against the black background and the part against the white background, the two half-rings will appear to be different in lightness. (To create a border, simply place a pencil along the division between black and white.) The border is necessary because the ring is perceived as a single "good" figure (see Chapter 11), and tends to appear homogenous in color; the border breaks it into figures that can each take on a different lightness (Koffka, 1935; see also Berman & Leibowitz, 1965).

Wallach (1948) tested simultaneous contrast by projecting a disc of light on a screen in an otherwise dark room. When the disc was shown in isolation, it appeared self-luminous; when it was surrounded by an annulus of light (of either lesser or greater intensity) the disc seemed to be white or gray. How light or dark it appeared was influenced by the annulus surrounding it; an annulus of higher luminance made the disc appear dark, and an annulus of lower luminance made it appear light. A second disc (of different luminance) surrounded by an annulus was shown on the other side of the display; the subject's task was to adjust the luminance of the annulus surrounding the second disc so that the second disc appeared the same color (lightness) as the first. Wallach found that the two discs appeared equally light when the ratios of their luminances to the luminances of their respective annuli were the same. For example, a 200-unit disc could exactly match a 100-unit disc if the former were surrounded by a 400-unit annulus, and the 100-unit disc by a 200-unit annulus. Similar findings had been reported in 1894 by Hess and Pretori.

The rule that the lightness of an object is given by the ratio of its luminance to that of its surround is quite attractive for its simplicity, and for the relatively direct way it can be related to the physiology of the visual system.

Another way to express the ratio rule is to say that we are responsive to the *contrast* of an image. When we discussed the concentric receptive fields of retinal ganglion cells (Chapter 6) and lateral geniculate neurons (Chapter 8), we emphasized that these cells respond to contrast. Increasing light in the center of a ganglion cell receptive field will tend to increase its response (increased inhibition is also an increased response), but light falling in the surround will decrease the center-driven response. The net response is therefore given by the balance of the light in the center and the light in the surround. This is the premise of lateral antagonism, which we discussed in Chapter 6; a moderate light appears dimmer if surrounded by bright light, and brighter if surrounded by darkness. It is safer to describe this phenomenon as lateral antagonism than by the specific receptive field structure by which lateral antagonism is achieved, for one would not expect the test discs in a psychophysical experiment to coincide exactly with the centers of receptive fields of ganglion cells. The principle that nearby light diminishes the responses in a particular area does, however, apply.

BOX 13–2 ▬▬▬▬▬▬▬▬▬▬▬▬

As we have already pointed out that the center and surround of a ganglion cell receptive field seem to interact subtractively (Rodieck & Stone, 1965; Enroth-Cugell & Pinto, 1970), one might wonder why a ratio rule should be expected. The answer lies in the fact that the firing rate of a ganglion cell in response to light is approximately proportional to the logarithm of the light intensity (Easter, 1968a; Levine & Abramov, 1975; Naka & Rushton, 1966). The logarithmic rule would apply in both the center and the surround of the receptive field; taking the difference between the responses in those two areas is therefore equivalent to subtracting the logarithms of the incident luminances. Subtracting logarithms is mathematically equivalent to taking a ratio, so the response of the ganglion cell is proportional to the logarithm of the ratio of the luminances in center and surround of the receptive field. Of course, this is an approximation and it does not hold for extreme ratios.

The ratio rule is simple but, not surprisingly, it does not work over large ranges. Heinemann (1955) studied the apparent brightness of discs surrounded by annuli over a wide range of luminances and ratios of luminances. When a test disc was surrounded by a much dimmer annulus, the brightness of the test disc was only slightly affected by the luminance of the annulus. Only when the luminance of the annulus was nearly the same as that of the test disc did the annulus make the test seem dimmer. When the annulus luminance surpassed that of the test disc, the test disc abruptly looked very dark.

An experiment that tested the ratio principle more directly was performed by Jameson and Hurvich (1961). They presented a display of five neighboring patches of known reflectances. The incident lighting illuminating the entire display was varied by a factor of about 10; at each illuminance level the ratios of the luminances of the patches remained constant (being given by the ratio of the reflectances) despite the difference in absolute luminances. Like Heinemann, Jameson and Hurvich had their subjects estimate the brightness of each patch by setting the luminance of an isolated matching patch, but here we can see the effects of changed luminance when the ratio of test to surround is constant.

If the brightness of the test patch were determined by the ratio of its luminance to the luminances of its neighbors, the brightness would be unaffected by changing the illumination; this is what happened when the ratio of test patch luminance to surround luminance was not too extreme. For that situation, the ratio rule worked perfectly (as it had for Wallach).

When the luminance of the test patch was either much greater or much less than that of the surround, however, the ratio rule failed. When the test patch was much lighter than its surround, its apparent brightness increased with increased illumination. In that case, it is possible that the patch was so much lighter than the surround that the surround was nearly irrelevant, and the patch was like a luminous source similar to the matching patch. In the limit, if the surround were perfectly black, the test patch and matching patch should be set to be physically identical.

The case in which the test patch is of considerably lower reflectance than the surround is rather interesting. Increasing the incident illumination seemed to cause a decrease in the apparent brightness of the test patch; more light on the patch made it darker! This is not as paradoxical as it seems, however, when one considers that the brightness is determined by the luminance of both the object and its surround. Increasing incident illumination increases the luminance of the test patch, but it also increases luminance of the surround. The brighter surround causes the dimmer test patch to appear blacker. When incident illumination is very low, everything appears a general gray; increased illumination brings out the surround and makes the patch appear relatively blacker (Hochberg, 1971a).

BOX 13–3

We should not overemphasize the failure of the ratio rule, for that may be an artifact of the relatively simple displays used in the experiments previously discussed. The ratio rule works quite well when the stimuli are more complicated (Arend & Goldstein, 1987).

The more complicated stimuli often used are made of various sized and shaped patches of shades of gray (or, in some cases, color). These stimuli are known as "Mondrians," after Piet Mondrian, the Dutch painter whose paintings these stimuli resemble. Mondrians are just abstract versions of the complicated images in the real world. The accuracy of judgment of lightness of patches in Mondrians under various conditions of illumination led Land and McCann (1971) to postulate a theory of lightness perception that they call the *retinex* theory. In this theory, lightness is built up from the ratios of luminances at the various borders. The light-

(continued)

(box continued)

ness of each patch buried within the pattern is computed by cumulating the differences at each border crossed as one goes from some reference point to the patch in question.

There is an added feature built into retinex theory to allow for the fact that luminance may change gradually across parts of an image; these gradients are what we encounter in a picture illuminated from one side. If they are gentle enough, the gradients may be imperceptible, for they represent extremely low spatial frequen-

cies. The retinex theory deliberately excludes gradients by postulating a threshold below which a change in luminance is imperceptible. We have already seen how gradients may be ignored compared to the edges of an image in the Craik-O'Brien illusion (Figures 6–6 and 10–12). Thus, the background gradient in the lower part of Figure 13–3 is ignored for the computation, and the retinex is "fooled" into seeing the circles as different in lightness. In fact, we are also fooled by gradients, as you can see in Figure 13–3. All the small gray circles are

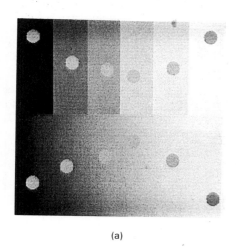

(a)

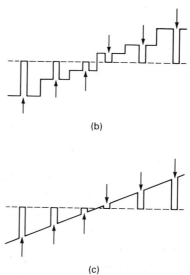

(b)

(c)

FIGURE 13-3   (a) Patterns in which identical circles appear different in lightness because of the background against which they are viewed. (b) Sketch of luminance versus position (through the centers of the circles) in the upper half of part (a). Arrows indicate the circles, with luminances matched to the horizontal dashed line. (c) Luminance profile for the lower half of part (a). From R. Shapley (1986). The importance of contrast for the activity of single neurons, the VEP and perception. *Vision Res*, 26:45–61. Reprinted by permission of Pergamon Press, Ltd. and the author.

(continued)

(box continued)

actually identical, but some are placed against a dark ground (so they appear light) and others against a light ground (so they appear dark). You can demonstrate that the circles are really identical by covering the picture with a sheet of paper with holes punched over each gray circle. The grays seen through the holes will be the same.

The retinex theory is satisfactory for the circles placed against a gradient, as in the lower part of Figure 13–3, but the borders of the steplike background in the upper part of Figure 13–3 should be well above the threshold. We should be aware of the steps against which the circles are seen. As a result, the reti-

nex theory predicts that all the circles in the upper part should be seen veridically; that is, they should appear to be equal in lightness. This is clearly not the case. Anomalies such as in Figure 13–3 have led some to question the retinex theory's reliance on the global changes in luminance. Shapley (1986) criticized retinex on these grounds, and proposed that the perception of lightness is based on the average contrast at the borders of each area being judged. As a result, the only contrasts of importance in Figure 13–3 are at the borders of the small circles. This way, their relative lightnesses are correctly predicted to be judged as different in both the upper and lower parts of the figure. A similar demonstration on a Mon-

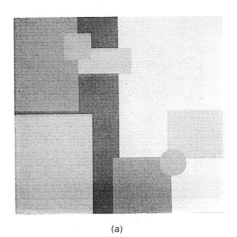

(a)

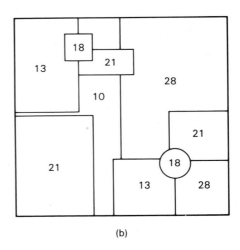

(b)

FIGURE 13–4 Mondrian pattern in which two patches of identical luminance appear different in lightness because of the surrounding patches. (a) The small square in the upper left is the same gray as the circle in the lower right. (b) Sketch of the pattern, with relative luminances of each patch indicated. From R. Shapley (1986). The importance of contrast for the activity of single neurons, the VEP and perception. *Vision Res*, 26:45–61. Reprinted by permission of Pergamon Press, Ltd. and the author.

(continued)

(box continued)

drian pattern is shown in Figure 13–4. Here, the square in the upper left is of the same luminance as the circle at the lower right, but appears lighter because of the darker surrounding boxes.

Notice that both the retinex theory and Shapley's contrast theory measure contrast at the borders. The difference is that retinex simultaneously includes *all* borders, while Shapley considers only the borders of the patch being judged. This closely parallels the older controversy of adaptation level versus simultaneous contrast. Both of those theories compared luminance in the patch being judged to an "average" background luminance; adaptation level considered *all* of the background, while simultaneous contrast considered only those parts near the patch being judged.

Cognitive Factors in Lightness and Brightness

It would be nice to be able to say that we can explain the perception of lightness and brightness from the physiology of the retina, and predict the apparent lightness of a surface by knowing the pattern of light on the retina. Lateral antagonism from areas surrounding the surface in question obviously plays a part in determining the lightness of the surface, but it would be misleading to end our discussion of lightness without pointing out that other perceptual aspects of a display affect the apparent lightness or brightness.

We have already seen an example of how higher processing of the image played a role in perception of lightness. A shadow appears darker when it is outlined (see Box 13–1), even though the outline is a minor part of the pattern on the retina. Similarly, the division of the ring in Figure 13–2 into two parts (by placing a pencil across the border) was necessary to show the effect of simultaneous contrast on the apparent grayness of each half.

A graphic demonstration of this point can be seen in Figure 13–5. This is a reversible figure similar to the ones we saw in Chapter 11; it may be seen as a tube with the opening to the right (so that the shaded crescent on the right is the inside of the tube), or with the opening to the left (so the crescent on the left is the inside). With a bit of concentration, it should be possible to see the tube in either configuration, just as Necker cubes could be seen in either of two configurations. The thing to notice here, however, is that whichever shaded crescent is seen as the inside of the tube appears slightly lighter than the other (mirror-image, but otherwise identical) crescent. Coren and Komoda (1973), who devised this figure, suggested that the reason for this is that the inside of a real tube receives less illumination than the outside; when the inside of a tube is seen as reflecting the same amount of light as the outside, the perceptual hypothesis is that it must be of higher reflectance (lighter in color) than the outside. Here, the pattern on the retina is absolutely unchanged as the figure reverses; the change in perceived brightness is a result of the interpretation of the pattern.

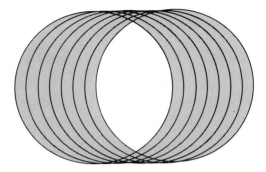

FIGURE 13-5 Ambiguous "tube" which may be seen opening to either left or right. Brightness of each shaded crescent depends on configuration seen. Figure 7.9 from *Sensation and Perception*, by Stanley Coren, Clare Porac, and Lawrence M. Ward, copyright © 1979 by Harcourt Brace, Jovanovich, Inc., reprinted by permission of the publisher.

Perceived depth can also affect the perception of lightness (Hochberg & Beck, 1954; Mershon & Gogel, 1970). Gilchrist (1977) provided a good demonstration of this effect. His observers looked through a peephole (to limit depth cues) into a room with a doorway that opened into a second, more brightly lit room (Figure 13–6[a]). On the far wall of the second room, visible through the doorway, was a piece of white paper; on the wall of the near (dimmer) room, partially overlapping the doorway, was a piece of black paper. The subject was asked to judge the lightness of the test, which was a piece of white paper fastened inside the doorframe. The test stimulus could be a square, overlapping the corner of the black paper so that it clearly was within the first (dimmer) room, as in Figure 13–6(b), or it could have two notches cut out of it so that it appeared to be behind the paper in the second (bright) room, as in Figure 13–6(c). When the test stimulus appeared to be in the near room, as it actually was, it was perceived to be of a light color; when it was incorrectly judged to be in the more brightly lit far room it was perceived to be a dark gray. The difference between the patterns reaching the observer's retina are slight; the lightness must have been determined in part by the interpretation given to the patterns.

BOX 13-4

In addition to the spatial factors that contribute to the perception of brightness, there is a temporal factor. Under certain circumstances, a flickering light can appear brighter than a steady light of the same mean luminance; this

phenomenon is known as *brightness enhancement*.

A light can be flickered (turned on and off regularly, as if viewed through the blades of a slowly turning fan) at any rate. If the rate is

(continued)

(box continued)

slow enough, the flicker is obvious, and it is easy to judge the brightness during the time the light is on. As the rate of flicker increases, it becomes harder to resolve that the light is actually flickering and not steadily on. For example, fluorescent lights flicker at a rate of 120 cycles/sec (a fluorescent tube becomes almost completely dark 120 times a sec), yet their light appears steady. Flicker at that rapid a rate is too fast to be detected; we say it exceeds the *critical fusion frequency*, or CFF, the rate at which a flickering light appears steady. The effective light coming from such a flickering light is the average amount of light in a cycle, or the average of the light half-cycle and the dark half-cycle.

When a light flickering at about 10 cycles/sec is compared to steady light of the same average luminance, the flickering light appears brighter (Bartley, 1938). The subject can easily detect the fact that the flickering light is not steady, but cannot correctly compensate and judge its brightness.

This phenomenon may be explained by recalling some characteristics of the responses of ganglion cells in the retina. The responses of the Y-type cells in particular are minimal in steady light; there is a peak of response when the light first comes on, and a much lower plateau of response while it is steady (see Chapter 6). A flickering light is continually re-exciting the peak response. On the average there is more activity in ganglion cells stimulated by a flickering light than in one stimulated by a steady light of the same average luminance, so the flickering light appears brighter (Walters & Harwerth, 1978). This enhancement has been demonstrated in single cell recordings in animals such as the cat (Enroth, 1952; Grüsser & Creutzfeldt, 1957; Hughes & Maffei, 1966) and the horseshoe crab, *Limulus* (Ratliff, Knight, & Graham, 1969).

SIZE CONSTANCY

Size constancy refers to our ability to judge correctly the sizes of objects despite the differences in the retinal images cast by them as they are viewed from different distances. The woman standing next to you projects a larger image on your retina than does the man across the room, but she does not seem larger than he. The size of the proximal stimulus (retinal image) is intimately related to the distance an object is from you, so it is clear that your ability to judge size is intimately related to your judgments of distance.

The relationship between size and distance is at the heart of the concept of *visual angle*. We have already made use of visual angles in speaking of eye movements and spatial frequencies, but here we must define it more carefully. The visual angle, θ, subtended by an object is the angle between the line drawn from the edge of the object through the center of the pupil of the eye and the line drawn from the opposite edge of the object through the pupil of the eye. The geometry is shown in Figure 13–7. Notice also that the projection onto the retina is defined by the same angle as the visual angle, for

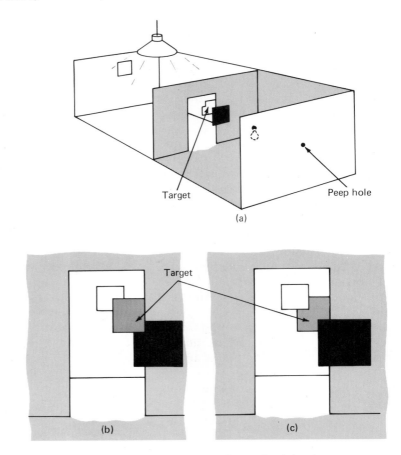

Target   Peep hole

(a)

Target

(b)   (c)

FIGURE 13-6 Demonstration of effect of perceived depth upon apparent lightness. After Gilchrist (1977) Perceived lightness depends on perceived spatial arrangement. *Science* 195:155–157. Copyright 1977 by the AAAS. Reprinted by permission of the publisher and author.

the rays from each edge of the object continue straight through the center of the optical system of the eye. The angle inside the eye is also θ, and the size of the image on the retina (a) is related to θ and y, the size of the eyeball. As the size of the eyeball (y) does not change as we view objects at various distances, the size of the retinal image depends only on the visual angle. We may therefore refer either to visual angle or to the size of the retinal image (proximal stimulus) and know that there is always a one-to-one relationship between them.

There is not a unique relationship between object size (distal stimulus) and visual angle, as the distance from object to eye can easily change. Consider Figure 13–8(a); two people are viewed from two different distances.

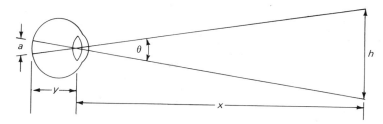

FIGURE 13-7 Definition of visual angle. An object of height h at a distance x subtends a visual angle θ; this angle uniquely determines the size of the retinal image, a.

The closer person (at position 1) subtends a larger visual angle (θ_1) than the equally tall person at position 2 (θ_2). Their heights are the same, but the distances are different; as a result, the visual angles subtended by them are different and the retinal images are not the same size. The retinal image of person 1 will be about three times as large as the image of person 2, but the observer will correctly judge them to be equally tall *if* he or she can correctly infer their relative distances.

Figure 13–8(b) illustrates the opposite situation. Here, the person standing in position 1 is only half the distance of the tree in position 2. He is also half the height of the tree, so the ratios of height to distance for each are the same: if the person is at distance x and is of height h, the tree is at twice the distance ($2x$) and stands twice as tall ($2h$). They subtend the same visual angle, and project identically high images upon the observer's retina. Nevertheless, the observer can correctly judge the tree to be twice the height of the person *if* he or she can correctly infer their relative distances.

The key to size constancy lies in the last phrase of the two preceding paragraphs: "*if* he or she can correctly infer their relative distances." The cues to distance were the subject of the previous chapter (Chapter 12); by making use of these cues, a distance is inferred, and perceived size follows directly from that inference. Of course, there is a certain amount of interaction, as the size of the proximal stimulus is also an important cue for determining the distance between an object and the observer. If the object has a readily known familiar size (see Chapter 12), the distance can be known from the ratio of the actual size to the size of the proximal stimulus. In general, what the observer must do is make a perceptual hypothesis (see Chapter 11) about the size *and* distance of the object, using all the available distance cues and size cues (such as known size of the object), to build a model of the visual scene somewhere within the mind. Built into this process, of course, is the hypothesis making that went into the determination of what was figure and what was ground, as well as actual identification of figure.

We must reemphasize here that the making and testing of perceptual hypotheses is an unconscious process. You do not look at a scene and think: "What could that be? Can I separate that set of lines into a closed figure?

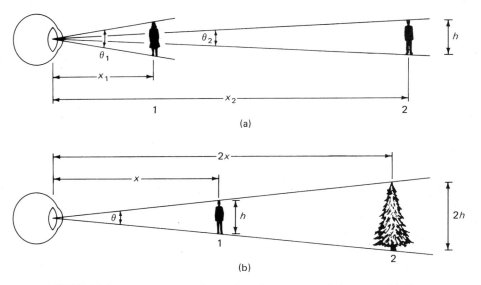

FIGURE 13-8   Relationship of visual angle to size and distance. (a) Two objects of the same height at different distances subtend different visual angles. (b) Two objects of different heights at different distances may subtend the same visual angle.

What figure is it? How far is it? Given that it is 500 m away and subtends a 21.8° angle, it must be, um, 500 times 0.4, or, ah, 200 m. Ok, it is a 200-m building 500 m away.'' Even when the inferences are wrong (as in optical illusions) and you are made *intellectually* aware of the actual situation, the misperception persists.

The classic experiment demonstrating the link between size estimates and perception of distance was performed in the corridors of Harvard University by Holway and Boring (1941). The subject was seated at the intersection of two corridors. Down one corridor was a disc whose size the subject was asked to judge. The disc could be at a number of different distances but whatever its distance, its size was selected so that it subtended exactly 1° of visual angle (Figure 13–9). Down the other corridor was a second (comparison) disc at a constant distance, whose size could be adjusted. The subject's task was to set the size of the comparison disc in the second hallway so that it appeared the same size as the 1° test disc in the first corridor.

There are two distinct ways a subject could do this. As the test disc subtended exactly 1° no matter what its distance from the subject, the size of the retinal images could be matched by always setting the comparison disc to subtend 1°. The comparison disc was always at the same distance, so its size would not change as function of the distance of the test disc. On the other hand, the subject could set the comparison disc to be the same physical size

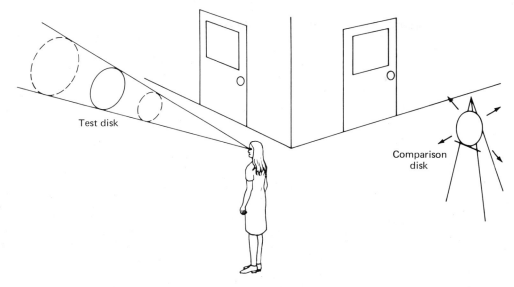

FIGURE 13-9 Experimental arrangement for study of size constancy used by Holway, A. H. and E. G. Boring (1941) Determinants of apparent visual size with distance variant. *Am. J. Psychol.* 54:21–37. Reprinted by permission.

as the test disc, making the comparison disc larger as the test disc was moved farther away (as the test disc was in fact made larger at farther distances in order to maintain the constant 1° angle).

The results of the Holway and Boring experiment for a number of different viewing conditions are shown in Figure 13–10. The predictions based on the two possible strategies outlined above are shown in dashed lines. If the subject matched visual angle, which was constant, the horizontal dashed line marked "constant visual angle" would result; if the size was correctly matched, the comparison disc would be made larger at larger distances, and the sloped line marked "size constancy" would result.

Consider first the circles, resulting from the relatively natural condition of viewing with both eyes. In this condition, the subject presumably had as much distance information as possible. Size constancy seemed to be the rule, although there was a tendency to overcompensate. (When the test disc was distant, it was seen as somewhat larger than it actually was.) As cues to depth were removed, size constancy worked less well. Thus, viewing with only one eye (removing all binocular cues) gave results in which the size was very slightly underestimated (triangles). A more drastic effect was obtained by having the subject view the discs through a peephole, a tiny pinhole (squares). The pinhole removed the depth cues of motion parallax (if the subject's head moved, the subject simply did not see through the pinhole)—see Chapter 12). With so few cues to depth, the subjects were nearly unable

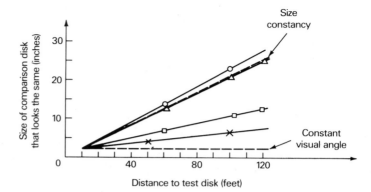

FIGURE 13-10 Results of size constancy experiment. Slanted dashed line represents perfect size constancy; horizontal dashed line represents judgments based on visual angle. Circles are for binocular viewing; triangles for monocular viewing; squares for viewing through a pinhole; Xs for viewing through a pinhole with curtains blocking stray reflections.

to determine the distance of the test disc, and tended to a compromise between size constancy and adjustment according to the size of the retinal image.

Finally, with the corridor darkened, curtains placed in front of doors to prevent any reflections, and viewing monocularly through the pinhole, the discs must have appeared as luminous circles of indeterminate distances. In that case, the subjects very nearly obeyed the law of constant visual angle, for there was nothing else on which to base size judgments. This is what is referred to as an *unstructured field*, meaning there is no structure or form to give cues to size or distance. Holway and Boring's subjects set the size of the comparison disc approximately according to the visual angle of the test disc (Xs), although there was still a hint of size constancy in their settings. Presumably, some depth cues still remained, and were potent enough to allow the subject to see the more distant test discs as somewhat larger. (In a 1950 experiment, Lichten and Lurie used screens that hid the shadowy structure of the corridor. The subjects were allowed to see only the stimuli, and based their settings of the comparison disc entirely on the visual angle of the test disc.)

There are two important lessons from Holway and Boring experiment. The first is that when a subject is allowed cues to the distance to an object, it is possible to compensate for the change of visual angle with distance and correctly judge the size. That is, within a reasonable range of distances, there is a law of size constancy. The second lesson is that when the cues to distance are removed, the subject cannot correctly judge size, and must base estimates mainly on the visual angle subtended by them (see also Hastorf & Way, 1952;

Zeigler & Leibowitz, 1957; Rock & McDermott, 1964). (Although perceived size is clearly related to perceived distance, the relationship is not perfect. If an object is moved to a new distance, the size may be correctly judged as the same but the new distance may be somewhat misestimated.)

BOX 13-5

That the perceived size of an object is related to its perceived distance may be conveniently demonstrated by noting the apparent sizes of afterimages. An afterimage can be generated by staring fixedly at a high-contrast pattern, such as a (not too) bright lamp, or a white shape on black paper (in bright illumination). Gaze away from the high-contrast pattern after fixating for about 30 sec to a minute, and stare at a blank (preferably gray) surface. After a moment or two, a reversed version of the original pattern should appear; this is because of local adaptation of the area of the retina that has been stimulated by the original pattern (see Chapter 7).

The afterimage has a constant retinal size, as it is created by the specific cells within the retina that have been adapted. It therefore subtends a constant visual angle, regardless of the distance to the surface against which it is seen. The afterimage appears as if it were floating on the surface it is viewed against; the farther away the surface is, the farther away the afterimage appears. An afterimage of a particular pattern viewed against a surface that is as far from the observer as the original pattern was will appear the same size as the original pattern. If the afterimage is viewed against a surface farther away (for example, the far wall of the room), it will appear considerably larger than the original pattern used to generate it. Conversely, if it is viewed against a near surface (a sheet of paper held close to the eye), it will appear smaller. The apparent size of the afterimage, which subtends a constant angle, depends on its apparent distance. This relationship between size and apparent distance of an afterimage is called *Emmert's law*.

Illusions of Size

We have already discussed some optical illusions in Chapter 11: optical illusions are those delightful gimmicks that fool and amuse us while teaching us something about how the visual system works. The largest class of optical illusions, the ones most often found on breakfast cereal boxes and in the pages of children's magazines, are the ones that give an erroneous impression of depth and therefore fool us about relative sizes. In these illusions, the apparent depth is not the same as the real depth, so the "constancy" of size is in error.

The most straightforward way to produce such an illusion is to create an impression of depth by using the cues of linear perspective. For example, the picture in Figure 13-11 shows an icy breakwater receding into the distance. All the cues (elevation, converging lines, fewer details, past experience with beaches) say that the end nearest the top of the picture is much farther away than the end at the bottom. The two ovals drawn on the picture are, in fact, identical in size and shape; they were drawn with the same template. They

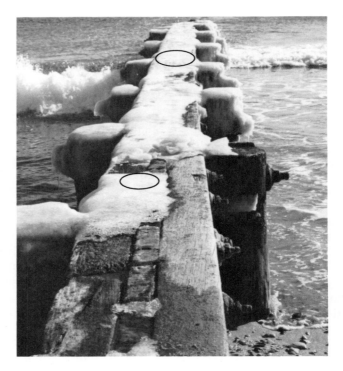

FIGURE 13-11   Demonstration of the corridor illusion. The two ovals drawn upon the breakwater are physically identical.

were drawn as if they were markings on the snow; the one nearer the top appears farther away than the lower one. As a result, the one nearer the top appears larger. Even after measuring the two ovals and understanding intellectually that they are the same size, the one nearer the top of the picture appears larger.

The illusion that the two ovals in Figure 13–11 are not the same size is an example of a variant of a group of illusions called the *corridor illusion*, because it is usually drawn as a long interior hallway. Any picture that gives the impression of receding into the distance can be used: a long hallway, a street, railroad tracks (an extremely popular one), a boardwalk. The distance cues include the converging lines, ever closer details, position in the frame, and change of focus (in photos). The more cues provided, the more compelling the illusion will be.

The illusion can also be achieved with only minimal cues. For example, if we strip away all the cues but the converging lines, and replace the ovals with circles, we obtain another illusion called the *Ponzo illusion* (Figure 13–12). (Actually, the Ponzo illusion is more often shown with the lines

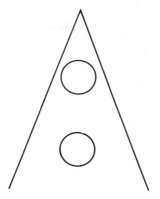

FIGURE 13-12 The Ponzo illusion. The two circles are identical.

converging to the side, rather than above the circles, as if the book was turned 90°; the argument about converging lines works in either case.) In the Ponzo illusion, the two lines converging toward a "vanishing point" may give the impression that the circle nearer this vanishing point is farther from the observer: it therefore appears larger. Demonstrate that the illusion is related to apparent depth by turning the Ponzo illustration (Figure 13–12) upside down. When the lines converge at the bottom of the picture, there is little sense to the perspective. The apparent depth is diminished, and the two circles appear essentially the same size.

A famous depth illusion designed by Adelbert Ames is called the *Ames trapezoidal room*. As the name implies, this is a room of trapezoidal shape such as the one in the illustration in Figure 13–13. An observer looks into the room through a pinhole in the front wall (remember, this prevents motion parallax, as well as enforcing viewing from a particular perspective and precluding binocular depth cues). The floor is trapezoidal, and slopes downward toward the corner at *A*; the rear wall is a trapezoid with trapezoidal windows. It is much larger at *A* (which is in fact quite far from the observer) than at *B* (which is fairly close). The trapezoids are arranged so that the view through the peephole gives the same proximal stimulus as a normal view of an everyday, rectangular room. Figure 13–14 shows the view from the pinhole.

Now, suppose two people are in the corners *A* and *B* (see Figure 13–14). They are essentially the same size, but the one in corner *A* is considerably farther from the observer at the pinhole than the one in corner *B*; he therefore subtends a considerably smaller angle. As the cues all indicate that the two are at the same distance, the perception is a difference in size (different visual angles at the same distance). This illusion is thus the converse of the corridor illusion, in which objects subtending the same visual angle appear

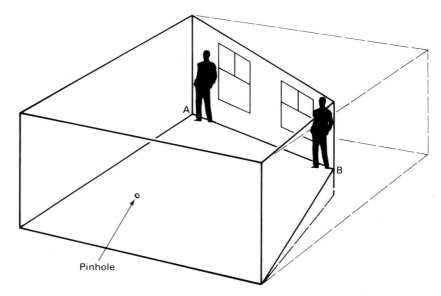

FIGURE 13-13   The Ames trapezoidal room, showing the actual configuration.

different in size because the cues indicate a difference in distance. The Ames
room demonstration is extremely compelling—it is most disturbing to see
two people in the actual room such that one is a hulking giant and the other a
midget, and watch each shrink or grow as they exchange places in the room.
It is interesting that in this case the familiar sizes of the people, and the expectation of constancy of size of each, is overridden by the illusion due to
apparent distance.

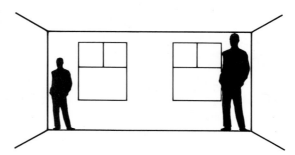

FIGURE 13-14   View through the pinhole into the Ames room
of Figure 13-13. From *Psychology: Themes and Variations*, by Wayne Weiten (Brooks/Cole Publishing
Company, 1989).

BOX 13-6

The illusions we have presented as illusions of distance can be explained in other ways. For example, the person on the right in Figure 13-14 may look larger simply by comparison to nearby features of the room. The "giant" is scrunched into a corner with the ceiling pressing his head, while the "midget" barely reaches the window. You would naturally judge a person huge who cannot fit into an apparently normal room, or car, or chair, without necessarily misperceiving distance. This is the trick used in movies to give the illusion of a miniature person; a normal actor is placed among mis-scaled props. Similarly, the upper circle in the Ponzo illusion (Figure 13-12) is "measured" by the closer lines near their vertex, and the ovals in Figure 13-11 are "measured" by the width of the breakwater.

At this stage, we are confusing size and distance. The ovals in Figure 13-11 are placed where the breakwater has different widths, but this is an inevitable result of linear perspective. If the breakwater did not change width, it would not appear to recede into the sea. We cannot state whether the illusion is due directly to the cues that also induce the impression of depth (as discussed in Chapter 12) or to the depth induced by those cues.

There are other illusions that may well depend on a misperception of distance that are not as directly perspective-related. One of these is called the *Hering illusion*; it consists of a starburst pattern of lines superimposed on two straight parallel lines (Figure 13-15). The straight lines appear bowed (you may have to convince yourself they are really straight by placing a ruler or the edge of a sheet of paper along each). It is possible that the explanation of this illusion is that the lines converging to a point suggest greater depth in the center of the figure; the parallel lines do not become closer (in visual angle) when they are "farther," and hence their separation

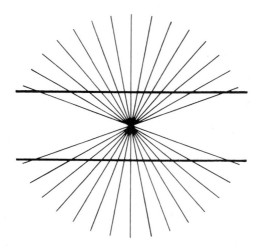

FIGURE 13-15 The Hering illusion. The 2 lines are straight and parallel.

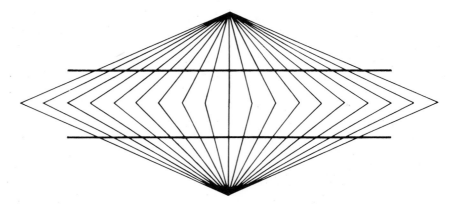

FIGURE 13-16   The Wundt illusion. The 2 lines are straight and parallel.

appears greater. On the other hand, presenting the illusion as a stereogram so that the parallel lines appear to be clearly in front of the converging lines does not disrupt the illusion (Kaufman, 1974), indicating a mechanism other than apparent depth. Perhaps there is a distortion of the apparent angles made with the lines, as in the Poggendorf illusion (Figure 11–22).

Similar to the Hering illusion is the *Wundt illusion*; in fact it is like an inside out Hering illusion. It is shown in Figure 13–16. Here, the radiating lines give the appearance of a flattened spheroid, like a flying saucer. The horizontal parallel lines appear to converge either because they appear closer to the observer at their midpoints, or because of the distortion of the angles made with the radiating lines.

BOX 13-7

The Hering and Wundt illusions are grouped with others in a class called "shape illusions," as opposed to the size illusions we have been discussing. Other shape illusions are shown in Figure 13–17. In the figure on the left, the radiating lines cause an apparent distortion of the regular shapes drawn on them. The square is actually a perfect square with straight edges (called the *Ehrenstein illusion*), and the circle is perfectly round (called the *Orbison illusion*). The figure to the right is called the *Zöllner illusion*; the long diagonal lines are actually straight and parallel. Like the Hering and Wundt illusions, these could be explained by

effects of apparent depth or perspective, or could be more closely related to distortions of angle such as seems to dominate for the Poggendorf illusion in Figure 11–22 (Brigell & Uhlarik, 1980).

Perhaps a hint as to whether these are really illusions of distance (depth), rather than relative size or angle, can be found by asking whether the illusions are present when depth is not salient. In Chapter 12, we presented several indications that the magnocellular system is essential for the perception of depth. The magnocellular system seems to be color blind; it cannot "see" a stimulus that is equiluminant

(continued)

(box continued)
(drawn in red and green such that the two are equally effective, and therefore indiscriminable by the magnocellular system). It was because equiluminant stimuli failed to produce a perception of depth that Livingstone and Hubel (1987b) concluded that the magnocellular system mediates depth. They also examined equiluminant versions of many of the illusions shown here, including the Poggendorf (Figure 11–22), the Ponzo (Figure 13–12), the Hering (Figure 13–15), the Zöllner (Figure 13–17[b]), and the Müller-Lyer (Figure 13–19). They saw no illusory effect at equiluminance in any of these. It thus seems that these illusions also require the participation of the magnocellular system. Of course, we cannot say whether they depend on the magnocellular processing of depth or on other functions of the magnocellular system.

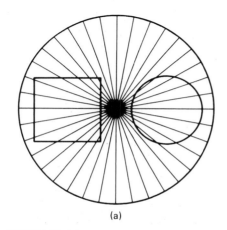

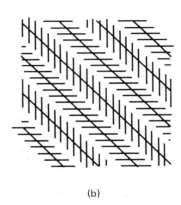

(a)   (b)

FIGURE 13-17   Shape illusions. (a) The Ehrenstein and Orbison illusions. (b) The Zöllner illusion.

An illusion that appears more distinctly depth-related is the *Jastrow illusion*, shown in Figure 13–18. The two arcs appear to be parts of rings lying on the floor; the one higher in the frame appears farther away and therefore larger. In fact, the two shapes are identical. (This illusion, like the corridor and Ponzo illusions, works less well if turned upside down.)

Now we come to the most famous, and perhaps most controversial illusion, the *Müller-Lyer illusion* shown in Figure 13–19. As everybody almost certainly has already been told, the two vertical line segments are equal in length (go on, measure them). Nevertheless, the one with the outward-splayed tails appears longer than the one with the inward-facing arrowheads. Why this is so has been the subject of considerable theorizing. Boring (1942) listed 12 different theories of the Müller-Lyer illusion presented in the first 12 years after it was devised! These include the possibility that the tails are

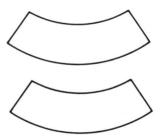

FIGURE 13-18 The Jastrow illusion. The two shapes are identical.

somehow included in the estimate of the lines, that the angles are misjudged (as with the Poggendorf illusion) and seem to point at a "false" line ending, that eye movements are greater when the tails face out than in, that lateral interactions at the intersections of the tails and lines affect the positions of the maximum excitations, or that the Müller-Lyer figure gives a false impression of depth that accounts for the apparent size difference. It is this last possibility we shall explore here.

The principal modern proponent of an apparent distance explanation for the Müller-Lyer illusion is R. L. Gregory, who likens the two figures to an exterior corner of a building and the interior corner of a room (see Figure 13-20). The exterior corner, which contains the arrows-in figure, should appear to approach the observer from the page, while the interior corner, containing the tails-out figure, should appear to be behind the page. The arrows-in figure should appear closer; because the visual angles are the same, the "closer" figure should appear smaller.

This explanation depends on the notion that the apparent depths of the straight lines in the Müller-Lyer figures are different. Gregory (1970; 1978) had subjects report the apparent depth of the figures by setting the apparent distance of a comparison spot, and found a depth difference commensurate

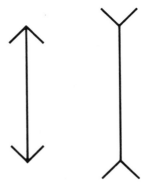

FIGURE 13-19 The Müller-Lyer illusion. The two vertical lines are equal.

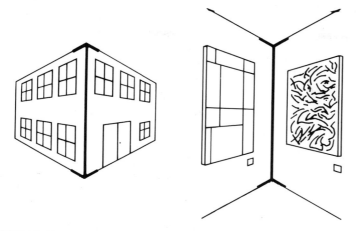

FIGURE 13-20 Drawing indicating how the Müller-Lyer figures could be perceived as indicating depth.

with the illusion. An even more potent test was to use stereograms of the Müller-Lyer figures and see if disrupting the apparent depth by an overriding binocular cue could disrupt the illusion. This was reported by Gregory and Harris (1975), who found a normal amount of distortion when the stereograms were appropriate to the differences in depth expected from geometric considerations, but a much diminished illusion when the stereograms were reversed so that the arrows-in figure appeared farther away than the tails-out figure (Figure 13–21[a]). In other words, a binocular cue that opposed the apparent geometric cue seemed to cancel the illusion.

BOX 13-8

The idea that there is a depth-related explanation for the Müller-Lyer illusion is accepted by many psychologists, but certainly not all. (For arguments against a size constancy explanation see Day, 1965; Massaro & Anderson, 1970; Waite & Massaro, 1970.) Even the demonstration that a stereogram depth reversal cancels the illusion does not settle the issue, for a depth reversal of the kind described by Gregory and Harris would be expected to give a size illusion that would cancel the illusion regardless of its actual origin. (The fact that the stereogram giving the appropriate depth rela-
(continued)

tionships did not enhance the illusion might speak against this argument.) A more appropriate test would seem to be one in which the stereogram causes the arrowheads to face the "wrong" way without affecting the apparent distances of the lines. Pitblado and Kaufman (1967) set up a stereogram in which the lines to be judged were unchanged in apparent depth but the arrows-in lines appeared to come toward the observer, and the tails-out lines appeared to recede. They found no disruption of the illusion in these circumstances, and con-

(box continued)
cluded that the Müller-Lyer illusion is not dependent on apparent distance.

A stereogram producing the effect that Pitblado and Kaufman found nondisruptive is shown in Figure 13–21(b); it should be compared to the apparently disrupting stereogram of the type used by Gregory and Harris, shown in Figure 13–21(a). The difference between the two is that in Figure 13–21(a) the ends of the wings are in the same plane as the fixation cross, while the horizontal lines lie in front of or behind that plane. In (b) it is the horizontal lines that are in the same plane as the fixation cross, while the wings extend in front of or behind the plane. (Both parts are set up so that the direction of the wings from the horizontal

lines is opposite that postulated by Gregory in explaining the illusion.) Note, however, that neither stereogram is so effective that you cannot convince yourself the illusion is either present or absent as desired.

There is a lesson here, which can be applied to a number of other experiments that claim to have "ruled out" one or another explanation of this (and other) illusions. The lesson is that perceptual hypotheses are based on all kinds of cues—there is no one cue that leads inevitably to a particular hypothesis. It is thus possible that under different circumstances illusions could be from different sources. It is probable that there is no single explanation for any given illusion (Fisher, 1970; Coren & Girgus, 1973).

Finally, we come to one of the most compelling illusions, one "devised" by nature rather than human beings. It is the *moon illusion*, in which the zenith moon (directly overhead) appears smaller than the horizon moon. (The same effect applies to the sun, but staring directly at the sun can permanently damage your eyes.) It may actually be a surprise to learn that the moon does *not* in fact change size as it travels across the sky; it always subtends the same visual angle (about $1/2°$) whether it is high overhead or serving as a huge harvest moon just over the treetops. It is *not* magnified by some strange effect of the more dense atmosphere near the horizon (it is slightly compressed in the vertical direction), nor is it actually closer to you at the horizon (it is very slightly farther away at that point). Nevertheless, the horizon moon appears larger than the zenith moon.

As with any good illusion, there are several theories to explain this one. Holway and Boring (1940) suggested that the zenith moon appears smaller because you must tilt your head back to see the moon overhead; this was shown not to be so by Kaufman and Rock (1962), who used mirrors to view horizon moons overhead and zenith moons straight ahead. They found that nearness to the perceived horizon was the essential cue to achieve the effect. Others (Restle, 1970) have argued that the illusion is explicable by the relative expanse of sky surrounding the moon. The size of a horizon moon is measured relative to the small stretch of sky separating it from the horizon, while the zenith moon is measured against the vast expanse of sky between it and the rest of the world.

The most interesting explanation for the moon illusion, and the one most commonly accepted, is that it is an illusion of apparent depth (Kaufman & Rock, 1962; Rock & Kaufman, 1962). The idea is that the moon is seen as if it were on the "surface" of the sky. If the sky were perceived as a hemispheric bowl, there would be no illusion; however, the sky is perceived as a flattened bowl that is closer at the zenith than at the horizon (as if it has gradually settled over the millennia). Clouds, when they are present, seem to heighten this flattened bowl effect, for clouds overhead are, in fact, closer than those at the horizon; and they appear closer in the sense that there is more visible detail in overhead clouds than horizon clouds. When thunderstorms roll in we seem to be sandwiched between two parallel planes, for the curvature of the earth is too slight to detect. Figure 13–22 shows a section of our clouded-over plane, indicating how the overhead clouds are actually closer than the distant clouds. We do not see the two planes extending to infinity with a gap

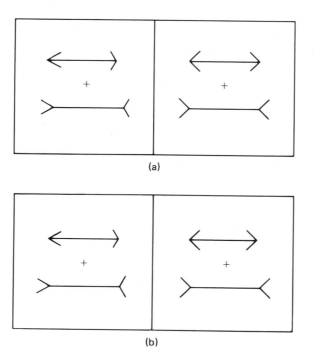

FIGURE 13–21 Stereograms that attempt to abolish the depth effects of the Müller-Lyer illusion. Note there is an illusion in each panel. Stereograms should be viewed according to the instructions on page ix. (a) The horizontal lines are displaced in depth; this should cancel the illusion. (b) The arrowheads are made to appear in the wrong depth for the interpretation in Figure 13–20; this should not affect the illusion.

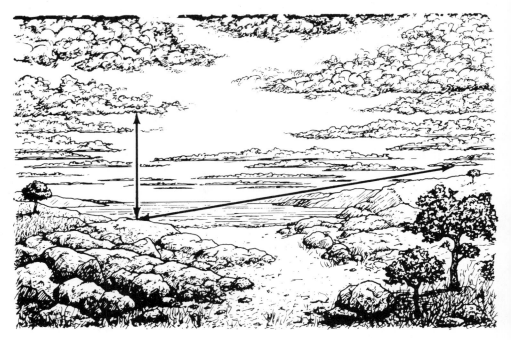

FIGURE 13-22 Indication of why the sky at the horizon should appear more distant than the zenith sky.

between sky and earth, however; the two seem to converge, and we idealize this as a flattened dome. Figure 13–23 shows the flattened dome of the sky with a truly hemispheric dome indicated in dashes.

The moon maintains a constant size in its travels across the sky; it is equivalent to moving a "moon-disc" along the true hemisphere (dashed). We perceive it as if it were traveling on the flattened bowl. (The projections of the moon in two positions are shown in Figure 13–23.) The moon appears larger at the horizon because it seems farther, and appears smaller overhead because it seems nearer, yet subtends the same visual angle. This idea is corroborated by the fact that afterimages also display the moon illusion when viewed against the sky (see Box 13–11).

There is a catch in this explanation, however. The horizon sky appears more distant than the zenith sky, but the horizon moon appears closer than the zenith moon. The low harvest moon seems to float above the treetops, practically within reach. If it appears closer, why does it not appear smaller? Kaufman and Rock recognized this problem, and have proposed that the judged distance to the horizon moon is influenced by its perceived size. That is, the horizon moon appears larger than the zenith moon because it appears to be on the more distant horizon sky; it then is judged to be closer than the zenith moon because it is apparently larger. In effect there are two distances: a "registered" distance that the perceptual system uses in gauging size, and a "judged" distance that is the overt estimate the observer would give of distance. (Rereading this last paragraph will probably not help you at all.)

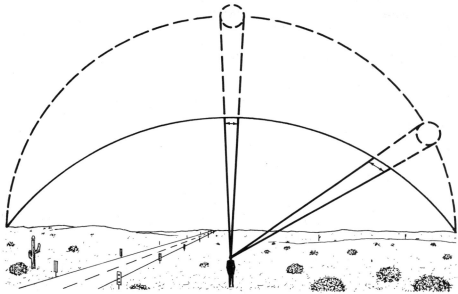

FIGURE 13-23 The moon illusion. The sky is perceived as a flattened dome (solid) against which the equal visual angle moon is projected. After Kaufman, L. and I. Rock (1962).

BOX 13-9

The two kinds of distance proposed by Kaufman and Rock are a form of parallel processing. Judged distance is the "output" of the distance system, the one we tap when we ask a subject how far away something is. Among its determinants are size; for example, your judgment of how high an airplane is when you are watching from the ground may be largely determined by your judgment of the familiar size of a plane of that type. Registered distance, on the other hand, is not available to your estimation apparatus; it is an internal datum used by the size-estimating system.

We have seen how the parallel pathways in the cortex may duplicate similar functions. For example, orientation selectivity is a property of both the magnocellular and parvocellular pathways at all levels above the lateral geniculate. Presumably, each requires this information for the tasks it performs, even though the two systems perform somewhat different tasks. Livingstone and Hubel (1987b) have argued that the movement-sensitive system displays orientation selectivity that is independent of the orientation selectivity evident in the texture or pattern system. Judged and registered distance may be an example of duplication in parallel pathways at another level of processing.

SHAPE CONSTANCY

The third kind of constancy we wish to discuss is called *shape*, or *object constancy*. It refers to our ability to perceive the shape of the distal object rather than the shape of the proximal stimulus.

Shape constancy is really a special case of size constancy. Distortions of the shapes of plane figures are caused by the fact that different parts of the figures are at different distances from the observer; those parts farthest away subtend smaller visual angles than corresponding parts of the same size that are nearer. When we speak of shape constancy, we really mean nothing more than the reconstruction of the correct relative sizes of the parts of a figure given their relative distances from the observer. To do this accurately, the observer must correctly infer the slant at which the figure is viewed.

To illustrate the kinds of distortions actually undergone by the proximal stimulus, we introduce the concept of the *frontal plane projection*. A frontal plane is like a window between the world and your eyes. If you traced the scene on that window, you would have a pretty good representation of the retinal image (like Magritte's painting in Figure 12–10). In fact, the photograph taken by a camera at the locus of your eye is a frontal plane projection of the scene. The advantage of referring to the frontal plane is that it allows us to demonstrate the geometry of objects viewed at different angles.

Figure 13–24 illustrates the frontal plane, and the frontal plane projections of a slanted circle and square. The circle is foreshortened into an ellipse, and the square becomes a trapezoid. These are the shapes of the proximal stimuli that are projected by those distal stimuli; note that there would be no difference in the shape of the pattern on the retina between a square seen from an angle and a trapezoid seen straight on. Shape constancy refers to the fact that a subject can perceive a square when the proximal stimulus is a trapezoid (and the distal stimulus is a square at a slant).

We might thus expect a relationship between the perceived slant of an object and the apparent foreshortening, just as there was a relationship between the size and the apparent distance (Koffka, 1935). This is, in fact, at least partially true, as shown by Beck and Gibson (1955). They showed subjects a display in which a triangle was mounted at 45° to a vertical background. On the background were two triangles, one of which was physically identical to the slanted one, the other of which was identical to the frontal plane projection of the tilted triangle. When the subjects viewed the display through a peephole so that they could not detect the slant of the test triangle, they chose the triangle with the same frontal plane projection as being the same as the tilted one. When the subjects viewed the display with both eyes, they chose the physically identical triangle as the same. The apparent shape was determined by the perceived slant.

Similar findings have been made with experiments in which the shape of tilted objects was to be judged (Thouless, 1931; Langdon, 1951; Miller & Bartley, 1954; Nelson & Bartley, 1956). As a general rule, the matched shape

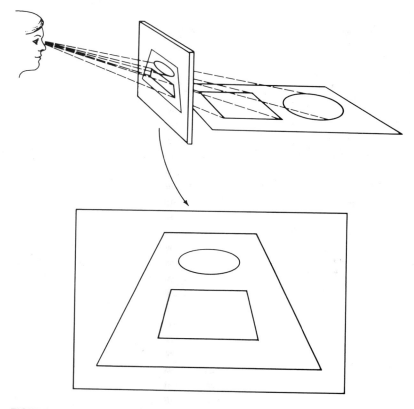

FIGURE 13-24 Frontal plane projection of objects at a slant.

lies between the frontal plane projection and the real shape. The more cues to the slant, the more like the real shape an object appears.

When an observer (not a trained artist) is asked to indicate the shape of a tilted object *as it appears in the frontal plane*, there is a tendency to draw a shape somewhat biased toward the actual physical shape. Thouless (1931) has called this "phenomenal regression to the real object." What that means is that you automatically correct for the registered tilt, just as perception of size includes an automatic correction for registered distance. This may explain the way children draw before they learn the rules of perspective. For example, Figure 13-25(a) is a "clear glass of water" drawn by a 6-year-old. Notice the overly round top and bottom of the glass; the child knew they were circular, and so drew them as nearly round. (Isn't this what Picasso does when he shows both a profile and frontal view of a face in the same picture?) Figure 13-25(b) provides an interesting comparison. It is a drawing of a glass made by a congenitally blind woman. Notice the same tendency to show the top and bottom as circular. The line down the middle represents the front of the glass, a "feature" not normally drawn by the sighted.

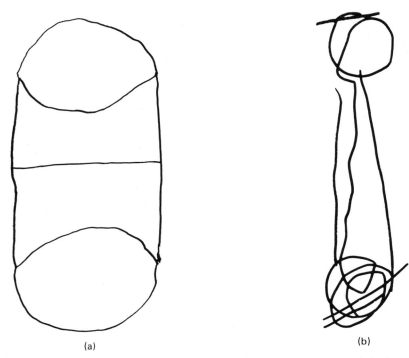

(a)   (b)

FIGURE 13-25   A "clear glass of water" showing exaggeration of the
circles at top and bottom. (a) Drawing by Matt Levine,
age 6. (b) Drawing by a congenitally blind woman,
from Kennedy, J. M. (1980). "Blind people recognizing
and making haptic pictures." In *The Perception of Pictures*, ed. M. Hagen pp.263–303. New York: Academic
Press. Reprinted by permission.

This apparent distortion of shape is not confined to our talents in drawing pictures. Coren, Porac, and Ward (1979) present an interesting demonstration, shown in Figure 13–26. The figure shows a drawing of a box; the
question is, could we lay a dime on the blank top of the box so that it would
not overlap any of the lines of the drawing? Most people think they can. If
you try, you will find that you were fooled into believing the top of the box
was a square, and therefore had more area than it really does.

Another demonstration is found in Figure 13–27. The fountain in the
center of the drawing is formed by a heavy ellipse. You can easily recognize
that it is an ellipse and not a circle (although the fountain appears circular).
Which of the ellipses to the right is the same shape as the heavy ellipse? You
will probably be surprised to learn that it is the second one down (check by
tracing it). Your judgment of the ellipse was affected by your perception of it
as a circle at an angle.

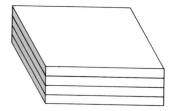

FIGURE 13-26 Demonstration of shape constancy. Will a dime fit on top of the box? Figure 14.2 from *Sensation and Perception*, by Stanley Coren, Clare Porac, and Lawrence M. Ward, copyright 1979 by Harcourt Brace Jovanovich, Inc., reprinted by permission of the publisher.

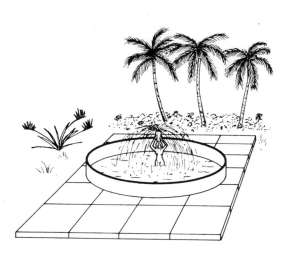

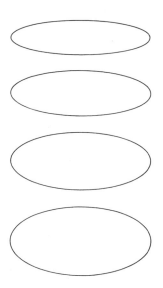

FIGURE 13-27 Demonstration of shape constancy. Which of the ellipses to the right is physically the same as the one that forms the top of the fountain?

BOX 13-10 ▬▬▬▬▬▬▬▬▬▬▬

When we think of regression to the real, we probably think that this carries an implication of some knowledge of the real object, based on past experience. Thus ellipses should look like circles, and trapezoids like squares; these are shapes that we are familiar with. It does *not* ap-
(continued)

pear that familiarity has a clear influence on shape constancy (Thouless, 1931; Nelson & Bartley, 1956). The only hint that familiarity might contribute to shape constancy comes from an experiment by Borresen and Lichte (1962). These workers used meaningless

(box continued)
shapes and found the amount of regression to the real. There was always some tendency to correct for the viewing angle, but the tendency could be increased somewhat if the subjects were first familiarized with the shapes that would be used.

At this stage, we should point out that the fact that there is a relationship between the perceived tilt and the estimated shape does not necessarily mean that there is a lawful compensation for tilt. In the physical domain, there is a trigonometric relationship: the height in the frontal plane is proportional to the cosine of the angle of tilt. The same is not necessarily true in the psychological domain. Nelson, Bartley, and Bourassa (1961) had subjects look at luminous circles and ellipses in an otherwise dark field; the subjects had to draw the shapes they saw and indicate tilt by setting a "tilt board"—a board on which their hands rested that could be moved to any angle in the manner of an automobile gas pedal. The subjects thus reported both the perceived shape and the perceived tilt. The relationship found was *not* exactly the cosine law relating physical tilt and the frontal plane projection; in fact, the exact law depended on the amount of texture in the pattern. On the other hand, when subjects set visual comparisons to both shape and tilt, shape and tilt are found to trade off as a true invariance (Kaiser, 1967). The point, however, is that the perceived tilt and perceived shape are not brought into a perfect trade-off. We already pointed out that the perceived size and judged distance also are not in an exact inverse relationship as real size and distance are.

Examples of illusions that depend on shape constancy are hard to single out, as shape constancy and size constancy are intimately related. After all, the former is a way of allowing for the shrinkage of the far edge of a figure that is viewed at an angle. The examples we can point to, therefore, can also be taken as examples of size constancy.

One such example is the Ames trapezoidal window, discussed in Chapter 11 (page 290). In that example, a window shaped like a trapezoid was rotated; because the larger edge always appeared closer, the window seemed to be rocking rather than rotating. We fooled our shape constancy mechanism into taking the trapezoidal shape as the frontal plane projection of a tilted rectangle. Alternatively, we could say that according to size constancy, we simply take the larger edge to be closer. In fact, both statements amount to the same thing.

We can summarize shape constancy by saying that it is the principle by which objects are seen as their correct shapes despite their being viewed at an angle. We judge the shape of an object by taking into account its tilt and not simply by the shape of its frontal plane projection. For this reason, photographs and paintings can convey correctly the shapes they portray despite the distortions of these shapes. We treat these representations as frontal plane projections, and perceive them as we would our own naturally occurring frontal plane projections. We also automatically compensate for the projected sizes of the images, and see objects in the picture in their appropriate relative sizes.

BOX 13-11

Pictures represent a remarkable second level of transformation that we can accept with no difficulty. A photograph is a frontal plane projection from the position of the camera. There is little problem understanding how, when we view a photo straight on, we can interpret ellipses as circles in the real scene (as, for example, the paper plates in Figure 13-28, which are ellipses in the photo but are obviously circular plates on the table). What is remarkable is that we can view the photograph from the side (not too extremely) and still correctly perceive the scene portrayed.

Actually, we do not compensate perfectly. Perhaps you have seen a portrait in which the subject is staring straight out of the frame. As you walk past such a painting, the eyes in the portrait seem to follow you as you move about the room. Objects such as eyes and pointing fingers in pictures fail to rotate because the point of view cannot change; Wallach (1987) invokes a compensatory mechanism that normally would prevent apparent rotation of real objects as we walk by them (a problem considered in the next chapter). Surprisingly, while the amount of rotation of objects in a painting may

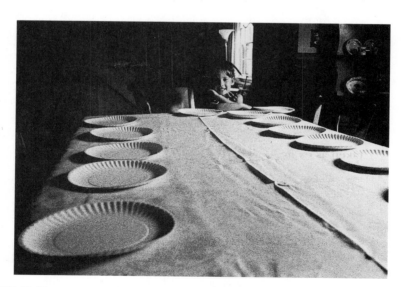

FIGURE 13-28   Child setting picnic table. Shapes are correctly perceived despite distortion into frontal plane of camera.

(continued)

(box continued)

differ, the spatial relationships among them do not seem to change (Goldstein, 1979).

The next level of abstraction is generally beyond our capabilities. Take a photograph of a photograph from one side, and the picture within the picture looks distorted. This is true even if the photograph of the photograph includes ample information about the way it was taken, as in Figure 13–29. Here we see what is obviously a scene in which the photo of Figure 13–28 is a part. We are unable to compensate for the distortion of the frontal plane represented by a photograph of it, and the scene in the photo-in-the-photo looks distorted. Now the images of the plates are in fact approximately circular, but look like strange ellipses.

We pointed out that the distortion caused by looking at a picture from an angle was automatically compensated for, up to a point. If the angle is really extreme, the process breaks down. This breakdown is the reason traffic instructions painted on the roadway must be made in such tall, stretched-out letters; they would not be legible in normal proportions. The distortions of extreme angles are also exploited in a form of painting called anamorphic art; some of these pictures were painted so that the subject could only be seen correctly when viewed at an extreme angle. An example is shown in Figure 13–30. To see the subject of this painting, you must look at it from the right side, with your eye practically touching the book.

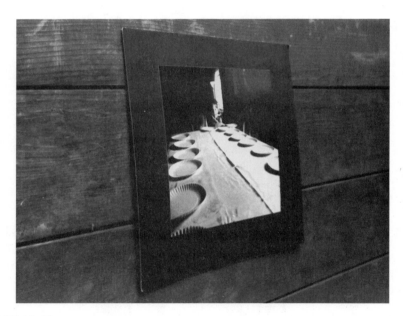

FIGURE 13-29   Photograph of a photograph. Notice the distortion of the objects in the embedded photo (which is Figure 13–28).

(continued)

(box continued)

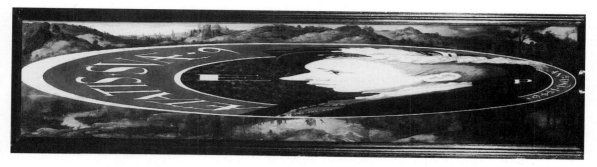

FIGURE 13-30   Anamorphic art. Viewed straight on the picture is quite distorted, but viewed from the right at an extreme angle (close one eye and let the other practically touch the page) it is a clear portrait of Edward VI. Reprinted by permission of The National Portrait Gallery, London.

SUGGESTED READINGS

There are several popular paperbacks available that concentrate on the illusions and constancies of vision. Two that are readable (although the reader is cautioned they are not without bias toward their author's positions) are by R. L. Gregory. One, *The Intelligent Eye* (McGraw-Hill, 1970) is noteworthy for its treatment of illusions and impossible or ambiguous figures, and for the inclusion of a large number of stereograms that can be viewed with the red/green goggles included in the book. The other is *Eye and Brain*, 3rd Edition, (McGraw-Hill, 1978), which includes somewhat more reference to the research literature. Another book of interest is *Visual Illusions*, by M. Luckiesh (Dover Publications, 1965; reprinted from a 1922 edition). Despite the fact that the book was written more than 50 years ago, the discussions of illusions and contrast are surprisingly up to date. The chapters of particular interest are: Chapter 4 (geometric illusions), Chapter 6 (angles), Chapter 7 (illusions of distance), and Chapter 8 (brightness contrast).

Surface Color Perception, by Jacob Beck (Cornell University Press, 1972) is devoted almost entirely to lightness and brightness perception. Much of the discussion is concerned with general theories of lightness constancy, with experimental evidence presented as it bears on theoretical positions. Of particular note is Chapter 7, which deals with anomalous illumination and shadows.

Chapter 8 of E. H. Gombrich's book *Art and Illusion*, 2nd Edition (Princeton University Press, 1961) deals with portrayal of depth and shape, and some illusions due to perceived depth. (We also recommended this book in Chapter 11 for its treatment of the principles of perception as applied to fine art.)

There are three pertinent *Scientific American* articles, all of which have been reprinted in the collection *Perception: Mechanisms and Models*, edited by R. Held and W. Richards (W. H. Freeman, 1972). They are: "Visual illusions," by R. L. Gregory (November 1968; offprint #517), which discusses illusions of depth (including the Müller-Lyer) and impossible figures; "The moon illusion," by L. Kaufman and I. Rock (July 1962; offprint #462), which presents their account of the moon illusion; and "The perception of neutral colors," by H. Wallach (January 1965; offprint #474), a discussion of simultaneous contrast and lightness perception. A more recent article is "Geometric illusions," by B. Gillam (January 1980); this article is reprinted in *The Mind's Eye* (introduction by J. M. Wolfe) (W. H. Freeman, 1986), and in *The Perceptual World*, edited by Irvin Rock (W. H. Freeman, 1990). This latter collection of *Scientific American* articles also contains Alan Gilchrist's account of how spatial relationships help determine the apparent lightness of a surface: "The perception of surface blacks and whites" (March 1979).

THE PERCEPTION
OF MOVEMENT

14

In this chapter, we will consider an important topic in visual perception: how we perceive the movement of objects through space. At first glance, this might seem to require only a straightforward extension of ideas that have been presented earlier; if we know something about form perception, object constancies, and the identification of objects that have depth associated with them, how much more do we have to know to understand how the same phenomena are perceived when moving? As usual, however, nothing is as simple as it seems. The perception of movement is actually a complex topic, at least partially because of the fact that observers (and their eyes) do not remain stationary while viewing the world. How the visual system differentiates movement that is caused by the external environment from movement caused by the organism is obviously a problem of importance and complexity. In addition, even when a subject is relatively stationary, eye movements are occurring during which the position of the entire visual world is shifted on the retina. How we avoid perceiving these shifts as large-scale movements in the world is another problem that students of motion perception must consider.

Human beings perceive motion either by detecting position shifts of the image of a stimulus on the retina, or by using eye movements to follow a moving object so that the object's image is maintained in approximately the same retinal location. R. L. Gregory (1978) has named the perceptual system that responds to movement of an image across the retina the *image-retina* system, while the system responsible for following the position of a stimulus with eye and head movements is called the *eye-head* movement system. In this chapter, we discuss both of these ways of detecting movement. In addition, we discuss the phenomenon of *apparent movement*, a class of events in which subjects report strong impressions of movement under conditions in which stimuli are actually stationary. This is in contrast to real movement, where the stimuli actually are moving in space.

THE MOTION-SENSING SYSTEMS

Image-Retina System

The most straightforward type of movement perception occurs when the subject is relatively stationary and the movement of the stimulus image across the retina is the critical event (Figure 14–1). In the studies that we will be discussing in this section, the subject's eye movements are rarely if ever controlled; however, most of the effects revealed by these studies would still be seen in the absence of eye movements. These experiments, therefore, investigate the properties of the image-retina movement system.

Motion thresholds   One of the first steps in characterizing a sensory system is to determine its thresholds, or limits of operation, as well as investigating factors that affect those thresholds. In most experiments investigating motion thresholds, the duration of the stimulus is held constant while the velocity of the stimulus is varied. Threshold velocities determined in this way have been named *isochronal* thresholds (Leibowitz, 1955a).

One of the most important determinants of motion thresholds is the location on the retina of the moving image. Objects whose images pass through the center of the retina have much lower movement thresholds than stimuli presented to the retinal periphery (Aubert, 1886); that is, much slower movements can be detected. This may seem somewhat surprising in view of

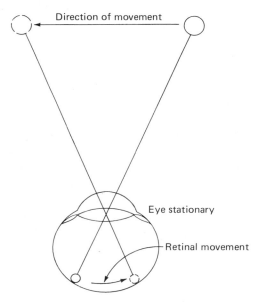

FIGURE 14–1   The image-retina system. As the stimulus moves, the image also moves across the retina. Adapted from Gregory (1978).

the fact that the periphery is often thought of as being selectively sensitive to novel or sudden movements, with a higher proportion of movement-sensitive ganglion cells than in the fovea. The absolute number of retinal cells in the periphery is much smaller than in the center, however; in addition, the size of retinal ganglion cell receptive fields grow with eccentricity, so a greater extent of motion may be necessary for it to be resolved. Leibowitz, Johnson, and Isabelle (1972) have shown that much of the deficit in peripheral movement perception is caused by optical factors that degrade images in this region of the retina. These investigators compared movement thresholds in the presence and absence of lenses that were designed to minimize peripheral refractive error. The results are shown in Figure 14–2; although movement thresholds rise as a function of eccentricity for both conditions, the effect is much greater in the condition in which refractive errors were not corrected. More recently, it has been found that when stimuli move at relatively fast speeds, the peripheral retina is actually superior to the fovea in detecting movement (Bhatia, 1975). This reversal in what portion of the retina is most sensitive to movement probably occurs at a stimulus velocity such that sustained ganglion cells (perhaps the X-cells that project to the parvo-

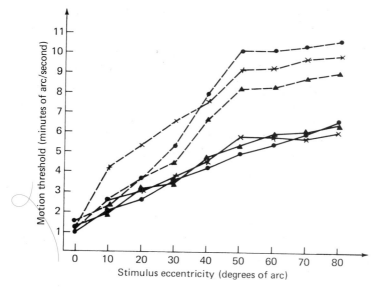

FIGURE 14–2 Motion thresholds for three observers as a function of stimulus eccentricity. Dashed functions are derived from experiments with no correcting lenses, solid functions come from experiments using lenses best to focus images in the retinal periphery. From Leibowitz, H. W., C. A. Johnson and E. Isabelle (1972) Peripheral motion detection and refractive error. *Science* 177:1207–1208. Copyright 1972 by the AAAS. Reprinted by permission of the publisher and author.

cellular system) are not effectively stimulated, but more transient ganglion cells are still quite responsive.

Other factors besides retinal position affect thresholds for detecting the motion of stimuli. One factor that has a large effect is the presence of reference points in the visual field; many studies have shown that thresholds obtained using a single stimulus in a homogeneous field may be much higher than when the field includes stationary reference points. It seems that this improvement only occurs under conditions when the stimulus duration is fairly long; for durations shorter than 4 sec, it does not matter whether reference points are present or not (Harvey & Michon, 1974). These data suggest that there might be different mechanisms responsible for the perception of motion of stimuli presented quickly and for those stimuli that remain for longer periods of time. Note, however, that this difference could also be partly due to drifts in eye position that would only be significant with the longer exposure times.

Motion aftereffects   In our discussion of retinal ganglion cells in Chapter 6, we described cells found in both the frog and rabbit retina that were selectively sensitive to movement. Cells were found that responded to movement of a stimulus in one direction but were completely unresponsive to movement in the opposite direction. In higher animals (cats and monkeys), ganglion cells are not generally sensitive to movement in a specific direction; however, many cells in the visual cortex are (see Chapter 8).

The presence of directionally selective cells in the human visual system could form the basis of the image-retina movement system. In fact, there is evidence for the presence of direction-specific movement detectors in the human visual system. The supportive evidence comes mostly in the form of investigations of a phenomenon called the *movement aftereffect* (MAE) (Figure 14–3). Most people who stare at a waterfall for a couple of minutes and then look away get an illusion of the objects they are looking at (trees, rocks, etc.) floating upwards. This effect is called the *waterfall illusion*, and is an example of an MAE. Other examples of MAEs abound in the natural world; for instance, a passenger sitting in a train that has come to a stop often has the feeling that the stopped train is moving backwards. Or if you watch all the closing credits on a video, and they scroll up the screen at a steady rate, the entire TV may seem to be moving downward after the credits have ended.

BOX 14-1

One of the most striking motion aftereffects is the *plateau spiral* illusion, which can be demonstrated using the spiral in Figure 14–3. Trace the spiral, cut out along the dotted line, and place it on the turntable of a record player. Stare at the spindle in the center of the spiral while the turntable is rotating for about 1 minute and then stare at a neighbor's face. There
(continued)

(box continued)
should be a striking impression of continual expansion of the person's face. What is most disconcerting is that the impression is one of continual expansion, even though the face does not change size.

The most common explanation for MAEs is that they are caused by adaptation of the motion-specific detectors that are tuned to the direction of movement of the stimuli in the scene being viewed. For example, in the waterfall illusion, all the detectors sensitive to downward movement are continuously stimulated while viewing the waterfall. If these detectors adapt and become less sensitive, when the viewer shifts gaze and looks at other objects, all the movement detectors in the other directions will be activated more than the downward motion detectors, resulting in an impression of the scene moving upward. Both the phenomena and this explanation of them are reminiscent of the figural aftereffects discussed in Chapter 10.

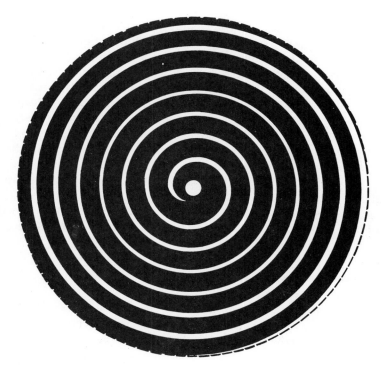

FIGURE 14–3 Stimulus for inducing spiral aftereffect. For instruction on how to get the illusion, see Box 14–1.

BOX 14–2

Motion aftereffects also apply to moving stimuli. On page 310, we discussed a kinetic depth effect in which a field of dots (the shadows cast by spots on a transparent sphere) presents a three-dimensional appearance when the sphere rotates. If the light source is far away (like the sun) so that the rays are parallel, it is impossible to tell from the shadow which dots are on the near side of the sphere and which are on the far side. The result is that the direction of rotation is ambiguous; you cannot say whether the sphere is rotating clockwise or counterclockwise. As with other ambiguous stimuli (see Chapter 11), the direction of rotation seems to reverse spontaneously.

Nawrot and Blake (1989) added an MAE to this ambiguity. They had their subjects adapt to an unambiguous rotating globe before showing them the shadow pattern of dots. As a result of the preexposure, the ambiguous pattern was always seen rotating in the opposite direction from that of the globe. This is what one would expect if adapting to a globe rotating, for example, in a clockwise direction adapted all the "clockwise" detectors, so the "counterclockwise" detectors prevail to determine the apparent rotation of the field of dots. Notice, however, that this is quite different from adaptation of left-moving or right-moving detectors: it is adaptation to a rotation in depth.

If MAEs are caused by adaptation of direction-specific motion detectors, perhaps we can get some idea of where in the visual system these detectors are located by varying the conditions under which the aftereffect occurs. If the detectors are retinal in origin, there should be no interocular transfer of the effect; that is, if one eye was presented with an adapting stimulus that moved continuously in one direction, no aftereffect should be present in a test field viewed by the other eye. When Mitchell, Reardon, and Muir (1975) performed this experiment, however, they found that MAEs were present under such conditions. This is strong evidence that the motion detectors being adapted by the adapting stimulus are not retinal in origin, but must be located at or after the point in the visual system at which inputs from the two eyes have combined: that is, the visual cortex. This conclusion was further strengthened by Mitchell *et al's* observation that subjects who were stereoblind (that is, had poor binocular vision and depth perception presumably because of lack of binocular cells) failed to show interocular transfer of the aftereffect.

BOX 14–3

In our discussion of depth perception in Chapter 12, we noted that presenting two eyes with distinctly different visual scenes resulted in binocular rivalry in which the information

from one of the eyes was suppressed. Lehmkuhle and Fox (1975) wondered if the motion detectors responsible for the MAE were located before or after the point in the visual system at

(continued)

(box continued)

which binocular suppression occurred. They tested this question by presenting a unidirectional adapting stimulus to one eye under conditions that suppressed that eye for varying lengths of time. They checked whether the length of time that the adapted eye was sup-

pressed affected the strength of the MAE. Their results showed that suppressing the adapted eye using binocular rivalry did not affect the MAE, indicating that the detectors responsible for motion aftereffects are before the level where binocular rivalry operates.

Other evidence for direction-specific motion detectors   There have been several experiments designed to yield more information regarding the properties of the motion detectors. Levinson and Sekuler (1975) presented a grating moving in one direction at a constant speed, and manipulated the contrast of the grating to find a threshold level for which the grating could just be seen. They found that this contrast level did not change when a slightly subthreshold grating moving in the opposite direction was added to the visual display. This is evidence that, like the spatial frequency channels discussed in Chapter 10, the direction-specific motion detectors are independent of each other. For a stimulus to be above threshold, therefore, it must activate a single detector above a certain level, and activation of a second detector (for example, with a grating moving in the opposite direction) will not affect the threshold of the first detector. Other studies have confirmed this observation (Sekuler & Ganz, 1963; Pantle & Sekuler, 1969).

Other studies have further extended our knowledge about the direction-specific motion detectors. Tynan and Sekuler (1975) were interested in whether a moving stimulus had to be continuous through a field to activate the motion detectors in that field; they presented subjects with a stimulus array similar to that shown in Figure 14–4, in which two sections of a moving grating were separated by a piece of black construction paper that covered the center of the grating. When subjects viewed this stimulus configuration, they reported seeing the grating continued through the construction paper, even though that portion of the array was completely blank. The "phantom grating" seen on the blank part of the field looked considerably dimmer than the actual grating on either side, but it was of the same spatial frequency and traveled at the same speed. When the grating stopped moving and was held stationary, the phantom grating disappeared, and subjects saw just the middle portion of the field as being blank. The illusion of a phantom grating seen when the grating was moving was therefore a product of a movement detection mechanism, rather than reflecting more general processes. When either the top or bottom portion of the grating was covered, the phantom grating was not seen; however, if the top portion of the grating was seen by one eye and the bottom portion seen by the other eye, the phantom grating was seen.

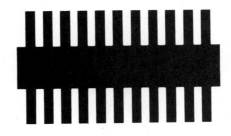

Direction of Motion of Bars

FIGURE 14-4 Stimulus used by Tynan and Sekuler (1975). From Tynan, P., and R. Sekuler (1975) Moving visual phantoms: A new contour completion effect. *Science* 188:951–952. Copyright 1975 by the AAAS. Reprinted by permission of the publisher and author.

This indicates that the location in the visual system in which the illusory moving grating is produced is after the point at which the information from the two eyes has combined; that is, the visual cortex.

The movement detectors responsible for producing the phantom moving gratings in this experiment are fairly global in nature; they cover a large area of the visual field and tend to fill in blank areas surrounded by movement all in the same direction. Weisstein, Maguire, and Berbaum (1977) performed an experiment that suggests that these are the same motion detectors that provide the basis for motion aftereffects. They presented the same type of stimuli as Tynan and Sekuler, a moving grating with an obstruction covering the center portion. After inducing the phantom grating pattern, they tested for a MAE in the area of the field in which the phantom grating had been seen. Their results showed that under all conditions that produced a phantom grating, a strong movement aftereffect was also seen. This is evidence that the detectors responsible for the movement aftereffects are the same ones that produced the phantom gratings described by Tynan and Sekuler.

Cortical motion detectors   Retinal ganglion cells that seem to act as motion detectors were discussed in Chapter 6. Similarly, we have seen (Chapter 8) that many cortical cells respond to specific velocities of motion or directions of motion. An MAE similar to that found psychophysically may be observed in cortical cells (Hammond, Mouat, & Smith, 1988; Hammond & Mouat, 1988). Thus, at least the simpler MAEs reflect the properties of cortical neurons.

Neurons in higher cortical areas have more complicated properties that are suited for detecting motion relative to a background. Cells in the lateral suprasylvian area in cat (probably homologous to MT in primates) respond best when a stimulus in the center of their receptive field moves in the opposite direction from a pattern of dots in the surround (von Grunau & Frost,

1983). Similar properties have been reported in MT of monkey (Komatsu & Wurtz, 1988b), and in tectum of pigeon (Frost & Nakayama, 1983). Such cells would recognize that the target is moving, rather than the eye sweeping across the target, because they respond to relative motion. They therefore are useful for recognizing the edges of an object moving among other objects or against a background and might help in deriving depth or shape from motion.

Eye-Head System

When we attend to an object moving through our visual field, our eyes generally do not remain stationary; instead, they follow the path of the object. This can occur either through the use of head and body movements, or be caused by movements of the eyes themselves. As we follow the movements of the object, its images on our retinae will remain in approximately the same positions on the foveas (Figure 14–5). Obviously, we are able to detect that a stimulus is moving under these conditions; just as obviously, the image-retina movement system cannot be responsible for this perception of movement. When we follow the movement of a stimulus using eye movements, the background tends to stream past in the direction opposite to the direction of movement of the stimulus, providing a potential cue for the image-

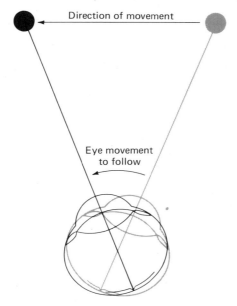

FIGURE 14–5 The eye-head system. When a stimulus moves, the eyes follow so that the image of the stimulus remains fixed on the retina. Adapted from Gregory (1978).

retina system to analyze. If we follow the movement of an illuminated stimulus against a dark background, however, movement is still perceived even though there is no moving background. This indicates that some other system must be operating under these conditions; Gregory (1978) has named it the eye-head movement system.

There are two major classes of mechanisms that might account for the operation of the eye-head system. One possibility is the *inflow theory* first suggested by Sir Charles Sherrington (1918); according to this theory, receptors in the eye muscles monitor the position of the eyes, and send this information to a hypothetical brain center that matches eye position with the information coming in from the two eyes (call it the eye-head center). The alternative way that eye position could feed into the eye-head center is known as the *outflow theory* of Helmholtz (1866). This theory suggests that it is not the receptors in the eye muscles that provide the necessary information on eye position, but the neural signals that are sent by the brain to control the state of contraction of muscles themselves serve as input to the eye-head center. Whichever way the system works, somehow the brain must be able to compare the signals coming in through the optic nerve with information about the speed and direction of movements of the eyes. These movements will often be caused by changes in the state of contraction of the eye muscles, but they do not have to be. For example, the world moves around us as we walk from place to place, with or without eye movements. The information from the skeletal muscles about where and how fast the body is moving must be integrated with the visual images that are moving across our retinae, or else we would see the visual scene moving past us, instead of us moving past the visual scene.

Experimental evidence seems to favor the outflow theory. Consider what happens when you change the position of your eye by shoving it with your finger (gently). If signals from your eye muscles were responsible for monitoring position, the world should remain stable, as they will accurately record position whether the movement was caused by the muscles or the external push from your finger. If you perform this experiment on yourself, you should note that the world does in fact seem to move when you move your eye with a finger. Sherrington's inflow theory cannot account for this movement; however, the outflow theory does predict that movement will seem to occur in this situation. If the neural signal to eye muscles carries the critical information, this information will not be affected by an external (that is, by way of a finger) movement of the eyes; therefore the eye-head system will treat the shift of images on the retina as being caused by movement of the world rather than the subject's eyes.

Another way to demonstrate the validity of the outflow theory is to paralyze the eye muscles of a subject and have the subject attempt to move the eyes. The neural signal to the eye muscles will be unaffected by paralyzing the muscles; as the eyes will not move, the image of the world on the retina will remain stationary. Therefore according to the outflow theory, it should seem that the eyes actually moved but that the world moved with them; in other words, the entire visual world should appear to jump from place to place. When the experiment was performed, this is exactly the result that was obtained (Howard & Templeton, 1966; Stevens, Emerson, Gerstein, Kallos, Neufeld, Nichols, & Rosenquist, 1976). If the system operated as suggested by inflow theory, the visual scene should seem to remain stationary. Still more confirmation for the outflow theory was provided by Brindley and Merton (1960). They covered the eye of the subject, anesthetized the surface of the eye and the tissue surrounding it, and moved the eye mechanically. The subject could not tell that the eye was moving, even though the inflow information that Sherrington proposed to be critical for such a task was still present.

The eye-head movement system has two related functions: it must be able to monitor eye movements to keep our impression of the visual world stable as our eyes move from one position to another, and it must provide information about the speed and direction of a moving stimulus that is being followed using eye and head movements. When your eyes follow the movements of a stimulus, they do so with smooth pursuit movements (discussed in Chapter 4). This type of eye movement only occurs when following a moving object; you cannot voluntarily make your eyes move in this manner. Saccadic eye movements, on the other hand, are under voluntary control and usually are not used to follow the movements of a stimulus; instead, they allow you to shift your attention from one aspect of the visual scene to another. When a saccadic eye movement occurs, therefore, the eye-head system can conclude that the images moving across the retina are a result of an eye movement and are not caused by the movement of a stimulus. Conversely, when a smooth pursuit movement is occurring, it will either be because of a moving stimulus in the visual field, or because the subject is moving through the field, and movement is perceived.

BOX 14-4 ▄▄▄▄▄▄▄▄▄▄▄▄▄▄

The movements of a retinal image during a saccadic eye movement do not correspond to movement of objects in the visual world, so it is to our advantage if our visual system has a way of ignoring them. One way that the visual system acts to disregard such moving images is to actively suppress the visual signals during a saccade. When visual sensitivity is tested during saccadic eye movements, it is found to be reduced by about a factor of three for a period of time shortly before, during, and after the *(continued)*

movement (Chase & Kalil, 1972); such an inhibition even occurs in complete darkness (Riggs, Merton, & Morton, 1974). This suppression of sensitivity during saccades probably occurs at several levels in the visual system; however, Adey and Noda (1973) have found that as early in the visual system as the lateral geniculate nucleus the responses of cells can be suppressed during occurrence of a saccade.

An alternative mechanism for suppressing visual information present during a saccade is

(box continued)

visual masking. Matin, Clymer, and Matin (1972) showed that subjects perceived a vertical slit of light as a horizontal smear when the stimulus was present only during a saccade. When the stimulus remained on after the saccade was over, however, the perception of a smear disappeared. Matin *et al* hypothesized that this was an example of backward masking, whereby the stationary visual scene in the period after the saccade masked the stimulus that was present during the saccade. More recently, Campbell and Wurtz (1978) have found that forward masking also acts to suppress visual responses during saccades.

Although experimenters have determined that the outflow theory of Helmholtz provides a good explanation for the operation of the eye-head system, the actual parts of the brain that integrate neural signals that go to the eye muscles and come from the retina have not been determined. Physiological studies have identified some areas that are involved in this system, however. Miles and Fuller (1975), recording in a part of the monkey cerebellum called the flocculus, found cells that responded only when the eyes were tracking a moving visual target. The firing rates of these cells were determined by the speed of the target; the faster the target moved, the faster the cells fired. Even when the monkey's head was mechanically moved by the experimenters while the animal was tracking a visual stimulus, the cells in this area of the brain were able to compensate for the head movements and respond in a way that accurately reflected the speed of the target. This area of the brain, therefore, is likely to be a part of the system that integrates visual and kinesthetic information to decide how objects in the physical world are moving.

Some of the integration of visual and extraretinal input can be seen in cells of the movement-sensitive MT. A class of cells called *pursuit cells* respond when the eye is following (tracking) an object in an otherwise dark room (Komatsu & Wurtz, 1988a). Since the retinal image is stable during slow pursuit of the target, these cells must be responding to the movement of the eyes. Some pursuit cells continue to respond even during eye blinks (Newsome, Wurtz, & Komatsu, 1988). These pursuit cells respond over a wide field, and prefer motion of a small stimulus in the direction opposite that of the pursuit (Komatsu & Wurtz, 1988b). Unlike the smaller field cells that probably direct the pursuit motion, these larger cells are probably concerned with the perception of motion of the target.

Illusions of the eye-head system   Our information about the position of a moving target often comes from the efferent signals sent to control the eye muscles. Under certain conditions, however, this system provides insufficient or incorrect information, resulting either in illusions of movement when in fact no movement has occurred, or in an inaccurate perception of the path of a moving object. One illusion resulting in a faulty perception of movement is called the *autokinetic effect*; it occurs when a subject fixates on a small stationary object against a dark or undefined background. Under such conditions, the subject will usually report that the stimulus begins to move somewhat randomly within the field.

There are two types of mechanisms that might account for the autokinetic effect, and both seem to operate to some extent (Hochberg, 1971a). One possibility is that involuntary eye movements change the position of the stimulus image on the retina. As the movements are involuntary, there is no outflow of signals going to the eye muscles that the eye-head system can compare with image position, so that a perception of movement results. Matin and MacKinnon (1964) performed an experiment using a stabilized image, so that the retinal image could not move. They found that under these conditions the magnitude of the perceived movements was reduced, indicating that involuntary eye movements are related to the autokinetic effect.

A second mechanism that may be partially responsible for the autokinetic phenomenon is one that involves changes in muscle tension during fixation on a stationary stimulus. While fixating for a relatively long period of time, the eye muscles may fatigue, causing a change in the position of the eyes. The proponents of this mechanism suggest that because of this change in eye position, a voluntary signal to correct the drift will be emitted. This signal will be interpreted by the eye-head system as resulting from the movement of the stimulus in space, as the system had no information regarding the change in eye position that preceded it (Bruell & Albee, 1955). The validity of this mechanism rests on the assumption that the visual system is unaware of movements of the eyes that are not the result of neural directives from the brain; as we have previously discussed in our comparison of the inflow and outflow theories, this assumption seems to be valid.

Even when motion is actually present in the visual scene, the eye-head system does not always accurately reflect this motion. Smooth pursuit eye movements are limited in velocity, a sometimes the positions of the eyes lag significantly behind the target (Puckett & Steinman, 1969). This lag can produce inaccuracies in a subject's judgments on the path that a moving object follows. Festinger and Easton (1974) presented subjects with a target that moved along a square path at a velocity that could be varied by the experimenters. At stimulus speeds so rapid that smooth pursuit movements could not occur, the subjects accurately described the shape of the path that the target was following. At slower speeds, however, subjects reported a distortion of the path that changed with stimulus velocity. Figure 14–6 shows two perceived paths of the target; the path in (a) is obtained when the target moves quite slowly, while the path shown in (b) is perceived when the target velocity is increased beyond a certain level. Both of the perceived paths are quite different than the actual path, which is a perfect square. This is a demonstration that the efferent information going to the eye muscles and

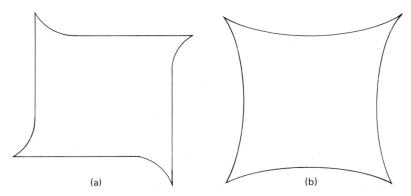

FIGURE 14-6   Perceived stimulus paths for a stimulus moving in a square path. (a) Slow stimulus movement. (b) Faster stimulus movement. From Festinger, L., and A. M. Easton (1974) Inferences about the efferent system based on a perceptual illusion produced by eye movements. *Psych. Rev.* 81:44–58. Copyright © by the American Psychological Association. Reprinted by permission.

feeding into the eye-head system does not always reflect the true position of a target in space.

When visual information is sparse, as in the previous experiments, eye movements can be an important determinant of apparent motion. When the visual field is rich with information, however, these movements seem to be accounted for by the visual shifts they induce. For example, you are not fooled by your own body movements, which can have even more dramatic effects on the aim of your eyes than your eye and head movements. Perhaps an even more compelling argument is that you can watch and comprehend a movie in which the camera is moving. You clearly do not control the way the camera pans or moves, nor do you receive any kinesthetic or vestibular feedback about the motions the cameraman underwent, but you have no difficulty seeing which things in the scene are moving and which motions are due to the change in camera angle.

PERCEIVED MOTION

What we are leading up to is the question of how you perceive that something moved in the world, rather than that you moved relative to the world. That is, you want to know about things changing spatial relationships with each other—or relative to you, as when something is flying toward your head. You are less interested in knowing that an image moved across your retina. But first, we shall digress to consider a case in which things seem to move, and there really was no motion.

Stroboscopic Movement

When you watch a movie or a television show, there is absolutely no doubt in your mind that the stimuli to which you are attending are physically moving. In reality, however, what you are seeing is a sequence of still pictures; the perception of movement comes from the fact that each picture is slightly different from the preceding one. Perceived movement caused by the presentation of two or more stationary stimuli presented in sequence is called *stroboscopic movement*, and has a long history in perceptual psychology.

The classic experiment on this subject was published in 1912 by the German gestalt psychologist Max Wertheimer; his method involved presenting in sequence two vertical lines placed close together. One line was exposed for a short time, a blank interval occurred, after which the second line was presented. By varying the length of the blank interval Wertheimer was able to produce a large number of different perceptual effects. If the blank interval was longer than 200 msec, the reported perception closely paralleled reality: subjects reported simply seeing two stationary lines with one being presented after the other. With blank intervals lasting between 30 and 200 msec, a variety of movement illusions was obtained. For intervals that lasted less than 30 msec, there was no illusion; instead, the two lines seemed to be presented simultaneously.

For intervals between 30 and 200 msec, the kind of movement reported depended on the exact interval length. When the interval was relatively short (about 60 msec), the line actually seemed to move from one location to the other. Wertheimer called this *optimal movement*, while others have named it *beta movement* (Kenkel, 1913). It is also what we have referred to as stroboscopic movement. At longer intervals, the lines did not appear to move from place to place, but an illusion of movement persisted. This type of movement has been named *pure movement* or *phi movement*. All of these illusions are collectively known as the *phi phenomenon*.

The world abounds with examples of the phi phenomenon. The signs that usher us into parking lots or movie theaters are often designed to produce stroboscopic movements. In addition, as we have already stated, all of the movements we see on television or in the movies are sophisticated examples of this illusion. It is perhaps not surprising, given the massive use by the entertainment and advertising industries, that much research has been devoted to determining the exact stimulus parameters that affect the illusion of stroboscopic movement. Korte (1915) found a number of specific relationships between stimulus parameters. He discovered that if the spatial distance between the two stimuli was increased, the blank interval also had to be lengthened in order to maintain the illusion at its optimal level. If the distance between the stimuli was kept constant but stimulus strength was varied, it was found that the length of the blank interval had to vary inversely with strength to maintain the movement illusion. In other words, as the stimuli became dimmer, the blank interval had to get longer. Finally, when the blank interval length was held constant and the interstimulus distance was varied, the strength of the stimuli had to be increased as the distance was increased. These stimulus relationships have been named *Korte's laws*, and have subsequently been confirmed and extended by a number of investigators. While it may seem that most of the parameters of Korte's laws imply processing of motion early in the visual system (perhaps even in the retina), the "interstimulus distance" includes distance in depth, not simply separation on the retina (Green & Odom, 1986). This implies processing at a higher level.

Is stroboscopic movement a special case of real movement, or are the two independent phenomena? Most models of motion detection are set up to respond to either type of motion, for the delays between stimulation at separate points would be the same whether or not the stimulus traversed the intervening space (see Sejnowski, Koch, & Churchland, 1988). Nevertheless, the question of whether they are really aspects of the same process remains. One indication that they may tap the same mechanisms is the finding that real motion in one direction can cancel apparent motion in the other (Gregory & Harris, 1984).

BOX 14–5

One of the more interesting aspects of the illusion of stroboscopic movement is what happens when the two stimuli in different positions are not identical, but differ either in color or in shape. It is easier to see stroboscopic movement between stimulus lights that are identical than between those that differ in shape, but motion is seen when the two stimuli are different (Shechter, Hochstein, & Hillman, 1988). For example, in Figure 14–7(a), the

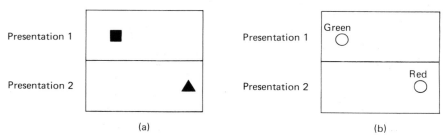

(a)   (b)

FIGURE 14–7   Transformations of movement and color. (a) Sequential stimulus presentations where the stimuli are different in position and shape. The perception is of a moving stimulus that smoothly changes shape from a square to a triangle. (b) Sequential stimulus presentations of two colored discs, one red and one green, each in a different location. The perception is of a moving disc that abruptly changes color in the middle of the path.

(continued)

(box continued)

stimulus in the first position is a square, while the stimulus that is presented after the blank interval is a triangle. When these stimuli are presented under conditions that evoke beta movement, and the two stimuli are not identical, subjects report that not only do they perceive seeing the stimulus move, but that it seems to change shape smoothly from one type of stimulus to the other (Kolers & Pomerantz, 1971). If the subjects are asked what the shape of the stimulus is at some point in between the two positions, they will report it looking more like the first stimulus if the point is near the position of that stimulus, and more like the second if the point is near that one.

If, however, the two stimuli differ in color instead of shape, no such smooth transformation takes place. Kolers and von Grünau

(1975; 1976) presented pairs of stimuli for which the first was green and the second was red (Figure 14–7[b]). They reasoned that if the visual system smoothly transformed shapes in the experiment previously discussed, perhaps it could transform colors in the same way. If so, as the stimulus appeared to move from one position to the other, it might continuously change color as it moved. When the experiment was performed, however, it was found that the stimulus stayed the same color as that in the first position until it passed the midway position between the two stimuli, where it abruptly changed to the color of the second stimulus. The fact that color changes abruptly while shape changes in a smooth manner suggests a major difference in the way that these two qualities are coded by the visual system.

Effects of Context on the Perception of Motion

In many cases, the perceived velocity of a moving stimulus or even its direction of movement depends on the context in which the stimulus is seen. Consider the two situations shown in Figure 14–8; in both cases, a continuous series of dark spots are moving downward within a rectangular framework. The only difference is that the framework on the right of the figure is twice as large as the framework on the left, as are the sizes of the spots and the physical distance between neighboring spots. If subjects are allowed to manipulate the speed at which the spots in the larger framework move, and are told to make the speeds in the two frameworks the same, they will tend to make the speed in the larger framework twice the speed of the spots in the smaller framework (Brown, 1931). Thus, in order to make the velocities in the two situations seem identical, the velocity of the larger stimuli must be increased in direct proportion to the size of the framework. This result makes sense if considered in light of our discussion on depth perception. If two stimuli of similar form but different size are presented together, the larger one often seems as if it is positioned closer to the observer than the smaller one. If, in fact, the larger framework is regarded as being twice as close to the observer as the small framework, the actual velocity of the stimuli in units of visual angle per unit time would have to be twice that of the spots in the smaller framework in order for them to seem equal.

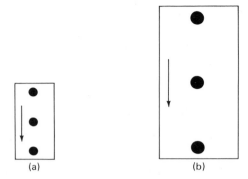

FIGURE 14-8 Stimuli similar to those used by Brown (1931). The spots in the larger frame must travel twice as fast to be perceived equal in velocity to the stimuli in the smaller frame.

Not only can the perceived speed of a moving object be affected by objects around it, but the perceived direction of motion can be changed as well. There are many situations in the physical world in which such effects occur; for example, consider a cloudy night sky with the moon ducking in and out of the drifting clouds. The moon is actually stationary relative to the clouds, but because clouds take up so much more room in the visual field than the moon, they appear to be stationary while the moon seems to move in the opposite direction from them. This is a phenomenon known as *induced movement*, where the apparent motion of the stimulus in question is "induced" by movement of surrounding objects (Wallach, 1959). An artificial example of induced movement is shown in Figure 14–9; if the small black square in the middle of the figure is kept stationary but the surrounding boundary is moved slowly to the right, the square will seem as if it is moving

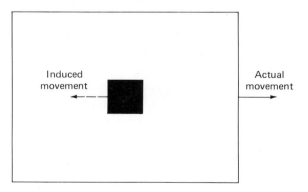

FIGURE 14-9 Stimulus situation to produce induced movement. If frame moves to the right, subjects will perceive the central square moving to the left.

to the left. Intuitively, it seems that the illusion of induced movement should have a strong experiential base; usually in the real world, smaller objects move relative to the larger surrounding field. The importance of experience in this illusion is illustrated by the fact that objects that are known from experience to be mobile (people, airplanes, and so forth), are often more susceptible to induced movement than are objects that are usually stationary (Brosgole & Whalen, 1967).

The importance of background in the perception of movement has also been emphasized by the work of James Gibson (1966; 1968). As an object moves through space, it successively covers different parts of the background and uncovers the portions through which it has just passed. Gibson calls this process *kinetic optical occlusion*, and sees it as an important way for the subject to discriminate between objects moving through space and movement on the part of the subject through a stationary world. When a single object moves through space, the change in the texture of the background is limited to the region directly in front of and in back of the object, while if the observer is moving, there is a transformation of the entire visual world according to the principles of motion parallax (see p. 307).

BOX 14-6

One of the classic movement illusions is called the *Pulfrich effect*, as illustrated in Figure 14-10. A subject viewing a pendulum swinging directly in front of the eyes sees the pendulum bob moving from side to side along the same path. However, when one eye is covered with a filter that attenuates the amount of light reaching that eye (a lens from an old pair of sunglasses will do), the pendulum bob seems to move in depth in an elliptical path that goes foward and away from the observer.

Most investigators consider this illusion to be caused by the fact that receptors in the eye respond more slowly to dim light than to bright light (Brauner & Lit, 1976; Gregory, 1978). The fact that the filtered eye receives less light from the stimulus causes it to respond more slowly, resulting in a delay in the transmission of signals from that eye. Therefore, at a given point in time, the position of the bob as seen from the filtered eye lags behind the position as seen from the other eye. A binocular disparity results that is consistent with a stimulus moving in an elliptical path such as that shown in the figure.

Where is the movement system in the brain? We have discussed the specialized motion cells in MT, which receives most of its input from the magnocellular pathway. In Chapter 9, we indicated the magnocellular pathway might be largely responsible for analysis of motion. If this is so, a stimulus that the magnocellular system cannot discriminate from the background should not appear to move (even though the parvocellular system can see the stimulus). Such a stimulus is one that is equiluminant with the background; for example, the magnocellular system presumably cannot "see" red against equiluminant green.

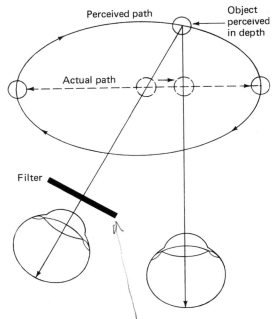

FIGURE 14-10   The Pulfrich phenomenon. The attenuated eye perceives the pendulum ball as lagging behind the position as seen by the unattenuated eye. This is consistent with the ball actually traveling in an elliptical path, as shown.

Livingstone and Hubel (1987b) tested this hypothesis for a number of movement demonstrations. They cited evidence that equiluminant stimuli appeared to move more slowly than those with luminance contrast (Cavanagh, Tyler, & Favreau, 1984), and observations suggesting that stroboscopic motion disappears at equiluminance. From their demonstrations, they conclude that the magnocellular system is responsible for motion effects.

On the other hand, a number of workers have found that MAEs can be obtained with equiluminant stimuli (Derrington & Badcock, 1985; Mullen & Baker, 1985), indicating a parvocellular motion system. Livingstone and Hubel counter that these effects may be the result of convergence of the parvocellular and magnocellular systems at higher levels, and do not imply that the parvocellular system itself encodes motion. Of course, we know that the two systems interact at a number of levels (see Figure 9–8), so some parvocellular influence should not be surprising.

SUGGESTED READINGS

A number of books have detailed and well-written chapters on movement perception. The chapter on movement in Rock's book *An Introduction to Perception* (Macmillan, 1975) is interesting and easy to read. For more detail on apparent movement and movement illusions, see Hochberg's chapter on space and movement in *Woodworth and Schlosberg's Experimental Psychology*, edited by J. W. Kling and L. A. Riggs (Holt, Rinehart, and Winston, 1971); for a more historical perspective, the place to go is C. H. Graham's movement chapter in *Vision and Visual Perception* (Wiley, 1965). Finally, the chapter on movement in L. Kaufman's *Sight and Mind* (Oxford University Press, 1974) provides the serious student an excellent in-depth discussion of the topics of real and apparent movement.

Hans Wallach's *Scientific American* article, "The perception of motion" (July 1959; offprint #409) gives good coverage of the topic of induced movement as well as other subjects, while Kolers' article, "The illusion of movement" (October 1964; offprint #487) is a very interesting article covering just what the title says. Also worth reading is Johansson's article "Visual motion perception" (June 1975; offprint #564), which covers a number of topics not discussed in this chapter, such as the phenomenon of biological motion. The perception of motion in the phi phenomenon, especially in cases in which the direction of motion may be ambiguous, is the topic of "The perception of apparent motion," by V. S. Ramachandran and S. M. Anstis (June 1986). Finally, Sekuler and Levinson discuss their research on direction-specific motion detectors in an article entitled "The perception of moving targets" (January 1977; offprint #575). The Wallach and Kolers articles are reprinted in *Perception: Mechanisms and Models,* edited by R. Held and W. Richards (W. H. Freeman, 1972), while the Johansson article is reprinted in *Recent Progress in Perception*, edited by Held and Richards (W. H. Freeman, 1976). The Ramachandran and Anstis article may be found in *The Perceptual World*, edited by Irvin Rock (W. H. Freeman, 1990).

COLOR VISION

THE PHYSICAL STIMULUS

We have been discussing the visual scene as if there were no more to the visual world than a quantification of light: more light, less light, light here rather than there. We also live in a world of colors. Color attracts attention, enhances contrast between objects of similar lightness, and even appeals to our aesthetic senses. Color may not be essential, but it certainly adds another dimension to visual perception. In fact, as we shall see, it adds two additional dimensions.

As real as color seems to us, it is, in fact, a purely psychological phenomenon. Light rays are not colored; they are radiations of electromagnetic energy of differing wavelengths. The attribute of color is entirely a fabrication of the visual system.

The physical stimulus for color vision, as for any vision, is light. Different wavelengths of light correspond to different colors, just as different energies correspond to different luminances. If you will recall from the beginning of Chapter 4, light may be described either as a wave phenomenon or a particle phenomenon. When we speak of colors, we will generally refer to the wavelength of light. Wavelengths are measured in nanometers (nm). One nm = 10^{-9} meters, or 1/1000th of 1/1000th of a millimeter, which is itself 1/1000th of a meter.

When we speak of light being absorbed by a photopigment, however, it is more convenient to count the number of quanta (photons) captured, and characterize each photon by its energy. Here, the energy of each quantum corresponds to the inverse of the wavelength of the light (see Chapter 4). Rather than speaking of the total energy of the light (number of photons times their individual energies), we count the number of photons.

The simplest kind of light to talk about would be one that is totally homogeneous—all the quanta of the same energy. Such a light would consist of a single wavelength only, and we could characterize it completely by its wavelength and total energy. A light of only one wavelength is as *pure* a light as possible, and is called *monochromatic (mono* = one, *chroma* = color).

It is quite difficult to produce a truly monochromatic light; when we refer to a light as being monochromatic, it generally contains all wavelengths within a very restricted spectral range. Natural lights, on the other hand, are *broad band*, the opposite of monochromatic. They contain significant amounts of a large portion of the electromagnetic spectrum. The light emitted by the sun contains nearly equal amounts of all wavelengths, and appears white to human observers. White is the least pure color there is.

Isaac Newton is credited with the first demonstration that sunlight is not qualitatively different from colored lights, but is merely the sum of all the colored lights. His demonstration is shown in Color Plate E on the inside cover; white light from the sun passes through a slit that restricts the light to a fine line. The line of light impinges on a prism, where the rays are bent by refraction. The amount of bending of the light depends on its wavelength; short wavelengths are refracted (bent) the most, long wavelengths the least. As a result, the light is spread out and arrayed by wavelength on the white screen. This display, the "spectrum," is a blurred rainbow of color, ranging from the longest wavelengths (red light at about 700 nm) to the shortest (violet light of approximately 400 nm). The spectral colors, in order, are: red, orange, yellow, green, blue, and violet.

Newton's prism decomposed white light into its spectral components; presumably, they could be recombined back into white light. Newton did this by using a lens to refocus the colors that had been dispersed by his prism, projecting a white circle in spite of the presence of the prism. In effect, the lens took the different wavelengths of light that had been spread out by the prism and projected them onto the same area of screen. It thus added the colors back together to produce a white light.

How are we to represent white light? Each of the colors of the spectrum may be represented by giving its respective wavelength, but white sunlight contains all wavelengths. Most lights contain a range of wavelengths, but in differing amounts. The usual way to represent the physical nature of any light is by graphing its *spectrum* (a slightly different usage of the word than the "rainbow" Newton's prism created). A spectrum is simply a catalog of how much energy there is at each wavelength in a given light—just as a spectrum represented contrast at each spatial frequency in Chapter 10. Graphically, it is a plot of energy versus wavelength, as shown in Figure 15–1. Monochromatic lights have spectra that are single spikes at the wavelength of the light. Figure 15–1(a) shows the spectrum of a yellow monochromatic light, wavelength = 580 nm. Part (b) shows a blue monochromatic light, wavelength = 480 nm. Part (c) shows an equal energy white light, with all wavelengths equally represented. Part (d) is the spectrum of a light that would appear yellow, although it clearly also contains wavelengths that by themselves would appear orange or red. Lights that are not monochromatic are represented by curves.

Newton wondered whether white light necessarily contained the entire spectrum or whether parts of it could be omitted. He tested by selectively blocking bands of the spectrum before re-adding the components. He found

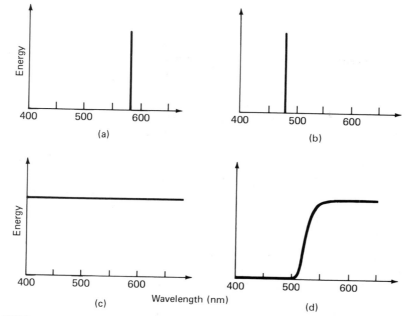

FIGURE 15-1 Spectra of various lights. (a) Monochromatic yellow light, wavelength = 580 nm. (b) Monochromatic blue light, wavelength = 480 nm. (c) Equal energy white light. (d) Yellow light such as you might obtain by passing sunlight through yellow cellophane.

that it was possible to block large amounts of the spectrum and still obtain white; he observed that if as few as three or four basic colors were present, white light resulted. Newton never bothered to see whether even fewer primary colors would be sufficient, because the situation already seemed too artificial to be of real interest. As we shall see, exactly three primary colors are necessary in general, and the implications of this fact are quite noteworthy.

COLOR MIXTURE

Newton devised a system by which he could categorize lights according to the spectral colors they looked like, with enough white added to make them less pure. The color itself is called the *hue*; the relative amount of color is the *saturation*. When two spectral colors are mixed, a new hue results. If the proportions of the two spectral lights are unequal, the mixture will be closer in hue to the wavelength that is represented in higher proportion.

Newton's system depends on the way the lights appear; that is, it is based on the psychological attributes of lights. The attributes of lights we introduced at the beginning of this chapter (wavelength, energy, and purity) are physical attributes. There is a rough correspondence between these: wavelength is a major determinant of hue, changes in energy have a great effect on the luminance (brightness), and purity is a determinant of saturation. But the terms cannot be used interchangeably. As we pointed out in Chapter 2, the hue of a given wavelength light depends somewhat on its energy (Bezold-Brücke hue shift), and the relative luminance of lights of the same energy depends on their wavelengths. Monochromatic lights (all of perfect purity), can differ in saturation.

Additive Mixture

At this point, it is best to clarify what is happening when colors are mixed. In visual science, the color mixtures we consider are *additive*, like the recombination of the spectrum into white. Additive color mixture is exactly what it sounds like: two (or more) lights are added to each other to make a new light.

There are several ways to add lights. Newton's was the most direct: projections of each color are superimposed on one screen. This is also how lights are usually added in the laboratory. There are three or four projectors (each like a slide projector) all aimed at the same screen. Each projector has a filter or some other means of selecting a single color from the white light emitted by its bulb. Each also has a control that allows the total amount of light it puts out to be changed. The light on the screen is the sum of the lights put out by each projector; for instance, if there are two projectors and each is fitted with so sharp a filter that it emits only a single wavelength, both wavelengths would be reflected from the screen. The spectrum of the light coming to the observer would be the *sum* of the spectra of the lights from each projector.

BOX 15-1

The laboratory apparatus actually used to present color mixtures is quite a bit more complex than described above. The "projectors" are more carefully made than the slide projector you may have at home, with optics that are precisely designed to avoid any distortion of the images. Each projector has neutral density (gray) filters that cut the light down to an appropriate level. Often, the control of color is by *monochromators*, instruments that select a narrow band of light to transmit, and block the rest.

The projectors do not aim at a screen, but combine optically through partially reflecting mirrors and project directly through the pupil of the observer's eye onto the retina. This kind of projection system is called a *Maxwellian* view system; it is the same principle as the eyepiece of a microscope or telescope that projects an image into the eye.

Another way to add lights is to place the colored lights side by side in close proximity. If the colored patches are small enough, the eye will be unable to resolve them separately. If several patches fit into each ganglion cell receptive field, the ganglion cells will be unable to distinguish between patches and diffuse overlapped lights, and so will respond as if the lights were superimposed. In fact, this is how a color television works. Examine the TV screen closely; it is made up of minute patches of red, green, and blue. Step back from the screen: the individual color patches merge, and what is seen is the additive mixtures of the three colors.

Another way to add colors is to present them in sufficiently rapid succession that they cannot be resolved as separate flashes. When a light flickers at a rapid enough rate, it is perceived as steady—for example, fluorescent lights shut off completely 120 times every second yet they give what appears to be steady light (see Box 13–4). If two colors were alternated (instead of alternating light and dark), their additive mixture would be seen. The mixture is additive because both colors would be in the mixture—as a time average. The result is the same as physical superposition. This is the principle used in the color wheel (Figure 15–2). The color wheel consists of a motor that rotates a disc at high speed. Sectors of colored paper are attached so that when it rotates, the sectors fuse and the additive mixture is seen. At any point, the colors are succeeding each other at a rapid rate, and they add.

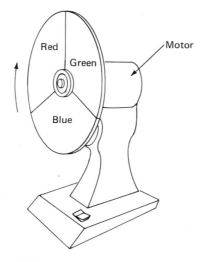

FIGURE 15–2 A color mixing wheel. Additive mixture of the color segments occurs when the wheel rotates rapidly.

The three primary colors of additive color mixture are generally taken to be red, green, and blue. For reasons that we will go into later in this chapter, those three are the colors most capable of being added to make any other color. They are the only three colors on a color television screen, and usually are the three on a color mixing wheel.

Yellow seems intuitively to be a primary color, but in fact an excellent yellow can be made by the additive mixture of red and green (see Color Plate F on the inside cover). White is also readily obtained from red, green, and blue. The additive mixture of all three, shown in Color Plate F, gives a white that cannot be distinguished from sunlight (a fact Newton stopped just short of discovering). If white is the sum of red + green + blue, however, it must also be the sum of yellow and blue, as red and green mixed make yellow. In fact, if we take the pure spectral yellow that is exactly matched by the mixture of red and green and add it to blue, white results. Alternatively, we could split the lights a different way, and point out that blue + green gives blue-green and blue-green + red add to make white. (This also works with a spectral blue-green + red.) Similarly, red + blue makes purple, and purple + green yield white (although there is no spectral light that appears purple). All these sums may be seen in Color Plate F.

BOX 15-2

The facts of color mixture will be clearer (and more believable) if you demonstrate them to yourself. We suggest you make a color wheel, as described below, and use it to try each of the mixtures as you read about them.

To make the wheel, take a piece of very stiff paper or cardboard and cut out a 6-inch diameter circle. (It is best to use a compass, as the wheel will work best if it is well balanced.) Cut six windows in the wheel as shown in Figure 15–3(a) make a hole in the center so the wheel will fit very snugly over a pencil (a bit of tape will help secure the wheel to the pencil). Obtain some clear red, green, and blue cellophane or acetate. If suitable candy wrappers or other packaging are not available, theatrical "gels" or artists' acetate or three of the colored report covers available in many stationery stores will do. Glue or tape a piece of cellophane over each window, as shown.

Hold the wheel up so you can see through the top window to a white wall or piece of paper. When the wheel is stationary, you will see the same color as the cellophane in that window. When the wheel is spun rapidly, you will see the additive mixture of the three colors. To spin the wheel, wind a piece of string around the pencil. Either hold the pencil loosely, or make a tube of cardboard for the pencil to fit into. Pull the string smoothly, as shown in Figure 15–3(b); the wheel will spin rapidly.

If the additive mixture is not white, it is because there is too much of one or two of the colors. To decrease the amount, tape a piece of paper over one of the windows of that color, as shown in Figure 15–3(c). If the mixture is pinkish, cover part of a red window; if it is greenish, cover part of a green window; with a little fooling around, a very good white can be made.

Look at a colored picture through the wheel. Look through a red window and there will be the red image only; look through a green or blue window and there will be the green or blue image only. Now spin the wheel: the additive mixture of the three separate images should recreate the full color figure, which is the additive mixture of patches of only three colors. (In fact, this method of producing color TV was patented, but lost out to the three color dot method now in use.)

You can also demonstrate that red + green

(continued)

(box continued)

make yellow. Completely cover the blue windows, and spin the wheel while looking at a white surface. The mixture should be yellow. If it is on the orange side, cover part of a red window; if it is on the pea-green side, cover part of a green window. By covering more and more of the red or green windows, the mixture can be varied from pure red, through orange and yellow, to pure green.

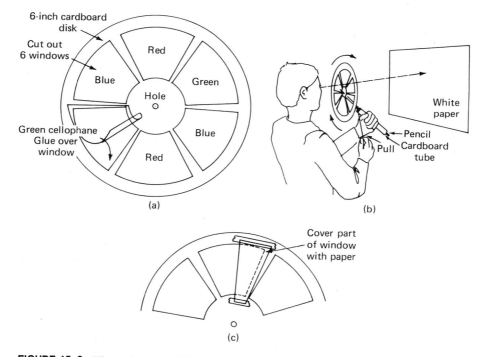

FIGURE 15-3 The color wheel for demonstrations, as described in the box. (a) The wheel. (b) How to view through the wheel. (c) Adjusting the relative mix of the colors.

The sums in additive mixtures do not depend on the actual spectra of the component lights. The yellow used to mix with blue to make white light could be a mixture of red and green, or it could be any yellow, including a monochromatic yellow. If we consider the addition of monochromatic yellow (580 nm) with monochromatic blue (480 nm), the resulting spectrum would consist of two points (the yellow and blue spectra are given in Figure 15–1; the result is shown in Figure 15–4). This mixture, although obviously quite different *physically* from the white shown in Figure 15–1(c), would appear white to a human observer; in fact, the two whites would be indistinguishable. Shown a white, you could not state whether it was equal energy, a mixture of 480 + 580, or any other mixture that makes white.

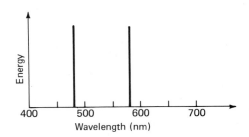

FIGURE 15-4   Spectrum of the white light made by an additive mixture of monochromatic blue light (480 nm) with monochromatic yellow light (580 nm).

Subtractive Mixture

Although additive color mixing is the type typically used in visual science, it is important to recognize that there is another more familiar kind: *subtractive* color mixing. Subtractive mixing is the exact opposite of additive mixing, in which lights are superimposed, so there is more light in the mixture than in either component; in subtractive mixing, light is successively removed, so there is less light in the mixture than in either component.

The simplest way to conceive subtractive mixing is by considering the stacking of colored filters. A colored filter is a piece of material (for example, cellophane) that selectively removes some wavelengths of light while transmitting others. A red filter makes white light red by removing all the short and medium wavelength light, leaving only the long wavelength light. A common type of yellow filter passes medium and long wavelength light but attenuates short wavelength light. It therefore makes equal energy white light look yellow (have a spectrum like that in Figure 15–1[d]), but has virtually no effect on long wavelength light, and appears opaque in deep blue light.

A simple way to make subtractive color mixtures is by stacking filters and making the light pass successively through two or more. Each filter blocks certain wavelengths while transmitting others; we can represent the characteristics of a filter by a plot called the *transmission curve*, which shows the percentage of incident light that gets through the filter (is transmitted) as a function of its wavelength. Transmission curves for yellow and blue filters are shown on the left in Figure 15–5 (b and d), which demonstrates the subtractive mixture of yellow and blue.

The mixture starts with white light containing all wavelengths (Figure 15–5[a]). It passes into the yellow filter, which has a transmission curve (Figure 15–5[b]) indicating it allows most of the long- and medium-wavelength light to pass through it, but it subtracts or removes (by absorbing) short-wavelength light. The result is yellow light containing long- and medium-, but not short-wavelength light (Figure 15–5[c]). The yellow light impinges on a blue filter (Figure 15–5[d]) that blocks long- but transmits short- and medium-wavelength light. The result shown in Figure 15–5(e) is light of medium wavelength only; the long wavelengths were removed by the blue filter and the short wavelengths by the yellow filter. The medium-wavelength light remaining appears green, which is the subtractive mixture of yellow and blue.

BOX 15-3

Demonstrate subtractive color mixing by using the remaining acetate left over from making your color wheel. Hold any two scraps together, and the subtractive mixture results. Notice that holding all three together results in a nearly opaque combination: each filter removes some light, and if the filters are good enough, nothing gets through. This is in contrast to the genera-

tion of white by adding the three additive primary colors.

Mixing yellow and blue to make green will be slightly awkward, as you may not have a yellow filter available. You can achieve the same result by looking at a yellow surface through the blue filter.

The resulting color in subtractive mixing is what is "left over" when each filter has removed certain wavelengths. The physical stimulus is what indicates the color—there are no surprises as with the mixture of monochromatic blue and yellow. In fact, the mixture that results depends on the inefficiency of the filters. If we stacked ideal yellow and blue filters (that passed monochromatic yellow light and blue light respectively), the mixture would not be green; it would be black, as *no* light could get through (Figure 15–6).

The mixture of colored paints is also subtractive, for paint is essentially a suspension of microscopic filters. When you paint a sheet of white paper green, you are covering it with a filter that prevents the reflection of long- and short-wavelength light, leaving only the medium wavelengths. When you mix paints, you are stacking the filters, and the rules of subtractive mixture apply. With each additional filter in the mixture less light is transmitted; mixing all the colors in the paint box gives a muddy brown because very little gets through.

PSYCHOPHYSICS OF COLOR

A large body of experimental data has been collected to define the laws of additive mixture. The fundamental law is that any colored light can be matched by a suitable arrangement using three primary lights. Any light, regardless of its actual spectrum, can be matched using only three primary

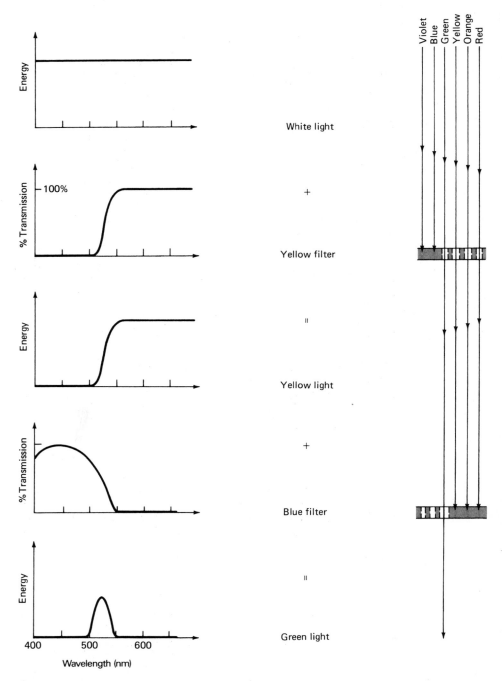

FIGURE 15–5 Subtractive mixture of yellow and blue to give green. Spectra or filter characteristics are shown to the left; a schematic of the process is seen to the right.

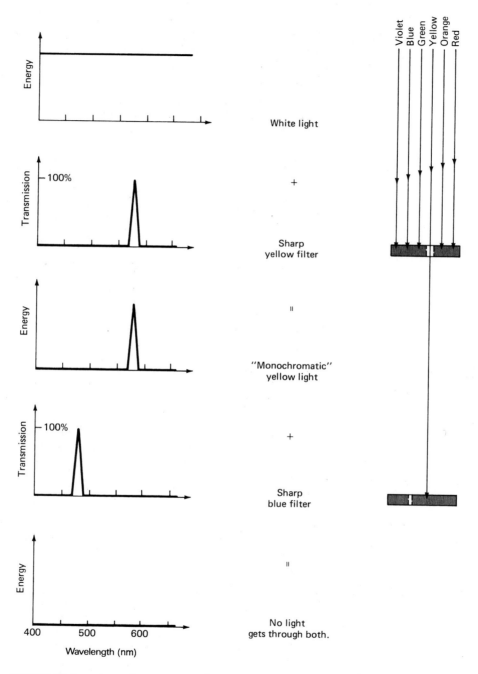

FIGURE 15-6 Subtractive mixture with an extremely selective yellow filter and an extremely selective blue filter to give no light (black).

colors; this includes white, spectral colors, or any other light there is. The primary colors themselves can, in fact, be almost anything—spectral (monochromatic) lights, or lights of some complex spectrum. The only restriction is that none of them can be matched by a mixture of the other two—if that were possible, there would actually be only two primaries.

Color matching is done by having the subject look at a "split field," a display with two halves (Figure 15–7). In one half of the field is the light to be matched, in the other is the sum of the three primary colors to be used to make the match. The subject adjusts the amounts of each primary color until satisfied that the two halves look identical. When the subject can detect no difference between the halves, a match has been made, and the amounts of each of the primary colors required can be recorded. The match is purely psychological, for the spectra of the halves can be quite different—they only *look* alike. Such a match is called a *metameric* match.

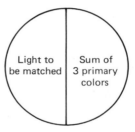

FIGURE 15–7   Stimulus display for metameric matching.

We have said that any three lights could serve as primary colors (with one restriction). Suppose we chose a system of primary colors in which the usual red was replaced with yellow. How could a subject match red light using only yellow, green, and blue? Suppose the light to be matched (the red) is on the left side of the split field; no matter how much yellow, green, or blue the subject adds to the right side, it can never become red. In particular, the more green that is added, the less red the field looks; what is needed is to put in less green. In fact, what is needed is less than none, a *negative* amount!

The physical correlate of negative light in a color match is light in the "wrong" half of the field. That is, the match is made by putting some green primary in the *left* field, where the color to be matched (red) is. The red and green add to make yellow, which is matched by the yellow on the right—the two half-fields appear identical. We cannot create (mix) any color, but we can make a metameric match to any color with three primary colors if we are allowed to use negative amounts of one or more of the primary colors. In other words, the two half-fields can be made to look identical when three primary colors are available to be added to either one. Notice the distinction between mixing and matching colors: to mix is to create a specific color of some description; to match is to make two lights look identical (but not necessarily like the original light to be matched).

BOX 15–4 ▄▄▄▄▄▄▄▄▄▄▄▄▄▄▄▄▄▄▄▄▄▄▄▄

Negative light sounds like cheating, but in fact it is a way of saying that metameric matching is like an algebraic manipulation. The split field is an equation in need of solution: on the left is some arbitrarily picked value, the light to be matched, which we can call X. On the right is the sum of the three primaries (1, 2, and 3), the amounts of which the subject will choose to satisfy the match. There are thus three values, a_1, a_2, and a_3, the amounts of each primary selected to make the metameric match. The equation balances when values of the three have been chosen to make the two half-fields look identical: that is to say

$$X = a_1 + a_2 + a_3$$

This "equation" should be interpreted to say

"light X looks like the additive mixture of a_1 of primary color 1 plus a_2 of primary color 2 plus a_3 of primary color 3."

Suppose the solution required a negative second primary color; that is, a_2 is negative:

$$X = a_1 - a_2 + a_3$$

In algebra, there would be no objection to rearranging this equation to read

$$X + a_2 = a_1 + a_3$$

the same is true in metameric matches. (The interpretation of the last equation is that there is a match when the light to be matched is added to a_2 of primary color 2 in the left field, and a_1 of primary color 1 is added to a_3 of primary color 3 in the right half-field.)

Color Space

The remarkable fact that three primary colors are sufficient for any and all metameric matches means that there is a simple way to represent any colored light. Think of the three primary colors in a matching experiment as the axes of a three-dimensional space (such as the one in Figure 15–8); every light is represented by a point in that space, for it can be matched by a certain amount of primary color 1, an amount of primary color 2, and some amount of primary color 3. We need three dimensions because we need three primaries. Any light's color (*not* its physical spectrum) can be completely specified by giving its location in the space; that is, by its *coordinates*.

The particular set of primary colors chosen was arbitrary. The only restriction was that no primary could be matched by a mixture of the other two. If a different set of primaries is chosen, the color space will look different; however, we can get back and forth between the two representations by noting that each primary in one space is a point in the other, and vice versa. The computations are tedious, but it is possible to get from any system to any other just by knowing the three colors used in each.

Three dimensions are a lot easier to deal with than the infinite number of color matches we might wish to describe, but drawing in three dimensions is

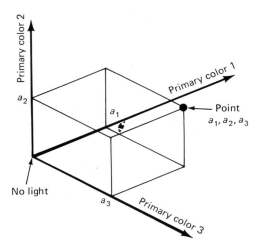

FIGURE 15-8   Location of a point in color space. The color is specified by the amount of each primary color required to make a metameric match to it.

difficult. It would be nice if we could represent color space as a two-dimensional plane, like a sheet of graph paper. Happily, we can do this with one simplification that can be made: we shall consider each of the primary colors as a proportion of the total energy. Then the sum of the three primary colors used in any match will be 1.0 (unity—note, however, that the proportion devoted to any one color could be greater than 1.0 because another might be negative). Since the sum is always unity, the system is reduced to two dimensions; the amount of the third primary color is completely determined by the amounts of the other two and the requirement that the three sum to unity. There are only two free variables, so we need only two axes. Another way to look at this is to note that the requirement of summing to unity means we are confined to a plane in the color space. This plane is shown in Figure 15–9.

The CIE Color Diagram

We now have reduced the three-dimensional color space to a plane by considering each primary color as a proportion of the total energy. It is important to remember that this two-dimensional plane still represents a three-color system. Each of the three primary colors is represented by a point in the plane, and the lines connecting these points (an equilateral triangle) are the axes of a color coordinate system (Figure 15–9[b]). Three axes collapse into two dimensions because they have been given the special relationship that the sum is a constant.

We could use the color plane in Figure 15–9(b), but we usually prefer to work with axes that are perpendicular to each other, not at 60°. If we imag-

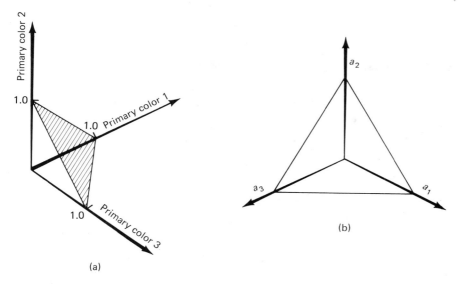

FIGURE 15-9   The unit plane in color space. (a) Location of the unit
plane in the color space of Figure 15–11. (b) Direct view
of the unit plane.

ine stretching the triangle in Figure 15–9(b) as if it were made of rubber, we
can straighten out the angle at a_3 until it is a right angle (this is a linear
transformation that is mathematically straightforward). We now obtain a nor-
mal-looking graph, shown in Figure 15–10. The vertical axis is a_2 (the
amount of the second primary color), the horizontal axis is a_1 (the amount of
the first primary color), and the third primary color is at the origin.

   We can put landmarks on this graph as soon as we define the three primary colors. There is a standard set of primary colors that is almost invariably
used, defined in 1931 by an international body called the Commission Internationale de l'Éclairage (International Commission on Illumination), or *CIE*.
Although the colors they chose may not be what we would pick today, all
color data have been displayed on a color map derived from their primary
colors (called the *CIE diagram*).

   The first thing we wish to see on the diagram are those lights it is easiest
to talk about, the monochromatic lights. On Figure 15–10 there is a curve,
called the *spectrum locus*, that traces the location of all the monochromatic
lights from 400 to 700 nm (some salient ones are indicated). The other interesting point is equal energy white, which lies near the middle of the picture (W).

   The CIE diagram summarizes all the facts of color mixture. To predict the
color of a mixture of any two colors, find the coordinates of each, and draw
the straight line that connects them. The mixture color lies on this line, at a
distance from each of them inversely proportional to the amount of it in the

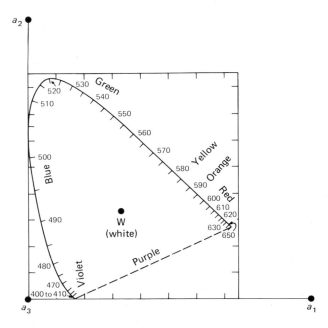

FIGURE 15-10 The CIE color diagram (unit plane), showing the spectrum locus and white. Appearances of colors are indicated.

mixture. (If lights were weights, and each weight sat on an end of the straight line, the appearance of the color mixture would be where the fulcrum would be for the seesaw to balance.)

As an example, suppose we mixed monochromatic green at 555 nm with monochromatic red at 620 nm. The line connecting those two colors is shown on Figure 15–11; in nearly equal mixture, the two exactly match monochromatic yellow (580 nm). That is, you cannot distinguish between monochromatic yellow and a mixture of monochromatic red with monochromatic green. Now consider a mixture of monochromatic yellow at 580 nm with monochromatic blue at 480 nm. In nearly equal radiant energies they are indistinguishable from equal energy white (see Figure 15–11). Of course, the monochromatic yellow is identical to a mixture of red and green; if the mixture yellow had been used instead, the same white would result from a sum of red, green, and blue. It can be seen that there are an infinite number of ways the identical white could be produced.

Now consider an equal mixture of 505 nm monochromatic blue-green with a monochromatic yellow-green of 550 nm, as shown in Figure 15–11. The mixture lies inside the spectrum locus, but is clearly not white. In fact, it is equivalent to (matches) a mixture of 520 nm green and white (with somewhat more of the green than the white). We may therefore say that the 505 +

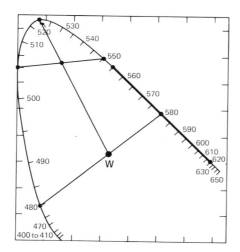

FIGURE 15-11 Color mixtures on the CIE diagram. Each line represents a color mixture discussed in the text.

550 mixture is like a mixture of 520 and white. We say that it is less saturated than monochromatic 520. The spectrum locus is the purest and most saturated of real lights of any particular hue; lights inside it are less saturated than the corresponding spectral hues. As you can quickly convince yourself, mixtures of spectral lights are never more saturated than the spectral light of the matching hue. In general, the spectrum locus is curved, so any mixture of two spectral lights is represented by a secant that lies within the locus (and is therefore closer to white than the locus itself). Except in the range from about 550 nm to 700 nm, the mixtures of spectral lights are less saturated than the matching hue; as more and more spectral lights are added the saturation declines, until all lights together yield the least saturated light, white.

As the purity of mixtures of spectral lights is never greater than 1, one may wonder if it is possible to achieve lights that are outside the spectrum locus—that is, more saturated than the spectral light of the same hue. The answer is yes, but not with real lights. The colors outside the spectrum locus may be matched by using negative amounts of some of the spectral colors. Such colors cannot actually be achieved as real lights, and are therefore called *imaginary*.

Now suppose that real colors are to be mixed with only three primary colors. Each primary color, if it is a real light, is represented by a point somewhere on or inside the spectrum locus. The three may be joined by a triangle; just as mixtures of spectral lights cannot extend outside the spectrum locus, mixtures of these three primary colors cannot extend outside the triangle connecting them. (This is assuming we are using these primary colors to create colors and cannot therefore make use of negative amounts of them.) This explains why the three colors chosen as primary for color television are red, green, and blue. They span the spectrum locus, which is the area of all real lights, as well as any three real colors possibly can. With any other choice, the triangle would be smaller, and some colors would be unobtainable.

Finally, consider the primary colors of the CIE diagram. All three are outside the spectrum locus; thus they are all imaginary. Primary color 1 is the "red"; it consists of red light, strengthened in its redness by negative green. Primary color 2 is the "green"; it has negative red. Primary color 3 (at the origin) is "blue"; it also has negative red in it.

The CIE diagram is only one possible diagram that we could draw, but any other would be remappable into the CIE. The diagram is simply a convenient, standard way to summarize the rules of color mixture. That it works for all the color mixing experiments that have been performed demonstrates that it is sufficient for the specification of colors.

IMPLICATIONS FOR COLOR THEORY

The color-matching experiments discussed in the last section showed that any arbitrary color could be exactly matched by an appropriate combination of three primary colors. This three-dimensionality of the human visual system was expressed formally by the CIE color space. It is reasonable to suppose that the tri-dimensional nature of our color vision is related to the fact that we have three different cone types in our retina. In order to demonstrate this relation, let us start with a color vision system consisting of only one receptor type, and work our way up to a three-cone system.

Monochromacy

Consider a visual system with only one type of receptor. Let us suppose that the absorption spectrum of the visual pigment in this receptor is as shown in Figure 15–12. From the figure, you can see that this receptor is most efficient at catching quanta (photons) when the stimulus is monochromatic light of 505 nm, with absorbance decreasing as wavelength gets longer or shorter than 505 nm.

How does a visual system with one type of receptor respond to lights of different wavelengths? Take as an example an equal number of quanta of 505 and 550 nm light. From Figure 15–12, we can determine that the receptor absorbs about 2 times more 505 nm quanta than 550 nm quanta. If we increase the number of available 550 nm quanta by a factor of 2, the receptor will then absorb equal numbers of quanta from the two lights. The receptor's responses to the two stimuli under these conditions will be identical; it has no way of distinguishing between the 505 nm stimulus and the (physically) much stronger 550 nm stimulus.

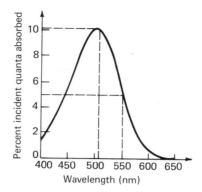

FIGURE 15-12   Percent absorption function for the visual pigment rho-
dopsin. From nomogram of Ebrey and Honig (1976).
New wavelength-dependent visual pigment nomograms.
Vision Res. 17:147–151. Reprinted by permission of
Pergamon Press, Ltd.

A similar relationship can be found for any other two wavelengths in the
spectrum. As a second example, from Figure 15–12 we can see that the receptor is equally good at catching quanta from lights of 550 nm and 445 nm.
Therefore 1000 quanta of 445 nm light impinging on the receptor will produce the identical response as 1000 quanta of 550 nm light. As far as our
single receptor can determine, the two lights would be identical.

The above examples are manifestations of the *principle of univariance*.
The principle may be stated in the following way: "Each visual pigment can
only signal the rate at which it is effectively catching quanta; it cannot also
signal the wavelength associated with the quanta caught" (Naka & Rushton,
1966). Therefore when we say that our single receptor is more sensitive to
505 nm light than to 550 nm light, we mean that it is better at catching 505
nm quanta than 550 nm quanta, and so will catch more of the 505 nm quanta
given equal amounts of each. Once a quantum is caught, however,
its effect on the receptor is completely independent of its wavelength. A receptor responds only on the basis of how many quanta it catches, with total
disregard for their wavelengths. Each photon absorbed—of whatever wavelength—results in a single isomerization, as discussed in Chapter 5.

It should be clear by now that a visual system based on one receptor type
will have no capacity to distinguish color per se. In fact, with such a system,
any one primary color can be made to match any colored light, simply by
manipulating the energy of the primary light to match the luminance of the
other color. Organisms that have this kind of visual system are called *monochromats*; such organisms have no ability to make discriminations on the
basis of wavelength. In human beings, some rare types of genetic disorders
result in people having monochromatic vision. This is the most severe form
of color blindness, and will be described in a later section.

A final point should be made regarding the visual capacities of mono-chromats. Not only will they confuse any two spectral colors, but they will also confuse any spectral color with white light. This is a direct consequence of the principle of univariance, as the receptor response only depends on the number of quanta absorbed; it does not matter whether these quanta are all of the same wavelength (as is the case for monochromatic light), or if the quanta are from a continuum of wavelengths (as may be the case for white light). The only effect that wavelength has is on the probability of any given photon being absorbed by the receptor.

BOX 15-5

What is the world like to a monochromat? You already know what it is like to see only gradations of luminance. When you watch a black-and-white movie, or look at a black-and-white photograph, your only clues to "color" are lightness and darkness. If three people in such a picture are wearing the same style shirt, but one is red, one is navy blue, and one is dark gray, you would be unable to say the shirts are not identical, because all three would come out the same shade of gray on the film.

Notice that becoming a monochromat (by looking at a black-and-white picture) did not mean you no longer had a normal visual system. As long as there is a reduction to one channel at any point in the pathway from stimulus to percept, the color information is lost. You do no better at judging the colors in a color TV transmission than in a black-and-white transmission, if all you have is a black-and-white TV set. It is thus possible for cells in the visual pathway to be monochromats, even though they receive information from more than one receptor type.

For several chapters, we have been present-ing arguments that depend on the magnocellular cells being monochromats. In particular, we have described demonstrations in which the magnocellular pathway was inactivated when equiluminant stimuli were presented. We then argued that whatever is lost in these conditions is a function of the magnocellular pathway (however, as you will soon see, some parvocellular cells are also monochromats).

An equiluminant stimulus is one in which colors may vary, but the energies are set so that the luminance is completely uniform across the entire image (Figures 9-10 and 9-11 are nearly equiluminant pictures). As a simpler example, imagine a square wave grating constructed of red bars alternating with green bars. If the energies of the red and green are adjusted so that they are equally effective for a monochromat, the monochromat cannot distinguish them and the field looks uniform. This is a direct consequence of univariance; the same number of quanta are absorbed from the green as the red, so they cannot be distinguished.

Dichromacy

Let us now consider a hypothetical *dichromatic* visual system; one with two different receptor types. Suppose that the two receptors have absorbance spectra as shown in Figure 15-13; receptor *A* has its maximum sensitivity at 500 nm, while receptor *B* has its sensitivity maximum at 600 nm. Individu-ally, each receptor obeys the principle of univariance; its response depends *only* on the number of quanta caught. In combination, however, the system becomes more complex. As long as the signals from each receptor system can be compared, we can no longer make one spectral light match any other simply by manipulating their energies. For example, let us look at the responses of each receptor to lights of 500 nm and 600 nm. Suppose each light is presented for one second at an energy such that 1000 quanta impinge on each receptor. From Figure 15–13, we see that at 500 nm, receptor *A* absorbs 9% of the incident quanta, while receptor *B* absorbs 2%. At 600 nm, however, receptor *A* absorbs only 1.5% of the incident quanta, while receptor *B* absorbs 9%. If each stimulus contains 1000 quanta, the number of quanta actually absorbed by each receptor of the two wavelengths would be as shown in Table 15–1.

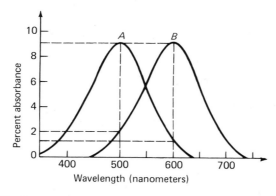

FIGURE 15–13   Percentage of absorption functions for two hypothetical visual pigments.

TABLE 15–1   The Number of Quanta of Two Wavelengths Absorbed by Each Receptor

	Receptor A	Receptor B
500 nm	90	20
600 nm	15	90

A brief inspection of this table should make it clear that 500 nm and 600 nm light will always cause different relative absorptions by the two receptors, no matter how the energy of either light may be varied. Equating the lights for one receptor must inevitably cause a large discrepancy for the other. On the basis of these two receptors, it would always be possible to distinguish 500 nm light from 600 nm light. Therefore a visual system based on two receptors is capable of making discriminations based on wavelength in a way that a monochromatic system cannot.

Dichromatic systems are two-dimensional; while color matching studies performed on normal human subjects require the use of three primary colors, a dichromat only needs two to match all spectral colors. In human beings, there are a number of genetic disorders (to be discussed later), that result in a dichromatic visual system.

Another feature that distinguishes a dichromatic visual system from visual systems containing three types of receptors is that one can always find a wavelength of light that dichromats will confuse with white light. This is called the *neutral point*. The explanation for the phenomenon is straightforward. A white light will excite both types of receptors, with the exact ratio of excitation determined by the spectrum of the white light. Therefore, a monochromatic light that excites both receptors in the same ratio as the white light will be indistinguishable from white. In most dichromatic systems, the wavelength that is confused with white will be fairly near the point at which the two receptor absorption spectra intersect; at that wavelength, the two receptors are excited in equal proportions. For receptors *A* and *B*, the intersection point is at about 550 nm; depending on the exact spectrum of the white light, therefore, a stimulus in this spectral region should be confused with the white light. Note that this is the *only* monochromatic light that would be confused with the white light. This property also distinguishes dichromats from monochromats, who will confuse all monochromatic lights with white light, as well as from trichromats, who do not confuse any monochromatic light with white.

Trichromacy

All of the color matching experiments discussed in the first part of this chapter were performed on *trichromatic* subjects; those whose color vision system is based on three receptors. We will therefore only briefly discuss trichromatic vision here. Figure 15–14 shows absorbance spectra for three hypothetical receptors comprising a trichromatic system. Several features of this figure should be noticed. First, no single wavelength of light will excite all three receptors in similar proportions to white light. Therefore no wavelength of light will be confused with white light. Second, the presence of three receptors that all absorb some light throughout most of the visual range implies that the system is three-dimensional; that is, we need three primaries to match a given light. This is, of course, the result obtained from the color-matching experiments.

BOX 15–6

In general, any colored light may be matched by a sum of the same number of primary colors as there are receptor systems in the eye of the subject doing the matching. To see why this is so, imagine that we will do a color-matching experiment in which three "primaries" are of-

(continued)

(box continued)

fered to the subject. The arbitrary light to be matched is called X. The amount of each primary color used to make the match (the variables over which the subject has control) are a_1, a_2, and a_3.

First consider monochromats; they have only one receptor system. The fraction of any light the receptor system will absorb is dependent on the spectrum of that light and the characteristics of the receptor; for any particular light, the absorbed fraction is simply a number. For this receptor system, called α, the fraction of primary color 1 it will absorb is denoted $R_\alpha(1)$; for X it is $R_\alpha(X)$, and so forth. The excitation of the receptor by any one light is the product of the amount of light and the fraction absorbed: for primary color 1 it is $a_1 R_\alpha(1)$, and so on. The total excitation is the sum of the excitations due to all lights in the field; X or the sum of the primary colors. For a match, the excitation from X equals that from the sum of the primary colors:

$$R_\alpha(X) = a_1 R_\alpha(1) + a_2 R_\alpha(2) + a_3 R_\alpha(3)$$

This is a single equation, so it has a unique solution only if there is a single unknown variable. It may be satisfied using only a_1 (all other a's = 0) no matter what X is, because

$$R_\alpha(X) = a_1 R_\alpha(1)$$

has a unique solution. It could equally well be satisfied using just a_2 or a_3. If there are more unknowns on the right, there are an infinite number of solutions.

Assuming the subject is not a monochromat, there will be more than one receptor system, and *each* must be satisfied by the match. Each will have an equation analogous to the equation for system α:

$$R_\beta(X) = a_1 R_\beta(1) + a_2 R_\beta(2) + a_3 R_\beta(3)$$

$$R_\gamma(X) = a_1 R_\gamma(1) + a_2 R_\gamma(2) + a_3 R_\gamma(3)$$

However many receptor systems there are, there will be that same number of equations. Because in general we can satisfy a set of simultaneous equations with a unique solution when the number of unknowns is the same as the number of equations, there should be the same number of primaries (unknowns) as receptor systems (equations).

As far as we know, trichromatic vision is the most sophisticated kind of color vision in the animal world. It would be perfectly possible, however, to construct a visual system based on four or more receptor types that would provide more information about the visual world than what is available to us. As Cornsweet (1970) has noted, an individual with a visual system based on four receptor types would be able to see through color camouflaging that would fool a trichromatic observer.

TRICHROMATIC THEORY

The preceding sections have presented evidence leading to the conclusion that normal human beings have a trichromatic color vision system. The development of this conclusion required only the analysis of some fairly simple psychophysical experiments and the use of our logical processes; no detailed

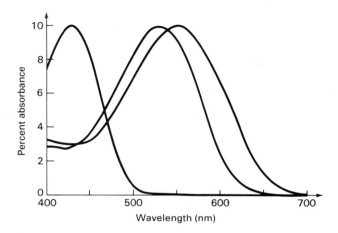

FIGURE 15–14 Percent absorption functions for three hypothetical visual receptors. These are the functions used by Smith, Pokorny, and Starr to model color mixing data. We assume 10% absorption at the peak of each. From Smith, et al. (1976) Variability of color mixture data—I. Interobserver variability in the unit coordinates. *Vision Res.* 16:1087–1094. Reprinted by permission of Pergamon Press Ltd.

knowledge of the structure or physiology of the human visual system was necessary. In fact, the same conclusion was reached in 1807 by Thomas Young, who proposed that there must be three fiber types in the human eye, one most sensitive to red light, one to green, and one to violet. He made this suggestion based on his observation that all colors could be matched by a suitable mixture of three primary colors, without any knowledge of the nature or number of human receptor types.

Young's trichromatic theory was formalized later in the nineteenth century by Helmholtz (reprinted 1924), who proposed hypothetical excitation curves for each of the three types of fibers (Figure 15–15). Helmholtz used these curves to predict quantitatively the abilities of human beings to make discriminations on the basis of wavelength.

The results of psychophysical experiments provided enough information for the general idea of trichromacy to become accepted doctrine. It was left to physiology, however, to provide the actual shapes of the absorbance spectra for the three receptor types. These measurements were made with a type of apparatus called a *microspectrophotometer*, an instrument that directs a finely focused beam of light onto a single isolated human cone. For each of a large number of wavelengths, the intensity of light transmitted through the single receptor was compared to intensity of the light prior to passing through the receptor. If the values were similar, not much light at that wavelength was absorbed by the receptor. If the values were very different, the

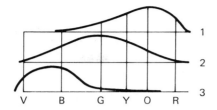

FIGURE 15-15 The hypothetical visual pigment absorption functions proposed by Helmholtz. From Helmholtz, H. C. F. (1924) *Physiological Optics*, Vol. 2. Reprinted by permission of the Optical Society of America.

receptor must have absorbed a significant proportion of the incident light. By measuring the exact amount of light absorbed for a large number of wavelengths of light, a curve was derived showing the relative absorbance of the receptor versus wavelength. This type of experiment was performed on the eyes of humans and other primates (Brown & Wald, 1964; Marks, Dobelle, & MacNichol, 1964); the investigators found that primate cones fall into three major groups, with absorbance maxima at 450 nm, 525 nm, and 555 nm. The shapes of the obtained absorbance functions of human cones are shown in Figure 15–16. These three curves provide a firm physiological basis for the trichromacy of human vision.

Notice that the three cone types represented by the absorption curves in Figure 15–16 do not correspond to the primary colors or fundamentals. The long wavelength-sensitive cone is *not* a "red" cone in any way. It is sensitive to longer wavelengths than the other two cone types, but its peak sensitivity is at 555 nm—a light that appears yellowish-green. It is no more sensitive to

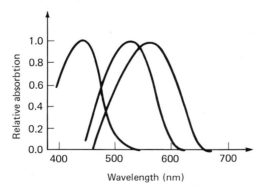

FIGURE 15-16 Absorption spectra for pigments in human cones. From Wald, G., and P. K. Brown (1965) Human color vision and color blindness. *Cold Spring Harbor Symp. Quant. Biol.* 30:345–359. Reprinted by permission of the author and publisher.

lights that appear red (around 630 nm) than to lights that appear blue (around 450 nm).

Figure 15–16 shows the absorbance characteristics of the pigments present in single human cones. In order to demonstrate that the absorbance characteristics of receptors are directly related to their response properties, the next logical step would be to find a way to record directly the electrical responses of single cones to lights of different wavelengths. This is of course not an experiment to be performed on humans; however, experimenters have been successful in recording the responses of single cones from a number of different animals. For the carp, a fish with trichromatic color vision, both spectrophotometric (Marks, 1965) and electrical response data (Tomita, Kaneko, Murakami, & Pautler, 1967) have been obtained. Figure 15–17 shows that the agreement between these two types of experiments is quite good, with both revealing the existence of three types of cones. Each individual cone contains only one of the three cone pigments. These results have recently been confirmed in single cones of the macaque retina (Schnapf, Kraft, Nunn, & Baylor, 1988).

Color Defects

Our entire discussion of color vision to this point has emphasized the trichromacy of the human visual system. There are many people, however, who either do not have trichromatic vision, or have trichromatic vision with a weakened ability to make certain color discriminations. These people are sometimes called *color blind*, although most of them do see colors and should more properly be called *color defective*. The only truly color blind people are the monochromats.

There are many different kinds of color blindness. An individual may possess trichromatic vision, but have one (or more) cone type that contains visual pigment with abnormal spectral absorbance characteristics. Such a person is called an *anomalous trichromat*; he or she will require the usual three primary colors to make a color match, but the relative amounts of each will be different than for a normal subject. In general, anomalous trichromats usually are poorer than normal at making wavelength discriminations in the red or green regions of the spectrum.

Dichromats

The most extensively studied color defects are those in which one of the three cone pigments is completely missing. There are three classes of dichromat, depending on which of the three pigments is absent: *protanopes* (lacking the long wavelength-sensitive pigment), *deuteranopes* (lacking the medium wavelength-sensitive pigment), and *tritanopes* (lacking the short wavelength-sensitive pigment).

Most dichromats are either protanopes or deuteranopes, two categories often grouped as "red-green defects." These are sex-linked hereditary de-

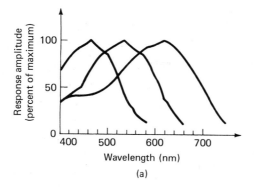

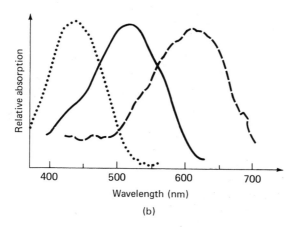

FIGURE 15-17 Absorption spectra and electrophysiological receptor response versus frequency curves for fish retina. (a) Responses from single cones. From Tomita, T., A. Kaneko, M. Murakami, and E. C. Pautler (1967) Spectral response curves of single cones in the carp. *Vision Res.* 7:519–531. Reprinted by permission of Pergamon Press, Ltd. (b) Absorption spectra. From Marks, W. B. (1965) *J. Physiol. Lond.* 178:14–32. Reprinted by permission.

fects, with genes for the long and medium wavelength-sensitive pigments located on one arm of the X-chromosome (Nathans, Thomas, & Hogness, 1986). Men have only one X-chromosome and women have two. When one normal gene is present, the person has normal color capability, so red-green color defects are rare in women (Nathans, Piantanida, Eddy, Shows, & Hogness, 1986). About 8% of all U.S. males have red-green defects (Piantanida, 1988). Tritanopia is much rarer, and is due to a defect on chromosome 7 (Nathans, Thomas, & Hogness, 1986).

We talked about the general properties of dichromatic vision earlier; these include the ability to make color matches based on only two primaries and the presence of a wavelength that is indistinguishable from white light (neutral point). All dichromats share these properties; they differ only in the actual values of the color matching and the placement of the neutral point.

The CIE chromaticity diagram provides a useful way to summarize the properties of the different types of dichromacy. Imagine that the short wavelength-sensitive cones are missing (a tritanope), so any discrimination that depends on the relative amount of stimulation of that cone type cannot be made. Since those cones are most sensitive to blue lights, you can visualize them as contributing a fundamental near the blue primary (lower left corner of the diagram). Of course, the other cones are also capable of detecting blue lights, so what is missing is not really a spectral color or a primary. Nevertheless, for simplicity, you can imagine that all the points on any line passing through the origin have the same ratio of green to red (the ratio is the slope of the line), and so differ only in the amount of blueness.

Two such idealized lines are shown on the CIE diagram in Figure 15–18. The actual place all such lines would intersect would not necessarily be at the origin; we show them passing through the origin in Figure 15–18 for the purposes of illustration. All the points a_1, a_2, . . . on one line have the same green/red ratio, and so would look alike to a person with only the long wave-

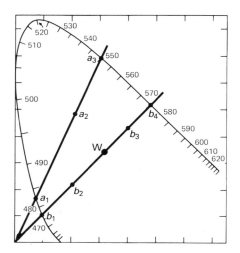

FIGURE 15-18   CIE chromaticity diagram. Stimuli marked with a's and stimuli marked with b's would be indiscriminable from each other if the blue fundamental were missing. We make the simplifying assumption that the blue fundamental is at the origin.

length- and medium wavelength-sensitive pigments. Similarly, the points b_1, b_2, . . . (and W) on the other line would look like each other to such a person, although they would look different from the a points.

A diagram of actual confusion lines for a tritanope is shown in Figure 15–19. (The confusion lines for tritanopes do not exactly converge at a point for reasons that we will not go into.) In this figure, all of the confusion lines radiate from an area near the blue end of the spectrum, as would be expected if the blue fundamental is missing. The line passing from the missing fundamental through W terminates near 570 nm. Therefore tritanopes confuse a 570 nm light with white light. A confusion line also lies almost parallel with the CIE curve from 460 nm to about 510 nm; this implies that wavelength discrimination is very poor for tritanopes within this region.

Figure 15–20 shows a chromaticity diagram with the confusion loci for a protanope drawn on it. All of the confusion lines emanate from the spectrum locus at 700 nm; the line that passes through the point W representing white) intersects the CIE curve near 495 nm; near 495 nm is a wavelength that a protanope will confuse with white light. Notice also that the CIE curve itself is almost straight from 700 nm to about 550 nm. This also constitutes a confusion line, and means that a protanope will confuse all spectral lights from about 550 nm to 700 nm.

Figure 15–21 shows the confusions made by deuteranopes. The confusion lines in this figure are quite similar to those obtained for protanopes;

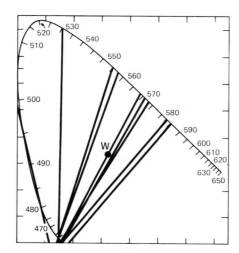

FIGURE 15–19   Confusion loci for a tritanope. From Wright, W. D. (1952) The characteristics of tritanopia. *J. Optical Soc. Am.* 42:509–521. Reprinted by permission of the Optical Society of America.

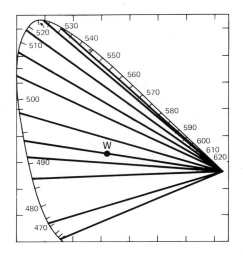

FIGURE 15–20 Confusion loci for a protanope. From Le Grand (1957) *Light, Color, and Vision*. London: Chapman & Hall Ltd. Reprinted by permission.

they emanate from a point in the lower right part of the diagram. The neutral point for deuteranopes as shown on this figure is near 500 nm, slightly longer in wavelength than that found for protanopes. Like protanopes, deuteranopes have a confusion line that lies along the CIE curve in the region of 700 nm to 540 nm. Deuteranopes, therefore, also cannot discriminate among colors in this spectral range.

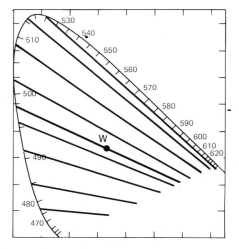

FIGURE 15–21 Confusion loci for a deuteranope. From Le Grand (1957). Reprinted by permission.

BOX 15–7

The fact that the spectrum locus is almost a straight line for wavelengths above about 550 nm also has important implications for normal human vision. Remember that the CIE diagram is a two-dimensional representation of a three-primary color system, with the added assumption that the total amount of all primary colors is constant. In this representation, a straight line means that you can match all spectral colors with two primary colors; all you have to do is choose as primary colors the two spectrum loci at each end of the line segment. All colors on the straight line between the two primary colors can be matched by varying the relative amounts of the primary colors. In this spectral range, therefore, the human visual system is only two-dimensional; in other words, we are all dichromats for wavelengths above 550 nm. Dichromacy results because the short wavelength-sensitive cones are almost totally unresponsive for wavelengths longer than 550 nm. If, as is the case for protanopes and deuteranopes, one of the other cone types is missing, the visual system will actually be monochromatic at longer wavelengths. The fact that a red-green confusion line runs along the CIE curve for wavelengths above 550 nm reflects this monochromacy.

Monochromats

A very small proportion of people have monochromatic visual systems. Most of these people lack all three cone types, leaving only the rod photoceptors to mediate the visual process. The characteristics of rod monochromats include those discussed earlier for monochromats; they can make *no* distinctions solely on the basis of wavelength. In addition, rod monochromats have the same characteristics we normally associate with scotopic vision, among which are poor visual acuity and a strong tendency to be dazzled by bright lights.

OPPONENCY

We have seen in previous sections that trichromatic theory accounts for many characteristics of human color vision. Both the results of color-matching studies and the lack of a single wavelength that is confused with white light are consistent with the hypothesis that color information is encoded by the relative responses of the three cone types. There is a whole class of other visual phenomena, however, that is not easily explained by this formulation. In this section, we will first describe the psychophysical results that are hard to explain on the basis of trichromatic theory, and then introduce another type of model that incorporates the trichromacy of human receptors and these additional data.

Turn to Color Plate C in the inside cover and stare for 30 sec at the cross in the center of the blue square (called an inducing figure). Then quickly transfer your gaze to a clean sheet of white paper. There should be the impression of a yellow square surrounding the cross on the sheet of white paper. (Allow a few seconds for the afterimage to appear.) Then follow the same procedure with the green inducing figure. After staring at the green square for 30 sec, you should see a red square when you stare at a clean sheet of white paper. These illusions of color are called *afterimages*. Staring at a green inducing figure produces a red afterimage (in conditions that favor the formation of negative afterimages—see Chapter 7); blue and yellow are paired in the same fashion. There is nothing in trichromatic theory that suggests a mechanism for this pairing.

Evidence that certain colors are paired with each other is present in, but not explained by, the CIE chromaticity diagram. Figure 15–22 shows a CIE curve with a family of lines that pass through the point W, the coordinate corresponding to white light. Any one of these lines intersects the spectrum locus at two wavelengths. From our previous discussion of the properties of color mixtures, remember that the coordinates corresponding to a mixture of two spectral lights falls somewhere on the straight line connecting them. Therefore an appropriate combination of the two lights connected by any one of the lines in Figure 15–22 would result in a light with the chromaticity coordinate of white light. White light can be produced by a combination of only two wavelengths; any pair that can be connected by a straight line drawn through *W* can be used for this purpose.

Pairs of colors that can be combined to produce white are called *complementary colors*. Blue and yellow are complementary, as are red and bluish-green, and reddish-yellow and greenish-blue. In fact, the same colors found to produce image-afterimage pairs also turn out to be complementary pairs. The fact that there is this kind of consistency across different experimental situations suggests that this pairing of colors is revealing something basic about human color processing.

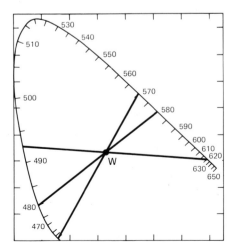

FIGURE 15-22   Three pairs of complementary colors, plotted on the CIE chromaticity diagram.

The experimental technique of color naming reveals another class of phenomena that is difficult to explain on the basis of trichromatic theory. This type of experiment involves the presentation of various monochromatic lights to human subjects, after which the subject is asked to assign a color name to each light. The experimenter provides the names that can be used, for example, restricting the subject to three colors such as red, green, and blue. In this case, the subject would have to name all spectral lights using these three colors in any combination: greenish-blue, bluish-red, reddish-greenish-blue, and so forth.

One interesting result to come out of this type of experiment is that subjects have a hard time naming the whole range of spectral lights using only three color names (Judd, 1951). No matter which three names are used, subjects are able to assign names to stimuli from some parts of the spectrum, but cannot satisfactorily name stimuli from other spectral regions. When the list is expanded to four names, however, subjects are able to name any spectral light. The satisfactory set of names is "red, yellow, green, and blue," which are also the "unique" colors. (You will encounter this set of four colors again when we describe the properties of color-opponent cells later in this chapter). When subjects use these names to identify colors, the names fall into pairs that seem to be mutually exclusive: a subject never describes a light as "reddish-green" or "bluish-yellow" (Boynton & Gordon, 1965). Studies of the evolution of color names in various cultures indicate that there is apparently a genetic predilection for dividing the spectrum in this way (Berlin & Kay, 1969).

The requirement of four color names is rather difficult for trichromatic theory to explain, as the theory postulates the existence of only three chromatic systems. The fact that four names is the minimum set for naming the entire visual spectrum suggests the possibility that, at some point in the human color vision system, four channels are present. (For a discussion of the biological significance of the color names, see Ratliff, 1976.)

To summarize, data accumulated from experiments on color afterimages, complementary colors, and color naming raise questions about the trichromatic model's ability to explain all color phenomena. Some of these problems were recognized in 1878 by Ewald Hering, who proposed an alternative model for the perception of color, called *opponent process theory*. The next section describes some of the basic characteristics of this theory (as modified by current investigators), and shows how it can account for the visual phenomena just discussed.

Opponent-Process Theory

Hering proposed that color vision is mediated by three complex "substances" such that one supposed "substance" accounts for perceptions of red and green, a second "substance" would be responsible for blue and yellow, and a third would be responsible for the white/black distinctions. These substances were postulated to be "opponent," in the sense that the red/

green substance might respond positively to red light but negatively to green light. Contemporary supporters of opponent theory refer to opponent processes rather than substances, and believe that the red/green and yellow/blue processes are built by subtractive combinations of the three cone types. In this conception, opponent processes are results of the way the different receptor types are "wired into" the retinal processing system. In later sections, we will discuss the physiological support for this model and indicate how receptor systems might interact to form opponent processes.

In modern opponent theory, the white/black process is built up by a combination of different cone types. Its purpose is to signal the brightness of a given light. The white/black process plays an important role in quantitative attempts to make the model account for various types of data; however, for now we will consider only the properties of the two chromatic processes.

The red/green opponent process is organized so that it responds in opposite directions to red and green lights. Therefore if we were to present a reddish stimulus, we should be able to null the response of the red/green process by adding some amount of green light. Hurvich and Jameson (1957) followed this line of reasoning to measure the strength of each opponent process as a function of wavelength. For example, to map out the red/green process, they presented subjects with a monochromatic stimulus, and asked them to add either green or red light to the stimulus until it looked "neither red nor green." If green light had to be added, the amount was recorded and assigned a positive sign; if red light was added, its amount was recorded and given a negative sign. If red light had to be added to the stimulus, Hurvich and Jameson reasoned that the original stimulus had evoked a green response from the red/green system, and that the amount of green excitation was related to the amount of red light that had to be added to cancel it. Similarly, if green light had to be added to produce a light that was neither red nor green, that meant that the stimulus before addition had evoked a red response from the red/green process.

Hurvich and Jameson plotted the relative amounts of green or red light that had to be added to the stimulus as a function of the wavelength of the stimulus; they called this the chromatic response function for the red/green process. They obtained the chromatic response function for the blue/yellow process in a similar way; that is, they measured the amount of blue or yellow light that had to be added to a stimulus to produce a light that looked neither blue nor yellow. These chromatic response functions are shown in Figure 15–23. The open circles represent the yellow/blue process, with positive numbers occurring when the process is signaling yellow, and negative numbers implying the process is signaling blue. The red/green process is represented by the closed circles, with positive numbers implying red and negative numbers implying green.

The chromatic response functions in Figure 15–23 explain many of the phenomena that were troubling for trichromatic theory. For example, Figure 15–23 shows why we need four colors to name all the colors in the spec-

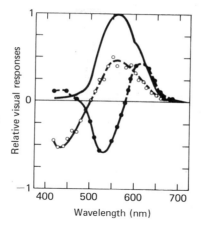

FIGURE 15-23 Psychophysically obtained chromatic response functions for one observer. From Hurvich, L. M., and D. Jameson (1957) An opponent process theory of color vision. *Psychol. Rev.* 64:384–404.

trum. The opponent processes model produces four different color responses. Even though these processes result from the activity of three cone types, there are four separable perceptual events.

Colored afterimages can also be explained by the opponent processes shown in Figure 15–23. As an example, suppose you stare continuously at a rectangle of 490 nm light (which appears bluish-green). The red/green opponent process will give a vigorous green response to this stimulus. As you stare at this stimulus, the middle wavelength-sensitive system (which is responsible for the vigorous response of the red/green system) will adapt, much in the way one adapts to a bright light. The adaptation of this system will cause it to become less sensitive. When you transfer gaze from the green rectangle to a white rectangle, the white light will cause the red/green opponent process to respond. White light would normally cause the two opponent processes both to be at their null points, but the fact that the middle wavelength-sensitive system has been adapted will shift the balance of the red/green process to favor the long wavelength-sensitive system. White light will then elicit the response normally associated with red light, resulting in a red afterimage. Other colored afterimages can be explained in a similar way. (Note that this explanation is virtually identical to the one given in Chapter 10 for aftereffects in which apparent size is affected. With a change in labeling of the axes, and the assumption that there is a subtractive comparison of the "channel" responses, Figure 10–18 could be used as an illustration for this paragraph.)

Physiological Evidence for Opponency

Although opponent process theory is an elegant explanation for a large variety of visual phenomena, it was criticized for many years because it required complex interactions for which there was no physiological evidence. More recently, however, the basis of this criticism disappeared with the discovery of cells in the visual system that behave in ways that are remarkably similar to Hurvich and Jameson's opponent processes.

Important physiological evidence for opponent processes came from the experiments of DeValois, Abramov, and Jacobs (1966). These investigators used microelectrodes to record from single cells in the LGN of the macaque monkey, an animal whose color vision capabilities are similar to those of humans (DeValois, Morgan, Polson, Mead, & Hull, 1974). The LGN cells were driven by illumination of the retina with diffuse monochromatic light at a number of wavelengths. DeValois and his co-workers found four types of color-coded cells. One type of cell responded with excitation to the presentation of yellow lights and inhibition to the presentation of blue light; it was designated as $+Y - B$. The converse of $+Y - B$ cells were also found; that is, cells that were inhibited by yellow light and excited by blue light $(+B - Y)$. The other two types were selectively sensitive to red and green lights; one was excited by red and inhibited by green $(+R - G)$, while the other was of the reverse sign $(+G - R)$. Similar results were obtained by Wiesel and Hubel (1966).

The average spectral response curves for the $+R - G$ cells and for the $+Y - B$ cells are shown in Figure 15–24. It is clear that the responses of these cells closely resemble the red/green and yellow/blue opponent processes obtained psychophysically by Hurvich and Jameson and shown in Figure 15–23. Hurvich and Jameson used their opponent process functions successfully to predict color-naming data, spectral saturation, and wavelength discrimination functions; therefore the responses of LGN cells should also be able to predict responses in the same experimental situations (DeValois, Abramov, & Jacobs, 1966).

These experimenters found spectrally opponent cells when recording from the LGN; in more recent experiments, other investigators have found evidence for opponency while recording from more peripheral cells. In the central area of the monkey retina, more than half of all ganglion cells may be spectrally opponent (Gouras, 1968; DeMonasterio, Gouras, & Tolhurst, 1975). These cells are organized in the typical center/surround manner that we discussed in Chapter 6; however, the center portion of the ganglion cell receptive field receives inputs from a different type of cone than the surround. Figure 15–25 shows an example of a color-opponent monkey ganglion cell. Stimulation of the center region of the receptive field results in excitation of this cell, with this region being more sensitive to long-wavelength light. Surround stimulation inhibits the cell, with the most effective stimulus being green light. Note, however, that since both chromatic mecha-

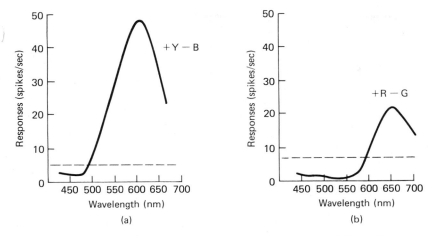

FIGURE 15–24 Spectral response functions for +Y − B (left) and +R − G (right) cells in the LGN of the macaque monkey. From DeValois, R. L., I. Abramov, and G. H. Jacobs (1966) Analysis of response patterns of LGN cells. *J. Optical Soc. Am.* 56:966–977. Reprinted by permission of the Optical Society of America.

nisms are broadband, *any* color light in the surround will inhibit the cell. If we stimulated this cell with diffuse light of any color, the responses would be similar to those seen for LGN cells. When the cell is illuminated with red light, the center region will be stimulated more than the surround, as it is selectively sensitive to long-wavelength lights. Therefore the response of the cell will be excitatory. Diffuse green light, on the other hand, will stimulate the surround more than the center, resulting in net inhibition of the cell. Thus, when diffuse light is used this cell closely resembles a +R − G LGN cell. When there is a luminance difference in the stimulus (for example, a grating of any color), this cell resembles a spatially antagonistic cell such as we discussed in Chapter 6. This cell will *not* respond well to an equiluminant grating (of the optimum spatial frequency for a luminance grating), for the center and the surround will be nearly matched.

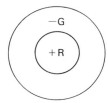

FIGURE 15–25 Schematic of a receptive field of a color opponent monkey ganglion cell.

BOX 15–8

In the visual cortex, more complicated color opponent cells have been described (Ts'o & Gilbert, 1988). Some cells, called Type I, are like those we just described for the retina and LGN. Others, called Type II, are spectrally opponent but not spatially opponent; that is, they are like the cell in Figure 15–25, but with center and surround of identical size. A "modified Type II" cell is very similar, but has a larger additional surround that suppresses firing when light of any color falls on it. Finally, some cells are *double-opponent* (Daw, 1968; Michael, 1973). Such a cell is shown in Figure 15–26. Both the center and the surround are color opponent; for any given color, the cell is spatially opponent. Notice that an equiluminant grating of the appropriate spatial frequency will have a strong effect on such a cell, unlike the Type I cell in Figure 15–25. There is some question about whether such cells are common (Michael, 1985) or rare (Ts'o & Gilbert, 1988) in V1.

The concentric color cells are found mainly in layers IVa and IVcβ (Michael, 1985), the layers to which the parvocellular cells of the LGN project. In the upper layers of the cortex, the color-sensitive cells are found in the cytochrome oxidase blobs (see Chapter 9), with each blob dedicated to a particular type of opponency (+R − G, +G − R, +B − Y, or +Y − B) (Ts'o & Gilbert, 1988). From the blobs, there is a strong projection to the thin cytochrome oxidase stripes in V2, where similar types of color coded cells are found (Hubel & Livingstone, 1987).

In addition to these color-specific cells, there are color-selective cells of the simple, complex, and hypercomplex types (Michael, 1979; 1981; 1985). These orientation-selective color cells are found in the interblob regions, with connections to the appropriately color coded blobs (Ts'o & Gilbert, 1988). They probably account for the color selectivity of the pale stripes in V2.

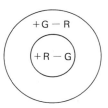

FIGURE 15–26   Schematic of a receptive field of a double opponent cell.

Spatially

Opponent cells such as the ones we have just discussed provide an explanation for many visual phenomena. For example, afterimages are a direct consequence of organization into opponent cells. Consider the monkey's ganglion cell whose receptive field is shown in Figure 15–25. If this cell is illuminated with bright, diffuse green light for a fairly long period of time, the receptors most responsive to such light will be the ones providing input to the surround. Therefore these receptors will also be the ones that will be adapted by the green light; that is, they will become less sensitive. Now suppose we turn off the green light and turn on a diffuse white light. This light will excite all receptors, but the receptors feeding into the surround will be desensitized and will be responding at a lower level. The response of this cell will therefore be dominated by the center mechanism, yielding an excitatory response that signals to higher centers the presence of red light. This is the same explanation for afterimages that was given in the discussion of Hurvich and Jameson's opponent-color model; the difference is that we are now able to assign specific functions to physiological substrates.

From Trichromacy to Opponency

The trichromatic theory and opponent-processes theory originally were considered two alternative explanations for the same phenomena: the phenomenological appearance of colors. Color matching is trichromatic in that three primary colors are required to match any color, and both theories account for this fact. The major difference is that in trichromatic theory the three fundamental processes of color vision are all sensitive to a broad range of wavelengths: one is most sensitive in the long wavelengths, one to middle wavelengths, and one to short wavelengths. In the opponent-processes theory, the three fundamental processes include one broadband system (the black/white) and two opponent systems (red/green and yellow/blue).

Modern opponent theory does not contradict trichromatic theory; it extends it. Hurvich and Jameson based their model on the existence of three types of cones, each with differing spectral sensitivities. The two opponent processes are formed by subtractive interactions among the three cone types. At the level of the cones there is trichromacy in exactly the form Young and Helmholtz suggested, as verified by spectrophotometry. By the level of the ganglion cells there are opponent processes in the form of spectrally opponent cells; they represent the way the nervous system "reads out" the information presented by the three sets of cones.

Given the spectral absorbance curves of the three cone types, we can attempt to determine the interactions that produce opponent processes. The actual details become quite involved, and there is considerable disagreement on a number of significant points. The fundamental idea that there is a subtraction of the responses of cone types is generally accepted, however.

To illustrate, let us consider the red/green process. Abramov (1968) demonstrated that the $+R - G$ and $+G - R$ cells in the monkey lateral geniculate nucleus receive inputs from only the long wavelength-sensitive and middle wavelength-sensitive cones. (Ingling [1977] and Wooten and Werner [1979], however, argue that a short wavelength-sensitive cone input is present under certain conditions.) The responses of these cells, which presumably comprise the monkey's red/green process, should therefore be derivable from the spectral sensitivities of the two cone types.

Figure 15–27(a) shows percent absorption as a function of wavelength for the long wavelength-sensitive and middle wavelength-sensitive cones. We assume that a $+R - G$ cell is excited by the long wavelength-sensitive

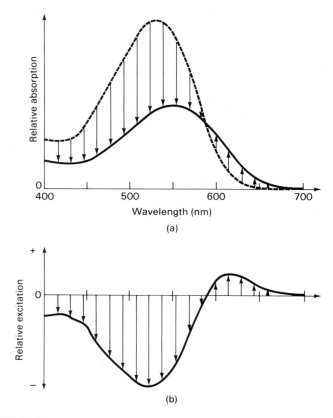

FIGURE 15-27   Demonstration of how chromatic response processes may be generated. (a) Relative absorption spectra for long and middle wavelength-sensitive visual pigments taken from long and middle wavelength-sensitive curves in Figure 15–14. The relative heights of the two functions have been scaled so that they cross at 590 nm. (b) Chromatic response function obtained simply by subtracting the absorbance of the middle wavelength pigment from that of the long wavelength pigment, at each wavelength.

cones and inhibited by the middle wavelength-sensitive cones. The response of a +R − G cell, relative to its maintained firing in the absence of light, is thus related to the difference between the number of photons absorbed by each of these cones. These differences are shown in Figure 15–27(a) as arrows between the two absorption curves; upward arrows mean the long wavelength-sensitive pigment absorbs more; downward arrows mean the middle wavelength-sensitive pigment absorbs more. The differences are plotted in Figure 15–27(b). A +G − R cell would be made by subtracting in the other order and would thus be represented by the same curve inverted.

If the curve in Figure 15–27(b) is compared with the red/green opponent process in Figure 15–23, it can be seen that this simple model provides a reasonable approximation for the way the red/green process may be made. In addition, compare it with the $+R-G$ cells shown in Figure 15–24; the curves in general correspond quite well. (The main difference is that the cells compress the negative portions—after all, they cannot fire at a rate less than zero.)

The yellow/blue process is also made from a difference between the responses of cones, but in a somewhat more complicated manner. There is almost unanimous agreement that all three cone types are needed to make a $+Y-B$ cell or a $+B-Y$ cell, but the question of which two oppose the third is not yet resolved.

The antagonism between responses of different cone types has the effect of sharpening the wavelength selectivity of the retina. In this way it is analogous to lateral antagonism, which sharpens borders. In lateral antagonism, responses of receptors from one area subtract from those in another area— the result is that ganglion cells are more selective for the position of a stimulus. Antagonism (differencing) between cone types results in a sharpening of the spectral responses of the ganglion cell—cones "from" one region of the spectrum subtract from those "from" another region. The sharpening can be seen in the curves in Figure 15–27. A $+R-G$ cell is excited only by wavelengths between 600 nm and 700 nm, as compared to the long wavelength-sensitive cones, which are excited to some extent by any visible light.

We have seen that the initial analysis of color is a two-step operation (at least). The three cone types are the first stage of processing. They provide the initial basis for the essential trichromacy of color mixing. The opponent cells are the second stage. Here, the selectivity of the system is sharpened by an antagonistic mechanism. The opponent processes explain the need for four color names, as well as the presence of complementary pairs and afterimages.

BOX 15–9

The chromatically opponent cells we have discussed are part of the parvocellular system in the cortex. Where are the nonopponent cells that account for the black/white system?

DeValois, Abramov, and Jacobs (1966), who described the four types of color opponent cells in the LGN, also found two classes of cells whose responses were of the same type regardless of the wavelength of light. One type always increased its firing when a light came on; the other always decreased its firing. They *(continued)*

called these cells L-type, for they assumed these were the cells that signaled luminance. Since L-type cells were found among the color opponent cells of the LGN, it is likely that these cells were also in the parvocellular layers.

Of course, we know of another type of cell that is not color-coded: the magnocellular cells. For a number of reasons, Lennie and D'Zmura (1988) reject the idea that magnocellular cells provide the achromatic signal. They argue that the opponent cells (which are the

(box continued)
majority of parvocellular cells) carry both the chromatic and the luminance information. We have already seen that a Type I cell (Figure 15–25) responds to either color or luminance

contrast. Lennie and D'Zmura suggest how different combinations of Type I cells could form both a luminance and a chromatic pathway at higher levels.

SURFACE COLORS AND COLOR CONSTANCY

So far, we have been dealing with the colors of isolated lights, or the two halves of a self-luminous display. Colors in the real world occur in complicated scenes. We really want to describe the colors of surfaces that are reflecting the light from some source of illumination, and we want those colors to be independent of the illumination. This, of course, is the same problem we discussed for the apparent lightnesses of surfaces that reflect light (see Chapter 13). We are now concerned with *color constancy*, the tendency for a surface to appear a particular color despite the illumination conditions. It is exactly analogous to lightness constancy, except that (as you now know) we must consider three reflectance parameters to satisfy trichromacy.

Boynton (1988) discusses a list of 11 basic colors. There are the four colors we encountered from opponency (red, yellow, green, and blue); there are three more "achromatic" colors that we encountered in Chapter 13 (white, gray, and black); and there are four additional surface colors (orange, purple, pink, and brown). These 11 are "basic" in that they are consistently recognized with minimal response times. The surface colors differ in their lightnesses; for example, brown is a darker version of orange. The 11 colors form clusters in a three-dimensional color space (Boynton & Montag, 1988).

In a complicated display, the color of a particular patch is strongly dependent on what surrounds it. Put another way, the color of a surface is poorly related to the spectrum of the light emanating from it. A red shirt appears red in sunlight, electric light, and even in colored party lights (although there may be subtle differences, as you know if you ever matched colors in a store with fluorescent lighting and were surprised when you got home and saw them in daylight!).

Some of the most compelling demonstrations of color constancy have been devised by Edwin H. Land in support of his retinex theory (see Box 13–3). In one, a colored scene (a still life with fruits, vegetables, and a wine bottle) was photographed three times in black-and-white through three different colored filters that roughly allowed only the long, the middle, or the short wavelengths to pass through. The three resulting uncolored slides were then projected through appropriately colored sharp filters and superimposed on a screen. This is a nonstandard way to achieve a three-color separation, and the final product was a good full-color reproduction of the scene. Now, by using only one projector at a time, Land was able to measure the amount of light in each of the three wave bands in any particular part of the picture (such as a red pepper). Not surprisingly, the image of the pepper was dominated by the long wavelength light. Land then put a neutral filter in front of the red projector, so that there were equal energies in all three wave bands at the pepper when all three projectors were on. Nevertheless, the pepper appeared red! Of course, the relative amount of red in all other objects in the picture was also greatly diminished. The lights from the three projectors could be adjusted so that there were equal energies in the three wave bands in any one of the objects, but all the objects always appeared to be of the correct color. These demonstrations provide evidence that color perception is not well tied to the spectral composition of the light emanating from each point in a complicated image.

BOX 15–10

Land is better known for an earlier color demonstration that may have inspired his development of retinex theory. In that demonstration, shown widely in the early 1960s, a still life was photographed only twice in black-and-white: once through a green filter and once through a red filter. The two images were projected in register, the "red" image through a red filter, the other with no colored filter. There was a surprising range of colors in the resulting image, even though it was dichromatic in that only two channels were used to encode it. (This two-color method is named for Land, but was actually in commercial use much earlier. From 1909 to the end of the silent movie era, color movies were produced by a process called "Kinemacolor." In Kinemacolor, alternate frames were projected with or without a red-orange filter, giving an additive mixture by their rapid superposition [Klein, 1936]).

Land's two-color demonstrations were intended to show that there is more to color perception than simple trichromatic matching, and that they did. However, the colors in these demonstrations are not perfect, and modern retinex theory invokes three-color systems. As one would expect, the colors available with the two-color system are confined to a plane in the three-dimensional color space (Land, 1986).

How can we explain color constancy? One appealing idea is that adaptation "readjusts" the color sensitivities of the system for an appropriate balance. If you view a scene lit by reddish light, the light reflected to your eyes from all the objects in the scene will be dominated by the long wavelengths. This will cause adaptation of the long wavelength-sensitive mechanisms (long wavelength-sensitive cones, $+R - G$ cells, and so forth), making your visual system less sensitive to longer wavelengths of light. The relatively weaker medium- and short-wavelength lights will thus be as effective as the powerful long-wavelength lights, restoring a balance similar to what would be achieved unadapted in white light. This is essentially an expanded (trichromatic) version of Helson's adaptation level theory for lightness constancy (page 329).

Unfortunately for this idea, detailed analysis of how adaptation should affect simple and complex scenes does not agree with the data on color constancy (Brill & West, 1986). Moreover, colors are perceived correctly with very brief exposures to an image, and adaptation would be expected to take considerably more time (Land, 1986; Brill & West, 1986).

Another suggestion is that the observer "knows" the illuminant of a scene, and therefore "discounts" it in evaluating the colors of objects in the scene (see Boynton, 1988). The illuminant might be known by the direct reflections from shiny surfaces (see Lennie & D'Zmura, 1988), or from the appearances of objects of known color. These mechanisms can be bypassed by presenting images of abstract, matte finish surfaces. The stimuli so devised are called Mondrians, colored versions of the stimuli discussed in Box 13–3. Mondrians are made as a collage of rectangular papers of various colors. When colored Mondrians are used, the apparent color of any given swatch is independent of the illuminant, just as for the still life images (Land, 1986). Even animals as simple as goldfish judge the true colors of Mondrian patches when the illuminant is colored (Ingle, 1985). In these cases, the observer clearly cannot be evaluating the illuminant by its effect on familiar objects.

In order to explain color constancy, we must invoke some computation across the entire image (Boynton, 1988; Churchland & Sejnowski, 1988). In the retinex theory, ratios of energies at each border are computed in each of three broad energy bands (Land, 1986). Another possibility that could be explored is a computation of the contrasts at the borders (see Box 13–3). There would be three contrasts to compute, presumably in one non-opponent and two color-opponent systems.

There is physiological evidence for these computations. While the second order color cells in LGN (Nothdurft & Lee, 1982) and V1 (Zeki, 1983b) respond to the spectral composition of the lights with no apparent regard for the surrounding regions, cells in V4 respond to the apparent color rather than the spectral composition of patches in Mondrians (Zeki, 1983b). V4 is an area that has been implicated in color processing (Zeki, 1973), being the main receiving area for the V2 thin stripes (which receive their inputs from the V1 blobs; see Figure 9–8). It thus seems reasonable to assign a third level process, in which colors are represented by their appearance and color constancy is maintained, to some cells in V4.

BOX 15–11

While there is appeal to the idea that V4 represents the color processor in a set of parallel pathways to perception, we know that is far too simple an idea. We have seen in Chapter 9 that in addition to the input from the thin cytochrome oxidase stripes, V4 receives input from the pale stripes of V2, and from V3 (which is in the magnocellular stream). It is a processor not only of color, but also of orientation and depth, providing information to the inferotemporal cortex from which a "what" identification may be made. It is therefore not too surprising that such an area, combining so many attributes, does not have an overwhelming concentration of color selective cells (Schein, Marrocco, & DeMonasterio, 1982).

It might be puzzling that some workers find the color cells in V4 unremarkable compared to those in the retina (DeMonasterio & Schein, 1982). These workers believe there are no significant differences in color processing between lower levels and "higher" cortex. Perhaps this finding is tempered by the stimuli used; V4 cells explored with simple stimuli are not asked to show the color constancy responses demanded with Mondrians. There are two important lessons that may be drawn: (1) The reported properties of a cell studied electrophysiologically can depend on the properties sought and the tests used. When you want to find line detectors, test with lines; when you want to find color constancy, test with Mondrians. (2) Individual cells may participate in more than one task. We have commented that the color opponent cells in the parvocellular stream may also carry information about luminance. Similarly, individual cells in V4 may play a role in all the various tasks in which V4 participates (see Lehky & Sejnowski, 1988).

SUGGESTED READINGS

A careful and painstaking account of color perception is given by T. N. Cornsweet in *Visual Perception* (Academic Press, 1970). Chapters 8, 9, and 10 are devoted to color, including color spaces, retinal physiology of color, and the psychological aspects of color. A somewhat briefer but slightly more technical account of the same topics may be found in Chapter 9 of *The Psychobiology of Sensory Coding*, by W. R. Uttal (Harper and Row, 1973).

An account of the physiological aspects of color vision, including details of cone pigment spectral sensitivities, can be found in a *Scientific American* article by E. F. MacNichol, Jr., called "Three-pigment color vision" (December 1964; offprint #197). A somewhat unorthodox view of color vision is presented by E. H. Land in "Experiments in color vision" (May 1959; offprint #223). The Land article is reprinted in the collection *Perception: Mechanisms and Models*, edited by R. Held and W. Richards (W. H. Freeman, 1972), pages 286–298. Land's theory is further elaborated in his article "The retinex theory of color vision" (December 1977; offprint #392). This article is reprinted in the collection *The Perceptual World*, edited by I. Rock (W. H. Freeman, 1990).

An account of the genetics of color pigments and color defects is given in an article by Jeremy Nathans in *Scientific American* (1989) 260 (2), page 42.

Chapter 5 of *Surface Color Perception* by Jacob Beck (Cornell University Press, 1972) includes a discussion of the appearance of colored surfaces illuminated by colored lights. The principal approach taken is to consider the perception of the hue of these surfaces as an extension of the ways we perceive lightness of a surface (this book was recommended among the readings for Chapter 12). Land's color theory is discussed within this framework.

There are two comprehensive books by leading researchers in color vision that cover most of what we have discussed in this chapter (plus several other aspects of color vision). These books are somewhat technical, but readable. They provide useful references on the CIE space and its fundamentals, and on specific forms of color defects, as well as presenting color-matching data and the physiology of color vision. *Human Color Vision*, by Robert M. Boynton (Holt, Rinehart, and Winston, N.Y., 1979) has a number of interesting demonstrations, and an appendix on the CIE space. *Color Vision*, by Leo M. Hurvich (Sinauer Associates, Sunderland, Massachusetts, 1981) is illustrated with a large number of color plates; this book has a more complete coverage of opponent process theory.

THE STRUCTURE OF THE AUDITORY SYSTEM

16

So far in this book, we have described (in some detail) the properties and capacities of only one sensory system, the visual system. With this chapter, we begin our discussion of audition, the second most extensively studied sense. Our treatment of audition follows lines somewhat similar to that of the visual system: the nature of the physical stimulus is discussed first, followed by a description of the physiological machinery that receives and processes the stimulus. We describe, insofar as is possible, how the auditory system functions to give us the psychological impressions of loudness, pitch, timbre, and localizations of specific sounds in space. Finally, we discuss an auditory analog of form perception: speech perception.

Differences between light and sound   Some of the differences between the sense of sight and the sense of hearing may be attributed to differences between light and sound. Both forms of energy travel as waves through space and allow us to sense what is happening at a distance. But light waves travel in straight lines, while sound waves bend around corners. This is because sound waves have a much longer wavelength than light waves, a difference that also limits the ability of sound waves to produce sharp images. This is both an advantage and a disadvantage; you cannot locate a predator precisely, but neither can it hide behind a rock if it is emitting sounds.

An important difference between light and sound is that we see most objects by reflected light, but we hear them by sounds they themselves produce. You see a cat by light from the sun or a lamp bouncing off her fur, but you hear her by the meows she makes. Distinctive sounds are therefore not dependent on the nature of some outside energy source in the way that the appearance of surfaces depends on the nature and amount of illuminant. Therefore, with sounds, we do not have the constancy problem that we encountered for vision (see Chapters 13 and 15).

On the other hand, sound does bounce off other objects in the environment and is therefore "colored" by the environment. Your voice sounds different in a small room, in a large lecture hall, or outdoors. The ways in which sound reflects and is distorted is another cue to the space around you. Just as you might shine a flashlight around a dark room, some animals (such as bats) emit squeals that allow them to "see" in the dark. Congenitally blind people are quite good at comprehending their surroundings from the sounds that reach them.

THE PHYSICAL NATURE OF SOUND

In contrast to light, which is a type of electromagnetic radiation, sound is a purely mechanical phenomenon. It is produced by the physical vibration of an object, which results in the alternate compression and rarefaction of matter surrounding the object. The slight changes in position of the molecules are propagated as a wave that emanates in all directions from the object, even though the positions of individual molecules may not change appreciably. In air, the presence of a sound wave is evidenced by slight changes in local air pressure or concentration of air molecules in a particular location. Figure 16–1 illustrates how the air molecules might be distributed about a regularly vibrating object (a loudspeaker). At any instant in time, there is an orderly and cyclical pattern of locations with high and low concentrations of air molecules. The speed at which the waves emanate from the source depends on the medium through which they are traveling. In air, sound waves travel at a velocity of approximately 340 m/sec; the velocity is considerably greater when sound waves travel through water, and even faster when traveling through metals.

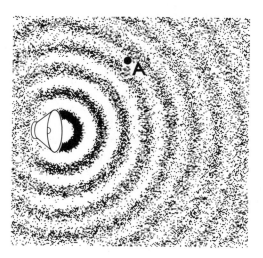

FIGURE 16–1 Schematic representing the cyclic rarefaction and compression of air molecules caused by a uniformly vibrating object (a loudspeaker). Notice the decline in amplitude with distance from the source, and the "shadow" behind the speaker.

One way of representing the sound produced by a given source is to graph the pressure changes that occur at a single point in space as a function of time. For example, if you measured the pressure changes at point *A* in Figure 16–1 caused by the vibrating loudspeaker in the left center of the figure, you might obtain a function such as that shown in Figure 16–2. The function shown in the figure is a sine wave; sounds that can be represented by sine waves are called *pure tones*. From both the physiological and the mathematical points of view, pure tones are the simplest types of sounds to deal with; therefore we shall be discussing them quite extensively. The period (*P*) of the wave is simply the amount of time between two successive maxima (or minima); that is, the length of time for one complete cycle to be carried out at a particular point in space. The *frequency* of the wave (*f*) is the reciprocal of the period; it is the number of cycles that occur in a 1-sec interval. The frequency is measured in units of cycles per second (cps), or *Hertz* (Hz), after the physicist Heinrich Hertz. The psychological attribute of sound that is most closely related to frequency is the pitch of the sound; the exact relationship between pitch and frequency and the other factors that influence the perceived pitch of a tone are discussed in Chapter 17.

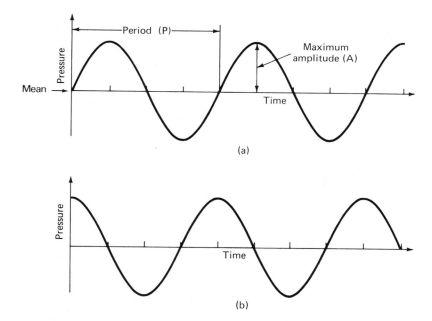

FIGURE 16–2 Two pure sinusoids, with the bottom wave differing in phase from the top wave by one-quarter of a cycle.

Besides the frequency of a pure tone, two other characteristics of the stimulus that are of importance to the auditory system are the *amplitude* and the *phase* of the signal. The amplitude (A) of the sound wave may be defined in units of pressure or of energy, and is related to the perceived loudness of the tone; the greater the amplitude, the louder the sound. As we will discuss later, however, loudness also depends on other factors, such as the frequency of the tone. The phase of the sound wave refers to the part of the cycle that is occurring relative to some fixed time. For example, the wave shown in Figure 16–2(b) is identical to the one in Figure 16–2(a) in all respects except the phase; when the curve in (a) is at a maximum, the curve in (b) is at the mean level. We can see that the two curves are out of phase by an amount of time corresponding to one-quarter of a cycle. Since a pure tone can be characterized as a sine wave, and one complete cycle of a sine wave is defined as 360°, a phase difference of one-quarter of a cycle can be alternatively described as a 90° phase difference. Phase becomes important to consider when we are interested in the response to a sound wave that is being detected at two different points in space; for example, at our two ears. Properties of sine waves were more fully discussed in the beginning of Chapter 10, and they are considered in more detail in the appendix.

Drawing the shape of a particular sound wave as a function of time is not always the most convenient way of representing the important characteristics of that sound. For pure tones, all you need to know to have a complete description of the sound are the frequency and amplitude of the signal. More complex sounds cannot be so easily described, however; the sound waves graphed on the left in Figure 16–3 cannot be represented by a single frequency and amplitude pair. We can use Fourier analysis to separate these types of sound waves into their component sine waves of varying frequency and amplitude, just as we did for complex spatial stimuli in Chapter 10. Complex sound waves can be expressed by their spectra, where the amplitudes of sine wave components are plotted versus the frequency of the components. You can see from the right side of Figure 16–3 that sound spectra can be broken into two general classes. Complex sound waves that are periodic in structure (wave forms that continuously repeat) will yield spectra that consist of a discrete number of specific frequencies with nonzero amplitudes; for example, see the spectra associated with the sound waves in Figures 16–3(a), (b), and (c); and Figure 16–5. Sounds that do not regularly repeat themselves are represented by spectra that are themselves continuous; that is, sine waves at all frequencies are represented in the signal to some extent. As examples, Figures 16–3(d) and (e) show the waveforms and Fourier spectra for a single pulse and a white noise stimulus, two nonperiodic signals. The spectra are continuous functions showing a range of frequencies for which there are nonzero amplitudes, in contrast to the spectra in (a), (b), and (c). Both periodic and nonperiodic complex sounds can be thought of as sums of pure tones with frequencies and amplitudes as expressed by their respective spectra. These are exactly analogous to the spectra that you have seen in Chapter 10.

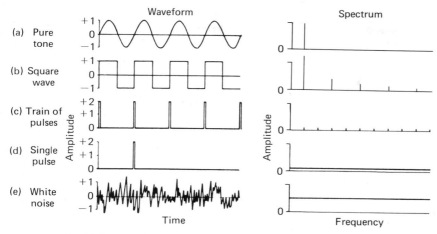

FIGURE 16–3 Fourier spectra of a number of different sound waves. From Moore, B. C. J. (1977) *The Psychology of Hearing*. London: Macmillan Press Ltd. Copyright © Brian C. J. Moore. Reprinted by permission.

Measurement of Sound Intensity

It is a general characteristic of sensory systems that discriminations on the basis of stimulus magnitude can be made over very large ranges of energy. We can make brightness discriminations over a range of approximately 11 log units, which corresponds to an energy ratio of 100,000,000,000:1. Similarly, our auditory system can respond differentially to stimuli the intensities of which vary over a 14-log unit range. Because of the immense range of auditory intensities that must be considered, a modified logarithmic scale called the *decibel scale* (dB) has been developed.[1] In this scale, one particular energy level is chosen as a reference intensity, and all other intensities are expressed as multiples of that reference level. The usual reference level is 10^{-16} watts per square centimeter, which is just barely audible for most people when the sound is a pure tone at 1000 Hz. (When a sound is specified using 10^{-16} W/cm² as a reference, the sound level is referred to as a sound pressure level, or SPL.) The decibel scale has been set up so that a difference of 10 dB corresponds to a 1-log unit (or factor of 10) change in sound intensity. Therefore an increase in intensity of a sound from 10 to 20 dB corresponds to a tenfold intensity difference, while an increase from 10 to 30 dB is a change in the intensity by a factor of 100. The formula relating decibels to the intensity of a sound is

$$dB = 10 \log\left(\frac{I}{I_{ref}}\right)$$

---

[1] The basic unit is actually the Bel (named after Alexander Graham Bell). 1 Bel corresponds to a change in intensity of a factor of 10, which is rather large. We therefore divide the Bel into tenths, and call the new scale *decibels*.

$$= 10 \log \left(\frac{I}{10^{-16} \mathrm{W/cm^2}} \right)$$

If, instead of measuring the intensity of a sound, we have measured the pressure changes associated with that sound, the formula for calculating decibels is different, because intensity is proportional to the square of the pressure:

$$I = P^2$$

Therefore the formula relating decibels to pressure is simply

$$\text{decibels} = 10 \log \left(\frac{P^2}{P^2_{\text{ref}}} \right)$$

$$= 10 \log \left(\frac{P}{P_{\text{ref}}} \right)^2$$

$$= 20 \log \left(\frac{P}{P_{\text{ref}}} \right)$$

From the above formula, you can see that a 20-dB change in sound pressure level corresponds to a 100-fold change in the intensity of the sound, but only a tenfold change in the pressure. The sound levels in decibels of some familiar everyday noises are presented in Table 16–1.

TABLE 16–1   Sound Levels in Decibels for a Number of Common Sounds

Sound	Intensity Level (dB)
Rocket launch (from 150 ft)	180
Jet plane take-off (from 80 ft)	140
Pain threshold	130
Loud thunder	120
Inside subway train	100
Inside noisy car	80
Normal conversation	60
Normal office level	50
Quiet room	30
Soft whisper	20
Absolute hearing threshold (for 1000-Hz tone)	0

Note: Levels are only rough guesses and may vary tremendously.

Pure tones come from sources that vibrate in a sinusoidal fashion. Most vibrating bodies, however, do not move in such a simple way. For example, when a guitar string is plucked, it will vibrate in a manner dependent on the nature of the string, the amount of tension applied to it, and the distance between the two ends of the string that are being rigidly held. Figure 16–4 shows some of the ways that a string can vibrate if it is being held at two points (1 and 2 in the figure). In (a) of the figure, the entire string is moving up and down in unison; the entire length of the string in this case corre-

sponds to one-half of a complete wavelength. A second cycle length that will
also have nonmoving locations at points 1 and 2 is shown in Figure 16–4(b);
in this case, the wave corresponds to one complete wavelength between the
two points, so that the wavelength is half as long as the wave in (a). In other
words, the frequency of the sound produced by the vibrations in (b) of the
figure will be double the frequency of the vibrations illustrated in (a). The
wave in (b) has an additional location besides the two endpoints at which
the position of the string is constant; point 3 in the exact middle of the string
is also immobile. The frequency of the vibration in (b) of the figure could
therefore have just as easily come from a string whose length was half the
distance between points 1 and 2. If you decrease the length of the string by
one-half, therefore, the lowest possible frequency will be exactly double the
previous lowest frequency. This is easy to demonstrate on any stringed musical instrument that is handy. Take any string and pluck it; touch the string at a
point exactly in between the two endpoints, and the observed pitch becomes
much higher. This change in pitch corresponds to a change in the primary
frequency of the vibrating string by a factor of two; in music, this change
corresponds to one octave.

There are infinite numbers of other waves whose cycle lengths would
conform to two stationary points at the end positions in Figure 16–4. Parts

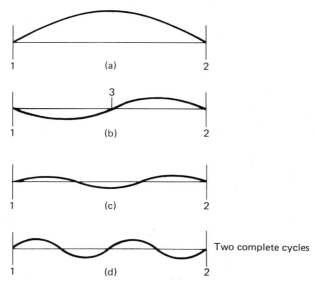

FIGURE 16–4 Four ways that a string fixed at two points can vibrate.
The wavelengths of the vibrations of the string in (b),
(c), and (d) are one-half, one-third, and one-quarter of
the wavelength of the vibration of the string in (a), respectively, giving vibrations with frequencies 2, 3, and 4
times that in (a).

(c) and (d) of the figure show two more examples of such waves; they possess wavelengths that are one-third and one-quarter the wavelength of the wave in (a). Therefore the sound produced by these movements of the string will be three and four times that of the frequency of the sound produced in (a). The set of frequencies that can occur with stationary positions at points 1 and 2 will have frequencies that are integer multiples of the lowest possible frequency; that is, the frequency of vibration of the string in (a). This lowest possible frequency is the fundamental frequency; all the higher vibrations that are multiples of this are harmonics of that frequency.

You have encountered harmonics before, during the discussion of spatial frequency in Chapter 10. In that chapter, we talked about how a square wave grating could be generated by a sum of sine wave gratings. Those sine waves included one that had the same frequency as the resulting square wave; this is the fundamental frequency for that square wave. All the other sine waves in the series were harmonics of that fundamental; they all had frequencies that were integer multiples of the fundamental frequency. Harmonics are also important in the generation of musical chords; pairs of notes that sound consonant (or harmonious) when played simultaneously almost always have fundamental frequencies that are related to each other by a ratio of small numbers. The two notes are harmonics of each other. In addition, although musical notes often sound "pure," they never are. Instead, they are composed of a fundamental frequency, combined with a large number of harmonic frequencies that are present in varying amounts. The fundamental is what determines the pitch of the note, whereas the harmonics are important in producing a quality that is called the *timbre of* the sound. Figure 16–5 shows the waveform of an "open" violin G string bowed with medium intensity, along with the spectrum of the waveform. The lowest frequency is the fundamental frequency, but there are also many harmonic frequencies present in the signal. In fact, the harmonics account for nearly all of the sound energy. These harmonics are generated by the vibrating string, but which are large and which are small depends on characteristics of the entire instrument. That is why a piano playing a G sounds different from the violin playing the same note. (Other differences are due to the rate of increase of the sound's amplitude, its duration, and its rate of decrease.)

STRUCTURE OF THE EAR

The ear can be divided into three fairly distinct components, according to both anatomical position and function. The *outer ear* is responsible for the gathering of sound energy and funneling it to the eardrum. Just past the eardrum, the *middle ear* acts as a mechanical transformer, and transmits the sound information to the *inner ear*, where the auditory receptors are located. In this section, we will start by describing the properties of the outer

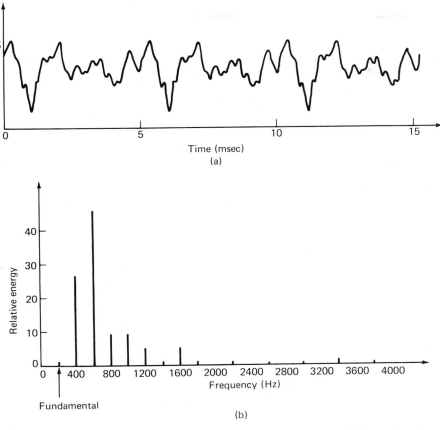

FIGURE 16-5 Sound wave (a) and Fourier spectrum (b) of a violin G string. After Seashore, C. E. (1938) *The Psychology of Music*. New York: McGraw-Hill. Reprinted by permission.

ear and then follow the passage of the auditory information through the middle ear and inner ear.

The Outer Ear

Figure 16–6 shows a sketch of a human ear. The *pinna* is the most peripheral portion of the ear; it is composed mostly of cartilage and is attached to the head by a number of ligaments and muscles. In many animals, the pinna is an effective sound gathering device, with the ability to change position as a function of the location of the sound source. This is comparable to the way we redirect the aim of our eyes within our heads to look directly at something. In humans, however, the pinna is immobile, and we must reposition our heads to aim an ear at a sound source (although there are some people who can slightly wiggle their ears). Our pinna is relatively smaller than the pinna of many other animals with well developed auditory systems. Although its function as a sound-gathering device may be minor in humans, its effectiveness can be increased by cupping a hand behind the ear. In addition, many studies have indicated that the shape of the pinna is important in the localization of sounds in space (Batteau, 1967; Freedman & Fisher, 1968). More will be said regarding auditory space localization in Chapter 18.

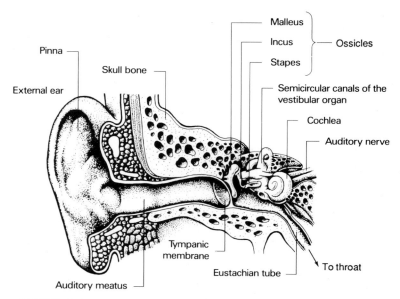

FIGURE 16-6 Anatomy of the ear.

The largest depression in the pinna leads into the *external auditory meatus*, the tunnel that leads to the eardrum, or *tympanic membrane*. The meatus is about 2.5 cm long, and its length can have some influence on the sounds that reach the eardrum. Because of its physical shape, the meatus improves the selectivity of the auditory system for sounds that have frequencies in the range of about 3500 Hz, close to the midpoint of the human auditory range (Gulick, 1971).

BOX 16-1

The outer ear ends at the tympanic membrane, a three-layered tissue that vibrates in response to pressure changes in the external meatus. The eardrum is stretched tightly across

(continued)

(box continued)
the inner end of the auditory meatus, and is pulled slightly inward by structures in the middle ear. Because the tympanic membrane is not a uniformly stiff tissue, its vibration patterns in response to incoming sound waves are often quite complex. At fairly low frequencies (below about 2400 Hz), the membrane vibrates pretty much as a whole, although there are distinct areas of maximum and minimum excursion of the eardrum. As the frequency of the input sound is raised, however, the vibration pattern changes so that different parts of the eardrum are vibrating somewhat independently of each other (Tonndorf & Khanna, 1970).

The Middle Ear

On the other side of the tympanic membrane is the middle ear, which is an air-filled chamber containing three connected bones called *ossicles*. You can see in Figure 16–6 that the tympanic membrane is connected to a bone called the *malleus* (Latin for hammer). The malleus is connected to the *incus* (anvil), which is a slightly larger bone that articulates with the *stapes* (stirrup). Movement of the final bone in this chain, the stapes, is the output signal of the middle ear. The stapes moves in and out of an opening in the cochlea called the *oval window*.

The function of the middle ear is to provide a mechanical transformer system that acts as an interface between the outer and inner ears. The reason for this interface is that the inner ear is a fluid-filled chamber, and so passage of sound information from the outer to inner ears involves a boundary between air and the fluid of the inner ear. You may have observed from personal experience that sound does not travel well across such an interface (try yelling at your pet goldfish, or talking to someone who is underwater); in fact, approximately 99.9% of the sound energy incident on an air/fluid boundary is reflected back within the air medium, so that only 0.1% of the energy is transmitted to the fluid (Wever & Lawrence, 1954). This is a decrease in energy of a factor of 1000, or a 30-dB difference. Such a reduction in energy between the inside and outside of the ear would make us very insensitive to sounds, unless an additional mechanism were present to counteract this reduction.

The middle ear provides two ways of doing so. The first has to do with the relative sizes of the tympanic membrane and the oval window into which the stapes moves. The effective area of the tympanic membrane is about 55 mm², while the oval window is on the order of 3.2 mm² (Békésy, 1960). Remember that intensity changes have been expressed in units of watts/square centimeter; if the total wattage remains constant, but the area in which it is expressed decreases, the intensity per unit area is proportionally increased. Put slightly differently, if the same force is applied to a large area and to a small area, the force applied to the small area will result in a bigger pressure change. This should not be too surprising; you can hit a wall with a hammer and only make a dent, but if you hit a nail with a hammer swung with the same force, all the force is concentrated at the small point of the nail, and it is driven into the wall. The tympanic membrane and oval window differ in area by about a factor of 17, so just by the difference in size of the two partitions, pressure (force per unit area) can be increased by this factor.

The other mechanism by which the middle ear transforms the auditory signal is the lever action of the three connecting bones: the malleus, incus, and stapes. Figure 16–7 shows how a lever system can increase the force of an incoming signal. In this figure, the lever is pivoting around a fulcrum at point C. The distance D_1 between the fulcrum and the point of the applied force is larger than the distance D_2 between the fulcrum and the position of the resultant force. The increase in force due to lever action is given by the following equation:

$$F_{\text{resultant}} = F_{\text{applied}} \left(\frac{D_1}{D_2} \right)$$

Therefore the closer the fulcrum is to the point where the output force is applied, the larger the resultant force will be. The ossicles of the middle ear are arranged so that they act as a lever in a way analogous to the simple lever discussed earlier. The length of the malleus corresponds to D_1, the distance between the applied signal and the fulcrum, while the incus acts as the lever portion between the resultant signal and the fulcrum. Measures of the lengths of these two bones indicate that the force of the incoming auditory signal is increased by the ossicles by a factor of about 1.3 (Wever & Lawrence, 1954; Fischler, Frei, Spira, & Rubenstein, 1967).

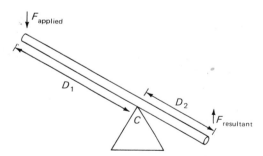

FIGURE 16–7   Lever amplification. If D_2 is less than D_1, then the resultant force will be greater than the applied force.

The combined effects of the difference in areas between the tympanic membrane and the oval window and the lever action of the ossicles produce an increase in the force of the auditory signal that can be measured experimentally. Békésy (1960) investigated the mechanical properties of the middle ear in human cadavers and found that it increased the sound pressure level by about 20 to 24 dB. The reduction in sound level caused by the fluid/air interface at the junction of the middle and inner ears is estimated to be about 30 dB; therefore the action of the middle ear approximately counteracts this reduction.

The middle ear has another function in addition to the mechanical transformation of the auditory signal. When the auditory system is subjected to very loud sounds that may be potentially harmful to the inner ear, two sets of muscles in the middle ear contract and reduce the magnitude of the auditory signal transmitted through the middle ear. One of these muscles, the tensor tympani, is attached to the malleus; when activated, it pulls the tympanic membrane so that its stiffness is increased, and the magnitude of vibrations from incoming sounds is reduced. Similarly, the stapedius muscle connects to the stapes, causing it to retract from its normal position when the muscle is activated. This has the effect of reducing the amount of movement of the stapes in response to an auditory input. Both of these muscles contract reflexively in humans in response to very loud noises and can cause reductions in sensitivity of the auditory system by as much as 30 dB (Reger, 1960). The combined responses of the tensor tympani and stapedius muscles are called the *acoustic reflex*.

BOX 16-2

The acoustic reflex has many parallels to the pupillary reflex of the eye. Each acts to reduce the sensitivity of a sensory system when stimulus magnitude exceeds a certain level, although neither can protect the system from the damaging effects of very sudden and intense stimuli. In addition, the pupillary and the acoustic reflexes are similar in that one cannot evoke either in just one eye or one ear. A stimulus presented to one ear that is loud enough to evoke the acoustic reflex in that ear will necessarily evoke the reflex in the other ear, just as causing pupil contraction in one eye will cause an equal contraction in the other eye. Of course, the eye also has a more effective protecting reflex, the blink.

The Inner Ear

The inner ear is a complicated structure encased in a *bony labyrinth*. Within the labyrinth are the *semicircular canals*, a series of fluid-filled tubes that are the primary receptor organs for the sense of balance. Continuous with the semicircular canals is the *cochlea*, a spiral-shaped structure that contains the cells that act as the auditory receptors. Figure 16–6 shows the relationship between the cochlea and the middle ear; the final bone of the ossicular chain, the stapes, transmits vibrations into the cochlea. The cochlea is filled with a fluid, which is incompressible, so movement of the stapes causes pressure changes in the cochlear fluid. It is these pressure changes that produce the movements that stimulate the primary auditory receptors.

Although it appears from the outside that the cochlea is a single coiled tube, closer investigation reveals that there are three separate compartments within it. This could be seen more clearly if we could unravel the cochlea, a process that is impossible in practice but easy on paper. (Bear in mind that the cochlea is a fluid-filled hollow in the skull, and not a structure unto itself.) As we shall see, the properties of the cochlea do not depend on its being coiled into a spiral; this particular configuration seems to be more a matter of economy of space than of function. Figure 16–8 shows what the cochlea might look like if it were unraveled; of the three cochlear compartments, two are continuous with each other at the very tip of the cochlea. The oval window separates the middle ear from a compartment called the *scala vestibuli*, which is filled with a fluid called "perilymph." The scala vestibuli connects to the chamber at the bottom of the unraveled cochlea called the *scala tympani*; as the two compartments are continuous, both contain the same fluid. This fluid, the perilymph, is essentially the same in its composition as the extracellular fluid bathing most of the nervous system. The two compartments connect at the very *apex of* the cochlea, through an opening called the *helicotrema*. At the part of the cochlea near the stapes, the scala tympani ends at a flexible membrane called the *round window* (Figure 16–6). When the stapes moves into the oval window increasing the pressure within the cochlea, the round window acts to release the pressure by moving outward toward the middle ear.

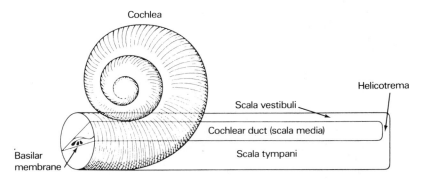

Cochlea

Helicotrema

Scala vestibuli

Cochlear duct (scala media)

Scala tympani

Basilar membrane

FIGURE 16–8   The cochlea unraveled.

The third compartment within the cochlea is called the *cochlear duct* or *scala media* (see Figure 16–9). It is separated from the topmost chamber, the scala vestibuli, by a membrane called *Reissner's membrane*. The structure separating the cochlear duct from the scala tympani is called the *basilar membrane*. The cochlear duct is completely distinct from the two other cochlear compartments, and contains a fluid (called *endolymph*) that differs from the fluid in those channels. Endolymph is very high in potassium, and low in sodium. Within this duct lies the sensory organ responsible for transducing pressure changes into neural impulses.

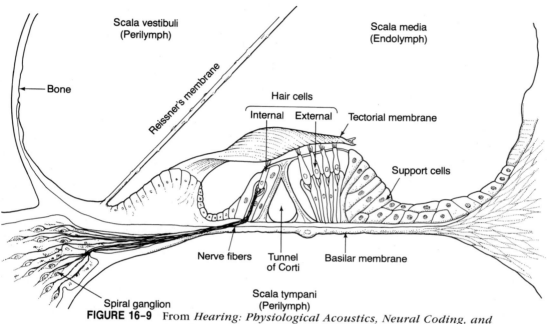

FIGURE 16-9   From *Hearing: Physiological Acoustics, Neural Coding, and Psychoacoustics* by W. Lawrence Gulick, George A. Gescheider, and Robert D. Frisina. Copyright © 1989 by Oxford University Press, Inc. Reprinted by permission.

Lying on top of the basilar membrane is a structure called the *organ of Corti*, which is the primary auditory receptor structure. Figure 16–9 shows in some detail a cross section of the unraveled cochlea with the organ of Corti. Just above the basilar membrane is a shelf of tissue called the *tectorial membrane*. On the basilar membrane sits a rigid inverted "V" known as *Corti's arch*. On either side of the arch are the receptor cells themselves, called *hair cells*. These cells are so named because of their ciliary projections, which are imbedded in the tectorial membrane. When the center of the basilar membrane moves in response to pressure changes in the cochlea, it produces lateral movements of the hair cell cilia. Through a transduction process, discussed in the following box, movement of the hair cell cilia results in a depolarization of the hair cells. The depolarization of the hair cells is the first neural signal in the auditory pathway.

BOX 16–3

The transduction of sound energy into neural energy is rather different from the way light is transduced in the rods and cones of the eye. The cilia of each hair cell form a fairly dense bundle. An extraordinarily fine filament apparently links the tip of each cilium to the flank of its neighbor (Pickles, Comis, & Osborne, 1984). The tips of the cilia are where there is a change induced by bending (Hudspeth, 1982). Although the process is considerably more complex than a simple trip cord, it is as if the filament directly opened channels on the cilium tip when the cilia are bent in the preferred direction (Hudspeth, 1985). Actually, the result is a change in the probability of the channels being open, and the channels each rapidly oscillate between open and closed.

The channels that open in the tips of the cilia are relatively nonselective about what ions they allow to pass through them (Corey & Hudspeth, 1979). However, potassium is very plentiful in the endolymph that bathes the cilia, so potassium is practically the only ion that actually flows through the channels. Usually, we expect a flow of potassium to hyperpolarize a cell, because potassium is in relatively high supply inside cells and flows out. In the case of the hair cells, endolymph is even higher in potassium, and the flow is reversed. Positive potassium ions *enter* through the channels and depolarize the hair cell (see Gulick, Gescheider, & Frisina, 1989). This depolarization leads to the release of chemical transmitter to the cells of the auditory nerve.

As in other synapses, the depolarization that leads to transmitter release acts through an intermediary: calcium. Depolarization opens channels in the base of the hair cell that allow calcium to enter the cell from the surrounding fluid (which is perilymph at the base of the

cell). Calcium is instrumental for the release of transmitter. In the hair cell, it has still another function: it opens special potassium channels, called the calcium-gated potassium channels. But if you think that means there will be even more depolarization, we have still another surprise for you. Potassium *leaves* the cell through these channels, because the perilymph on the other side is low in potassium. Think of the hair cell as a potassium lock in a canal. The channels in the cilia are bathed in high-potassium endolymph, so when they open, the potassium flows in. The channels at the base of the cell are bathed in low-potassium perilymph, so when they open, the potassium flows out. Overall, potassium flows from endolymph to perilymph.

In any case, the potassium *leaving* the hair cell through the calcium-activated channels in the base results in repolarization of the cell, just as potassium channels throughout the nervous system normally lead to hyperpolarizing currents. This acts to "quench" the depolarization caused by bending of the cilia. Bending lets potassium in, causing depolarization; depolarization opens calcium channels, letting calcium in to release transmitter and open the potassium channels in the base; these potassium channels let potassium out, ending the depolarization (Hudspeth, 1985).

Calcium may play still another role in the hair cell. The channels at the tips of the cilia are not very selective, and calcium can enter through them. Since calcium enters less readily than potassium, it may "clog" the channel, so there is less depolarization when calcium is abundant than when it is rare (Corey & Hudspeth, 1983). This is similar to an effect calcium has in the rod outer segments (see Box 5–5). In addition, calcium apparently affects

(continued)

(box continued)
the abilities of the channels to open, allowing
it to make hair cells less sensitive (Corey &

Hudspeth, 1983). In these ways, calcium may
play a role in sensory adaptation, as it seems to
in visual receptors.

Hair cells can be found on both sides of Corti's arch. Receptors on the side of the arch where the tectorial membrane arises are called *inner* hair cells, while the *outer* hair cells are located on the other side of the arch. Inner hair cells are arranged in a single row down the entire extent of the cochlea; all told, there are about 3500 inner hair cells in the human cochlea. The outer hair cells are arranged in rows on the other side of Corti's arch; the total number of outer hair cells has been estimated at about 20,000 (Goldstein, 1974). There are some structural differences between the inner and outer hair cells. Inner hair cells have about 40 hairlike cilia protruding from each cell, while outer cells have about 140 hairs (Moore, 1977). This may or may not account for the fact that outer hair cells are considerably more sensitive to weak auditory stimuli than are the inner hair cells, and are also more susceptible to damage on exposure to very loud sounds. There have also been suggestions that the two groups of receptors differ in how they respond to stimuli of a particular frequency (Billone & Raynor, 1973; but see Dallos, Santos-Sacchi, & Flock, 1982); how the auditory system as a whole codes the frequency of sounds is the subject of the next chapter.

The Auditory Pathway

The hair cells themselves do not have axons, but synapse within the organ of Corti on the dendrites of auditory nerve fibers. Like rods and cones in the retina, hair cells do not fire action potentials, but release transmitter substances when they are depolarized (see the previous box). The innervation patterns of the inner and outer hair cells seem to be somewhat different. It seems that only about 10% of the auditory nerve fibers synapse on the outer hair cells, with 90% synapsing exclusively upon the inner hair cells (Spoendlin, 1970). One fiber will only make contact with one inner hair cell, while each inner hair cell may contact up to 20 auditory nerve fibers. In contrast, the outer hair cells receive much less innervation; a given fiber may be contacted by up to ten outer hair cells, with each hair cell synapsing onto only about four auditory nerve fibers (Goldstein, 1974). The innervation of inner and outer hair cells has been shown to be completely independent by Kiang, Rho, Northrop, Liberman, and Ryugo (1982). Even though there are more outer hair cells, and each one is more sensitive than an inner hair cell, more information from the inner hair cells is transmitted to central auditory centers, because of the more extensive innervation of inner hair cells.

The auditory nerve fibers leaving the organ of Corti have their cell bodies in a structure called the *spiral ganglion*. (A ganglion is defined as a group of nerve cell bodies outside the central nervous system.) The spiral ganglion is so named because it is situated right next to the cochlea and winds around in a spiral fashion just as the cochlea does. Approximately 30,000 auditory nerve fibers have their cell bodies in the spiral ganglion; this number is slightly greater than the total number of inner and outer hair cells in the cochlea. This is unlike the visual system, in which there are far fewer retinal ganglion cells than receptors. The axons of cells in the spiral ganglion leave the ear and enter an area of the brain called the brain stem. Within the brain stem, almost all fibers in the auditory nerve synapse on cells in the *cochlear nucleus*. The relationships of the cochlear nucleus and higher auditory centers in the auditory processing system are shown in Figure 16–10.

Most of the axons of cochlear nucleus cells cross from one side of the brain to the other. As a result, most of the auditory information processed by each half of the brain comes from the ear on the other side of the head. This is in contrast to the visual system, where ganglion cell fibers cross from one side of the brain to the other or stay on the same side of the brain in nearly equal proportions. (Of course, this is also because our eyes look forward and our ears aim to the sides; animals whose eyes aim to the sides show a crossing for optic fibers as well as for auditory). Both crossed and uncrossed fibers from the cochlear nucleus synapse in an area of the brain called the *superior olivary complex*. This is the first location in the ascending auditory system to receive inputs from both ears, although most of the presynaptic fibers come from the contralateral ear.

From the superior olivary complex, axons travel one of two routes. Some fibers synapse in the *nucleus of the lateral lemniscus*, but the majority of them pass directly through this nucleus and synapse in an area of the brain called the *inferior colliculus*. At this level, there is another major pathway allowing information to pass from one side of the brain to the other, so that by this nucleus and higher up in the auditory system, information from the two ears is almost equally represented on both sides of the brain. In addition to the pathway from one hemisphere to the other, fibers leaving the inferior colliculus project to the *medial geniculate nucleus* of the thalamus. This nucleus is a close neighbor of the LGN, the location of first synapse that the visual system makes within the brain. The structure of the auditory system is therefore not closely analogous to the visual system; while the visual system has a high level of neural processing carried out at the external sense organ, the auditory system has only one synapse before going into the brain. Before the auditory system reaches the equivalent level within the brain as the visual system, however, it passes through a sequence of up to five synaptic levels. Thus the auditory system performs many functions centrally that in the visual system are carried out in the periphery.

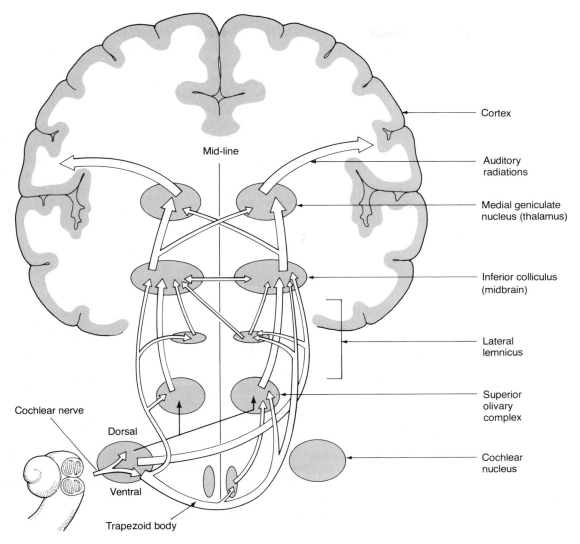

Cortex

Auditory
radiations

Medial geniculate
nucleus (thalamus)

Inferior colliculus
(midbrain)

Lateral
lemnicus

Superior
olivary
complex

Cochlear
nucleus

Mid-line

Cochlear nerve

Dorsal

Ventral

Trapezoid body

FIGURE 16–10   From *Hearing: Physiological Acoustics, Neural Coding, and Psychoacoustics* by W. Lawrence Gulick, George A. Gescheider, and Robert D. Frisina. Copyright © 1989 by Oxford University Press, Inc. Reprinted by permission.

Just as lateral geniculate fibers project to the visual cortex, so do medial geniculate fibers project to the auditory cortex, whose location on the surface of the brain is shown in Figures 16–11 and 19–15. Auditory cortex bears some resemblances to the visual cortex. Most cortical cells within auditory cortex receive input from both ears, just as most cells in visual cortex are binocular. In addition, a spatial map of sorts is represented on the surface of the cortex; as one records from cells in different areas, one finds a systematic relationship between the spatial positions of cells within the cortex and the frequencies of sounds to which those cells are sensitive (Neff, 1961). This relationship is known as a *tonotopic map* and will be discussed in more detail in the next chapter. Some cortical cells require more specific stimulus parameters than just a particular frequency; many cells respond only to sounds coming from a particular location in space, while others respond only to onset or offset of a stimulus (Brugge & Merzenich, 1973).

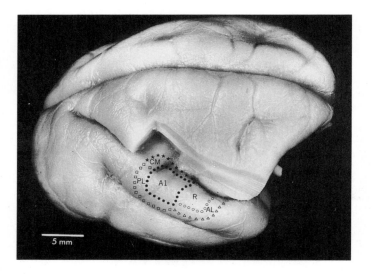

FIGURE 16-11   Monkey brain partially dissected to show the areas of auditory cortex. From Imig, T. J. et al. (1977) Organization of auditory cortex in the owl monkey. *J. Comp. Neurol.* 171:111–128. Reprinted by permission.

In the tonotopic map, there is a systematic change in preferred frequency as you move along the cortex. If you move in the orthogonal direction, you will find another map on the auditory cortex. This map encodes the amplitude of the sound (Suga & Manabe, 1982). Within any vertical penetration through the cortex, you find columns of cells with similar response preferences in frequency and amplitude. This arrangement is quite similar to the arrangement described for visual cortex (see Chapter 9), in which the orthogonal column systems code for ocular dominance and preferred orientation, rather than for amplitude and frequency.

BOX 16–4

We have described how the auditory system transmits information from the cochlea through a complicated processing system to the auditory cortex. There is another system, however, that follows a similar path through the brain, only in reverse. This is the descending auditory system, whose function is presumably to allow such phenomena as selective attention to favor input from one ear over the other. The final cell in this descending system has its cell body in the spiral ganglion of the cochlea and sends axons to synapse directly on the hair cells. The contacts that descending cells make with the hair cells are more diffuse than those of the auditory nerve fibers; one descending fiber will synapse on a relatively large number of hair cells. Thus this system provides a way of affecting a large portion of the receptor population, rather than affecting small numbers of cells separately from the rest of the cells in the cochlea.

Investigators have studied this system by electrically stimulating different nuclei that send descending fibers, and looking to see what effect this stimulation has on activity of the auditory nerve. It was found that stimulation of the descending pathway could reduce responses in the auditory nerve by an amount equivalent to a reduction in sound level of 18 to 25 dB (Desmedt, 1960).

The existence of a descending auditory system is not actually a difference from the visual system. We mentioned in Chapters 8 and 9 that there are descending pathways from cortex to LGN, and from "higher" cortex to primary cortex in the visual system. There even may be an analog of the fibers that go to the cochlea: fibers that descend from brain to retina. Such fibers are well known in lower vertebrates (Dowling & Cowan, 1966; Witkovsky, 1971), and may be present in mammals as well (Brooke, Downer, & Powell, 1965), although their existence is still not clear (Rodieck, 1973).

SUGGESTED READINGS

Suggested readings for this chapter are included with those for Chapter 17.

FREQUENCY CODING IN THE AUDITORY SYSTEM

17

In the previous chapter, we discussed the properties of the auditory stimulus and briefly described the structure of the auditory pathway. With this material as background, we are now ready to examine how the auditory system extracts features from the incoming stimulus to provide us with information regarding the pitch, loudness, and location in space of the stimulus. The physical characteristic of the input stimulus that is most closely related to perceived pitch is frequency. In this chapter we consider how the auditory system gets its information about the frequency of a sound, as well as how this information is transmitted through the auditory pathway.

THE BASILAR MEMBRANE AS A FREQUENCY ANALYZER

In Chapter 16, we described the position of the basilar membrane within the cochlea without going into detail about its physical characteristics. These characteristics, however, form the basis for our sophisticated ability to discriminate between sounds on the basis of pitch. As the auditory hair cells respond to physical movement, and these cells are located on the surface of the basilar membrane, early auditory theorists had long been concerned with the role of this structure in the response to sound.

One early theory was that the entire basilar membrane vibrated in unison with the incoming sound wave, acting in a way similar to the diaphragm in a telephone. According to this theory (now called the *telephone theory*), hair cells located in all positions along the basilar membrane would be stimulated in synchrony, and the frequency of the incoming sound wave would be signaled by the pattern of hair cell responses. Other theorists, one of whom was the great German physiologist Helmholtz (whom we have already encountered as a pioneer of color theory), hypothesized that each location on the basilar membrane was independent of other locations, with each separate segment differentially sensitive to a very small range of frequencies. According to this view (known as the *place theory*), information about the particular frequency of an incoming sound wave would be coded by which segment of the basilar membrane vibrated in response to that sound, and therefore which subpopulation of hair cells was activated. As we shall see in this chapter, both of these types of theories are still invoked to explain auditory pitch perception, although both theories have been significantly modified over the years.

Place Theory

We begin our discussion of auditory theories with the place theory. Helmholtz's idea was that neighboring regions of the basilar membrane are not connected to each other; he assumed that each section is under varying amounts of tension so that it resonates at a specific characteristic frequency when stimulated (in the same way that tuning forks or guitar strings vibrate at specific resonant frequencies). When a sound is presented with a frequency near the characteristic frequency of a particular section, that section would be set vibrating, and thus stimulate those hair cells attached to it. We now know, however, that the basilar membrane is a continuous structure that is not under tension. Its response to incoming sounds of a given frequency is due in part to its continuity, as well as the fact that its mechanical properties vary considerably from the base of the membrane (near the stapes) to the apex (near the helicotrema). At its base, the basilar membrane is fairly narrow and stiff, but as one investigates areas of the membrane farther away from the base, one finds that the membrane gradually becomes floppier and wider. This transition from a narrow stiff structure at the stapes to a wide and floppy structure at the helicotrema has great implications for the processing of sounds of different frequencies; a vibrating system that is light and stiff will tend to vibrate at higher frequencies than one that is floppy. The basilar membrane can therefore be expected to vibrate more strongly at its basal end when the input sound is of high frequency, and vibrate relatively more at its apex when the sound is of a lower frequency.

Georg von Békésy was the first scientist actually to observe the movements of the basilar membranes of humans, and he found that different portions vibrated more or less according to the frequency of the input stimulus. Békésy (1947) exposed the basilar membranes of human cadavers and measured the displacement of the membrane at many locations along its length. He found that an auditory stimulus produced a *traveling wave* on the basilar membrane that traveled from the end near the stapes to the apex. Although the waves originate near the stapes, their direction of travel does not depend on the origin of the stimulus for the wave. The movement of the stapes into the oval window causes a virtually instantaneous pressure change in the entire scala vestibuli; therefore the effect of stapes movement is the same all along the basilar membrane. The increased pressure in the scala vestibuli will cause the entire membrane to be pushed downward toward the scala tympani, the partition below the cochlear partition. It is this downward force exerted over the entire membrane that is the stimulus that causes the traveling waves to be generated. This can be demonstrated by the fact that even when pressure changes are artificially initiated at the apex, traveling waves still go from the stapes to the apex on the basilar membrane.

Figure 17–1 shows the response of the basilar membrane to a steady pure tone, measured at four instants in time. The continuous curves show the displacement of the basilar membrane as a function of distance from the stapes (only the last one-third of the basilar membrane is shown); the entire membrane participates in the traveling wave. That this wave actually travels down the membrane can be observed by comparing the continuous curves; the displacement patterns displayed by the lighter curves represent sequential states of the membrane at very short times before the instants during which the patterns displayed as the heavier continu-

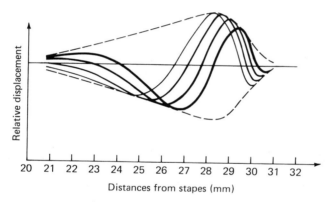

FIGURE 17–1 Displacements of the cochlear partition in response to a 200-Hz tone. The solid curves represent the patterns of displacement at four successive instants; the darker the line is drawn, the later in time that configuration occurred. The dashed curve is the envelope of maximum displacements. Note that the vertical displacements have been greatly exaggerated in this figure in order to make them visible; on the same scale as the horizontal axis, the vertical displacements would be less than 1/1000th as large as they appear here. After Békésy, G. (1947) The variation of phase along the basilar membrane with sinusoidal vibrations. *J. Acoust. Soc. Am.* 19:452–460. Reprinted by permission.

ous curves were recorded. You can see that the entire pattern moves to the right, causing a change in displacement of all points along the basilar membrane. If the traveling waves in response to this same steady tone were measured at many instants in time, you could generate a function of all the maximum displacements of the membrane as a function of distance along the membrane. Such a function is shown by the dashed curves. For this particular steady-tone input, the magnitude of the maximum membrane displacement increases gradually the farther one goes from the stapes. At a region of the membrane about 28 mm away from the stapes, the displacement reaches its maximum and then decreases rather abruptly at distances greater than 28 mm. The function relating maximum amplitude of displacement to position along the basilar membrane is called the *envelope* of the waves evoked by the stimulus.

Although the waves are traveling along the basilar membrane, the motion of the membrane itself is up and down. If you were sitting in a small boat at anchor in a sea with long, slow swells, you would see waves moving past you but your boat would just move up and down. If your boat were sitting on a giant's basilar membrane, each wave would grow as it approached some region, and then shrink as it passed away. How much your boat moved up and down would depend on how near to that maximum point you had "anchored"; the envelope is nothing more than a map of the vertical excursion at each point. As the envelope is symmetric (that is, you go as far down in the troughs as you went up on the peaks), only the top half of it need be shown.

The envelope of the wave displayed in Figure 17–1 shows an area of maximum displacement at a certain position along the basilar membrane; the particular location of the maximum of a given envelope will depend on the frequency of the input sound wave. As the membrane is stiff and narrow near the stapes, high frequency sounds will produce envelopes that have maxima closer to the stapes, while the responses to low frequency sounds will be maximized closer to the apex. This is the physiological basis of the place theory. Figure 17–2 shows the envelopes of patterns of vibration on the basilar membrane in response to a number of pure tones of different frequencies. The top curve shows the envelope for a very low frequency tone; at this frequency, the entire membrane moves as a unit, but the location of maximum vibration is at the apex of the cochlea. The rest of the figure shows the responses to a series of stimuli of increasing frequency. As the frequency of the sound wave gets higher, the location of the displacement maximum moves closer to the stapes. The shape of the envelope also changes, becoming narrower as frequency increases. For fairly high-frequency tones, therefore, only a small portion of the basilar membrane moves to any significant degree, while the entire membrane responds to low tones.

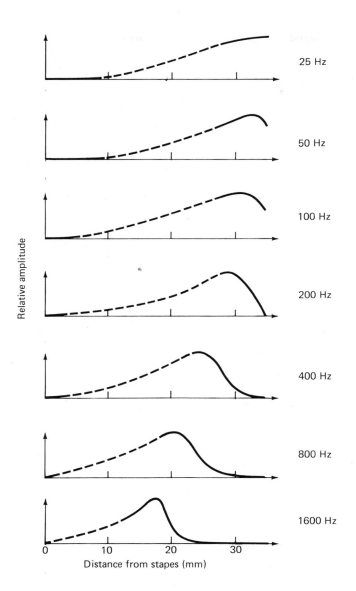

FIGURE 17-2 Envelopes of vibration patterns on the basilar membrane for pure tones of different frequencies. Note the envelope for 200 Hz, the rightmost third of which was shown as the dashed curve in Figure 17–1. From Békésy, G. (1960) *Experiments in Hearing*. New York: McGraw-Hill. Reprinted by permission.

BOX 17–1

The techniques that have been used to measure the vibration of the basilar membrane deserve some mention. When Békésy (1928; 1942) first performed his experiments on human cadavers, he obtained recordings of the position of the basilar membrane by viewing the entire cochlea using a light microscope under stroboscopic illumination. Thus he could photographically record the position of the entire membrane during a given instant. The major problems with this method were that it could only be used with dead preparations, and the light microscope did not give high enough resolution to see the vibrations produced by anything but very loud sounds. These problems were resolved with a technique that involved placing a small amount of radioactive material directly on the basilar membrane, and measuring the changes in the radiation emitted by the material when a sound wave caused vibration of the membrane (Johnstone, Taylor, & Boyle, 1970). For those of you with a physics background, this technique involves measuring the Doppler shift for emitted radioactivity; it allows much finer resolution of movement of the basilar membrane than is possible using a light microscope.

Instead of measuring the maximum displacement of the entire basilar membrane in response to a particular sound wave, it is possible to measure the maximum displacement of a single point on the membrane in response to a large number of sounds of different frequencies. Figure 17–3 shows a series of such functions, with each curve derived from responses of one particular location along the membrane. These functions are called *resonance curves*; they are a useful way of looking at the response of the basilar membrane to sound, because they show how a single hair cell located at one position along the membrane will be stimulated by tones of different frequencies. The resonance curves in Figure 17–3 contain the same information present in the envelopes of basilar membrane vibrations shown in Figure 17–2. In the first case, responses are measured for single frequencies at all points along the membrane, while in the latter case, responses at a single point on the membrane are measured as a function of frequency. The two types of curves are simply alternate ways of displaying the same thing. For example, the second curve from the left in Figure 17–3 peaks at about 200 Hz. From Figures 17–1 and 17–2, we can see that the part of the basilar membrane most sensitive to vibrations at 200 Hz is about 28 mm from the base (or about 6 mm from the apex); this curve must therefore correspond to that position on the basilar membrane. Similarly, the second curve from the right in Figure 17–3 peaks at about 1600 Hz; from Figure 17–2 we can estimate that it corresponds to a position about 17 or 18 mm from the base (just about halfway from base to apex).

The resonance curves displayed in Figure 17–3 have a number of important features. For example, at any particular point on the basilar membrane, one frequency will maximally excite that point. This fact is of crucial impor-

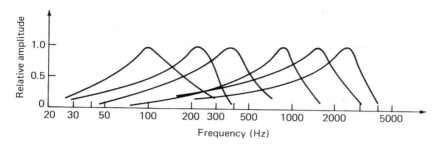

FIGURE 17-3   Resonance curves at six different positions along the basilar membrane. From Békésy (1960). Reprinted by permission.

tance; it means that the mechanical properties of the membrane allow the auditory system to distinguish one frequency from another by the location on the membrane that is maximally excited by a particular frequency. Thus if the response of the auditory hair cells at a particular location along the basilar membrane is directly related to the amplitude of vibration at that location, the auditory system can get information about the frequency of a pure tone by attending to which hair cells are responding more than their neighbors on either side.

Another feature of the basilar membrane resonance curves that deserves mention is the fact that the curves are asymmetrical. For any given location on the membrane, the curve decays more gradually on the low-frequency side of the preferred frequency for that location than on the high-frequency side. Thus a tone that is lower than the preferred frequency will produce a larger displacement than a tone that is an equivalent amount higher. This is consistent with the shapes of the envelopes of maximum basilar membrane vibration shown in Figure 17–2; lower frequencies cause the entire membrane to vibrate, so that any given location will tend to respond to a wide range of tones that are lower than the preferred frequency for that location.

BOX 17-2 ▬▬▬▬▬▬▬▬▬▬▬▬

Τhe asymmetry in which all parts of the cochlea respond better to frequencies lower than their best frequency than to higher frequencies is a common property of oscillators. Imagine a simple oscillator in which a weight is hung by a spring, as shown in Figure 17–4 (you can try this yourself with a weight such as a pair of scissors hung by a rubber band). When the system is "driven" slowly (the hand moving up and *(continued)*

down in a slow sinusoid, as shown at the top), the spring stays the same length, and the weight also moves up and down. As the rate of motion increases, the spring starts stretching on the upward pulls, and contracting as the weight is still rising when the arm starts down. At the frequency that gives the maximum motion of the weight (middle of the figure), the weight and hand are completely out of phase. At even

(box continued)

higher frequencies, the spring just stretches and contracts, and the weight never actually moves at all (bottom). The maximum motion of the weight is at the resonant frequency (middle). Notice that there is motion at lower frequencies (top), but not at higher (bottom).

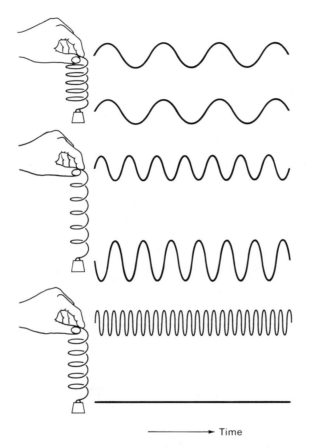

→ Time

FIGURE 17-4   Action of a simple oscillator: a weight hung from a spring, driven by sinusoidal motion of the hand.

The previous discussion presents strong evidence that the basilar membrane is involved in a frequency-to-place conversion for pure tone stimuli. How does this system respond to more complicated stimuli—for example, a combination of two pure tones? If the two tones are quite far apart in frequency, the response of the membrane to the combination will be two essentially separate patterns of displacement. There will be two local vibration maxima along the basilar membrane, with the locations of the maxima identical to where they would be if the tones were presented singly. In this way, the basilar membrane takes a complex tone combination and breaks it down into its component frequencies. For combinations of tones fairly far apart in frequency, then, the auditory system acts as a Fourier analyzer in the same way that the visual system may analyze the frequency components in a grating stimulus (see Chapter 10). For tones that are close together in frequency, however, the response of the basilar membrane is more complex. If the two frequencies are quite close together, there will no longer be two discrete maxima; instead there will be one fairly broad maximum that encompasses the locations at which each tone presented singly would produce its maximum response. This will occur even though the auditory system as a whole may be perfectly capable of discriminating between the two sounds when each is presented separately. Possible mechanisms by which the auditory system can resolve such stimuli will be discussed in a later section.

Neural Correlates of a Place Theory

In the preceding section, we presented evidence supporting the hypothesis that the basilar membrane is involved in a frequency-to-place conversion for any incoming sound wave. As most auditory nerve fibers synapse on one hair cell only, the response of a given fiber should reflect the frequency selectivity of the location on the basilar membrane from which it comes. In fact, when microelectrodes are used to record the responses of single axons within the auditory nerve, such frequency selectivity is usually found. There are several ways in which the frequency selectivity of single fibers can be displayed. One is to present to a single fiber a wide range of stimuli at different frequencies but identical intensity; the function generated when the responses to the stimuli are plotted against the frequency of each stimulus is called an *iso-intensity contour* (Rose, Hind, Anderson, & Brugge, 1971). Figure 17–5 shows a family of such contours for a single fiber in a monkey auditory nerve; each curve was generated using a different intensity level of the stimuli. Although at high intensities the contours are quite broad, for moderate intensities they reveal a single well-defined frequency maximum that corresponds to the location on the basilar membrane from which the fiber originated.

Another way to display the tuning characteristics of individual auditory nerve fibers is to employ a sensitivity measure rather than the response measure of the iso-intensity contour. (The usefulness of sensitivity measures over response measures was discussed in Chapter 7.) Figure 17–6 shows a set of functions called tuning curves, showing how the threshold intensity for a given fiber varies as a function of stimulus frequency. Each curve is generated by determining, for a single fiber, the lowest intensity of a pure tone that will

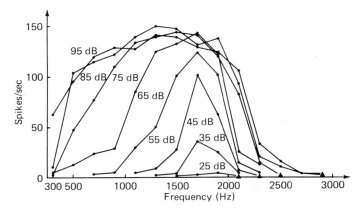

FIGURE 17-5   Iso-intensity contours for a single auditory nerve fiber in the monkey. From Rose, J. E., J. E. Hind, D. J. Anderson, and J. F. Brugge (1971) Some effects of stimulus intensity on response of auditory nerve fibers in the squirrel monkey. *J. Neurophysiol.* 34:685–699. Reprinted by permission.

produce a detectable response, for an entire series of pure tones. The frequency of the tone for which the threshold of a given fiber is lowest is called the *characteristic frequency* of that fiber.

Neural interactions in the auditory system   Single locations on the basilar membrane and single auditory nerve fibers each respond selectively to a limited range of stimulus frequencies. It is important to know, however, whether the responses are quantitatively similar to each other, or if neural interactions in the auditory periphery act to modify the signal leaving the cochlea. One way to investigate this question would be to generate tuning curves for both basilar membrane responses and auditory nerve fibers and to present them on the same coordinate system. Weiss (1964) combined the data from experiments by Békésy (1942) on the mechanical responses of the basilar membrane, and by Kiang, Pfeiffer, Warr, and Bakus (1965), who recorded from single auditory fibers. The mechanical and neural tuning curves are shown in Figure 17–7; although the curves are qualitatively similar, there are substantial quantitative differences. In particular, the neural tuning curves are narrower than the curves generated from the mechanical responses of the basilar membrane. In other words, the auditory nerve fibers are more finely tuned with respect to frequency than are specific locations of the basilar membrane. This suggests that some sort of neural interactive network acts to sharpen the frequency response before the level of the auditory nerve fiber.

One mechanism that would act to sharpen the neural response to pure tones would be a lateral inhibitory system analogous to that found in the

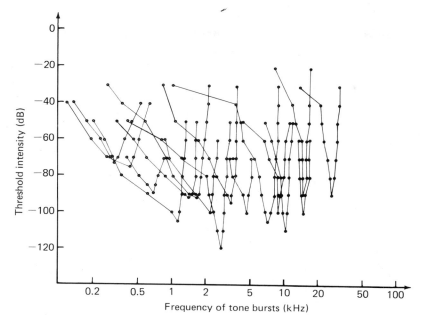

FIGURE 17-6 Tuning curves for 16 auditory nerve fibers in the cat. From Kiang, N. Y.-S., T. Watanabe, E. C. Thomas, and L. F. Clark. (1962) Stimulus coding in the cat's auditory nerve. *Ann. Otol. Rhinol. Laryngol.* 71:1009–1025. Reprinted by permission of the publisher and author.

visual system. The antagonistic interactions between the center and surround of a retinal ganglion cell allows the visual system to enhance spatial borders; investigators interested in the auditory system reasoned that the same type of interaction between cells located at different positions along the basilar membrane could enhance the selectivity to certain frequencies. In fact, the phenomenon of lateral antagonism has been demonstrated in the auditory system. Recording from cells in the cochlear nucleus, onto which auditory nerve fibers synapse, Rose, Galambos, and Hughes (1959) showed that the response of a cell to a stimulus at its characteristic frequency could be inhibited by a presentation of another stimulus of another frequency. This is illustrated in Figure 17–8, where response of a cochlear nucleus cell is plotted as a function of time. A steady tone at this cell's preferred frequency (5300 Hz) is continuously presented, while a second tone (at 4500 Hz) is presented for short time periods at regular intervals. The effect of the second tone presentation is to abolish completely the response of the cell, even though the preferred tone is still present.

Other experiments involving recording from neurons in the cochlear nucleus have provided more details regarding the extent of this lateral interaction. Greenwood and Maruyama (1965) recorded from cells in the cochlear

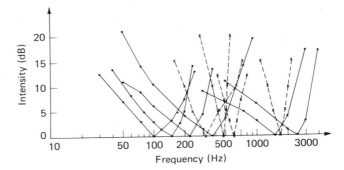

FIGURE 17-7   Comparison of mechanical tuning curves (basilar membrane, shown by solid lines) and neural tuning curves (dashed lines) from similar areas of the basilar membrane. From Weiss, T. F. (1964) A model for firing patterns on auditory nerve fibers, Technical Report No. 418. *Research Laboratory of Electronics, M. I. T.* March 2, 1964, p. 58. Reprinted by permission.

nucleus that possessed an ongoing maintained discharge in the absence of stimulation. They found that cells could be found that responded with increased firing to stimuli within a restricted frequency range, but actually reduced their firing below the maintained level when they were presented with stimuli just outside that range. Figure 17–9 shows an example of a cell

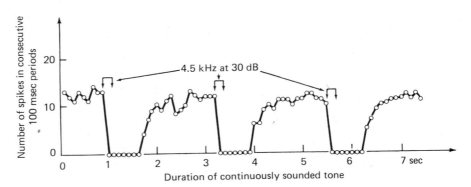

FIGURE 17-8   Demonstration of lateral inhibition along the basilar membrane. A 5300-Hz tone is presented continuously, with bursts of a 4500-Hz tone superimposed on the continuous tone. Firing is markedly reduced when 4500-Hz tone burst is presented. From Rose, J. E., R. Galambos, and J. R. Hughes (1959) Microelectrode studies of the cochlear nuclei of the cat. *Johns Hopkins Hosp. Bull.* 104:211. Reprinted by permission.

with these inhibitory sidebands. The dashed line in the center of the figure represents the tuning curve using a threshold criterion response; the extent of this curve shows the frequency and intensity ranges within which stimuli caused the cell to increase its firing. The shaded areas show the frequencies for which stimuli reduced the firing of the cell. The analogy of this type of cell to a retinal ganglion cell is striking; there is a center region on the basilar membrane within which stimulation will cause excitation of the cell, but there are areas just bordering on the excitatory center, activation of which will cause the cell to decrease its firing. This type of interaction within the visual system resulted in the sharpening of spatial borders; enhancement of border responses along the length of the basilar membrane should result in increasing frequency selectivity of the system. (The analogy breaks down on close inspection, as the same frequency stimulus can cause either excitation or inhibition, depending on the intensity of the stimulus.)

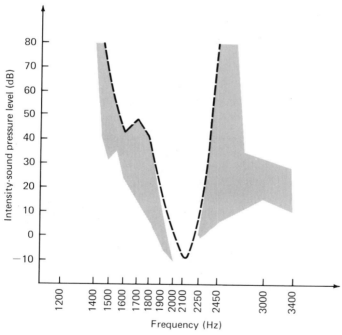

FIGURE 17-9 Representation of excitatory and inhibitory response areas for a neuron in the cochlear nucleus of the cat. Dashed line in the middle of the figure is the excitatory tuning curve for the cell. Shaded regions show the inhibitory regions for this cell. Adapted from Greenwood and Maruyama (1965). Excitatory and inhibitory response areas of auditory neurons in the cochlear nucleus. *J. Neurophysiol.* 28:863–892. Reprinted by permission.

While the presence of lateral inhibition in the auditory system has been demonstrated, the mechanism underlying this interaction is still a matter of speculation. One possible mechanism is suggested by the fact that the auditory system possesses two distinct subpopulations of receptors, with only one of the subpopulations providing the primary input to the auditory nerve. Although the outer hair cells greatly outnumber the inner hair cells, they provide less than 10% of the synaptic inputs to the auditory nerve. In addition, they are considerably more sensitive to weak stimuli than the inner hair cells are. The question therefore arises as to their function, with many experimenters suggesting that outer hair cells interact with the inner cells in some way to sharpen the frequency response characteristics of the latter (Evans, 1975; Ryan & Dallos, 1975; Strelioff, Sitko, & Honrubia, 1976).

BOX 17-3

Recently, a method has been developed by which the functioning of inner hair cells could be studied in the absence of outer hair cells. Kiang, Moxon, and Levine (1970) found that when cats were treated with the antibiotic kanamycin, both inner and outer hair cells completely degenerated over large areas of the basilar membrane. While these investigators did not note a differential effect of the drug on inner and outer hair cells, Dallos and Harris (1978) found that it attacked outer hair cells preferentially over inner hair cells in the chinchilla. In animals treated with kanamycin, large sections of the basilar membrane could be found having inner hair cells that appeared to function normally with no outer hair cells present.

Dallos and Harris found that they could record from auditory nerve fibers coming from areas on the basilar membrane where no outer hair cells were present. They found that such fibers did respond to sound in a frequency se-lective way, but that the shapes of their tuning curves were markedly affected. The sensitivity of individual cells was much reduced, and the shape of the tuning curve was broadened, particularly on the low-frequency tail of the curve. Their conclusion was that the outer hair cells acted on the inner hair cells in some way to enhance the sensitivity of the cells in a frequency-dependent way. The interaction between inner and outer hair cells thus could be the neural mechanism that sharpens the frequency response of auditory nerve fibers.

This conclusion is called into doubt by more recent work indicating that the tuning of inner and outer hair cells is quite similar (Dallos, Santos-Sacchi, & Flock, 1982). For the outer hair cells to affect the tuning of the inner hair cells by a neural mechanism, their tuning might be expected to differ. Even more recent suggestions implicate a mechanical action of the outer hair cells (see the following).

Nonneural mechanisms of frequency tuning While there clearly is a lateral inhibitory mechanism in the auditory system, many now consider that its importance was originally overstated (see Zwislocki, 1981). When the tuning of a healthy basilar membrane is compared to the tuning of the corresponding auditory nerve fibers, the difference is not as great as originally thought (Khanna & Leonard, 1982). While the best fiber is more finely tuned than the best hair cell, the ranges show considerable overlap (Dallos, Santos-Sacchi, & Flock, 1982).

Why did the difference seem so great earlier? One possible reason is that the early mechanical measurements were done on cadavers. There's a reason cadavers are colloquially known as "stiffs." Among other things, their basilar membranes may be less compliant than that in living tissue.

An overlooked mechanism is that the hair cells themselves may be electrically tuned. That is, their neural responses need not necessarily mirror the mechanical vibration. The neural responses could be sharpened electrically if the depolarization at the peak of the cycle caused some compensating hyperpolarization; depending on the time-course of this hyperpolarization, it could either amplify or reduce the response. An intrinsic negative feedback of this type has been found in hair cells (Hudspeth, 1985), and is described in Box 16–3.

Still another factor has also been found: the hair cells change their mechanical properties in response to commands from the descending auditory pathways (see Chapter 16) and in response to sound. The cilia can actually exert force against the tectorial membrane, and thereby affect their own vibration (Hubbard & Mountain, 1983; Brownell, Bader, Bertrand, & Ribaupierre, 1985). Unhealthy (or dead) hair cells would not produce this response, and so the mechanical properties of the basilar membrane in such preparations might not be tuned in the same way as in a healthy preparation. Since the mechanical response depends on the electrical responses, this kind of mechanism could allow for tuning by coupling the mechanical and electrical properties of the hair cells (Weiss, 1982).

Frequency Coding in Higher Centers

If auditory nerve fibers coming from particular locations on the basilar membrane project in an orderly fashion onto the cochlear nucleus, we might expect to find that cells within this nucleus have preferred frequencies that vary as a function of their position in the nucleus. This is, in fact, the case; there is an orderly representation of preferred frequencies along the surface of the nucleus that is called a *tonotopic mapping*. Cochlear nucleus cells seem quite similar to auditory nerve fibers in their frequency characteristics; in fact, cells from all major nuclei in the auditory pathway are similar in their frequency selectivities (Goldstein, 1974).

This same tonotopic organization is also maintained in higher auditory centers. Just as there is a retinotopic representation of the visual world on the surface of the visual cortex, different positions along the basilar membrane are found to be projected systematically to specific locations along the surface of the auditory cortex (Merzenich, Knight, & Roth, 1975). Figure 17–10 shows a map of the surface of the primary auditory cortex. The numbers shown are the characteristic frequencies of the cells encountered at each particular location. Going from left to right on the figure, the characteristic frequencies of the cells encountered progressively decrease. The dashed lines that run almost vertically within the figure are called iso-frequency contours; along those lines, the preferred frequencies of the cells remain approximately constant. Left-to-right movement in the figure corresponds to forward-to-back movement on the surface of the brain. Thus within the auditory cortex, the preferred frequency of the cells decreases from the front to the back of the head.

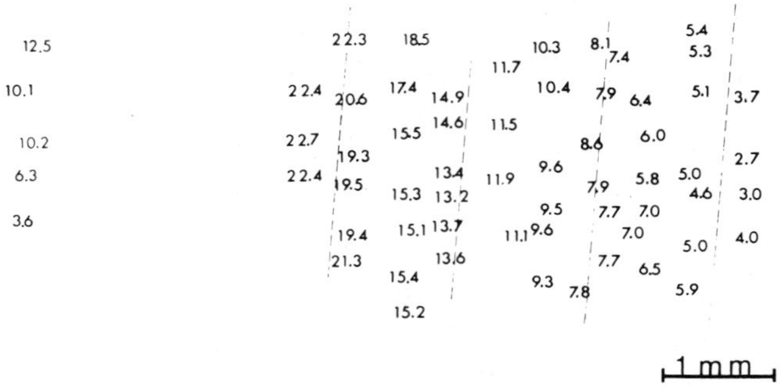

```
12.5          22.3   18.5        10.3  8.1      5.4
                             11.7     7.4       5.3
10.1     22.4 20.6 17.4 14.9    10.4  7.9 6.4   5.1  3.7
                  15.5 14.6 11.5
10.2          22.7   19.3            8.6   6.0       2.7
 6.3          22.4 19.5  13.4 11.9  9.6  7.9  5.8 5.0
                     15.3 13.2              4.6     3.0
 3.6                            9.5   7.7 7.0
              19.4 15.1 13.7 11.1 9.6     7.0   5.0  4.0
              21.3       13.6             7.7 6.5
                    15.4         9.3          5.9
                                    7.8
                    15.2
```

1 mm

FIGURE 17–10 Tonotopic map on the surface of the auditory cortex. Numbers reflect the best frequencies (in KHz) of cells encountered at that location. From Merzenich, M. M., P. L. Knight, and G. L. Roth (1975) Representation of cochlea within primary auditory cortex in the cat. *J. Neurophysiol.* 38:231–249. Reprinted by permission.

We have been speaking (here, and in Chapter 16) of a tonotopic map on the surface of the auditory cortex, implying that such an arrangement could simply be a consequence of the tonotopic mapping in the cochlea. Our discussion of the cochlea as a frequency analyzer suggests that, in accordance with place theory, different positions along the basilar membrane correspond to different frequencies. Thus, a map of the cochlea on the cortex would retain the tonotopic characteristics of the cochlea itself. We might then refer to this as a *cochleotopic* map, just as the retinotopic map in visual cortex also represents visual space.

BOX 17–4

In fact, the tonotopic map encodes the pitch of the stimulus. If complex stimuli are used, the location of the maximum response on the auditory cortex corresponds to the pitch, not the frequency components, of the stimulus (Pantev, Hoke, Lütkenhöner, & Lehnertz, 1989). Since the mechanical vibration of the cochlea is purely dependent on frequency,

(continued)

(box continued)

there must be a transformation to what we recognize as pitch between cochlea and cortex.

Another way to demonstrate that pitch depends on more than the location on the cochlea is by directly stimulating the cochlea at locations that are inappropriate for the frequency of the stimulation. When Tong, Dowell, Blamey, and Clark (1983) did this on humans, they found two components, both interpreted as "pitch." One component corresponded to the location of the stimulation in the cochlea; this is the "place" pitch. The second component corresponded to the *frequency* of the

stimulus, independent of where it was applied within the cochlea. If it is correct that cortical cells do not show phase-locked firing (Brugge & Merzenich, 1973; Merzenich, Knight, & Roth, 1975), these signals must be somehow "finding" the appropriate tonotopic locations in the cortex, despite their original cochleotopic locations. The important point is that the temporal frequency of the stimulus is not lost when it is inappropriately "placed" on the basilar membrane. Some mechanism other than position on the basilar membrane must encode the temporal frequency. The next section discusses such a mechanism.

There is strong evidence that the auditory system processes information about the frequency of an incoming sound wave according to which location along the basilar membrane is maximally activated. The neural signals coming from the basilar membrane reflect the existence of mechanisms that act to make the tuning curves of individual neurons sharper than would be expected solely on the basis of the properties of the membrane. After the level of this interaction, however, auditory neurons do not undergo a noticeable neural sharpening process; tuning curves in the medial geniculate nucleus look quite similar to the tuning curves for auditory nerve fibers. In addition, the conversion from frequency to position that originates at the basilar membrane is maintained all the way up to the auditory cortex, where there is a clear tonotopic mapping of frequency onto the surface of the cortex.

EVIDENCE FOR TEMPORAL FREQUENCY CODING IN THE AUDITORY SYSTEM

Although the evidence for the place theory is compelling, there is some question about whether the tuning curves obtained for neurons in the auditory system provide a mechanism for frequency discrimination that is fine enough to account for the behavioral data. Humans can detect remarkably small differences in frequency; for a 1000-Hz frequency at a moderate intensity, people can detect a difference that is as small as 3 Hz (Moore, 1977). The narrowest tuning curves that were presented in the preceding section still seem to be too broad to account for such resolution. An alternative to the place theory that might account for our well-developed abilities to discriminate between nearby frequencies was suggested many years ago by Wever and Bray (1930). They proposed that the entire basilar membrane vibrated in unison in response to a pure tone, with the vibration of the membrane matching the input frequency. They further suggested that the auditory receptors responded in such a way that the *temporal pattern* of the basilar membrane vibration was reproduced in the firing of the auditory nerve. This alternative theory has been named the "telephone theory," because the basilar membrane is hypothesized to act in a way analogous to a vibrating diaphragm in a telephone.

From the early work of Békésy, we know that the basilar membrane does not act precisely in the way proposed by Wever and Bray; however, it is still possible that some frequency information could be present in the pattern of particular auditory nerve firings. Wever and Bray proposed that if the frequency of the pure tone stimulus were low enough, auditory nerve fibers would respond by firing one or more action potentials at the same time in every cycle of the pure tone. Thus the response pattern of an individual nerve fiber would accurately reflect the frequency of the sound wave. As neurons cannot fire much faster than, say, 500 action potentials per second, however, this type of mechanism would seem to be limited to transmitting information about low-frequency tones only. Criticisms that a telephone theory would only be able to account for perception of low-frequency tones led Wever and Bray (1937) to modify their theory, and suggest that for higher frequency sounds, an individual auditory nerve fiber would not fire in a way that would give an exact reproduction of the pattern of the sound.

For frequencies of the input signal high enough that an individual nerve fiber could not fire fast enough to follow the signal, Wever and Bray proposed the operation of the *volley principle* illustrated in Figure 17–11. In this figure, the sound wave illustrated at the top is of too high a frequency for a single auditory fiber to follow. According to the volley principle, however, a given fiber will fire only at a certain point in each cycle of the sound wave, even if the fiber does not respond to every cycle. In the figure, the eight fibers displayed are responding somewhat irregularly to the incoming signal. Even though every cell does not fire during every cycle of the sound wave, they are all responding in phase; that is, if on any cycle a given auditory nerve fiber does fire, it does so in the same relative position within the cycle. If auditory nerve fibers do respond in such a fashion, and the important signal for higher auditory centers is the ensemble or combination of the responses of many fibers, then we should look at the combined response of all the fibers that are responding to a given sound wave. The bottom trace in Figure 17–11 shows the combined responses of the eight auditory fibers displayed in the rest of the figure; while none of the individual fibers could fire fast enough to reproduce the pattern of the wave, the combined responses of all cells is sufficient to reproduce accurately the frequency of the incoming signal. Thus according to the volley principle, frequency of the sound is coded by the response pattern of an ensemble of auditory nerve fibers.

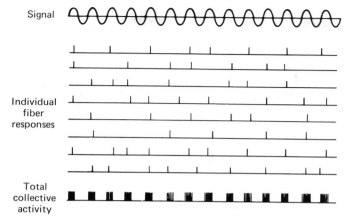

Signal

Individual fiber responses

Total collective activity

FIGURE 17-11 The volley principle. The ensemble of fiber responses shown at the bottom has a pattern of responses that corresponds to the input sound wave, even though individual fibers may not be firing fast enough to follow the pattern of the stimulus. Adapted from Wever, E. G., *Theory of Hearing*. Copyright © 1949 John Wiley & Sons, Inc. Reprinted by permission.

Our discussion of how response pattern could act to code the frequency of a sound wave has so far been entirely hypothetical; it is now time to see if there is any physiological evidence for such a mechanism. Such evidence has been found in the responses of single auditory nerve fibers in the monkey. Rose, Brugge, Anderson, and Hind (1968) stimulated the monkey auditory system with pure tones of different frequencies, and constructed *inter-spike interval* histograms for each stimulus presentation. An inter-spike interval histogram is generated by taking all the times between successive action potentials and collecting them into bins according to their durations. Thus all the intervals that were between 2 and 3 msec in duration would be thrown into the same bin; all the intervals between 3 and 4 msec long would be thrown into the next bin, and so on. After this binning procedure is finished, we can plot the number of intervals that are in any particular bin as a function of the average duration of the intervals that went into that bin.

Figure 17–12 shows six inter-spike interval histograms, generated using stimuli of different frequencies. On the horizontal axis is plotted the length of the interval, while the number of intervals is plotted on the vertical axis. In (a), the stimulus was a tone of 408 Hz; if a single fiber fired one action potential at the same time during every cycle of the stimulus, the interval between each action potential would be $1/408 = 2.45$ msec. If the neuron were firing at the same time every second cycle, the interval between successive spikes would be twice the interval length calculated above; that is, 4.9 msec. A cell firing at every third cycle would show inter-spike intervals of

7.35 msec, and so on. The histogram shown in (a) has a concentration of intervals that would be expected if the cell were firing at every cycle, as well as many intervals of lengths that are even multiples of the interval expected if the cell were firing to every cycle. This cell, therefore, sometimes fires on consecutive cycles, sometimes fires every other cycle, every third cycle, and so on. Thus its firing pattern is an accurate reflection of the frequency of the incoming sound wave, just as the telephone theory would predict.

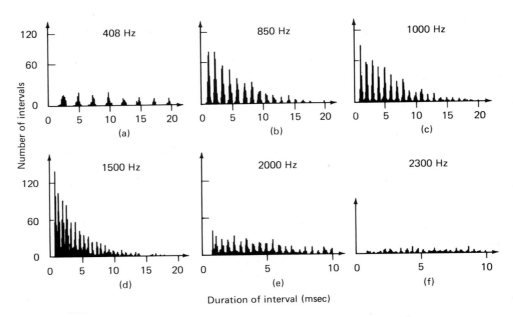

FIGURE 17-12   Inter-spike interval histograms for a single auditory neuron in the monkey, for tones of different frequencies. From Rose, J. E., J. F. Brugge, D. J. Anderson, and J. E. Hind (1968) Patterns of activity in single auditory nerve fibers of the squirrel monkey. In *Hearing Mechanisms in Vertebrates*, eds. A. V. S. de Reuck and J. Knight. London: Churchill. Reprinted by permission.

The other parts of Figure 17–12 show inter-spike interval histograms of the same cell in response to different frequency sound waves. In (c), the stimulus is a tone of 1000 Hz; the volley theory would predict that most of the inter-spike intervals would be either of length $1/1000 = 1$ msec, or even multiples of 1 msec. This prediction is borne out in the histogram; there are large numbers of intervals at 1 msec, but there also are concentrations at 2 msec, 3 msec, 4 msec, and so on. The firing pattern of this cell accurately reproduces the frequency of the sound wave for all of the stimuli in this figure except the 2300-Hz stimulus whose histogram is shown in (f). This is because the auditory fiber being recorded from has its origin fairly close to the apex of the basilar membrane, and is therefore insensitive to high frequencies. Remember that although we are now presenting evidence for temporal patterning as a way of transmitting frequency information, the place theory is also valid.

Auditory nerve fibers have been found that code frequency by the pattern of their response for frequencies up to 4000 or 5000 Hz (Rose, Brugge, Anderson, & Hind, 1967). Above that level, the variability inherent in all neuronal firing becomes too great for such fine patterns to be resolved. Above the 5000-Hz level, therefore, frequency is probably coded solely by the place theory; remember that it is at these high frequencies that auditory nerve fiber tuning curves are at their narrowest, to give the finest discrimination on the basis of place. Below this frequency level, the preceding discussion raises the possibility that frequency may be coded using temporal pattern—as well as place—information, as proposed by Wever in 1949. We should note that there is no direct evidence that the auditory system actually uses the temporal pattern information present in the auditory nerve fibers. In fact, it is unclear how the "higher" centers would extract this information. In later sections, we will discuss some perceptual phenomena, such as auditory localization of sounds in space, that suggest that different mechanisms may be responsible for the perception of frequency above and below 5000 Hz.

BOX 17–5

The histograms in Figure 17–12 were each generated from a long record of the firing of a single neuron during the presentation of a sustained pure tone. Gathering enough intervals for the pattern to emerge may require many seconds of firing. Our auditory systems can detect the pitch of a tone from a much shorter sample, a fraction of a second. In that time, one cell might produce only about a dozen intervals, so the histogram from that one neuron would have only a few scattered bins with intervals in them.

The reason that the nervous system can determine pitch from a much shorter sample is that it has available the firing of a larger number of fibers. If we made a histogram from the intervals produced by a thousand neurons, we could obtain a picture like those in Figure 17–12 in 1/1000th of the time. We can record the activity of the whole auditory nerve, but notice that if we could not keep straight which cell was producing which action potential it would do us no good. The phases would be different for different neurons (remember, this is a traveling wave, so it stimulates different cells at different times), and the volley would be smeared out. The nervous system must have a way of taking account of these phase shifts.

Remember that the higher centers in the auditory system can make use of the information from a large number of single cells. This is a point we sometimes overlook when we seek to understand a whole system from the activity of single cells. When we perform an operation like generating the histograms in Figure 17–12 we are averaging over time, and we implicitly assume that the statistics of any individual over a long time are the same as those of the ensemble at any moment.

THE PERCEPTION OF FREQUENCY

So far in this chapter, we have discussed various possible mechanisms by which the auditory system might abstract frequency information from a sound stimulus. It is now time to consider what kinds of discriminations people can actually make on the basis of frequency, as well as the effect that variations in frequency can have on the auditory percept. There are two psychological qualities that are affected primarily by the frequency content of a given auditory stimulus; they are the *pitch* and the *timbre* associated with the sound. Pitch is a sound quality that is closely related to the frequency of a pure tone or the fundamental frequency of a complex tone containing many harmonics. Pitch is not identical to the frequency of a tone, however, just as the color of a light is not identical to its wavelength. Timbre is a sensation that is related to the quality of the sound. Two sounds can be judged equal in pitch but may sound quite distinct because of differences in the timbre. This sensed quality is what accounts for the difference in sound of, for example, a woodwind instrument and a violin playing the same musical note. Differences in timbre between two sounds of identical pitch are usually ascribed to differences in the harmonic content of the two sounds, while pitch is a function of the fundamental frequency.

The Perception of Pure Tones

Pitch versus frequency   Pitch is the sound quality most closely related to the frequency of a pure tone. High-frequency tones are perceived as being of high pitch, while low-frequency tones are said to be low in pitch. The relationship between pitch and frequency is not a simple linear one, however. In order to make more precise statements about how the two are related, an arbitrary unit called the *mel* has been defined as the unit of pitch. The pitch of a 1000-Hz tone at 40 dB has been given a fixed value of 1000 mels, and psychophysical scaling techniques have been used to determine the number of mels that are associated with different frequency tones. This is done using the method of magnitude production discussed in Chapter 2; a subject is presented with a 1000-Hz tone and told that its pitch is 1000 mels and then is asked to manipulate the frequency of a variable frequency tone until that tone has a pitch that is one-half as high as the 1000-mel tone. That tone is assigned a value of 500 mels. The subject can then find a frequency that is half the pitch of the 500-mel tone; such a tone should be assigned a value of 250 mels. In this way, an entire function relating frequency to mels can be generated.

Figure 17–13 shows an example of such a function. Frequency of the tone is shown using a logarithmic scale for the abscissa, while mels are displayed as the ordinate. This curve shows that pitch is not related to frequency

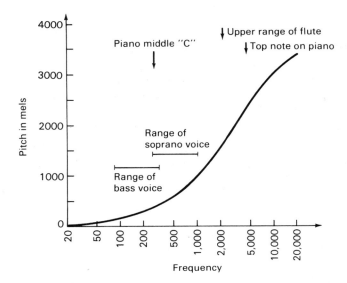

FIGURE 17-13 Pitch in mels plotted versus frequency of an auditory stimulus. Fundamental frequencies of some musical reference points are indicated. Remember that one octave is represented by a doubling of the frequency. From Stevens, S. S., and J. Volkmann (1940). The relation of pitch to frequency: A revised scale. *Am. J. Psychol.* 53:329–353. Reprinted by permission.

in either a linear or a logarithmic fashion. Rather, the relationship is more complex.

Differential sensitivity People can hear and assign pitch values to pure tones having frequencies that range from about 20 Hz to 20,000 Hz. The range is largest in young children and decreases systematically as age increases. Below 20 Hz, a stimulus at high enough sound levels will still be perceived as present, but a subject will not be able to assign it a pitch. Rather, the perception a person has of an extremely low-frequency tone may be a "chugging" sound (Geldard, 1972), with discrete sounds being heard at every cycle.

Although we perceive sounds as having specific pitches within the frequency range of 20 to 20,000 Hz, we are not equally good at making discriminations between different frequencies throughout all portions of this range. By measuring the difference threshold (limen), or smallest frequency difference for which two pure tones can be discriminated, and repeating this measurement for a large number of reference tones, a function relating this difference threshold to the frequency of the reference tone can be obtained.

Figure 17–14 shows a set of these functions, with each curve generated by using stimuli of a different loudness level. For a considerable portion of the auditory range, the difference threshold is about 1 to 3 Hz for moderate loudness levels; that is, humans can discriminate between two tones that differ in frequency by 3 Hz or less.

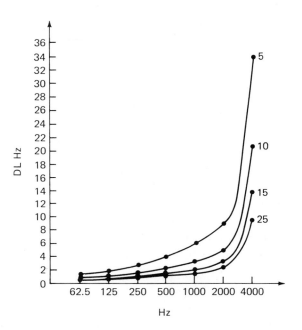

FIGURE 17-14   The difference limen for pitch as a function of frequency, for four different loudness levels. From Harris, J. D. (1952) Pitch discrimination. *J. Acoust. Soc. Am.* 24:750–755. Reprinted by permission.

It is this very well-developed ability to make discriminations on the basis of frequency that caused some auditory theorists to conclude that the auditory system must be making use of information present in the pattern of auditory nerve firings, in addition to place information. The fact that the size of the difference threshold starts increasing rapidly for frequencies above 4000 to 5000 Hz further strengthened this contention, as this is the frequency range in which auditory nerve fibers stop being capable of patterning their responses as a function of input frequency. If both pattern and place information were present in the auditory nerve signal for frequencies below 5000

Hz, but only place information was available for higher frequencies, such a decrease in differential frequency sensitivity could be easily explained.

Pitch versus intensity In Chapter 2, we discussed the phenomena of static invariances; for example, in the Bezold-Brücke hue shift, two lights of somewhat different wavelengths could be made to have the same hue by manipulating the intensities of one of the lights. There is an analogous auditory phenomenon: pure tones change in perceived pitch as their loudness is increased or decreased. Gulick (1971) showed this effect by presenting subjects with a standard tone of fixed frequency and intensity and asking them to match the pitch of the standard by manipulating the frequency of a comparison tone of a fixed intensity. He found that when the standard tone was above about 2500 Hz, very loud comparison tones had to be of a lower frequency than 2500 Hz in order to match the standard. In other words, as loudness increases, the perceived pitch increases. For standard tones lower than 2500 Hz, perceived pitch decreases with increasing intensity; that is, when the standard tone is of low frequency, loud comparison tones had to be of higher frequency than the standard in order for their pitches to match. Figure 17–15 shows the changes in perceived pitch as a function of intensity for nine different frequencies. The abscissa is the change in frequency required for the comparison stimulus to match the pitch of the standard, at the intensity shown by the ordinate. For a very high-frequency tone (7000 Hz), the pitch shift can be quite substantial; when the comparison stimulus is much louder than the standard, its frequency may have to be more than 100 Hz lower than the standard in order for a match to be made.

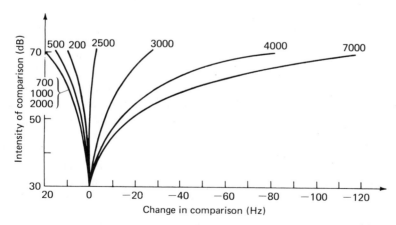

FIGURE 17–15 From *Hearing: Physiological Acoustics, Neural Coding, and Psychoacoustics* by W. Lawrence Gulick, George A. Gescheider, and Robert D. Frisina. Copyright © 1989 by Oxford University Press, Inc. Reprinted by permission.

BOX 17-6

You might think that the fact that perceived pitch of a pure tone changes with intensity might cause severe problems for writing and playing music. As different frequency tones are shifted in different directions, it would seem that the entire melody of a musical piece would be affected by the loudness at which the piece was played. Fortunately for those of us who appreciate music, however, the pitch shift only seems to occur for intensity changes of pure tones. The sounds produced by musical instruments all have extensive harmonic structures; it is these structures that account for the different sounds among different instruments playing the same note. The presence of these harmonics is the reason that a musical note has the same pitch whether it is played loudly or softly. The reason that the auditory hue shift does not occur with complex sounds is not known.

THE PERCEPTION OF COMPLEX TONES

Beats

If you are presented with a combination stimulus consisting of two pure tones of similar but not identical frequency, a phenomenon known as beating occurs. To the listener, the stimulus does not remain at a constant loudness but seems to vary at a rate that depends on the frequency difference between the two tones. The reason that beats occur is illustrated in Figure 17–16. When two tones are close in frequency, the relative phase difference between them will vary slowly in time. In the left side of the figure, the two tones (shown by the top two sinusoids) are exactly in phase; when combined, the stimuli add together to produce a wave that is the sum of the amplitudes of the individual tones (bottom). At some points, however, the stimuli will be out of phase with each other, so that when one wave is at a maximum, the other is at a minimum. When the tones are combined under these conditions, they will tend to cancel each other, as is shown in the middle of the bottom trace in Figure 17–16. The amplitude of the total sound wave is very small at this time, so that the combined stimulus will seem quite soft.

The rate at which the perceived loudness of a combination of two tones will wax and wane depends on the frequency difference between them. For example, if a 500-Hz and a 501-Hz tone were presented together, the beat frequency would be exactly 1 Hz; that is, the combination stimulus would have one loud period and one soft period every one second. For these types of combination stimuli, the perceived pitch is somewhere in between the pitches of the two components when presented separately.

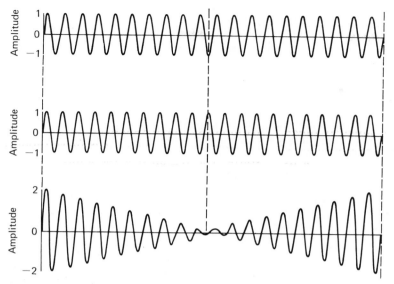

FIGURE 17-16 Two pure tones of similar frequency adding together to produce beats. Top two traces show the individual waves, bottom trace is their arithmetic sum. Dashed vertical lines facilitate comparisons of phase.

Periodicity Pitch

Combination stimuli that produce beats have perceived pitches that are similar to the pitches of the components. For other complex combinations, however, the pitch of the complex tone may not be at all close to the pitches of *any* of the components. Moore (1977) presents the example of a stimulus consisting of a sequence of very short clicks, occurring at a rate of 200 clicks/sec. The pitch of such a stimulus will be very close to that of a 200-Hz pure tone, even though the click stimulus contains significant amounts of energy at the harmonics of 200 Hz; that is, 400 Hz, 600 Hz, 800 Hz, and so on. Using electronic filtering techniques, it is possible to remove from this signal all of the 200-Hz component; in this case, the pitch of the remaining signal will still be that of a pure 200-Hz tone. In fact, it is possible to remove all but a small number of high-frequency harmonics, for example 2200 Hz, 2400 Hz, and 2600 Hz, without changing the perceived pitch of the stimulus. The timbre of the stimulus will change greatly as extra harmonics are added or subtracted, but the pitch remains remarkably constant. This phenomenon is known as *periodicity pitch*, or the perception of the *missing fundamental* (see also Chapter 10).

Several explanations for periodicity pitch have been proposed. According to one theory, nonlinear properties of the basilar membrane cause vibrations to be set up at the place on the membrane corresponding to the fundamental frequency of the sound, whether or not that fundamental was actually present. This hypothesis can be fairly conclusively rejected, however, as experiments have shown that the missing fundamental will still be perceived even when the portion of the membrane most sensitive to the fundamental has been inactivated. Licklider (1956) presented the high harmonics of a low-frequency tone simultaneously with a wideband low-frequency stimulus that completely saturated the locations on the basilar membrane sensitive to low frequencies. Even under these conditions, the low-frequency pitch corresponding to the fundamental was heard.

BOX 17–7

Many experiments have been performed that have attempted to determine the critical features that determine the pitch of a complex of high-frequency tones. A question that has received considerable attention is whether the observed pitch is due to the difference in frequency between the tones in the complex or whether other factors are also important. Schouten, Ritsma, and Cardozo (1962) investigated the changes in perceived tone that occurred when the frequency differences between the component tones were kept constant while the absolute frequencies were varied; they found that the relative frequency differences were not the only important factors in determining the perceived pitch. If a complex tone with frequency components at 1800, 2000, and 2200 Hz is presented, the difference in frequency between the tones is 200 Hz, and the subjective pitch is similar to the pitch of a pure tone at the fundamental frequency of the series, 200 Hz. Now consider what happens if a constant frequency is added to each tone, so that the individual components are, say, 1840, 2040, and 2240 Hz. The frequency differences have not changed, but the tones are no longer the consecutive harmonics of a pure tone at 200 Hz. In this case, a low-pitch sound is still heard, but the perceived pitch is not a pure 200-Hz tone. Instead, the pitch is slightly higher, and it can be matched by a tone of approximately 204 Hz. Thus neither the difference in frequency between the successive tones nor the presence of a fundamental frequency can completely account for the effect of periodicity pitch.

SUGGESTED READINGS

For a more detailed look at auditory physiology, T. Glattke's chapter in *Normal Aspects of Speech, Hearing and Language*, edited by F. Minifie, T. Hixon, and F. Williams (Prentice-Hall, 1973) is a good place to start. Those looking for an even more complete treatment should turn to the chapters by M. H. Goldstein and V. B. Mountcastle in Mountcastle's *Medical Physiology*, 13th edition (C. V. Mosby, 1974). The auditory periphery is also extensively and rigorously examined in P. Dallos' book *The Auditory Periphery* (Academic Press, 1973). Those interested in the particulars of frequency coding in the auditory system might try reading Békésy's *Experiments in Hearing* (McGraw-Hill, 1960). Another good (and quite readable) discussion of this topic may be found in Chapters 3 and 4 of B. Moore's *Introduction to the Psychology of Hearing* (University Park Press, 1977).

A somewhat more advanced treatment of all the topics in Chapters 16 through 18 may be found in *Hearing: Physiological Acoustics, Neural Coding, and Psychoacoustics* by W. L. Gulick, G. A. Gescheider, and R. D. Frisina (Oxford University Press, 1989).

Scientific American articles relevant to the topics discussed in this and the previous chapter are numerous. They include Békésy's "The ear" (August 1957; offprint #44), Warren and Warren's "Auditory illusions and confusions" (December 1970; offprint #531), and Oster's "Auditory beats in the brain" (October 1973; offprint #1282). The articles by Oster and by Warren and Warren are reprinted in *Recent Progress in Perception* (W. H. Freeman, 1976), while Békésy's article is reprinted in *Perception: Mechanisms and Models* (W. H. Freeman, 1972).

PERCEPTION OF LOUDNESS AND SPACE

18

In the last chapter we discussed in some detail how the auditory system made discriminations on the basis of the frequencies of the incoming waves. In addition to pitch, there are numerous other aspects of sound that we are capable of perceiving. This chapter is devoted to two of these properties: loudness and stimulus location in space. Although the perception of loudness may seem like a simple task, it is complicated by interactions between the perceived loudness and the frequency of a given tone, as well as the fact that the components of complex tones sometimes act as if their loudnesses add to, and sometimes act as if they are inhibited by, each other. The perception of the location of a given sound is also a complex phenomenon, with the final percept resulting from a combination of monaural and binaural cues.

THE PERCEPTION OF LOUDNESS

The loudness of an auditory stimulus is a psychological, not physical, attribute of the stimulus. As such, it depends on the characteristics of the observer, as well as on those of the stimulus. The physical attribute of sound that is most closely correlated with loudness is intensity; however, because humans are not equally sensitive to sounds of all frequencies, the perceived loudness of a tone will depend on its frequency as well as its intensity. In this section, we discuss how we perceive the loudness of pure tones, and then move on to the loudness of more complicated stimuli.

Pure Tones

Absolute thresholds The minimum sound intensity that can be heard varies greatly as a function of stimulus frequency. People are most sensitive to tones of frequencies around 3000 Hz, with sensitivities decreasing for tones that are either higher or lower in frequency. Many investigators have obtained functions relating absolute auditory threshold to stimulus frequency, using a number of different experimental techniques. One method involves delivering the stimuli using loudspeakers and measuring the sound pressure at the entrance to the auditory meatus. A threshold measured in this way is known as a *minimum audible field* (MAF). In contrast, when sounds are delivered through headphones, and sound levels calibrated using artificial ears, the threshold measure is called the *minimum audible pressure* (MAP). MAF thresholds are plotted as a function of frequency in Figure 18–1. From this figure, you can see that threshold is minimized in the region from 2000 to 5000 Hz and rises steeply for frequencies above and below these levels. We should note here that many other animals (for example, dogs, bats) can detect frequencies far higher than those detectable by people. That is why dogs can respond to whistles that humans cannot hear at all.

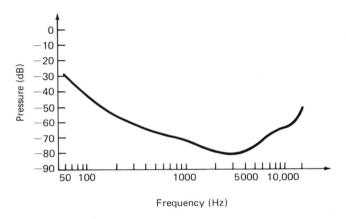

Frequency (Hz)

FIGURE 18–1   Auditory thresholds as a function of frequency. After Sivian, L. J., and S. D. White (1933) On minimum audible sound fields. *J. Acoust. Soc. Am.* 4:288–321. Reprinted by permission.

The threshold sound levels displayed in Figure 18–1 produce extremely small physical displacements at both the tympanic and at the basilar membranes. Wilska (1940; as reported by Geldard, 1972) found that for sounds of frequencies to which the human auditory system is maximally sensitive, threshold sound levels caused movements at the eardrum that were on the order of 0.01 nanometers in total excursion. When you consider that the wavelengths of visible lights range from 400 to 700 nanometers, you can more fully appreciate what small movements the eardrum is making. Stevens and Davis (1938) have extrapolated from data on tympanic membrane movements to suggest the physical response of the basilar membrane to near threshold sounds is even smaller, or on the order of 0.001 nm. Such movements are significantly smaller than the diameter of a single hydrogen atom! The sensitivity function shown in Figure 18–1 is a valid representation of the sensitivity of the human auditory system only for one particular group of humans: young people. As we grow older, we become less sensitive to stimuli of all frequencies, but the maximum hearing losses occur for high-frequency tones. The progressive loss of hearing sensitivity with age is known as *presbycusis* (or *presbyacusia*); the details of this effect are shown in Figure 18–2. In this figure, hearing loss (measured from a standard scale) is plotted as a function of frequency for each of two groups of people. The dashed line shows the auditory capabilities of a group of young men ranging in age from 18 to 30 years (0 dB means no difference from "normal"); the solid black curve was derived from a group of men all of whom were more than 65 years old. This group is at least 7 dB less sensitive than the younger group throughout the entire frequency range, with the maximum difference in sensitivity occurring for frequencies greater than 1000 Hz. For frequencies above 5000 Hz, the older group is as much as 50 dB less sensitive than the younger group. Whether this age-related hearing loss is directly caused by some aging process, or if it is the result of cumulative exposures to very loud sounds and illnesses, is a question that has not yet been resolved.

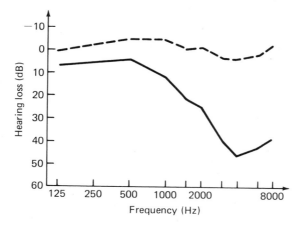

FIGURE 18–2   Hearing loss as a function of frequency. The dashed curve shows losses for men ranging in age from 18 to 30; the solid curve shows losses for men over the age of 65. From Weiss (1963).

BOX 18–1

It should not come as a surprise that most hearing losses are in the high frequencies. The frequencies lost are the ones for which the vibrations are essentially restricted to the base end of the basilar membrane (see Chapter 17).

They are therefore detected by a small subset of hair cells. Moreover, that subset of hair cells responds to all frequencies (see Box 17–2), and are therefore the ones most likely to be "worn out" with age.

$dB = 20 \left(\frac{P}{P_0} \right)$

Equal loudness contours   One of the most common problems in psycho-physics is relating a subjective quality such as loudness to a physical quantity such as sound pressure level. Equal loudness contours provide a way of studying the details of this relationship: they are generated by taking a 1000-Hz tone at a specific intensity, and determining the sound levels at other frequencies that are subjectively equal in loudness to the 1000-Hz tone. For example, a subject might be presented with a 1000-Hz standard tone at 60 dB and then asked to manipulate the intensity of a 2000-Hz comparison tone until it matched the loudness of the 1000-Hz tone. The same 1000-Hz tone would then be compared with a 3000-Hz tone, the intensity of which would be manipulated until this tone was equal in loudness to the standard tone. In this way, intensities of tones at a variety of frequencies could be obtained so that all the tones matched the loudness of the 60-dB 1000-Hz tone. These intensities could then be plotted as a function of frequency, yielding an equal loudness contour. All the tones with intensities and frequencies as given by the contour will be subjectively equal in loudness; these sounds are assigned a loudness level of 60 *phons*. For any equal loudness contour, the loudness level in phons is defined as the decibel level of the subjectively equally loud 1000-Hz tone.

A series of equal loudness contours is presented in Figure 18–3. For low loudness levels, the shapes of these curves closely resemble the sensitivity function shown in Figure 18–1, as would be expected by the fact that a threshold intensity versus frequency curve is really just an equal loudness contour. As loudness level increases, however, the contours change in shape, becoming much flatter than at lower levels. This means that the rate at which loudness grows with increasing SPL varies as a function of frequency. For example, the difference in sound level between two 1000-Hz tones at 60 and 70 phons is 10 dB (by definition). For a 30-Hz tone, however, two stimuli that are 60 and 70 phons respectively will only differ in sound level by about 3 dB. Clearly, we must know frequency as well as amplitude to determine loudness, just as we must know intensity as well as frequency to determine pitch.

The family of equal loudness contours displayed in Figure 18–3 show that we are relatively more sensitive to low-frequency tones at high loudness levels than at low loudness levels. Because of this, certain sounds that are identical in their frequency and phase components may sound different simply because of variations in loudness. For example, voices appear to have much greater low-frequency components when heard from a loudspeaker at full volume, giving them a quite "boomy" sound (Moore, 1977). In addition, musical recordings that are made at a relatively high volume and then played softly often seem as if they are lacking in the amount of bass. This is because at low volumes we are relatively less sensitive to those low tones. Many stereos compensate for this effect by having a "loudness" switch that adds extra bass at low intensity levels.

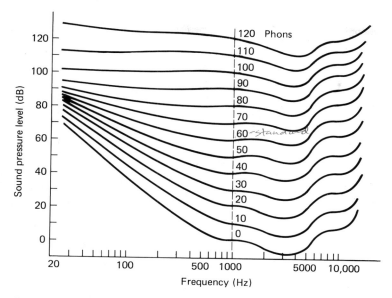

FIGURE 18-3   Equal loudness contours. The curve marked 0 reflects
the absolute sensitivity of the human auditory system.
From Berrien, F. K. (1946) The effects of noise. *Psych.
Bull.* 43:141–161.

Loudness scaling   Using equal loudness contours, we were able to generate the phon scale, which relates subjective loudness level of an arbitrary
tone to the intensity of a pure 1000-Hz tone that matches the arbitrary tone in
loudness. A more direct way to create a scale for subjective loudness is to use
the direct magnitude production techniques developed by S. S. Stevens and
discussed in detail in Chapter 2. Stevens and Davis (1938) defined the *sone*
as the unit in such a loudness scale; one sone is arbitrarily assigned to be the
loudness of a 1000-Hz tone at 40-dB intensity. To obtain a tone with a loudness of 2 sones, a subject is asked to manipulate the intensity of the stimulus
so that the loudness is exactly twice that of the 1-sone sound. Similarly, a 0.5-
sone stimulus is one that is perceived to be exactly one-half the loudness of
the original tone. Loudnesses that are not even multiples of the original 1-
sone sound are obtained by bisection; that is, a 3-sone tone is one that is
perceived as midway between the loudness of a 2-sone and a 4-sone stimulus.
    Stevens (1957) obtained loudness estimation data from a large sample of
subjects and determined that loudness (in sones) was related to the sound
intensity of a sound by a power law of the form

Loudness = $k \cdot$ (intensity)$^{0.3}$

The relationship between decibels and sones is shown in Figure 18–4; the
straight line is obtained because sones are plotted on a logarithmic, instead
of linear, scale.

BOX 18-2

Stevens' power law, represented in Figure 18-4, can be restated in a slightly different way: loudness doubles for every 10-dB increase in stimulus intensity. This statement sometimes misleads students into believing that 10 dB represents multiplication by two. You recall, of course, that 10 dB actually represents a tenfold change in intensity (see Chapter 16).

To understand why the power relationship implies a doubling of loudness for each 10-dB change in intensity, take the logarithm of the power relationship:

$$\log (\text{loudness}) = \log (k) + 0.3 \log (\text{intensity})$$

Then, for every log unit change in intensity (which is 10 dB), there is a 0.3 log unit change in loudness. The antilog of 0.3 is 2 ($\log[2] = 0.3$), so 10 dB represents a doubling of loudness. You can also read that result from Figure 18-4: if you mark off a doubling of loudness on the y-axis (say from 1 to 2 sones), you will see a 10-dB change in intensity (in this case, from 40 to 50 dB).

Although we have been talking exclusively of pure tones, Stevens (1972) and others have proposed models that allow more complex sounds to be scaled according to their perceived loudness. These models all involve breaking up the stimulus into a number of narrow frequency bands, and obtaining some values for the SPLs within each band. The sone level of the total stimulus is then determined by summing the loudness of the individual bands. The complex tones whose scaled loudnesses are displayed in Figure 18-4 were obtained in this way. According to the data presented in this figure, the loudness of a rock band is approximately three times greater than the noise of a nearby truck, which in turn is about thirty times louder than the . sound of a quiet conversation.

BOX 18-3

Before we leave the topic of loudness scaling, we should note that not everyone agrees that the function shown in Figure 18-4 is truly an appropriate way to relate sound intensity to perceived loudness. Replications of loudness estimation experiments often yield power law exponents significantly different than 0.3 (Reynolds & Stevens, 1960; Warren, 1970), with great individual differences commonly being observed. In addition, the loudness esti-

mation technique is susceptible to bias, with results depending on many factors such as the range of stimuli presented, the loudness of the first stimulus, the range of responses that the subject is permitted to make, and others (Moore, 1977). An example of such a bias effect is that individual subjects have a tendency to limit their responses to the middle of the range that the experimenter makes available (see Chapter 2).

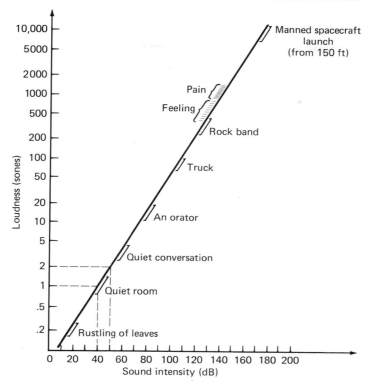

FIGURE 18-4 Graph relating loudness in sones to the intensity level of a stimulus. Figure 5–10 from Human Information Processing, Second Edition, by Peter H. Lindsay and Donald A. Norman, copyright © 1977 by Harcourt Brace Jovanovich, Inc., reprinted by permission of the publisher.

The coding of loudness changes In the first parts of this chapter, we have considered the psychophysical relationships between the intensity of a given auditory stimulus and its perceived loudness. From the data displayed in Figures 18–3 and 18–4, it is clear that the intensity range over which the human auditory system is capable of making loudness discriminations is about 130 dB (an energy range of more than $1:10^{13}$). In this section, we will briefly discuss how the auditory system might act to allow us to detect loudness changes over this extremely large range.

One possible way that the auditory system could code loudness changes is for individual auditory nerve fibers to respond differentially to sound levels throughout the entire intensive range. When Kiang (1968) recorded from single cat auditory nerve fibers, however, he found that they showed dynamic response ranges that were on the order of only 40 dB. In other words, the difference in intensity between a threshold stimulus and a stimulus that will produce a maximal response from the nerve fiber is about 40 dB. Figure

18–5 shows the responses of an auditory nerve fiber as a function of sound level of the stimulus. For this cell, threshold is at about 25 dB, and the cell responds maximally for all sounds greater than about 65 dB.

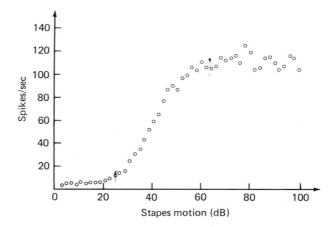

FIGURE 18-5   Intensity response function for a single auditory nerve fiber in the cat. The stimulus is a pure tone at the characteristic frequency of the neuron. From Kiang, N. Y.-S. (1968) A survey of recent developments in the study of auditory physiology. *Ann. Otol. Rhinol. Laryngol.* 77:656–675. Reprinted by permission.

If single nerve fibers do not respond across the entire range of auditory intensities, then perhaps different fibers have quite different auditory thresholds, so that loudness could be coded by simply noting which subpopulation of fibers were active. When a large sample of auditory fibers was examined from the cat auditory system, however, it was found that the variation in thresholds among the fibers in the sample was no greater than 20 dB (Kiang, 1968), for fibers with the same characteristic frequency. Thus if loudness of a pure tone stimulus was coded only by fibers with characteristic frequencies equal to the frequency of the stimulus, the range of intensities over which subjects could make loudness discriminations would only be about 60 dB (20-dB threshold variability and 40-dB dynamic range). The fact that the human range is more than 100 dB implies that fibers for which the stimulus frequency is not equal to their preferred frequency are also involved in the perception of loudness for that stimulus.

In our discussion of basilar membrane vibration in Chapter 17, we noted that a pure tone stimulus produced vibrations over a large area of the membrane, and that these vibrations are reflected in the responses of the hair cells. Thus a pattern of excitation is produced in the auditory nerve such that fibers with characteristic frequencies close to the input frequency are firing more strongly than those fibers whose characteristic frequencies are much different than the stimulus. A way in which the auditory system might code loudness differences that would be consistent with the preceding data is that the shape of this excitation pattern might change as a function of the intensity of a stimulus. Figure 18–6 gives an example of how such a mechanism might work. A pure tone with an intensity of 80 dB might produce a pattern of neural excitation along the basilar membrane that resembles the solid function in Figure 18–6. Let us make the hypothesis that the neurons most excited by this stimulus are firing at their maximum level; therefore increasing the intensity of the stimulus will not cause an increase in firing by these cells. The cells with characteristic frequencies either higher or lower than the stimulus frequency are not firing at their maximum level, however, and increasing the stimulus intensity should cause these neurons to increase their response levels. The effect of increasing the stimulus intensity should therefore be to broaden the excitation pattern, as is shown by the dashed curve in Figure 18–6; the firing in cells whose characteristic frequencies are near the input frequency is not changed, but cells with characteristic frequencies that are farther away from the input frequency will increase their response. Thus loudness would be coded by how broad the excitation pattern might be to a given stimulus. At the present time, this hypothesis seems best to fit the available physiological and psychophysical data on the perception of loudness.

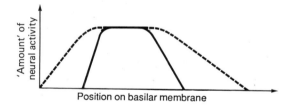

FIGURE 18–6 Proposed mechanism for the coding of loudness. For high-stimulus levels, further increases in stimulus intensity result in a change in the excitation pattern within the entire auditory nerve (dashed pattern), without changing the firing rates of the neurons most sensitive to the stimulus. After Moore (1977). Reprinted by permission.

Adaptation and fatigue In the course of our everyday experiences, we are exposed to sounds of many different loudness levels. Given this situation, a question that immediately arises is whether the auditory system—like the visual system—is capable of changing its sensitivity as a function of the level of ambient stimulation. The answer is an unequivocal yes; however, while all changes in visual sensitivity as a function of lighting conditions fall under the general category of adaptation, scientists interested in the auditory system have distinguished between two types of sensitivity changes. *Auditory fa-*

tigue occurs in response to quite intense stimulation, and is usually measured after the fatiguing stimulus has been removed (Hood, 1972), while adaptation is the reduction in sensitivity that occurs during the presentation of more moderate sounds.

To measure auditory fatigue, a fatiguing stimulus is presented for a certain period of time, and auditory thresholds are measured at various times after the original stimulus has been turned off. In the experiment for which data are shown in Figure 18–7 (Postman & Egan, 1949), a 115-dB white (broadband) noise was presented for several minutes, and the thresholds at different frequencies were measured at various times after the extinction of the fatiguing stimulus. The reduction in threshold is plotted versus the frequency of the test stimulus in Figure 18–7; hearing loss is greatest shortly after the fatiguing stimulus is turned off, with thresholds returning to near normal within 24 hours. Even though the original stimulus included components at all frequencies, the hearing loss is much greater for high frequencies than for low ones; one-half minute after the stimulus was turned off, thresholds were less than 10 dB higher than normal at 500 Hz, but were 50 dB higher than normal at 3000 Hz. The fact that fatigue is greatest for high frequencies may be related to the phenomenon of presbycusis, whereby we become progressively less sensitive to high-frequency tones as a function of age. Perhaps this permanent hearing loss is caused by the cumulative effects of auditory fatigue.

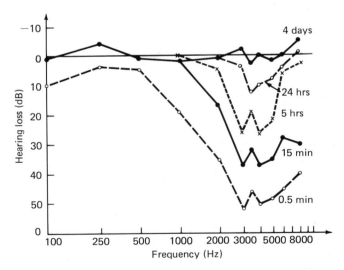

FIGURE 18-7   Audiograms showing the changes in auditory sensitivity following exposure to intense stimuli. Figure from *Experimental Psychology* by L. Postman and J. P. Egan. Copyright 1949 by Harper and Row, Publishers, Inc. Reprinted by permission of the publisher.

Auditory adaptation effects are usually measured while the adapting tone is still physically present. The technique most commonly employed is called the *simultaneous dichotic loudness balance* (SDLB); it involves presenting the adapting stimulus to one ear, and asking the subject to manipulate the intensity of a tone presented to the other ear until it matches the loudness of the adapting tone. The intensity of the comparison tone thus serves as a measure of the loudness of the adapting tone. Using the SDLB technique, investigators have found that if an adapting tone is turned on and left on for a long period of time, its perceived loudness decreases rapidly during the first two minutes of exposure, and reaches an asymptote by three to seven minutes (Moore, 1977). The more intense the adapting tone, the greater the decrease in perceived loudness. In contrast to the phenomenon of fatigue, adaptation occurs approximately equally to both low and high frequencies (Jerger, 1957); in addition, adaptation is maximized when the adapting and comparison tones are of the same frequency.

Complex Tones

Our discussion has thus far centered around how the auditory system codes information regarding the loudness of pure tones. The auditory world is full of more complicated stimuli, however, and it is important to know whether such complex sounds are treated differently from pure tones. In general, the answer to this question is yes; the auditory system responds quite differently to combinations of tones than it does to the individual components. In this section, we will discuss some of these differences.

The loudness of complex tones and the concept of the critical band

Suppose we perform an experiment in which a subject is presented with a complex stimulus consisting of equal intensities of stimulation for all frequencies between two limits. This type of stimulus is called band-limited; it is narrow band if the two limits are close together, and wideband if they are far apart. The *bandwidth* of such a stimulus is defined as the range of frequencies between the two frequency limits. If a subject is presented with a series of band-limited stimuli, with the bandwidth varying but the total energy of each stimulus remaining constant (Figure 18–8), the subject's perception of the loudness of the stimulus will depend on the bandwidth. For narrow band stimuli at moderate intensities, the subject will judge the loudness of the stimulus to be the same as a pure tone of the same energy, the frequency of which is at the center of the frequency range of the stimulus. As the bandwidth is gradually increased with energy kept constant, the perceived loudness will also remain constant; however, beyond a particular width, loudness will start to increase with further increases in bandwidth.

This phenomenon is shown graphically in Figure 18–9, where the loudness of a series of band-limited stimuli with frequencies centered around 1000 Hz are displayed as a function of the bandwidth of the stimuli (Zwicker

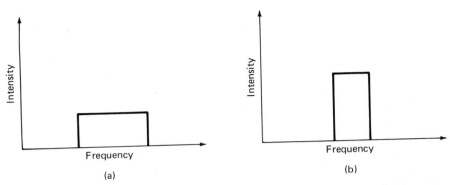

FIGURE 18-8   Graphs showing two types of band-limited noise having equal total energy.

& Feldtkeller, 1956). Look for the moment at the 60-dB function; the loudness stays quite constant as stimulus bandwidth varies from 50 to 160 Hz, but it begins to rise steadily as bandwidth is further increased. The other functions show how the loudness of sounds of different intensities varies as a function of bandwidth; they show the same general properties, with loudness remaining constant for bandwidths below 160 Hz, and increasing as the bandwidth becomes greater. The lone exception to this rule is the function for the 20-dB stimulus, for which loudness is completely independent of bandwidth.

This experiment suggests that if a complex tone consists of a fairly small

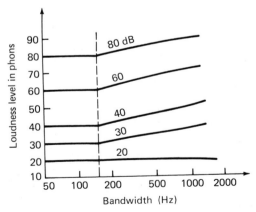

FIGURE 18-9   Graph showing the loudness levels for bands of noise centered at 1000 Hz, as a function of bandwidth. The five different curves show the loudnesses for five different total energies. From Zwicker, E. and R. Feldtkeller (1956) *Das Ohr als Nachrichtenempfänger*. Stuttgart: S. Hirzel Verlag. Reprinted by permission.

range of frequencies, it will not be perceived as being as loud as a stimulus of the same total energy, but with frequency components that are spread over a greater range. Experiments using combinations of pure tones instead of band-limited stimuli also lead to the same conclusion. If two pure tones of similar frequency are presented together, the loudness of the combination stimulus will be less than if the two tones were quite different in frequency (Scharf, 1961; 1970). The only exception to this rule occurs when the two tones are very weak, so that either tone presented alone might be below auditory threshold. In this case, the two tones would be perceived as louder if they were similar in frequency than if they were very different (Gässler, 1954).

Complex tones of moderate or high intensity are perceived as louder when their components are not similar in frequency. In contrast, very soft complex tones seem to be louder when their frequency components are similar than when they are not. From these and other types of data, it is clear that complex stimuli are treated differently by the auditory system when they are restricted to a narrow range of frequencies than when the components are spread over a wider area. These considerations have led to the development of what is called a *critical band theory*, which suggests that the auditory frequency range is divided into a number of bands, and that combinations of tones that fall within a critical band are treated differently than combinations whose components fall in separate bands. The critical bands in audition are analogous to the visual spatial frequency channels discussed in Chapter 10.

According to critical band theory, two tones that fall in the same band will interact with each other, while tones in separate critical bands are treated essentially independently by the auditory system. When two fairly intense tones that excite the same critical band are presented together, they tend to inhibit each other, so that the total loudness of the combination is less than one would otherwise expect. If the two tones were different enough in frequency so that different critical bands were excited, then the interactions that reduced the perceived loudness in the first case would not be present, and the loudness of the combination stimulus would be greater.

The situation is somewhat different when the two tones in the combination stimulus are weak enough so that they are either near or below threshold when presented alone. In this case, tones close enough in frequency to excite the same critical band will sum their effects, so that a suprathreshold stimulus will be perceived, even if the two components each produced subthreshold excitations when presented alone. If the tones are far apart in frequency so that they excite different critical bands, however, neither band may be excited enough to signal the presence of a stimulus, and the combination may not be heard at all. This reasoning accounts for the fact that the 20-dB function shown in Figure 18–9 does not show the increase in loudness as a function of increasing bandwidth that is reflected in the functions derived from the more intense stimuli. At this level of intensity, the components within the same critical band do not inhibit each other, so that increasing the bandwidth to excite other critical bands does not reduce the amount of inhibition.

BOX 18-4

Our discussion of critical bands agrees well with the explanation of the coding of loudness represented in Figure 18–6. If the frequencies of both tones are well within the range represented by the solid curve, the added energy of the second tone cannot raise the solid curve further; any tendency to broaden the curve (as a more intense single tone would) is offset by inhibitory interactions between the two tones. On the other hand, if the second tone is of sufficiently different frequency, it widens the area of stimulation, mimicking the dashed curve. For disparate frequencies, there is thus an increase in width of the curve, and therefore an increase in loudness.

When the tones are weak, on the other hand, the excitation is low. That is, the individual fibers are still within the range in which they can encode increases in stimulus by increases in firing (the sloped portion of the curve in Figure 18–5). Adding energy in a nearby frequency to which the fiber is receptive increases the firing of the fiber. As a result, weak tones sum their effects within the critical band.

In Figure 18–9, the loudness of a band-limited stimulus centered at 1000 Hz is shown to be independent of bandwidth as long as the bandwidth is smaller than 160 Hz. Above this level, the perceived loudness increases as a function of increasing bandwidth. This implies that the size of the critical band centered around 1000 Hz is about 160 Hz; by performing the same experiment with band-limited stimuli centered at different frequencies, we can obtain estimates of the sizes of the critical bands at different frequencies. Zwicker, Flottorp, and Stevens (1957) performed this experiment, and obtained the results shown in Figure 18–10. From this figure, you can see that the size of a critical band increases with frequency, going from about 100 Hz wide at low frequencies to more than 2000 Hz wide for frequencies greater than 10,000 Hz. Thus at low frequencies stimuli that are fairly close together in frequency may excite different critical bands and therefore be treated somewhat independently by the auditory system, while high-frequency tones the same distance apart in frequency may excite the same critical band and mutually inhibit each other.

Notice that above about 1000 Hz the curve in Figure 18–10 may be approximated by a straight line with a slope of unity. Since this plot is on log-log coordinates, a slope near one implies that the width of the critical band is simply proportional to the mean frequency (see appendix). For those frequencies for which there is a relatively narrow place of excitation on the basilar membrane, width of the critical band is proportional to frequency; at lower frequencies (when the basilar membrane vibrates as a whole), the width of the critical band is essentially constant.

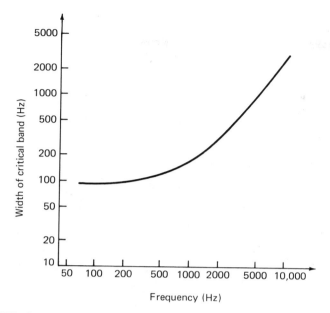

FIGURE 18-10 Width of the critical bands as a function of center frequency. From Zwicker, E., G. Flottorp, and S. S. Stevens (1957) Critical bandwidth in loudness summation. *J. Acoust. Soc. Am.* 29:548–577. Reprinted by permission.

In the preceding discussion we may have led you to the conclusion that two tones that stimulate different critical bands are always treated separately by the auditory system. If so, this is a misconception. As we shall see in the next section, two tones of very different frequencies can interact with each other, which raises the possibility that critical bands may extend over greater ranges than were indicated by the previously described experiments. In addition, critical bands are almost certainly not discrete, but rather are a series of extensively overlapping regions, like the overlapping receptive fields of retinal ganglion cells.

Auditory masking   For suprathreshold stimuli, two tones presented simultaneously that excite the same critical band should interact with each other to reduce the perceived loudness of the combination tone, much in the way that visual stimuli with similar spatial frequency components will mask each other (see Chapter 10). Another group of experiments that provides support for the concept of the critical band makes use of auditory masking. In these, the minimum intensity necessary just to hear a pure tone is determined both in the presence and in the absence of a continuous masking stimulus, which may or may not be similar in frequency to the pure tone. If the threshold intensity of the pure tone is increased by the presence of the masking stimulus, we say that the stimulus has masked the pure tone by an amount equal to the difference in thresholds between the masked and unmasked situations. Usually, the louder the masking stimulus is, the more it will increase the threshold for the pure tone.

Figure 18–11 shows the results of a typical masking experiment (Egan & Hake, 1950). Here the masking stimulus was a narrow band of noise centered at 410 Hz. (Band-limited noise is often used as the masking stimulus to avoid the presence of beats, which would occur if the masking stimulus and the test stimulus were similar in frequency.) For a given intensity of the masking stimulus, the threshold intensities for pure tones of various frequencies are determined (test stimuli), and the difference between the masked and unmasked thresholds is plotted as a function of frequency. For all intensities of the masking stimulus, the amount of masking is greatest when the frequency of the test stimulus is equal to the center frequency of the masking stimulus, and the amount of masking increases as the intensity of the masking stimulus increases. In fact, when the center frequency of the masking stimulus and the frequency of the test stimulus are the same, a 10-dB increase in the intensity of the masking stimulus produces a 10-dB increase in its masking effectiveness.

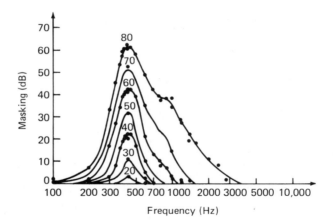

FIGURE 18-11 Amount of masking plotted as a function of frequency, for seven different masking intensities. Masking stimulus was a narrow band stimulus centered at 410 Hz. From Egan, J. P., and H. W. Hake (1950) On the masking pattern of a simple auditory stimulus. *J. Acoust. Soc. Am.* 22:622–630. Reprinted by permission.

As the test stimulus becomes more and more separated from the masking stimulus in frequency, the effectiveness of the mask decreases. For example, from Figure 18–11, an 80-dB masking stimulus centered at 410 Hz will increase the threshold of a 410-Hz pure tone by more than 60 dB, but will increase the threshold of a 300-Hz tone by only about 35 dB. Notice also that the function relating masking effectiveness to frequency of the test stimulus is asymmetrical; the amount of masking decreases much faster as the test stimulus becomes lower in frequency than the masking stimulus, as opposed to when the test stimulus becomes higher in frequency. In other words, a masking stimulus is better at masking tones that are of higher frequency than the mask than those that are of lower frequency than the mask. This asymmetry makes intuitive sense when we consider how the basilar membrane responds to sounds of certain frequencies. Figure 18–12 shows the response of the basilar membrane to a 1600-Hz tone; as discussed in the last chapter, the response on the low-frequency side of the point of maximum vibration decays much more rapidly with distance along the membrane than the response on the high-frequency side. If masking effects are at all related to interactions of responses on the basilar membrane, we would therefore expect that a stimulus on the high side of the masking stimulus would be more affected by the mask than a stimulus on the low-frequency side.

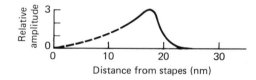

FIGURE 18-12   Shape of the response pattern along the basilar membrane in response to a pure tone of moderately high frequency. (This was the bottom curve in Figure 17–2.)

The asymmetry of the masking functions in Figure 18–11 also seems to become more pronounced as the intensity of the masking stimulus is increased. In other words, the slope of the masking decay on the high-frequency side becomes much shallower with increasing masking intensity, while the shape of the function on the low-frequency side remains much the same. This change in the shape of the masking curve with masking intensity provides the explanation for some everyday perceptual effects. For example, if a human voice is recorded and then played back at a higher intensity, it generally becomes much less intelligible. This is because as loudness of the total stimulus is increased, the low-frequency components of human speech tend to mask the higher components more and more. As important information is carried by these higher components, decreasing their audibility will make human speech less understandable (Moore, 1977). Speech perception is discussed further in Chapter 19.

AUDITORY SPACE PERCEPTION

In addition to the information we receive regarding the loudness, pitch, and timbre of an auditory stimulus, we are remarkably good at locating the position from which a sound originates. In order to do this, we depend in part on differences in stimulation at the two ears, just as binocular disparity is an important cue for visual depth perception. As we will see, however, information from only one ear (monaural cues) can also aid us in deciding the direction from which a sound is coming. In this section, we will present psychophysical data that quantitatively describe human localization abilities, as well as physiological data showing how individual cells in the auditory system respond to sounds from different locations. We will then describe some of the cues used in making decisions about the location of a sound, and see what happens when those cues are removed from the auditory environment.

Psychophysical Data

In one early study, Stevens and Newman (1934) investigated how accurately subjects could localize the direction of pure tones that were gradually turned on and off. They found that subjects were good at distinguishing sounds coming from their left sides from sounds originating on their right sides but that the subjects often could not tell the difference between a sound in front of them and its mirror image behind them. They excluded front-back errors, and plotted the amount of uncertainty of direction localization as a function of the frequency of the stimulus. The results are shown in Figure 18–13; localization is quite accurate for both low- and high-frequency sounds, but stimuli in the region of 3000 Hz are often local-

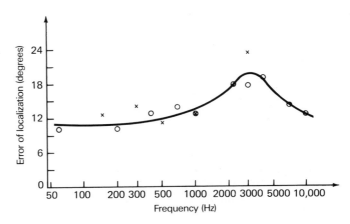

FIGURE 18-13   Sound localization errors as a function of frequency. From Stevens, S. S. and E. B. Newman (1934) The localization of pure tones. *Proc. Natl. Acad. Sci.* 20:593–596.

ized inaccurately. When this experiment was repeated using more modern techniques (Sandel, Teas, Fedderson, & Jeffress, 1955), the same type of function was again obtained, although the frequency for which localization was worst was about 1500 Hz. As we shall see, the shape of this function is directly related to the physical nature of the cues used by the auditory system to localize the position of a sound source.

Physiological Data

In recent years, investigators have begun to look at how the responses of single cells within the auditory system change as the position of a stimulus in space is varied. In the owl, an animal that relies greatly on its ability to identify the location of noise sources, cells have been found in the midbrain and in the primary auditory cortex that respond only to sounds in very specific locations. Knudsen, Konishi, and Pettigrew (1977) recorded from cells in the auditory cortex of the owl and found cells with spatial receptive fields like the one shown in Figure 18–14; for this cell, responses are only obtained

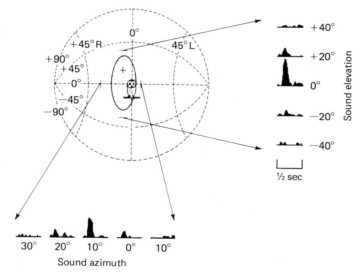

FIGURE 18–14 Receptive field of an owl auditory neuron. Stimuli located within the oval will result in responses, while those outside will not. The cell's responses to stimuli moved vertically and horizontally across the receptive field are shown along the right and lower portions of the figure, respectively. From Knudsen, E. I., M. Konishi, and J. D. Pettigrew (1977) Receptive fields of auditory neurons in the owl. *Science* 198:1278–1280. Copyright 1977 by the AAAS. Reprinted by permission of the publisher and author.

when the stimulus is within a restricted region just to the right of center. As is usually the case for auditory receptive fields, the vertical dimensions of the field are considerably broader than the lateral dimensions; in other words, the cell is more specifically tuned to lateral position than to vertical position.

Within an auditory nucleus of the owl's midbrain, Knudsen and Konishi (1978) found cells that were also sensitive to stimulus position. Unlike the cortical cells discussed in the previous paragraph, however, these receptive fields of midbrain cells had both excitatory and inhibitory regions. That is, if a stimulus was located within a central area, the cell responded with excitation; however, if the stimulus was placed just outside this region, the response of the cell was to suppress the maintained activity. The receptive field of such a cell is shown in Figure 18–15; in many ways, the receptive fields of these cells seem to be auditory analogs to the spatially antagonistic receptive fields of retinal ganglion cells.

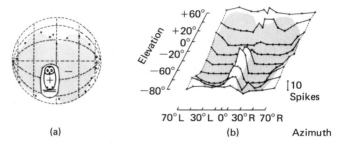

(a)   (b)   Azimuth

FIGURE 18–15 Center/surround receptive field of an auditory neuron in the owl. (a) Shows the receptive field; area within the oval is excitatory, while shaded area is inhibitory. (b) Shows the responses of this cell to stimuli placed in different locations within the receptive field. From Knudsen, E. I., and M. Konishi (1978) Center-surround organization of auditory receptive fields in the owl. *Science* 202:778–790. Copyright 1978 by the AAAS. Reprinted by permission of the publisher and author.

BOX 18–5

The auditory maps in the midbrain are aligned with visual maps. Eric Knudsen has studied the ways in which the two maps develop in register, and how they depend on each other. In one experiment (Knudsen, 1983), he plugged one ear in baby barn owls, so that the auditory cues to position would be shifted (see the discussion of "intensity differences" in the next section). When the birds matured, the auditory and visual maps in the tectum were in agreement. That is, the cells had overlapping visual and auditory fields. He then removed the

(continued)

(box continued)

earplugs, restoring a normal intensity balance (abnormal for the particular owl, who had grown up with an earplug). The visual map was unaffected, but the auditory map was significantly misaligned. These results were interpreted to indicate that the alignment of the two maps depends on experience in the two sensory systems.

In a later experiment, Knudsen (1988) did the converse operation: he raised owls with normal hearing but with their eyes closed. After 60 days, the eyes were opened, and the visual and auditory fields of cells in the tectum were analyzed. Although the owls had had no visual experience, their visual fields were essentially normal. Apparently, the visual system in birds does not require experience to maintain its function and mapping. The auditory maps, however, were crude and degraded, even though the birds had had normal auditory experience. The visual map must be essentially innate (in owls), and the auditory map must be actively aligned with it. The visual system must be active to guide the fine-tuning of the auditory map.

Cortical cells with receptive fields that are specific to the position of the stimulus have also been found in the cat. Morrell (1972) has found cells in association areas of the cortex that respond to both visual and auditory stimuli. For such bimodal cells, the receptive field within which visual responses are evoked completely overlaps the auditory receptive field. To maximize the response of such a cell, we would simultaneously present appropriate visual and auditory stimuli that originate from the same location in space.

Although the neural circuit that is involved in the ability of animals to localize objects in space is unknown, studies have shown that, at the very least, an intact auditory cortex is necessary for animals to perform tasks that require object localization. Neff and Casseday (1977) destroyed the cochlea of one ear in each of a number of cats, and then trained the cats to perform a task involving auditory localization. After the animals had learned the task, the experimenters produced a lesion in the auditory cortex either ipsilateral or contralateral to the functioning ear. They found that when the auditory cortex contralateral to the good ear was destroyed, cats were unable to localize objects, although they were able to perform the task when only the ipsilateral auditory cortex was destroyed. Cells in the inferior colliculus have also been implicated in localization of sounds in space (Kuwada, Yin, & Wickesberg, 1979).

Cues for Auditory Space Localization

In this section, we will consider what kinds of information are available in the auditory signal that can be used to allow us to determine where the signal is coming from. Binaural cues, or cues that require the presence of two ears, will be considered first.

Intensity differences In Figure 18–16, a sound source is shown positioned at an *azimuth* (lateral position) of 30° left, relative to the observer. That means that the left ear is directly in the path of the sound waves, but the right ear is somewhat blocked by the subject's head. There are two ways that the sound can reach the subject's right ear: it can either bend around the head, or it can pass through the skull on the way to the ear. Low-frequency (long wavelength) sounds have little trouble bending around an object the size of a human skull and will therefore reach the right ear without being significantly blocked by the head. High-frequency sounds, however, will not bend around the skull, with the result that the head acts to cast an "auditory shadow" in which the right ear lies. The only way that the sound will be able to get to the right ear if it is of high frequency is by passing through the head itself; in doing this, the head will act as a filter and reduce the amount of the stimulus reaching that ear. A high-frequency sound coming from the left side will therefore sound softer at the right ear than at the left ear. This difference in intensity between the two ears can serve as a cue for perceiving the azimuth of the stimulus. A sound originating exactly in front or in back of a subject would produce sounds of equal intensities at the two ears, with the intensity difference increasing as the sound source moves to either side.

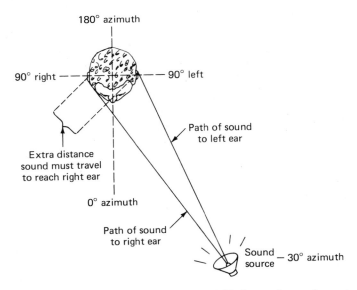

FIGURE 18-16 Different paths that noncentrally located sounds must take to reach the two ears.

Let us now reconsider Figure 18–13, showing the uncertainty that people have in localizing sounds as a function of frequency. As we go from moderate frequencies (1500 to 3000 Hz) to high frequencies (>5000 Hz), the errors in localizing sounds decrease. This improvement in our ability to localize sounds is easily understood if intensity differences between the two ears are used as cues, as it is at this frequency range that the differences become apparent. The fact that accuracy also increases for low-frequency tones implies that other cues are more important in the low-frequency end of the auditory spectrum.

Timing differences   The sounds received by the two ears of the subject in Figure 18–16 differ in more than just their relative intensities. The ears, each being at different distances from the noise source, will receive the stimulus at slightly different times. For a pure tone, this means that the stimulus may be somewhat out of phase at the ears; that is, the signals at the two ears will look much the same except that one signal will appear to lag behind the other by a certain fixed fraction of a cycle. The amount that one signal will lag behind the other will depend on the difference in path length of the sound to each ear; the farther the stimulus is from being equidistant from the two ears, the greater the path difference. For example, if the sound source in Figure 18–16 were 45° left instead of 30° left in its azimuth, the path difference between the ears would be increased.

The phase differences between the two ears for a pure tone input can only give useful information about the position of the sound if the wavelength of the tone is longer than about one-half of the distance of the path that the sound must travel around the head to go from one ear to the other. For shorter wavelengths, a given phase difference could be produced by a stimulus at a number of different locations in space. As the maximum distance (90° azimuth) is the distance between the ears (about 23 cm), a wavelength of 11.5 cm would be about the shortest wavelength that provides useful information about sound location. This corresponds to a frequency of about 1500 Hz as the highest frequency tone for which phase information is useful.

BOX 18-6

Notice how well matched our neural mechanisms are to the constraints of the physical world. Phase information is useful only to about 1500 Hz. How would phase information be encoded? Presumably in the timing of the volleys of action potentials hypothesized by the volley theory (see Chapter 17), which is effective for frequencies up to about 2000 Hz. Information about higher frequencies is encoded by the place theory, which would not be expected to retain phase information. Of course, phase is less useful at these higher frequencies, where relative intensity is a more potent indicator of position.

Information about the location of a pure tone is available from phase differences between the two ears for frequencies below 1500 Hz and from intensity differences at frequencies above this level. In the region between

1500 and 3000 Hz, however, neither cue provides unambiguous information, so that judgments of stimulus location are the most inaccurate at these frequencies. This is the explanation for the bulge in the localization curve shown in Figure 18–13.

We have so far been writing about how pure tones that were turned on and off gradually are localized in space; however, more complicated stimuli provide other cues that may be used by the auditory system. For sounds that are continuously changing in intensity (most everyday sounds), there will be small timing differences between the arrivals of the transient changes in intensity at the two ears, and these transients seem to play an important role in our localization abilities. Experiments have been designed to evaluate this factor in the absence of other cues such as head movements or intensity differences; this has been accomplished by presenting the signal through headphones so that intensity differences are eliminated and head movements are irrelevant. The signal going to one of the ears can be delayed by some particular amount of time to produce any timing difference between the two ears that the experimenter desires.

In order to assess how good human subjects are at perceiving timing differences between the two ears, Klumpp and Eady (1956) presented various types of stimuli through headphones and determined the minimum perceivable timing difference for each. They found that this minimum perceivable difference was smallest when the stimulus was band-limited white noise, which changes continuously over time. When the stimulus was a 1000-Hz pure tone, a slightly greater time difference was required, while an even greater difference was necessary for a 1-msec click stimulus. The minimum perceivable difference for the white noise was about 9 µsec; clearly short enough to be of use in the detection of timing differences due to differences in path length. (For example, the time difference caused by a sound at 90° azimuth is about 700 µsec. A 9-µsec difference in a distant source under optimal conditions means you could detect a displacement from straight ahead of less than a degree—a movement somewhat greater than from edge-to-edge of the moon!) It seems therefore that transients that occur within a stimulus reaching the two ears at slightly different times can aid in the perception of location of an acoustic stimulus.

Head movements   If human ears were just holes on either side of the head, the cues of intensity and timing differences just discussed would still provide useful information about the location of an auditory stimulus. We would not have an unambiguous idea of where a stimulus was, however. Rather, there would be a whole range of locations that would produce identical timing and intensity differences between the two ears. Figure 18–17 shows such a "cone of confusion"; anywhere on the surface of this cone, the difference in path length between the stimulus and the two ears will remain unchanged.

The timing differences between the ears will therefore also remain the same, and, if we assume that the head is perfectly spherical, the intensity differences will also not change. The subject therefore may not be able to distinguish changes of position of the stimulus as it moves from one point to another on the surface of the cone. A subject would be able to tell that sounds at locations 1 and 2 in Figure 18–17 were both on the left side of the head, but might not be able to say that one point was toward the front of the head while the other was toward the back.

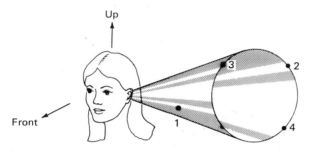

FIGURE 18–17   A possible cone of confusion. Adapted from Mills (1972). In Foundations of Modern Auditory Theory, Vol. II, J.V. Tobias (Ed.). Florida: Academic Press. Reprinted by permission.

One way that a subject gets information regarding the position of a stimulus on a cone of confusion is through the use of head movements. For example, by moving the head forward slightly, the stimulus should become slightly louder if it is at location 1, but softer if it is at location 2. Similarly, tilting your head in one direction or the other will help distinguish between sound locations 2 and 4 on the figure, which differ only in the vertical dimension. Head movements will also result in changes in the relative loudness between the two ears, providing an additional cue to the position of the stimulus.

Monaural space perception   In the previous section, all of the cues that we discussed involve slightly different auditory information reaching the two ears. Even with only one ear, however, we are still able to make discriminations about the location of a sound source. Head movements are one way of obtaining information about the position of a stimulus using one ear. Another factor that also seems to be important is the shape of the pinna, the external auditory structure. Batteau (1967) made plaster casts of human pinnas, and inserted a microphone where the eardrum would be. Sounds picked up by the microphone were presented to a subject through earphones. Using this artificial ear, subjects could make some discriminations about the position of a stimulus relative to the plaster pinna; however, if the microphone was taken out of the cast and placed in open space, the subject no longer had any impression regarding the position of the noise source. This experiment clearly shows, therefore, that the pinna can aid the perception of location of a sound source, even if only one ear is being used.

Harris and Sergeant (1971) attempted to measure the abilities of subjects to make localization discriminations monaurally in the absence of head movements. Subjects were told to keep their heads as still as possible, and were presented with white noise and pure tone stimuli both monaurally and binaurally. The measure used was the *minimum audible angle* (MAA), or the smallest angle of movement of the source that was necessary for the subject to detect a change. The experimenters found that the MAAs for binaural and monaural presentations of white noise were equal, although the binaural condition was superior to monaural when pure tone stimuli were used. We can conclude from this experiment that monaural cues are sufficient to make accurate discriminations of differences in the locations of sound sources.

The perception of movement of a sound source is detectable through other monaural cues. As a moving audible object comes close, it naturally tends to sound louder. This change in intensity may act as a cue for the movement of that object. Another cue for detecting a moving object is called the *Doppler shift*; it provides information about movement when a high-velocity sound source moves past. The Doppler shift is a change in the perceived pitch of a sound, depending on whether it is moving toward you or away from you. As a pure tone source moves toward you, it is emitting sound waves at a constant frequency. The origin of each cycle, however, is constantly moving, so that every successive cycle is produced at a location closer to you than the preceding cycle. This will cause the waves to pile up in front of the source, so that they are closer together than they would be if the source were stationary. The fact that the cycles are closer together means that the frequency of the sound will be higher. Just the opposite occurs as the sound passes you and heads away; each cycle of the sound wave will reach you slightly later than it would if the source were stationary, resulting in a lowering of the perceived frequency. The Doppler shift is the reason that a train whistle sounds high-pitched as the train comes toward you, but sounds much lower as it trails away.

SUGGESTED READINGS

B. C. J. Moore's *Introduction to the Psychology of Hearing* (University Park Press, 1977) has good chapters on both auditory space perception and the perception of loudness. A somewhat more detailed look at the topic of space perception can be found in A. W. Mills's chapter in *Foundations of Modern*

Auditory Theory, Vol. II, edited by J. V. Tobias (Academic Press, 1972). These topics are also covered in Chapters 12 and 13 of *Hearing: Physiological Acoustics, Neural Coding, and Psychoacoustics*, by W. L. Gulick, G. A. Gescheider, and R. D. Frisina (Oxford University Press, 1989).

Scientific American articles relevant to the topics discussed in this chapter include M. R. Rosenzweig's "Auditory localization" (October 1961; offprint #501) and G. Oster's "Auditory beats in the brain" (October 1973; offprint #1282). The Rosenzweig article is reprinted in Held and Richards' *Perception: Mechanisms and Models* (W. H. Freeman, 1972), and the Oster article in Held and Richards's *Recent Progress in Perception* (W. H. Freeman, 1976).

SPEECH PERCEPTION

19

Our discussion of vision progressed from the sensory aspects to the perceptual, from physiology and psychophysics to pattern recognition. Similarly, the preceding chapters on audition have moved from the physiological to the psychophysical; in this chapter, we address one of the pattern recognition problems faced by the auditory system.

Like the visual system, the auditory system recognizes particular patterns in the incoming stimuli. It does so without our conscious intervention, working from cues that lead to perceptual hypotheses. The visual system recognizes spatial shapes and objects, and reconstructs a visual scene with objects corresponding to the proximal stimuli. The auditory system also recognizes particular things in the environment: bells, sirens, voices, thunder, slamming sounds, music, and so forth.

We discussed visual pattern recognition as a result of the location of features (edges, borders) in a two-dimensional space, the frontal plane. In audition, the relevant features are sound waves of particular frequencies. They lie along a one-dimensional line, the sound frequency range. In fact, frequencies are physiologically arranged along a line—the distance from the base to the apex of the cochlea. This would make an excellent analogy to the two-dimensional plane of the retina were it not for the complication that the analysis of sound also includes patterning according to the volley theory. Nevertheless, there are tonotopic representations of frequencies on the auditory cortex (see Chapter 17) that we may consider as analogous to the retinotopic maps on the visual cortex (see Chapter 9).

We might think of the auditory recognition problem as a one-dimensional version of the two-dimensional visual recognition problem, except that there is an essential second dimension to sound analysis: time. Sound patterns consist of frequency components shifting in time; freezing a sound into an unchanging tonal pattern would completely destroy its identity (unlike freezing a visual pattern, say, by taking a photograph, which does not make it unrecognizable). Of course, visual patterns can also be in motion. We have tended to ignore visual patterns that change in our discussion of pattern recognition because there is a wealth of interesting material in static patterns, which are less complicated. We did, however, mention some of the difficulties of perceiving motion in Chapter 14.

Of all the pattern recognition problems faced by the auditory system, perhaps the most interesting and complex is the problem of recognizing the words spoken by our fellow human beings (many a musician would argue with that statement!). This is where much of the research in auditory pattern recognition has been done, and it is the only problem we shall consider in this chapter.

Although it is clear that the perception of speech is a form of perception that is auditory, we should note that it is really distinct from other forms of auditory perception. The perception of doors slamming, dogs barking, or sirens wailing represents a form analogous to visual perception in that the perceptual system is analyzing features of the world to determine what is "out there." In speech perception, however, the listener is charged with getting the semantic message that another human (or a machine) has encoded in a very stylized way, reflecting the peculiarities of the human vocal apparatus (see Liberman and Mattingly, 1989).

Several kinds of evidence indicate that the perception of speech invokes a special mode of auditory perception, called the phonetic mode (Liberman & Studdert-Kennedy, 1978; Liberman, 1982). Sounds that are heard as speech when embedded in a stream of speech sound like chirps, whistles, or clicks when they are isolated (Liberman, Delattre, & Cooper, 1952; Mattingly, Liberman, Syrdal, & Halwes, 1971; Whalen & Liberman, 1987). The way in which speech is analyzed in the brain bears a stong relationship to the way it is produced (Liberman, Cooper, Shankweiler, & Studdert-Kennedy, 1967; Dorman, Raphael, & Liberman, 1979), even to the extent of sharing some of the same parts of the brain (Ojemann & Mateer, 1979; Geschwind, 1972, 1979; Zurif, 1980). Moreover, as you will learn at the end of this chapter, much of speech production and perception are functions of the left half of the brain (Studdert-Kennedy & Shankweiler, 1970; Geschwind, 1972; Kimura, 1973). It may therefore be distinct from auditory perception in general, even though the initial processing is handled by the same sensory system.

SPEECH SOUNDS

The first thing we must do in order to discuss the perception of speech is to examine the stimuli that are being perceived. A large part of this chapter will be devoted to defining the units of speech, both in cognitive and acoustical terms. In fact, a large part of the study of speech perception is the study of speech itself.

It might seem that the sounds of speech are obvious. If you speak a phrase such as "to catch pink salmon," you may think you are producing a sequence of discrete sounds, just as the written phrase is made of a sequence of individual letters. You might think that in saying "to catch pink salmon" you first made a "t" sound, then "oo," then "k," and so forth, as you might do if speaking absurdly slowly. As you will see later in this chapter, however, the sounds of speech come in a continuous and indivisible stream. You cannot take a tape recording of the phrase "to catch pink salmon" and chop it into letter-sized pieces that you can resplice into a different phrase; neither can you play the tape backwards and expect it to sound like "nah-mass knip ch-tak oot." We shall first discuss the apparent units of speech, but you will find later that these units cannot actually stand alone.

Classification of Speech Sounds

The basic units of speech that correspond roughly to letters are the *phonemes*. Phonemes are those sound units that, by their differences, convey differences in meaning. Within a given phonemic class are sounds that are easily perceived as different but convey the same significance; differences in the perceived sound are called *phonetic* differences. For example, the sound of the "A" in the word "bad" is not the same when spoken normally, when whispered, or when spoken by someone who has a stuffed nose. Nonetheless, these phonetically different sounds are all part of the same phonemic class. We shall be speaking of phonemes in this chapter, but we shall only deal with their normally spoken phonetic versions.

Now a word about notation. The International Phonetic Association (IPA) has devised an alphabet by which sounds may be transcribed into writing. (If you recall the way Professor Higgins transcribed Eliza's speech into apparently meaningless hieroglyphics in Shaw's *Pygmalion*—or *My Fair Lady*—he was presumably using the IPA notation.) If you read further in linguistics or speech perception, you will find that this notation is used throughout. We feel, however, that learning IPA notation for the sake of reading this one chapter involves more effort than it is worth. It also will hamper understanding, because you will probably have to keep looking back to decipher the notation. We therefore will use the following, more cumbersome notation: we will print the letters representing the sound in question in boldface within a word that tells you how to pronounce it. Thus "*b**A**d*" should be read as "the sound of the 'a' in the word 'bad.'" (The IPA symbol for the phoneme *b**A**d* is æ.) Those who do further reading will have to deal with the IPA notation, which is summarized in many secondary sources (for example, Liberman, 1977).

The phonemes of English are generally divided into two classes: vowels and consonants. It is hard to explain the phonetic difference between them, although you undoubtedly already have a feeling for what is meant by vowels and what is meant by consonants.

BOX 19-2

It is difficult to state a rule for determining which sounds are vowels and which are consonants (Studdert-Kennedy, 1976). The one difference that is generally valid is that vowels contain more sound energy than consonants (Lieberman, 1977). Nevertheless, the consonants seem to convey the bulk of the meaning in a sentence. Consider, for example, the following sentence with all its consonants omitted: "A _oo _e _e _e i_ _a_ _ _o _i_ _, a_ _ _a_ _e_ _o _a_ _e." Quite a puzzle. The same sentence, however, with the vowels omitted and consonants included is not impossible to read: "_ g_ _d s_nt_nc_ _s h_rd t_ f_nd, _nd h_rd_r t_ p_rs_." It seems odd that the main energy is going into the least informative parts of the speech. Quite possibly, the vowels convey other information, such as the stress, tone, or emotional content of the utterance (Lehiste, 1976). Box 19-7 will deal further with this possibility.

The vowels may be further classified according to the way they are produced. Vowels are *voiced* in normal speech; that is, the vocal cords vibrate while the vowel sound is being produced. The differences among the vowels are produced by the way in which the articulatory apparatus (particularly the tongue and lips) are positioned. Hold your mouth slightly open and make the prolonged sound a-a-a-a-a (*sOd*). While doing this, bring your tongue upward so that it touches your upper teeth on each side (but not your palate). The sound will change into a prolonged eeee (*bEAd*); lower your tongue slightly and you get 'eh' (*bEd*). Go back to the relaxed position (*sOd*), then purse your lips as if for a kiss; the sound changes to oooo (*tOOth*). In all of these manipulations, you have changed the vowel sound by changing the position of your lips and tongue, without any particular change in what your vocal cords were doing. In fact, if you hold a vibrating instrument (such as an electric shaver) to your throat and silently make the manipulations suggested above, you will hear the razor "saying" the vowels.

The vowels of English can be classified according to the position the tongue takes when they are made. Most (not all) of the vowels fall along a continuum from tongue forward in the mouth and high (*bEE*), through tongue low in the mouth and far back (as if being swallowed) (*sOd*), then higher again though far back (and with the lips pursed) as one goes from *jAW* to *tOOth*. We can plot some of these sounds on a graph in which tongue position (high or low in the mouth) is the ordinate and the point where the tongue narrows the passage the most (near the front or back of the mouth) is the abscissa (Figure 19-1); this is called the IPA vowel "quadrilateral."

This method of classifying vowel sounds was pioneered in the nineteenth century by Melville Bell. It is a valid classification in that the maneuvers described do produce the appropriate sounds, although modern x-ray studies of the vocal apparatus during speech have shown that these maneuvers are not necessarily the way the sounds are produced (Ladefoged,

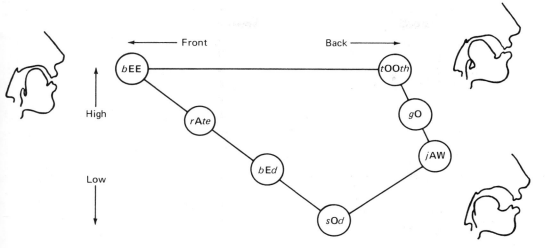

FIGURE 19-1 The vowel "quadrilateral," showing how the different vowel sounds depend on tongue position. After Lieberman, P. (1977) *Speech Physiology and Acoustic Phonetics*. New York: Macmillan Publishing Co. Inc. Reprinted by permission of the author.

DeClerk, Lindau, & Papcun, 1972). The same sounds can be produced in different ways, and different speakers may use different strategies for generating the same phonemes. The classification scheme is based on maneuvers that may not in fact be performed; nevertheless, this scheme provides a good framework for classifying speech sounds.

The consonants are somewhat more complicated than vowels, as they vary along more dimensions. Like the vowels, consonants may be produced with the major constriction of the articulatory pathways near the front, middle, or back of the mouth. We can list a number of places of constricting: the lips as in **P**it, **B**it, **M**e, or **W**e; the lips and teeth as in **F**an or **V**an; tongue and teeth, as in **T**ip, **N**ip, or **TH**in; teeth alone, as in **S**in or **Z**oo; tongue near the middle of the mouth, as in **G**em, **T**op, **CH**urch, or **D**ay; or tongue near the back of the mouth, as in **G**et or **C**ow; or without any particular constriction, as in **H**at.

In addition to the position of the constriction, consonants differ in how they are formed. A major distinction is between those made with the vocal cords vibrating and those made without vocal cords vibrating; the former are voiced and the latter *unvoiced*. For example, the differences between **F**an and **V**an or between **S**in and **Z**oo is that in the first member of each pair the consonant is unvoiced, in the second it is voiced.

Another distinction is between the consonants that are *plosive* and those that are not. A plosive consonant is one in which the air from the lungs is bottled up by a restriction and suddenly released in a little puff. If the lips provide the restriction, we hear **P**it (unvoiced) or **B**it (voiced); if the tip of the tongue provides the block, we get **T**ip (unvoiced) or **D**ay (voiced); if the back of the tongue stops the passage, we hear **C**ow (unvoiced) or **G**et (voiced).

Another possible way to make consonants is by restricting the airway so that air gets out in a noisy hiss, rather than being completely stopped and then released. Sounds made in this way are called *fricatives*. As the point of constriction moves from the lips to farther back in the mouth we have a progression of unvoiced fricatives: **F**an, **TH**in, **S**in, and **SH**ow. The equivalent progression with voicing is: **V**an, **TH**en, **Z**oo, and *bei***GE**.

There are a number of other consonant types. *Nasals* are made by restricting the mouth and allowing the sound to come through the nose, as in **M**an (lips closed) or **N**ose (tongue to palate). *Laterals* are made by restricting one side of the mouth more than the other, as in **R**oad. *Glides* involve a relatively slow change from one sound to another, as in **Y**ell or **WH**at.

ACOUSTICS OF SPEECH

The previous section outlined the nature of speech sounds in terms of the articulatory actions required to produce them; we now wish to know the characteristics of the sound waves conveying speech to the ears. In the course of an utterance many different sounds are emitted in rapid order; the sounds produced by the speaker change in frequency. In other words, the stimulus for speech is a pattern of sound frequencies that changes with time. Before we can consider the acoustic characteristics of speech sounds, we will need a way of representing these stimuli graphically on the pages of this book. The graphical representations of speech sounds that we will be using are called *spectrograms*; they are produced by a machine called the *sound spectrograph* (Koenig, Dunn, & Lacy, 1946). The next section is intended to explain what a spectrogram is, so that you can interpret the spectrograms in the remainder of the chapter.

The Spectrogram

To understand what a spectrogram is, we must consider what it is intended to display. We wish a representation that will show the component frequencies of a sound—this, of course, is a spectrum of the sound. We have already encountered spectra of spatial frequencies in visual displays (Chapter 10), and of continuous sounds (Chapter 16), so the idea of representing component frequencies should not be new. The special problem here is that the spectra of speech sounds are not continuous in time, but are in constant flux. A tone generated by an oscillator is unchanging; we can look at its spectrum at any time while it is present and see the same picture as at any other time. We now wish to represent spectra that are changing—the spectrum a moment after the sound starts can look different from those taken a few moments later, which can look different from ones taken still later.

For example, consider the sound made by a single ring of the telephone. A spectrum of the sound just as the ring begins is shown in Figure 19–2(a). This is an ordinary spectrum, just like those in Chapters 10 and 16, showing the energy in each band of frequencies as a function of frequency. We see considerable energy in the region below 1000 Hz, and a smear of energy (noise) in the region above about 1100 Hz. There is a tendency for there to be somewhat more energy in the regions of 1200, 2500, and 3400 Hz.

The second part of Figure 19–2 shows the spectrum of the sound about halfway through the ring. Now a great concentration of energy is in the region of 1200 Hz; most of the general noise has died and the spectrum shows four distinct bands of energy (four harmonics). The third part of the figure shows the spectrum after the actual ring has ended. All that remains is the relatively pure tone of the gradually fading vibrations of the bell, at about 1200 Hz.

If we took sample spectrograms every few milliseconds and leafed rap-

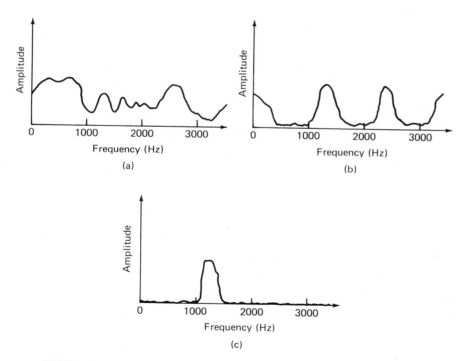

FIGURE 19–2 Sound spectra of the ringing of a telephone. (a) Spectrum taken just after the ring begins. (b) Spectrum taken near the middle of the ring. (c) Spectrum of the sound after the ring has ended and the vibration is dying down.

idly through them, we would have a movie of the spectrogram as it shifted and changed in time. This would be a fine representation of the spectrum in time, but it would be impossible to print in a book, and difficult to quantify or describe. We need a better way of representing these successive pictures.

Suppose we took each spectrum and cut it out of heavy cardboard. We could then paste the cardboard spectra together to make a three-dimensional model of the sound. Figure 19–3 shows a perspective view of this kind of model, with the three frames of Figure 19–2 drawn in heavier lines. Each sketch is a spectrum at a given moment. As you move your attention along the time axis (toward you, out of the page) you go from earlier to later spectra. You thus see the spectra evolving in time. Each of the four major harmonics (less than 500 Hz, 1200 Hz, 2500 Hz, and 3400 Hz) can be traced from the time it first appears until it disappears at the end of the ring.

Figure 19–3 is a sketch of a three-dimensional graph. Instead of using time as the third dimension (as in showing the successive spectra as a movie), we have drawn a third axis coming out of the paper. The problem is that three-dimensional graphs are hard to draw and not that easy to interpret. What we want is a two-dimensional picture like all the other graphs in this book.

A function plotted on a three-dimensional graph is a surface, rather than a curve. In Figure 19–3 there is a surface representing the amplitude of sound energy (the height or elevation) at any point specified by its frequency (left-right direction) and the time (into or out of the paper direction). This surface is like the surface of the land—ridges of mountains that happen to run parallel to the direction into and out of the paper. Our problem is how to represent this mountain range on a flat piece of paper.

We can collapse a three-dimensional graph into a two-dimensional graph by sighting along one of the axes. If you sighted along the amplitude axis— looked down from above in Figure 19–3—you would see the layout of the mountain range. In effect, you would be looking at a map, only the compass directions would be frequency (instead of North) and time (instead of East). We wish to represent the elevation of the mountains at each point on this map—we can do this by using a "gray scale." We make the map darker when the elevation is higher; for the sound we make the paper darker when there is sound energy at that frequency and time. The dark parts of this picture, which is the spectrogram, show the locations of the components of the sound. It is as if you flooded the mountain range in Figure 19–3 to the level indicated by the dashed line on the rearmost spectrum. The spectrogram is then a map of the mountain peaks (islands, in black) in the newly flooded sea (white).

A spectrogram of a telephone ringing is shown in Figure 19–4. In fact Figures 19–2 and 19–3 were based on this spectrogram, and it should be easy to see how we arrived at each of them. (The times at which the three spectra shown in Figure 19–2 were taken are indicated by the letters *A, B,*

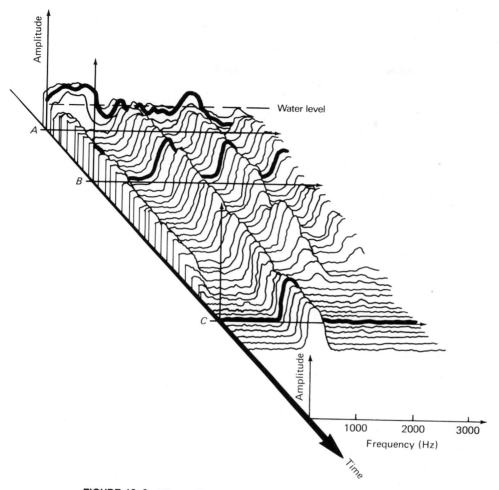

FIGURE 19-3 Three-dimensional graph of the sound of a telephone ringing. The three spectra in Figure 19-1 are indicated by heavier curves.

and *C* in Figure 19-4.) This spectrogram, a plot of frequency versus time, shows us the location and history of each of the components. We can see the 1200-Hz component, for example, starting rather weakly (a faint gray line with gaps) but growing to become the strongest component (darkest) and eventually outlasting the other three. We also see that this "component" is really a range of frequencies (a single frequency would be a narrow line, not a band) and that it becomes louder and softer (the band gets quite light at points), presumably because of beats among the individual frequencies in the band (see Chapter 17).

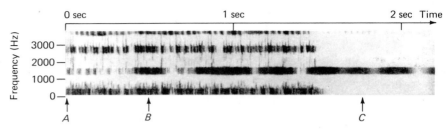

FIGURE 19-4   Spectrogram of the sound of a telephone ringing. The times of the three spectra in Figure 19–1 are indicated by arrows. From Koenig, W., H. K. Dunn, and L. Y. Lacy (1946) The sound spectrograph. *J. Acoust. Soc. Am.* 17:19. Reprinted courtesy of Bell Laboratories.

BOX 19-3

How do you create a spectrogram? The machine that does it, the *spectrograph*, performs what amounts to a continuous spectral analysis. Sound enters through a microphone and is converted to an electrical signal. In effect the electrical signal is fed to a bank of filters—electronic devices that select specific narrow-frequency bands, somewhat like the channels we spoke of in Chapter 10, but far more selective. If the sound contains the frequencies a particular filter is tuned to, it gets through, and there is a signal coming through the filter. If it does not contain the right frequency, nothing comes out of the filter. An amplifier looks at the output of each filter; if it finds a signal, it sends an instruction to a pen corresponding to that filter to make a mark on the spectrograph paper as it moves through the machine. It is as if there were a bank of pens, each placed at a position corresponding to the frequency of the filter feeding it, writing on the moving paper. Therefore the position of a mark on the paper corresponds to a frequency and a time: the frequency of the filter associated with the pen and the time that part of the paper was under the pen. The darkness of the mark corresponds to the amount of energy (amplitude) in that frequency band at that moment.

Physical Characteristics of Speech Sounds

Now we shall consider what the physical stimuli are that correspond to each of the speech sounds. Let us take a phrase and see what its spectrogram looks like. The top part of Figure 19–5 shows the spectrogram corresponding to the spoken phrase "to catch pink salmon." It probably looks like a bunch of blobs, but those who are accustomed to the reading of spectrograms can point out its very specific patterns. An idealized version of this one is shown below it. You can probably see where most of the dark patches in the ideal version correspond to blotches in the actual spectrogram, although the emphasis may not be exactly what you would have come up with had you been asked to idealize the spectrogram. Nevertheless, the ideal version is easier to deal with, so let us discuss the features in it.

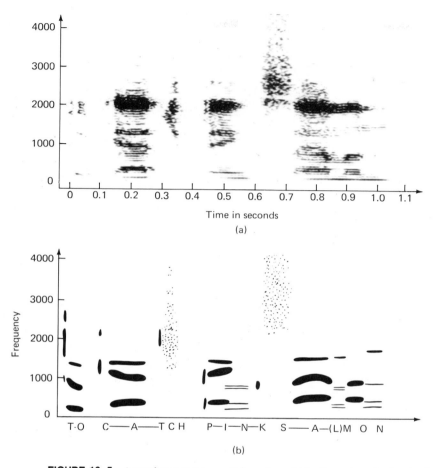

FIGURE 19–5   Actual spectrogram (above) and ideal version (below) of the phrase "to catch pink salmon." From Liberman, A. M., P. C. Delattre, and F. S. Cooper (1952) Perception of the unvoiced stop consonants. *Am. J. Psychol.* 65:497–509. Reprinted by permission.

BOX 19–4

The idealization of the spectrogram in Figure 19–5 has removed a feature that can be seen in the original. That feature is the horizontal banding evident in the vowel portions of the records. These are caused by the harmonics of

the vibrations of the vocal cords. The vocal cords vibrate at a rate determined by the air flow through the pharynx, size of the vocal cords, and tension placed on the cords (this last is how you vary the pitch when you sing). The

(continued)

(box continued)
vibration of vocal cords, however, at least in the lower frequencies used in speech, is not sinusoidal. In fact, the waveform of the sound waves produced by the vocal cords is more nearly a triangle wave, containing energy at various higher harmonics of the fundamental frequency (see the spectrum of a triangular waveform in Figure 10–7). The remainder of the vocal tract (lips, tongue, teeth) emphasize some of these harmonics while attenuating others, but the basic pattern of fundamental and harmonics remains (see Lieberman, 1977). Because the production of speech depends more on the articulation of the vocal tract than actual shifts in the frequency of the vocal cord vibrations, these are the more interesting features, and we can ignore the "stripes" caused by the harmonics of the vocal cord vibrations. We are more interested in which stripes are emphasized, and which are absent.

As an analogy, consider a flute playing a particular note; the sound emitted by the flute is complex. Now consider the difference in how the flute would sound at the end of a long cave; the sound made by the flute is the same, but which of its components reach you will depend on the properties of the cave. The cave will act like an organ pipe to amplify frequencies whose wavelengths are integer multiples of the cave's dimensions; other frequencies will be absorbed within the cave. If we wish to know something about the cave, we have to analyze what frequency regions are enhanced and which attenuated—not the pattern of harmonics that tells us it is a flute and not a violin in the cave. Similarly, when we wish to see what the articulatory apparatus has done to the sound made by the vocal cords, we are not interested in the fact that the original sound came from vocal cords, and not from one of the artificial vibrators used by people who have lost their vocal cords to disease. We therefore ignore the stripes and look for the frequency regions that are emphasized in the spectrograms of speech.

For the moment let us consider only the vowels. Notice that for each one there is a pattern consisting of three-component frequency bands. These components are called *formants*, and are numbered first, second, and third starting from the bottom (lowest frequency). Peterson and Barney (1952) did a classic study of the formants of English vowels and found that the first two formants contain enough information to allow identification of the vowel sounds. (The third formant is generally of smaller amplitude than the other two, and seems not to change as much from vowel to vowel.) Ideal spectrograms of some of the vowels including those shown in Figure 19–1 are given in Figure 19–6; (a) shows the spectrograms averaged from 33 adult male speakers in the Peterson and Barney study, while (b) shows the average spectrograms of 15 children speaking the same vowels. The width of the lines indicate the relative strengths of the formants (*not* the range of frequencies in each, as a real spectrogram would).

Each vertical slice of Figure 19–6 represents a single-vowel spectrogram

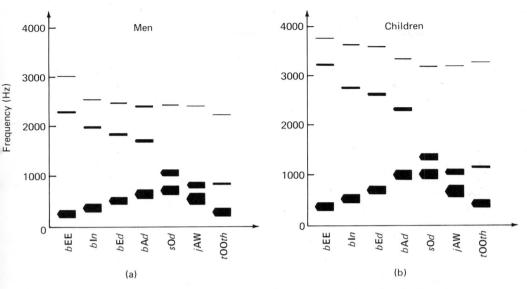

FIGURE 19-6   First three formants of vowels spoken by men (left) and
children (right). The width of each formant indicates the
relative energy it contains (*not* its bandwidth). Based on
data of Peterson and Barney (1952). Control methods
used in a study of the vowels. *J. Acoust. Soc. Am.*
24:175–184. Reprinted by permission.

(except that the width of each formant does not imply the bandwidth). On
the left, corresponding to the "high tongue near the front" in Figure 19–1 is
the sound *b*EE. We progress around the quadrilateral to *s*O*d* with the first
and second formants approaching each other. Having approached, they now
move downward together as we follow the quadrilateral upward from *j*AW to
t OO*th*. Notice that the changes in the way the two formants progress occur
at the same phonemes as the corners of the quadrilateral.

　　If we compare the left part of Figure 19–6 with the right half, we can see
the differences between adult males and children. Not surprisingly, the children's voices are higher in pitch, although the increase in frequency is not
the same for all formants. A child's voice is not exactly the same as a man's
voice with all the components shifted upward in frequency; speeding up a
tape (which would increase the frequencies of all sounds equally) gives a
"chipmunk's" voice not a child's. The vowels at the extremes of the range
(high tongue positions on the quadrilateral—that is, *b*EE and *t*OO*th*) show
the greatest differences between the second formants of man and child; vowels near the middle of the range (low tongue, as *s*O*d* or *b*A*d*) show approximately equal shifts in the first two formants.

BOX 19–5

We said we would just deal with vowels for now, but before we leave Figure 19–5 too far behind, let us make a comment about consonants. Notice that the consonants in "to catch pink salmon," particularly the **T**o, **CH**eck, and **S**in, are encoded by higher frequencies than the vowels. Since the third formant seems unimportant for identification of vowels, most of the vowel energy is below about 1200 Hz. Many of the consonants, on the other hand, depend on frequencies upward of 2000 Hz.

The fact that many consonants are signaled by high frequencies has an interesting consequence. You may recall from Chapter 18 that as we age we lose our sensitivities to the higher frequencies (presbycusis). As a result, older people may develop difficulty in hearing consonants, even though they can still hear. But consonants carry a large part of the information in speech (see Box 18–1). Older people may therefore have trouble understanding speech, simply because they miss many of the consonants. Unfortunately, this is sometimes interpreted as a mental decline with age, and can lead to psychological problems (Zimbardo, Andersen, & Kabat, 1981).

Synthesized Speech

Looking at spectrograms is a good way to see what the components of a speech sound are, but it has its limitations. One difficulty is that we are limited to the sounds that speakers actually make. If we cannot get a speaker to make a sound part way between *b***EE** and *b***I***t*, we cannot tell how it will be perceived; nor can we tell what would happen if there were some slight juggling of only one of the formants. The second problem is that it is hard to say how realistic the idealizations based on the spectrograms are. For all we could say, the gray stuff between formants might be the important things to the ear, and the formants just a big artifact.

Fortunately, there is a way to work the spectrograph backwards, to take a pattern painted on paper and generate the sound corresponding to it. The machine that does this is called the *pattern playback*, or *vocoder* (Liberman, Delattre, & Cooper, 1952). A large body of what we know about the perception of speech was derived by experiments performed at the Haskins Laboratories using this device (Cooper, Delattre, Liberman, Borst, & Gerstman, 1952; Liberman, Delattre, & Cooper, 1952; Liberman, Ingemann, Lisker, Delattre, & Cooper, 1959).

The pattern playback is effectively a reverse spectrograph. An ideal spectrogram painted on paper can be fed into the machine, and the sound corresponding to that spectrogram will be produced. A single horizontal line of paint will produce a single continuous tone. A small splash will cause a short burst of sound. A pattern like the one in the lower part of Figure 19–5 will cause the machine to say, quite distinctly, "to catch pink salmon."

Peterson and Barney (1952) had surmised that only the first two formants would be sufficient for the identification of vowels. This in fact proved to be the case; ideal "vowels" consisting of the first two formants were readily recognized as the appropriate vowels (Liberman, Delattre, & Cooper, 1952).

Consonants

So far so good: distinct patterns of formants uniquely determine the vowel phonemes they represent. The next question is what will happen when we consider consonants. Liberman, Delattre, and Cooper (1952) asked this question for the consonants **P**it, **T**ip, and **C**ow (the unvoiced plosives made with lips, tip of the tongue, and back of the tongue, respectively). They found that these consonants, when preceding a vowel, could be generated by a brief burst of relatively narrow band sound. Played alone, such bursts sound like clicks, but in conjunction with a succeeding vowel they sound like the plosive consonants. Here we see a hint of what is to come: the same sound in two different contexts may be perceived either as the (nonspeech) sound of a click, or as a consonant.

Figure 19–7 shows a typical stimulus used by Liberman *et al.* (1952). In this pattern, the noise burst was centered at about 1440 Hz,. and lasted 15 msec. It was followed by the first two formants of the vowel *s***O**d. This particular stimulus would give the sound of the plosive **C**ow followed by the vowel *s***O**d, so the sound heard should be identified as the nonsense syllable **CO***p*.

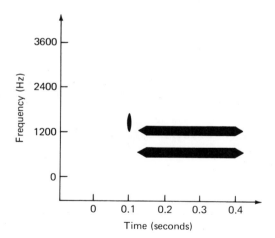

FIGURE 19-7 Ideal spectrogram used in the pattern playback to produce the syllable **CO***p*. Typical of the stimuli used by Liberman, Delattre, and Cooper (1952). The role of selected stimulus variables in the perception of the unvoiced stop consonants. *Am. J. Psychol.* 65:497–516. Reprinted by permission.

A noise burst of the same width and duration could be positioned at several different frequencies in front of any of seven different vowels (first two formants). For each stimulus, subjects were asked to identify the nonsense syllable they heard. Figure 19–8 shows a map of which plosives were perceived, as a function of which vowel patterns ensued. The x-axis lists the vowel phonemes, as in Figure 19–6; the ordinate is frequency. The black bars show the locations of the vowel formants, as if each slice were a short piece of spectrogram. Superimposed on this picture are the regions in which a particular consonant was perceived when the noise burst placed at that frequency preceded that vowel. Open circles represent the consonant **T***ip*, solid dots represent **P***it*, and diagonal lines represent **C***ow*. Larger symbols mean the judgments were more firm and reliable; smaller symbols (or blank area) mean the stimuli were ambiguous.

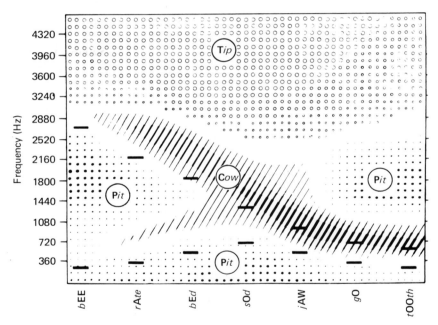

FIGURE 19-8 Map of the areas in which the judgment of the phonemes **P***it*, **T***ip*, or **C***ow* prevailed when a noise burst preceded vowel formants. Vowel formants are shown as horizontal bars, and indicated below the abscissa. From Liberman, Delattre, and Cooper (1952). Reprinted by permission.

We see that the **T***ip* sound always resulted when the noise burst was at a high frequency, regardless of the following vowel. Bursts above about 3000 Hz were almost invariably perceived as **T***ip*. The **P***it* sound was not as constant: **P***it* was heard when there was a medium-frequency burst followed by one of the high tongue vowels, but required a low-frequency burst when the burst was followed by a low tongue vowel. *Cow* also was very dependent on the following vowel: the further to the back of the mouth the constriction was in generating the vowel, the lower the frequency of the burst that was heard as *Cow*. The *Cow* part of the syllables **CA***pe* or **KE***pt* was generated by a burst centered at about 2600 Hz: the *Cow* part of **CO***de* or **COO***p* was generated by a burst centered at 800 Hz. If we follow the progression of syllables heard as noise bursts of increasing frequency are placed before the formants of the vowel *rAte*, we would hear the progression of syllables **PA***in*, **CA***ne*, **PA***in*, **CA***ne*, and **TA***le*. (Follow vertically above *rAte*.)

We may look at this another way. The same physical stimulus, a tone burst at, say, 1400 Hz, will be heard as different consonants depending on the vowel by which it is followed. As we trace from left to right in the figure, we would hear the same burst generate the series **PEA***t, **PA***te, **PE***t, **CO***p* (this is the stimulus in Figure 19–7), **CAU***ght,* **PO***ny* and **POO***l.* The perception of the sound depends on the context in which it is heard.

BOX 19–6

The importance of succeeding sounds does not depend on the fact that these are artificially produced speech sounds. Schatz (1954) cut up tapes of speakers saying words like *keep, cop, coop,* or *heap, hop, hoop,* and spliced the leading consonants from the first three words onto the vowels from the last three. This caused no change in the **K***id* sound, but if the **SK***ip* of *ski, ska,* or *school* was used, the perceptions were dependent on the following vowel to which they were spliced. In fact, the pattern of perceived consonants as a function of the fol-

lowing vowel in the spliced tape (not the vowel originally used when the **SK***ip* was recorded) was reminiscent of the map in Figure 19–8. The reason the experiment worked with the **SK***ip* sound is that there is a brief silence following this sound and preceding the vowel; the tapes could be cut during this (unperceived) silence. In the first series (*keep, cop, coop*) there is no such silence; the consonant included enough of a cue to the following vowel that subjects could correctly identify the consonant despite the ensuing splice.

The plosive consonants are perceived in context; there is a dependency on the ensuing vowel. Other consonants also depend on the vowels with which they are associated, in ways that are even more revealing of the kinds of relationships involved. For example, Liberman, Delattre, Gerstman, and Cooper (1956) studied rapid-frequency shifts in the second formant that were the cues to certain consonants. These shifts, which would be heard as rapid glissandos or chirps if they were not imbedded in speech, are called *transitions.*

Consider the series of spectrograms in Figure 19–9. The same two formants are present (the vowel is *yEt*), but each is approached from a lower frequency with an abrupt rise in frequency. The low point at which each pattern starts is the same, and is called the *locus* of the transition. What differs in these three patterns is the time it takes to get from the locus to the position of the vowel formants. When the transition is brief, as in the left figure, the consonant heard is **B**ed. When the transition lasts longer, the consonant becomes **W**et; at the longest durations, it changes into a shifting vowel (the subjects heard two vowels shading into each other). This series would be heard as **BE**d, **WE**t, cr**UE**t. A similar series is shown in Figure 19–10; in this case, the three sounds would be heard as **GE**t, **YE**t, and v**IE**t.

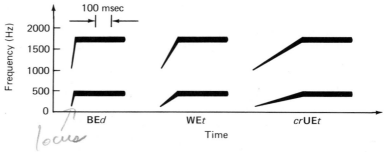

FIGURE 19–9   Series of syllables in which the duration of the second-formant transition varies. The three would be perceived as **BE**d, **WE**t, and cr**UE**t. After Liberman, Delattre, Gerstman, and Cooper (1956).

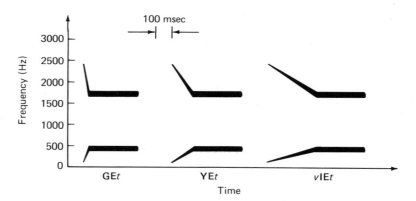

FIGURE 19–10   Series of syllables of varying second-formant transition duration. The three would be heard as **GE**t, **YE**t and v**IE**t. After Liberman, Delattre, Gerstman, and Cooper (1956).

The locus of the transitions is constant, regardless of the following vowel. The second formant transition for **BE**d, for example, starts at a locus near 1000 Hz; the transition proceeds to about 1800 Hz, the second formant of b**E**d. The optimal duration of **B**ed was about 20 msec, so the rate of change of frequency was about 40 Hz/msec. Had the vowel been *b*EE, whose second formant is about 2700 Hz, the rate of transition would have to be more than twice as rapid—about 85 Hz/msec—to get from 1000 Hz to 2700 Hz in 20 msec. Nevertheless, the significant factor seems to be the duration of the shift, not the rate of change of frequency. The locus and duration of the second formant transitions was the same when *B*ed was perceived before any vowel.

The locus of the second formant transition is the necessary cue for a number of consonants (Delattre, Liberman, & Cooper, 1955); however, this can manifest itself in somewhat unusual ways. Consider, for example, how *D*ig is generated in front of various vowels. The locus for the second formant transition for *D*ig is at about 1800 Hz; this can be seen in Figure 19–11, which shows the series: **DEE***d*, **DA***te,* **DE***nt,* **DO***t,* **DO***g,* **DO***pe,* **DO**. Notice that in **DE***nt* there is no transition to the second formant, for the second formant is itself at about 1800 Hz, which is the locus. In **DEE***d* and **DA***te* the second formants are above the locus, so there is an upward transition; in the remainder of the syllables the second formant is below the locus and the transition is downward. What all these transitions have in common is that they originate at the same locus.

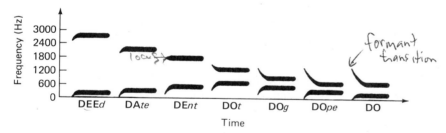

FIGURE 19–11   Series of syllables in which the initial consonant is perceived as **D***ig*. Second-formant transitions point to a locus at 1800 Hz. From Delattre, P. C., A. M. Liberman, and F. S. Cooper (1955) Acoustic loci and transitional cues. *J. Acoust. Soc. Am.* 27:769–772. Reprinted by permission of the publisher and author.

The transitions do not always start at the locus, however; they just point toward it. In fact, if the entire transition, starting from the locus, were given, the consonant would sometimes not sound like **D***ig* at all. Data on this point are shown in Figure 19–12(a). The transitions actually tested are shown, all originating from 1800 Hz. When the transition was extreme upward, the consonant was perceived as **B***ed*; when it was moderate downward, the consonant was **G***ot*. If the first 50 msec of the transitions were erased, however, as shown on the right, the consonant **D***ig*, was always perceived. The dotted portions of the transitions show how they point at, but do not reach, the locus at 1800 Hz.

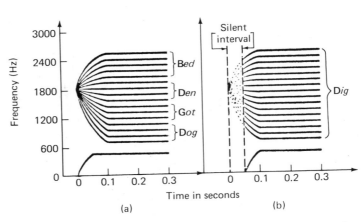

FIGURE 19-12 Demonstration of the importance of the time of onset of second-formant transitions. The series on the left have second-formant transitions starting at 1800 Hz but may variously be heard as **B**ed, **D**en, or **G**ot. The series on the right have the identical second formants, except that the first 50 msec of each transition has been deleted; the first formant has been shifted 50 msec to start simultaneously with the second formant. All the stimuli to the right are perceived to have the same initial consonant **D**ig. From Delattre, Liberman, and Cooper (1955). Reprinted by permission.

The Units of Speech

In the previous few pages, we talked about the perception of phonemes and treated the phoneme as the unit of speech. On the other hand, we have been discussing the perception of syllables, and have seen that the consonant simply cannot stand without an attached vowel. We also know that we cannot chop up a tape into phoneme-size pieces and splice them together to make words.

The size of the basic acoustic unit of speech perception is approximately that of a syllable (Studdert-Kennedy, 1976). There are a number of arguments indicating that this is probably the case, but one of the most convincing was given by Huggins (1964) and based on an observation made by Cherry (1953). A subject is asked to follow a stream of speech played through headphones. At a regular rate, the stream of speech switches back and forth from ear to ear. If the alternation was very fast (say, 20 switchovers per second) or very slow (one per second), the subjects had little difficulty following the gist of the speech. But at intermediate rates, comprehension became poor; the alternation from ear to ear made it nearly impossible to hear what was being said.

The relevance of this study can be best understood if we borrow an analogy from Neisser (1967). Consider the effect of alternation on the written word. If a line of text were chopped up and alternate segments displaced downward, it would look like one of the patterns in Figure 19–13. The top pattern has been cut at a slow rate—relatively large chunks stay together before the next alternation. The bottom row shows text cut at a high rate; part of each letter is on the original line and part on the displaced line. Neither of these forms is illegible. Consider, however, the texts chopped at medium rates. The rate of alternation is very nearly the same as the size of the basic units of the text, the letters. Each letter is fractured, and the line is difficult or impossible to read.

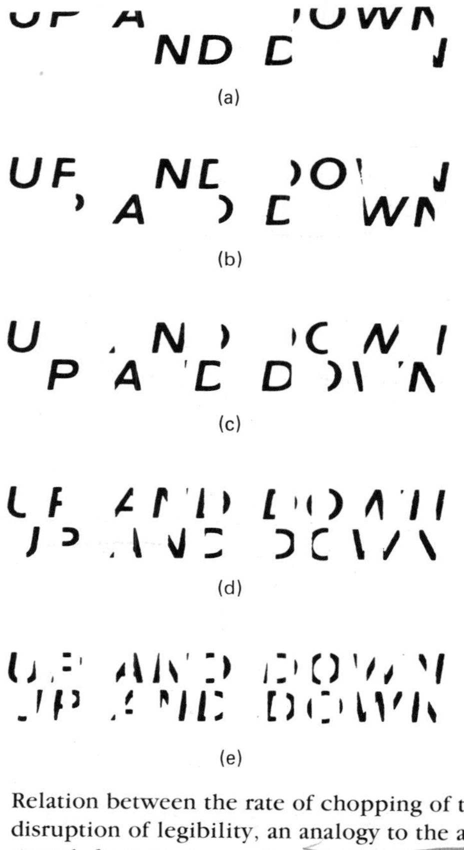

(a)

(b)

(c)

(d)

(e)

FIGURE 19–13 Relation between the rate of chopping of text and the disruption of legibility, an analogy to the alternation of speech from ear to ear. See text. From Neisser, U. *Cognitive Psychology*, © 1967, p. 186. Reprinted by permission of Prentice Hall, Inc., Englewood Cliffs, New Jersey.

The rate of alternation of speech in headphones that was most disruptive, therefore, would be the rate at which the segments were somewhat smaller than the perceptual units. In fact, the most disruptive rate corresponded to a size about 60% the length of the average syllable; the syllable would appear to be about the right size for the acoustic unit of speech.

There is also evidence that speech perception involves larger units as well. Miller, Heise, and Lichten (1951) found that the intelligibility of syllables masked by noise was greatly improved by imbedding the syllables in meaningful words or sentences. Fodor and Bever (1965) asked subjects to identify where within a spoken text a click was superimposed. Not only was the click always perceived as occurring between syllables (even when it actually was superimposed on an unperceived silence within a syllable), but the reported position of the click was often shifted more than 100 msec to fall between meaningful elements of the speech.

BOX 19-7

An aspect of speech that is encoded in pieces larger than a syllable is the *prosodic* element, also known as the *suprasegmental features*. These refer to qualities such as intonation, stress, emphasis, and ''punctuation'' (the spoken equivalents of periods, commas, and question marks). These important aspects of understanding spoken words are indicated by patterns that extend across syllables, words, and phrases (Darwin, 1975).

As an example, stress does not correspond to any single acoustic feature. Stressed words are judged as louder, but physical measurements do not show this to be so. The physical correlate of stress seems to be the *effort* put into the word by the speaker—not a single particular attribute of the sound produced (Lehiste, 1976). When we speak of the motor theory of speech perception (following), we will find other examples of cases in which the percept corresponds to a motor activity of the speaker rather than to a single acoustic feature of the utterance.

In natural sentences, the fundamental frequency of voicing (rate of vocal cord vibration—see Box 19–2) falls toward the end of the sentence. Questions are distinguished from statements by the fact that the fundamental frequency does not fall at the end of the utterance. The decline in frequency is a result of the drop in pressure of the air being expelled from the lungs as the speaker prepares to inhale and renew the air supply for the next sentence. There are other, less automatic ways in which some speakers produce this effect artificially by other maneuvers, however (Lieberman, 1977). In any case, the suprasegmental features are apparently conveyed by the vowels, which carry most of the voicing energy (see Box 19–2).

In order for us to be able to analyze these larger units of speech we must have stored information about the speech signal over a period of time, for the parts of an utterance are not present simultaneously. Just as visual pattern recognition depends on the net effect of a large number of features distributed in space (see Chapter 11), speech perception depends on features distributed in time. At least two types of memory have been postulated specifically for the immediate storage of the continuously arriving features in an utterance (Studdert-Kennedy, 1976).

BOX 19-8

Although we have been discussing the perception of phonemes as if they were the clearly perceived units of speech, normal conversational speech arrives in a continuous stream in which whole phrases run together. The division of this continuum into individual words is the responsibility of the listener; in doing this, perceptual hypotheses are made that are guided by the context of the conversation.

A striking demonstration of the way in which context influences speech perception is given by Prof. Ronald Cole of the Carnegie-Mellon Institute. To appreciate the effect fully, you should have a friend try it on you. Ask your friend to read the two phrases printed upside down on page 538; they should be read in a fast conversational tone, not distinctly enunciated. Listen as they are repeated several times; chances are, you will be unable to discern the words, and it will sound like gibberish. Now ask your friend to read the hint printed with them. The hint gives the context of the phrases—you may now be able to know what the phrases said just from your memory of the sounds. If not, ask to hear the phrases again, and see whether they make sense. If they still do not, read them to yourself. Once you know

what the phrases are, you will hear them distinctly each time they are read to you, even though the acoustic signal is just as poor as when you were unable to make head nor tail of them. That is why the demonstration is best performed without your knowing the phrases in advance; once you know what they are, they do not sound like gibberish.

This is a case in which there is clear perception of a stimulus that defied decoding until some guidance was given as to how to make a perceptual hypothesis; it is exactly like the perception of the hidden faces in Figure 11-17. When you first saw that figure, it looked like some abstract blobs, but once you were shown what it really was, it made sense. If you look back at that figure now, you will probably see the faces with little trouble—it may even be hard to imagine why the figure made no sense before you had looked at Figure 11-18. Just so, the phrases on page 538, are perfectly intelligible once we know how to make the right perceptual hypotheses about the acoustic signal; it is hard to believe your friend is not pronouncing the words more distinctly now than when you first heard the phrases.

SPEECH PERCEPTION

How do we actually do the analysis implied by the discussion of all the acoustic features of speech? What are the neurophysiological and cognitive mechanisms involved?

To begin with, we should note that our ability to perceive spoken words is quite extraordinary. We are not dealing with a sound equivalent of an alphabet (as we have seen); we have an intricately encoded signal to decode. Despite the intricacy of the code, it is so deeply ingrained that we can recognize and correctly categorize speech sounds that are drastically different from the norm.

When we identify a sound generated on the pattern-playback machine as one phoneme or another, we are merely categorizing it. Is our ability to discriminate these sounds somehow related to the categories into which we place them? Apparently so, for we are far poorer at discriminating sounds that are categorized as the same phoneme than we are at discriminating between sounds that are categorized as different phonemes (even though these two sounds may be acoustically more similar) (Liberman, Harris, Hoffman, & Griffith, 1957; Liberman, Harris, Eimas, Lisker, & Bastian, 1961; Lieberman, 1977). As an example of better discrimination of stimuli that are acoustically more similar than those not discriminated, consider the left part of Figure 19–12. The four stimuli with the lowest frequency second formants lead to perception of the consonant sound **D**og (the syllable is probably something like **DO**g). The fifth stimulus leads to a consonant perceived as **G**et; you would expect subjects to be far better at discriminating between the fourth and fifth stimuli than between the first and fourth, even though the first and fourth are physically more disparate.

We might think of these discriminations as a matter of learning, but infants also can make some of these distinctions (Cutting & Eimas, 1975). Interestingly, when only the second formant is presented the distinctions are *not* sharpest at the phonemic boundary (frequency at which the second formant would begin to signal a different phoneme). Infants presented second formants without first formants are no better at discriminating the transition associated with **D**og from that associated with **B**it than any other equally different pair within the one category or the other. The effect of a boundary is only found when a first formant (that is the same between stimuli) is present as well (Cutting & Eimas, 1975). The same seems true for adult listeners (Mattingly, Liberman, Syrdal, & Halwes, 1971). Apparently then, the phoneme boundaries are not specified by inherent preferences of the auditory system, but they are specific to the perception of speech.

We might have guessed that the definition of the boundaries was not innate, for they vary somewhat from language to language (see Lieberman, 1977). In fact, some of the pronunciation difficulties we encounter when speaking a non-native language may be because the phonemic boundaries can be slightly different. Two sounds distinguished as different phonemes in one language may be categorized as the same phoneme is another language, and so not be differentiated by a person raised in the second language who attempts to speak the first. For example, if you make a continuous "zzzzz" sound, and bring the tip of your tongue close to your front teeth, the sound will change into a prolonged **TH**en (a demonstration best not done in public). The distinction between **Z**oo and **TH**en is in the tongue position; the exact locus at which the sound changes from **Z**oo to **TH**en (the boundary) can be different in different languages. Thus native speakers of French make sounds that to their ears have crossed the boundary into **TH**en, but which to the ears of native speakers of English remain on the **Z**oo side; the French say they will ride in "ze car."

In short, categorization seems to be affected by learning, but either the learning begins very early in infancy, or it modifies a biological predisposition. We should note that categorization of this kind is apparently not confined to the perception of speech (Cutting & Rosner, 1974; Pastore, Ahroon, Baffuto, Friedman, Puleo, & Fink, 1977). It also is not confined to spoken language (Poizner, 1981), or even human languages (Nelson & Marler, 1989).

BOX 19-9 ▬▬▬▬▬▬▬▬▬▬

One possible way that experience could modify biological predisposition is by pruning out those categorizations that are not used. As we noted, very young infants make phonemic distinctions, with boundaries similar to those found for adults. Surprisingly, they not only make the distinctions their parents make, they also "recognize" boundaries that are used in foreign languages to which they have never been exposed (Werker, 1989). As children mature, they lose the ability to make distinctions across those phonemic boundaries they do not encounter, so that by about one year of age (roughly the time children begin to understand spoken language) they make discriminations only across those boundaries that are appropriate for their native language (Werker, 1989).

If this interpretation of how categorization arises is correct, we can conclude that there are a number of possible phonemic boundaries inherent in our nervous systems. Each human language draws on a subset of these boundaries, grouping all sounds within any boundary that is used as a particular phoneme. Since a somewhat different choice of boundaries may be used by different languages, there are sometimes similar phonemes in two languages with a different boundary to the next phoneme. A newborn infant has the capability of making any of the phonemic discriminations, but only those that are exercised are retained.

Now we come to the question of how the nervous system might analyze the acoustic signals presented to it during a speech pattern. We have reviewed various features that might be extracted: patterns of formants, transitions, and noise bursts. Recordings have been made in the auditory cortex of monkeys while playing various acoustic signals (Wollberg & Newman, 1972). Many cells responded to a wide range of stimuli, but there were some cells that seemed highly specific to certain monkey vocalizations. Similarly, quite specific cells were found in cat cortex (Whitefield & Evans, 1965), bullfrog (Frishkopf & Goldstein, 1965), and bat (Suga, O'Neill, & Manabe, 1979). Selective cells (for human speech sounds) have even been found in trained mynah birds, which mimic speech (Langner, Bonke, and Scheich, 1981). These feature-specific cells are somewhat reminiscent of the "bug detectors" in frog retina (Chapter 6); it is hard to say how seriously to take the claim that they are truly detecting the specific features claimed.

Feature detection theory (handwritten marginalia)

An interesting demonstration of feature detection in the auditory system comes from studies of the adaptation of the presumed detectors. Just as we could demonstrate spatial frequency detection channels by adapting to specific frequencies and thus desensitizing the channels selective for those frequencies (see Chapter 10). Eimas and Corbit (1973) showed that listening to a long series of syllables within a phonemic category could affect the identification of a syllable near the boundary (see also Miller & Eimas, 1977). For example, the voiced plosive made by the lips (**B***it*) and the unvoiced plosive (**P***it*) differ in the duration of the transition from locus to vowel second formant. If the entire transition is used, **B***it* is heard; if most of the transition is silent, **P***it* is heard. With a moderate length of transition, a subject might hear either consonant. Let us select a transition that tends to favor **B***it*, but is ambiguous. After a subject listens to a series of repetitions of the syllable **BO***nd*, the same slightly ambiguous **B***it* can be tested; it will more likely sound like **P***it*. The boundary has apparently shifted closer to the "ideal" **B***it*, because of fatigue of the **B***it* detector.

BOX 19–10

Refer to Box 19–8, and try the experiment before reading the phrases below.

Phrase 1: "In mud eels are."

Phrase 2: "In clay none are."

Hint: The phrases answer the question, Where can eels be found?

In addition, the adaptation effect is apparently central and not caused by simple fatigue in the auditory periphery, for adaptation to syllables played in one ear can affect categorization of syllables played into the other ear (Eimas, Cooper, & Corbit, 1973). Note also that these feature detectors are not simply linked to a single aspect of the acoustic signal (such as the duration of the transition), for changing other cues to the identity of the phonemes (such as the rate at which the sounds are produced) affects the positions of the boundaries (Repp, Liberman, Eccardt, & Pesetsky, 1978). The feature detectors seem to be specific to complex auditory cues that might be associated with phonemic features; however, nonspeech sounds can also affect these detectors (Samuel & Newport, 1979).

Motor Theory

We have considered how speech sounds might be recognized by feature detectors that pick out specific patterns in an auditory signal. Now we face the same problem we had to face in visual perception: how can there be enough feature detectors to recognize all the possible speech sounds and their variants? Despite differences in emphasis, voicing, and differences among speakers, we can quickly and effectively interpret the sounds of speech, arriving

at the awesome rate of 30 phonemes per second (Liberman, Cooper, Shankweiler, & Studdert-Kennedy, 1967).

We have already encountered a hint of a further difficulty: the acoustic
features associated with certain sounds can be specified in terms of transition
locus, onset delay, and so forth, but these do not seem to be "natural" things
to use as cues. The series of transitions perceived as the sound **D***ig* in Figure
19–11 shows a definite tendency for all second formant transitions to point at
the 1800-Hz locus; however, the truncated initial segment makes it hard to
imagine how we would recognize this as the locus being pointed at in **DEE***d
or* **DO**. An even more glaring example was presented by Delattre, Liberman,
and Cooper (1955) in a figure showing the second formant transitions responsible for the sound **G***et*. Liberman (1957) emphasized the significance
of the problem: there is a change in locus between the sounds **GO***t* and
GAU*ze* (Figure 19–14). As we progress from **GEE***se* to **GO***t*, there is an ever-
increasing second-formant transition, pointing to a locus near 3000 Hz. But
the next sound, **GAU***ze*, has a minimal transition, and the subsequent series
through **GOO** show small transitions from a locus near 1200 Hz. There is an
abrupt change in locus that has no corresponding shift in the phonetic value
of the sound heard: the **G***et* sound is the same in all of these syllables.

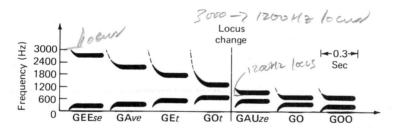

FIGURE 19–14 Series of syllables in which the initial consonant is
always perceived as **G***et*. Note the change of second-
formant transition locus between the syllables **GO***t* and
GAU*ze*. From Liberman, A. M. (1957) Results of research on speech perception. *J. Acoust. Soc. Am.*
29:117–123. Reprinted by permission of the publisher
and author.

There is, however, another "dimension" on which there is no change
between the sounds **GO***t* and **GAU***ze*. There is no difference in the articulatory maneuvers the speaker makes to produce the **G***et* in each case. We perceive as the same those phonemes that were made by the same motor activity
(a voiced plosive from the rear of the mouth), even though the physical
sounds seem to be in different classes. Evidence of this kind led Liberman and
his co-workers (Liberman, Cooper, Shankweiler, & Studdert-Kennedy,
1967) to formulate a *motor theory* of speech perception. According to this
theory, the acoustic cues are taken in syllable-size chunks, and these chunks

are "decoded" by determining what motor behavior must have been necessary to produce such a sound. In effect, the listener "knows" the motor behaviors that produce the various phonemes in conjunction with each other; when a syllable arrives in the ears, the listener builds a model of it based on the motor activity that would be made to produce that sound. (Of course, the listener does not actually make the sound, just determines the motor action that would make it.)

This model should remind you of the analysis-by-synthesis models of visual perception. In fact, a somewhat more explicit version of a motor theory called analysis-by-synthesis has been proposed (Halle & Stevens, 1959; Stevens, 1973). In this model, feature analyzers perform a preliminary analysis of the speech sounds and pass the digested version to a central processor. The central processor may find that the features presented (including the context, or other sounds it has previously been presented) are sufficient for classification. If classification is ambiguous, a "guess" (perceptual hypothesis) is made, and a synthesizer generates an internal model of the sound corresponding to the guess. This is compared with the memory of the features of the actual sound, and if it matches satisfactorily, the guess is taken to be correct. The point of all this is to generate an internal model of the articulatory gestures that would have led to the sound pattern received; this model then represents the utterance made by the speaker. It is analogous to the internal model in visual perception (Chapter 11) that we presumably build by making perceptual hypotheses about what distal stimulus could have been responsible for the proximal stimulus on our retinae. In speech, the distal stimulus is the articulation of the speaker, and the proximal stimulus is the acoustic pattern.

BOX 19–11

The motor theory was devised to explain how disparate acoustic stimuli could represent the same phoneme. The discontinuity in the acoustic stimuli for **GO**t and **GAU**ze is a striking example of a case in which the percepts are in accord with the articulatory maneuvers that made the sounds, rather than the acoustics of the sounds emitted. Another example is found in the interposition of brief silences in a spoken sentence. If a tape is made of the sentence, "Please say shop," and a silence of about 50 msec is inserted after "say," the sentence becomes "Please say chop" (Dorman, Raphael, & Liberman, 1979). This makes sense for the articulatory gestures required to say "Please say chop": to produce the sudden burst of sound for **CH**op requires closing the airway briefly, thereby creating a brief silence. Dorman *et al.* carried this one step further: they made a tape in which a female voice said "please say" to which was spliced a male voice saying the word "shop." In this case, a silence between "say" and "shop" made no difference to the percept—the final word was always (correctly) heard as "shop." The perception of the acoustic stimulus for "shop" depended in a very complex way on the perceived capabilities of the human vocal tract; when there were

(continued)

(box continued)

two different speakers, the silence was treated as irrelevant. From this and a number of other observations on the perception of speech with

interposed silences, Dorman *et al.* concluded that speech perception is closely related to the perceiver's knowledge of the capabilities of the human vocal apparatus.

One possible difficulty with a motor theory of speech perception is that it might imply the ability to speak is needed for one to be able to perceive speech. One would not expect a human, speechless from birth because of a defective vocal tract, to be unable to comprehend speech, however. Moreover, we know that speechless animals are capable of discriminating the sounds of human speech; this is true for monkeys (Morse & Snowden, 1975) and even for a rodent, the chinchilla (Burdick & Miller, 1975; Kuhl & Miller, 1975).

These objections are not as problematic as they might seem. Animals can learn to discriminate speech sounds, but we cannot say that they therefore perceive speech in the same way as humans do. They might simply be learning a set of auditory cues, just as you could learn to make various responses to different tones in a set of signal whistles but would not say the whistles were "speaking." As for the speechless human, the important thing might be the biological capability for speech, even in the absence of experience with a functioning vocal apparatus. In this regard, it is interesting that electrical stimulation of certain sites in the human brain leads to the facial gestures of speech and also affects the perception of phonemes (Ojemann & Mateer, 1979). There is a relation between speech perceiving and speech producing in the brain; this relationship would not necessarily be disrupted by damage to the vocal tract.

It also appears that the development of the ability to speak is intimately associated with the perception of speech. Human infants who are born deaf do not learn to speak when normal infants would; they babble appropriately for about six months, then gradually stop vocalizing (Mavilya, 1972). Similarly (perhaps), certain species of song birds fail to develop their species-specific songs unless allowed to hear an adult version of the song during a critical period in their development (Marler, 1975). In the absence of appropriate role models, inappropriate songs develop, although there are certain features that remain. Marler (1975) suggested that the critical thing needed for the development of speech is a set of "modifiable auditory templates" that serve both for categorical recognition of speech sounds and for motor control of the production of speech. Studdert-Kennedy (1976) takes this idea further by suggesting that there are both auditory and articulatory (motor) templates that develop hand-in-glove as the individual learns to speak and understand a language.

BOX 19–12

A motor theory of speech implies a bimodal process, for the auditory and motor systems must be linked. There is also a linkage to the visual system, for speech is easier to understand when you can watch the speaker's face. (Many hearing impaired people make use of this fact, partly lip-reading what they cannot quite hear.) The link between the facial expression and the sound is, of course, the articulatory maneuver by which the speech is produced. You can infer this maneuver from the sound (motor theory) or by direct observation. When both kinds of information are available, you can "hear" better than with only one. If the two are inconsistent (as in watching a dubbed movie), confusion may arise (McGurk & MacDonald, 1976).

The correspondence between sight and sound is also made by infants. If an 18- to 20-week-old infant is simultaneously shown two videos of the same face saying two different syllables, and hears one of the syllables through a loudspeaker placed directly between the video screens, the child gazes at the video face corresponding to the audible signal (Kuhl & Meltzoff, 1982).

With the motor theory of speech perception we have closed a circle, for we may now redefine the feature detectors of speech with the speech sounds with which this chapter began. The features in speech perception are aspects such as voiced versus unvoiced, plosive versus nonplosive, fricative versus nonfricative, front, middle, or back of mouth, and so on. These features are constant when the perceptions are of the same phoneme, even though there are discontinuities in the acoustic properties of the sounds representing them. This means that the features of speech are very complicated in their acoustic definitions, although there are relatively few of them. In vision, such features as edges, lines, and so on, are easy to define but do little to explain perception, while such higher order percepts as "jack o'lantern" or "mother-standing-at-the-stove" are not only complicated but far too numerous to be represented by specific "detectors." In speech perception, there is a very limited number of complex features to be detected, for the features of speech are limited by the capabilities of the human vocal apparatus.

SPEECH AREAS OF THE BRAIN

We have been discussing the perception of speech without much reference to the brain or specific neural mechanisms. However, scientists have been studying the anatomical basis of speech and speech comprehension for more than 120 years, and more is known about the neurology of language than most other brain processes.

For the vast majority of people, language is largely a function of the left hemisphere of the brain. This is true for virtually all right-handed people, and for the majority of left-handed people as well (Kolb & Whishaw, 1985).

For most of us, virtually the entire right half of the brain could be removed without causing any significant deficit in language abilities. A similar segregation of language specialization has been observed in monkeys (Heffner & Heffner, 1984), for the perception of species-specific vocalizations. Nevertheless, this specialization is another indication that speech perception is a "special" kind of auditory perception.

Within the left hemisphere, there is a specific circuit that must be intact for normal speech and language comprehension. Figure 19–15 shows the locations of the two major cortical components of this circuit. The first brain area found to be crucial for normal language is in the lower part of the frontal lobe. This area is called *Broca's area*, after the French physician Paul Broca, who noted in 1861 that patients with markedly decreased speech output proved (on autopsy) to have damage in this area. Broca's area is connected by a fiber tract (the *arcuate fasciculus*) to *Wernicke's area* in the temporal lobe. Damage anywhere in the pathway, including Broca's and Wernicke's areas, produces speech defects characteristic of where the damage is. These speech deficits are collectively known as *aphasias*.

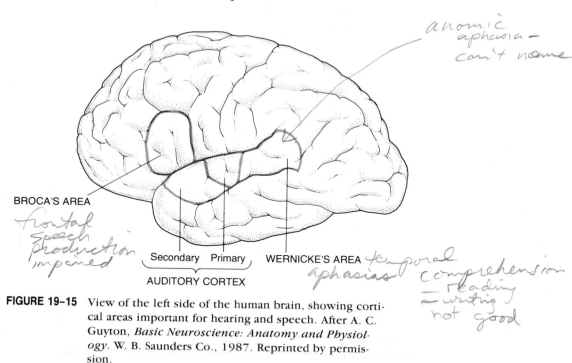

[handwritten annotations: anomic aphasia — can't name; frontal speech production impaired; temporal aphasias; comprehension — reading — writing not good]

FIGURE 19–15   View of the left side of the human brain, showing cortical areas important for hearing and speech. After A. C. Guyton, *Basic Neuroscience: Anatomy and Physiology.* W. B. Saunders Co., 1987. Reprinted by permission.

Damage to Broca's area produces a clinical syndrome called *Broca's aphasia*. Patients with Broca's aphasia have a severely reduced speech output. The words produced are usually correct and meaningful, but they are produced with great effort, often at a maximum rate of only 10 words per minute. The problem is not simply in the forming of sounds, for grammatically important words that link the concepts together are noticeably lacking. In contrast, comprehension seems to be only mildly impaired. The defect appears to be in the output of meaningful speech, not in its perception.

Damage to Wernicke's area produces a spectrum of language defects that are quite different from Broca's aphasia. Wernicke's aphasics are quite fluent in their speech output, often producing words at a normal rate. Their grammar may be correct, and the inflection and flow is like normal speech. But the words make no sense when put together, and may even be nonsense words. The patient speaks fluent gibberish, such as "Mother is away here working her work to get her better, but when she's looking the two boys looking in the other part. . . ." (Geschwind, 1979, page 111). In marked contrast to Broca's aphasia, comprehension in *Wernicke's aphasia* is grossly abnormal; patients are often unable to understand even simple, one-step instructions. Not surprisingly, both reading and writing are impossible for a patient with Wernicke's aphasia.

Another interesting speech deficit is known as *anomic aphasia*. Patients with this syndrome speak fluently, and have normal comprehension of speech; however, when they are asked to name objects, they perform poorly. They are exquisitely aware of their problem, and often try to hide it with phrases such as "that thing," or "whatever it's called." They often exclaim "it's on the tip of my tongue" (as we all do sometimes!). Anomic aphasia may be associated with Alzheimer's disease or any diffuse damage in the left hemisphere, but also may result from local damage near the top of Wernicke's area.

SUGGESTED READINGS

A very readable paperback account of the production and perception of speech is *The Speech Chain*, by P. B. Denes and E. N. Pinson (Anchor Books, 1973). It includes chapters on physics and psychophysics of sound, neurophysiology of hearing, physiology of speech production, acoustic characteristics of speech, speech recognition, and linguistics. Each chapter stands as a complete account of a topic, with little cross-referencing between chapters, so one can read any part as desired.

A considerably more technical account, but very readable, is given by P. Lieberman in *Speech Physiology and Acoustic Phonetics: An Introduction* (Macmillan Inc., 1977). This book spends considerable effort introducing the basic physics needed to understand the nature of the sounds produced in speech, and the spectral analyses of them. There is a detailed discussion of the principles of the spectrograph, with practical information on how to use it and interpret spectrograms. There is also a good discussion of the perception of speech.

SOMATOSENSORY SENSATION AND PAIN

In preceding chapters, we have gone into considerable detail about how our visual and auditory systems provide us with information about the world around us. Of course, human beings have other ways of receiving data regarding both our internal and external environments. Although perhaps not as developed as in some other animal species, our chemical senses of smell and taste provide us with very important information about the outside world. Similarly, the somatic senses of touch and proprioception allow us to gauge the positions of our limbs in space and to perceive stimuli that directly contact our bodies. In this chapter and Chapter 21, we will discuss how the somatic and chemical senses are organized and how they extract the relevant features we perceive as touch, taste, and smell.

SOMATIC SENSATION

Our first task in discussing the somatic senses is to describe a set of primary modalities. The sense of touch is obviously not unitary; the feeling of a feather tickling your skin is clearly different than the scratch of a dog's claws. Similarly, although a pin prick, a hot iron, a headache, and a punch in the nose can all be classified as painful, they are by no means the same sensations. However, by correlating anatomical and psychophysical studies, four primary somatic submodalities have emerged:

1. Proprioception: the sense of position of your body and limbs in space.
2. Tactile sensation: the sense elicited by nonpainful stimuli placed against the body surface.
3. Nociception (pain): the sense elicited by noxious stimuli applied to the body.
4. Temperature: the sense elicited by stimuli that are either warmer or colder than the body surface.

Although there is some overlap, these four submodalities are subserved by essentially different populations of receptors and follow one of two major pathways from the periphery to the brain.

Receptors

Many different types of receptors provide input into the somatic sensory system. Except for temperature receptors and one type of nociceptor, however, they are all mechanoreceptors; that is, their activity changes in response to mechanical deflection of their cell membranes. In this sense, they are similar to the hair cells of the auditory system, which become depolarized when their external processes, or hairs, are moved by sound waves. The actual mechanism by which membrane deflection results in membrane depolarization is not completely understood. However, in response to mechanical stimulation, ion channels selective for sodium and potassium are opened, resulting in a graded local depolarization called a receptor potential. The receptor potential is propagated in decremental fashion within the cell to an area capable of generating action potentials. This area, called the trigger zone, is where action potentials are produced with a frequency that depends on the size of the receptor potential (see Chapter 3). As will be discussed in detail in this chapter, different receptor types are connected to axons of varying conduction velocities, which travel to the spinal cord and then, by well defined pathways, to the brain.

Proprioception   One could conceive of at least four different ways that the somatic sensory system could get information about the position of the body and limbs in space. One way does not require the use of peripheral receptors at all. Since the position of the body is determined by muscle contractions, which are in turn controlled by the motor system of the brain, perception of movement and position could derive from the motor system itself. In other words, motor commands for voluntary movement could be directly sent to proprioceptive centers elsewhere in the brain. According to this view, proprioception would be the result of one part of the brain monitoring the commands issued by another part, rather than arising from the activity of peripheral receptors. This hypothesis, known as the outflow theory, was proposed by the famous German physiologist Hermann Helmholtz, in the last part of the 19th century (see Kandel & Schwartz, 1985). However, if this mechanism were important in the perception of limb perception, one would expect that a limb moving passively without a motor command would be perceived poorly or not at all. In fact, passive movement can be perceived with exquisite sensitivity; passive movement at the ankle joint can be estimated to within 2 to 3 degrees (Berenberg, Shefner, & Sokol, 1987).

The outflow theory may not account for how we perceive the position of our limbs in space, but it seems to be a good explanation for how we know where our eyes are pointing. As we discussed in Chapter 14, the brain obtains information about the direction of gaze by monitoring the level of activity of the output to the various eye muscles. Even if the eye muscles are paralyzed, the outflow of the motor nerves to the eye muscles will be used to estimate the position of the eyes within the head (see page 374).

BOX 20-1

Another phenomenon that seems to be well explained by the outflow theory is phantom limb movement. Very often, after someone has had a limb amputated, that person will report a very striking feeling of the limb not only being present, but being in active motion. While initially disturbing, this sensation evoked by the phantom limb is probably very useful when a patient tries to incorporate a limb prosthesis into a complex activity like walking. It is easy to see how Helmholtz' idea that motor commands from the brain provide proprioceptive input could explain how someone could perceive movement in a limb that no longer exists.

If position sense is usually not a direct result of the proprioceptive system monitoring commands issued by the motor system, then there must be peripheral receptors specialized to gather information about joint position. Cutaneous receptors located in the skin around joints could signal joint position by responding to changes in skin stretch. Such receptors do exist, and probably do provide important information about joint position. If the major nerves to the hand are inactivated with a local anesthetic, the forearm muscles that control hand movement are still functional, but sensation in the hand is abolished. Under these conditions, subjects will report that they cannot tell whether their fingers are moving or not. Moreover, when their fingers are moved for them, position is correctly estimated only at the extremes of joint position (Moberg, 1983). Under these circumstances, both cutaneous sensation and any possible sensation from joint receptors has been abolished. Receptors located within joints are called *tendon organs*; they respond in direct proportion to tendon tension and are therefore good candidates to mediate joint position sense. However, when tendon organ response characteristics were carefully studied, it was found that they respond almost exclusively to extremes of movement and are very insensitive to changes in position within most of the normal range of motion of an individual joint (Burgess, Wei, Clark, & Simon, 1982). Moreover, when they are completely removed, as happens when artificial joints are surgically implanted in the knee or hip, position sense in the artificial joint is nearly normal (Grigg, Cinerman, & Riley, 1973). Thus, cutaneous receptors probably are important for the perception of joint position, and joint receptors probably do not play a major role.

Another class of peripheral receptors important for detecting joint position are the muscle spindles, whose responses were shown in Figures 3–12 through 3–15. These receptors are composed of two types of specialized muscle fibers, called the nuclear bag and the nuclear chain. Free nerve endings are wrapped around both types of fibers (see Figure 20–1). When an entire muscle is stretched, the muscle spindle is also stretched; the mechanical deflection causes a change in membrane potential in the free nerve endings. This in turn results in an increase in the rate of firing of action potentials in the sensory fibers to which it is attached. Muscle spindles are sensitive to changes in joint position over the entire range of motion for an individual joint. Some of the sensory fibers that are excited by muscle spindle stretching fire in direct proportion to the actual length to which the muscle spindle is stretched; the responses of these fibers is said to be *static*, because it does not depend on how fast the muscle is stretched. Other fibers respond in a *dynamic* fashion; that is, they respond preferentially to change in the stretch of the muscle, and little or not at all when the length of the muscle remains constant. Thus, the brain receives information about actual joint position from the static fibers, and information about joint movement from the dy-

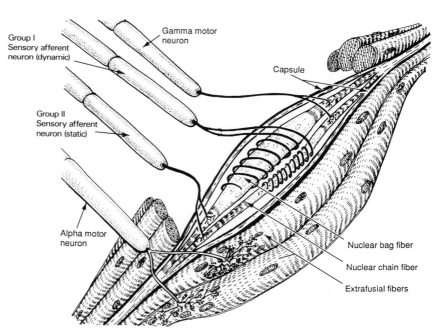

FIGURE 20–1 Drawing of a muscle spindle, including a nuclear bag fiber and a nuclear chain fiber.

namic fibers. This should remind you of the sustained and transient fibers in the visual system.

BOX 20-2

Figure 20–1 shows the locations of the static and dynamic afferents from the muscle spindle. There are two components to the spindle: the nuclear bag fiber and the nuclear chain fiber. Group I axons emanate from the central region of both fibers, and project to the spinal cord. These Group I fibers are fast conducting and are thought to be dynamic fibers, responding preferentially to change in stretch. Group II fibers arising in secondary endings along the periphery of the spindle extend more slowly conducting axons to the spinal cord, and are thought to be static fibers.

Both bag and chain fibers also receive signals from the spinal cord via neurons called *gamma motor neurons*. Activation of gamma fibers causes an increase in tension of the muscle fibers within the muscle spindle. This, in turn, will cause a change in the baseline level of activity of the Group I and II afferents, thus changing the response characteristics of these nerve endings to external stretch. By increasing the activity of the gamma system, therefore, the brain can alter the sensitivity of the muscle spindle to different types of movements.

Tactile receptors   The sense of touch comprises all the sensations caused by stimulation of the skin that are not painful or temperature specific. *Glabrous* skin—hairless skin found on the palm and fingertips—contains the four types of receptors shown in Figure 20–2. *Meissner corpuscles* and *Merkel cells* are located in the superficial layers of the dermis, while *Pacinian corpuscles* and *Ruffini endings* lie more deeply in the skin. Each of these receptors has a specialized terminal process that in part determines its response properties. The Pacinian corpuscle consists of a free nerve ending encapsulated by concentric layers of non-neural connective tissue. When pressure is applied to the skin over a Pacinian corpuscle, this outer capsule is deformed and the free nerve ending within is excited. However, the concentric layers of tissue accommodate to the pressure in such a way as to reduce the stimulation of the nerve ending. The response to a steady stimulus is thus a burst of initial activity, which rapidly decays. If the connective tissue layers are somehow removed, the remaining free nerve ending responds to a steady stimulus with a sustained level of activity (Lowenstein & Mendelson, 1965). Thus, the Pacinian corpuscle is a fast adapting receptor by virtue of its non-neural accessory structure.

The other rapidly adapting receptor in the skin is the Meissner corpuscle, which lies more peripherally than the Pacinian corpuscle. Perhaps due to its location closer to the surface of the skin, the receptive fields of the Meissner corpuscles are considerably smaller than those of Pacinian corpuscles (Johansson & Vallbo, 1983). With a smaller receptive field, the Meissner

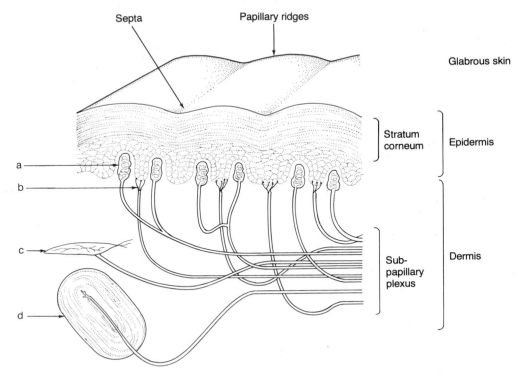

FIGURE 20-2   Drawing of a section of hairless skin, with different types of mechanoreceptors. Near the surface are Meissner corpuscles (a) and Merkel cells (b), while Ruffini endings (c) and Pacinian corpuscles (d) lie more deeply in the dermis. From Light, A. R., and E. R. Perl (1984) Peripheral sensory systems. In *Peripheral Neuropathy*, Dyck, P. J., P. K. Thomas, E. H. Lambert, R. Bunge (Eds.) Philadelphia: W. B. Saunders, p. 216. Reprinted by permission.

cell is better able to provide information that can be used in making fine spatial discriminations. Not surprisingly, these receptors tend to be located in areas such as the fingertips where spatial discrimination is best.

Two other kinds of tactile receptors tend to give sustained responses to steady stimuli, and are called slowly adapting receptors. The Merkel receptor lies peripherally in the skin, as does the Meissner corpuscle, and thus has a smaller receptive field than the deeply placed Ruffini ending. In contrast to the Merkel receptor whose receptive fields are relatively round, those of the Ruffini endings are longer in one dimension than the other, and respond differentially to skin stretch in one direction (Johannson & Vallbo, 1983).

BOX 20–3

By carefully considering the response properties of the receptors just described, one can make good guesses regarding the specific functions they subserve. We have encountered the distinction between tonic and phasic cells before in the visual system when we discussed X and Y retinal ganglion cells. In the visual system, we saw that these two types of cells provided the input for distinct systems, one of which may have been responsible for orientation to new stimuli, and the other for providing more detailed spatial information. In the so-matic sensory system, a similar division of labor may also take place. Moreover, there are some tactile stimuli, such as vibration, that are predominantly phasic in nature. The rapidly adapting receptors are particularly well suited to respond to this kind of stimulus. Conversely, in order to hold a delicate glass, you need information about the steady-state level of force you are exerting against the glass. Slowly adapting receptors would be particularly important in providing that kind of tonic information.

Pain receptors   From a consideration of your personal experiences with painful stimuli, it might not seem obvious that pain is mediated by different receptors than those that process touch and temperature. Pain often seems simply to be an excess amount of a stimulus. For example, a blunt object placed against the skin will become painful only as the pressure it is exerting against the skin exceeds a certain level. Similarly, a pleasantly warm stimulus becomes painful as a certain threshold temperature is exceeded. However, in the early 1970s it became possible to record from single afferent fibers in peripheral nerves, at which time individual fibers were found that responded only to noxious stimuli (Burgess & Perl, 1973).

Cutaneous receptors that respond selectively to noxious stimuli do not have distinctive terminal specializations as do the receptors for touch. Instead, they are simply free nerve endings located at varying levels within the skin. Some are responsive preferentially to painful mechanical stimuli and are called nociceptors. Others respond well to hot stimuli but not to pressure, while a separate group is multimodal, responding both to noxious mechanical and thermal stimuli (LaMotte, Thalhammer, Torebjork, & Robinson, 1982).

Temperature receptors   Anatomically, receptors sensitive to thermal stimuli are free nerve endings, like nociceptors. Their response properties, however, are quite selective. There are separate receptors for heat and cold, with receptive fields each about 1 mm in diameter (Kenshalo & Duclaux, 1977; Duclaux & Kenshalo, 1980). Hot and cold receptive fields are non-overlapping, creating punctate hot and cold spots on the skin. You can demonstrate cold spots on yourself by gently poking the back of your hand with a pencil point; at certain locations, the point will feel cold. Another illusion that illustrates the presence of localized cold spots is that of paradoxical cold. If a very hot stimulus is applied to a cold spot, the stimulus is not experienced as hot, but as cold. This is because cold receptors have two response ranges, one between temperatures of 10 degrees and 30 degrees C, and another at temperatures above 45 degrees (Long, 1977). At such high temperatures, cold receptors respond with increased activity, and the stimulus is interpreted as cold. The reverse phenomenon also exists: subjects will occasionally report a paradoxically hot sensation when presented with a stimulus that rapidly changes from warm to cold (Hamalainen, Vartiainen, Karvanen, & Jarvilehto, 1982).

Primary Afferent Fibers

The different classes of receptors just discussed transmit their information to the spinal cord by way of primary afferent fibers. In most cases these are simply the axons of the receptor cells themselves; however, at least one receptor type appears to have a peripheral synapse onto a separate primary afferent fiber. Different types of primary afferent fibers carry signals from specific receptor types to specific locations in the spinal cord, with each type transmitting action potentials at a characteristic conduction velocity. As discussed in Chapter 3, axons conduct action potentials at speeds that are direct functions of their diameters. When anatomists looked at the distribution of diameters of primary afferent fibers, they found that four distinct groups of fibers could be isolated. The smallest axons are named C fibers—they are unmyelinated and conduct action potentials slowly, at a rate of about 1 m/sec. A-delta fibers are the next smallest; they are thinly myelinated and conduct at a rate of about 5 to 30 m/sec. A-beta and A-alpha fibers are also myelinated, and their larger diameters allow them to conduct action potentials at rates of 35 to 75 m/sec and 80 to 120 m/sec respectively.

The large variation in primary afferent fiber conduction velocities means that information from peripheral receptors can arrive at the spinal cord at significantly different times. For example, if your toe is pinched and the information is carried along C-fibers, it would take about 1 second for the signal to reach the spinal cord. However, if A-alpha fibers were to carry the signal, the information would reach the spinal cord in about 10 msec, 100 times faster than the C-fibers.

As might be expected, different receptor types do not randomly transmit signals along all fiber types; instead there is an orderly relationship between receptor and type of primary afferent fiber. The receptors of proprioception—muscle spindles and joint receptors—need to send their information to the spinal cord as quickly as possible, so that movements can be coordinated. Accordingly, their signals are transmitted along A-alpha and A-beta fibers. All of the tactile receptors are connected to A-beta fibers as well. In contrast, the free nerve endings that mediate temperature and pain have axons that are either C-fibers or A-delta fibers.

The fact that pain fibers transmit action potentials slower than tactile fibers should correspond to your own personal experience. Everyone has stubbed a toe at some time. At such an unfortunate time, your first sensation is probably a nonpainful sense that your foot had struck something. After a noticeable delay, you start to feel a distinct sense of pain, which often far outlasts the specific feeling of something touching your toe. The delay in the sensation of pain is a direct result of the slow conduction velocities of the C-fibers transmitting the information. The persistence of pain long after the actual stimulus has ceased is due in part to the fact that, in addition to external stimuli, pain receptors also respond to chemical substances released locally into tissues in response to a noxious stimulus. These substances may remain in the area around the pain receptor long after the actual physical stimulus has been removed.

If you have ever stuck yourself with a pin, you may have noticed that different types of pain reach your awareness at different rates. The first pain sensation in response to a pin prick is a quite sharp and well-localized feeling that is easily recognized as pain. This sensation is transmitted to the spinal cord along A-delta fibers. Shortly thereafer, a less well-localized sensation, perhaps best characterized as burning pain, becomes apparent. One reason that the sensation of burning pain comes later than sharp pain is that receptors mediating this feeling transmit information along C-fibers, the slowest conducting primary afferents. As will be seen later, however, this is not the whole story, as the central pathway for burning pain is slower and more circuitous than that for sharp pain.

Central Pathways for Somatic Sensation

We have seen so far that there are different receptor types that selectively respond to different somatic sensations, and that the axons of these receptors can have distinctly different fiber diameters and thus conduction velocities. As we follow the pathways of somatic sensation from the spinal cord to the brain, we will see that the pathways for different kinds of sensations remain distinct. Before starting to describe these pathways, however, we must first know something about the general organization of the spinal cord. The spinal cord is divided into 29 distinct segments. Each segment receives sensory information via a single pair of sensory roots, one from the right and one from the left side of the body. A pair of motor roots goes out from each spinal segment as well. As shown in Figure 20–3, the sensory roots enter the spinal cord on the side of the cord closest to the back. Each sensory root is composed of a large number of primary afferent fibers, the cell bodies of which lie outside of the spinal cord in the *dorsal root ganglion*. The cell bodies located here belong to the peripheral receptors that we discussed earlier in this chapter. Note that, even though the motor fibers from the ventral root also pass near the area of the dorsal root ganglion, their cell bodies are in the spinal cord, not in the ganglion.

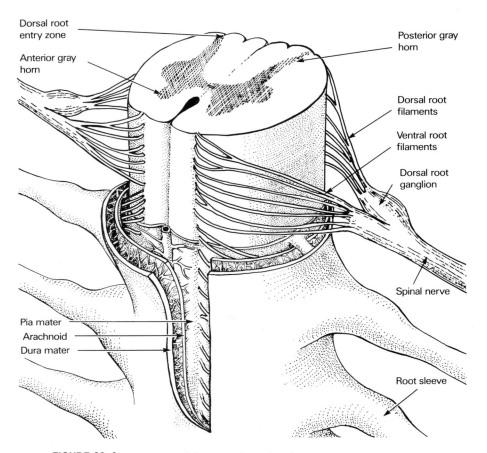

FIGURE 20-3 Drawing of the spinal cord and roots.

A single primary afferent fiber may follow a rather involved route to reach the spinal cord. In the periphery, it joins a peripheral nerve, containing both motor and sensory fibers. This peripheral nerve contains primary afferent fibers that will eventually enter the spinal cord at different segments. As a peripheral nerve gets close to the spinal cord, the sensory and motor fibers separate, and distinct spinal roots are formed.

Each spinal root contains sensory fibers from a certain area of the body. An area of the body that is innervated by a single spinal root is called a *dermatome*. Figure 20–4 shows a map of the dermatomes of the human body. There are 29 dermatomes on each side of the body, one for each pair of spinal roots that enter each segment of the spinal cord. The letters associated with each dermatome refer to the level of the spinal column from which the associated nerve root exits. "C" stands for cervical, "T" for thoracic, "L" for lumbar, and "S" for sacral.

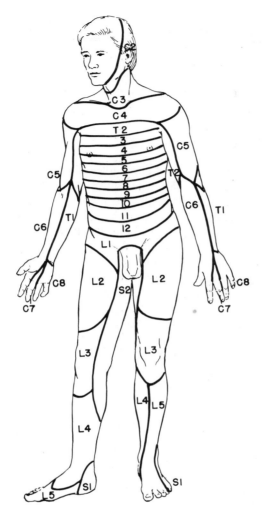

FIGURE 20-4 A dermatome map.

BOX 20-4

You might wonder how a map such as that shown in Figure 20–4 could be produced. There are actually a number of ways experimenters have used, with different methods producing slightly different maps. One way is to examine a large number of patients with a dis-

ease called shingles, caused by the same virus that causes chicken pox. This virus lies dormant in cell bodies of primary afferent fibers, often just in one dorsal root ganglion. For unknown reasons, at certain times the virus becomes activated and travels down the primary

(continued)

---

afferent fibers to the periphery. The area of skin in the region around the affected receptors erupts in a rash known as shingles. The distribution of the rash is precisely the dermatome of the spinal segment from which the virus came. By looking at the rashes of a large number of patients with shingles, maps such as the one in Figure 20–4 are generated.

Once entering the spinal cord in the dorsal root, primary afferent fibers may follow a number of different routes. As is shown in Figure 20–5, fibers can either synapse with spinal cord neurons within the gray matter of the spinal cord, or they can join one of a number of fiber tracts that form the white matter of the cord. Some primary afferent fibers do both; that is, they divide into collateral fibers, one of which synapses in the gray matter, while the other joins a fiber tract and ascends to the brain.

It is convenient to divide the white matter of the spinal cord into two regions. The *posterior columns* consist of the fiber tracts that lie between the two dorsal horns of gray matter, as shown in Figure 20–5. The fibers that lie in this region are mostly those that mediate proprioception and tactile sense. The *anterolateral columns*, which lie mostly along the lateral side of the cord, contain fibers that mediate pain and temperature.

Even from this elementary discussion, it should be clear that sensory input to the spinal cord is exceedingly orderly. Fibers are separated into dermatomes according to their origin on the body surface. Within the cord itself, primary afferent fibers are separated into distinct fiber tracts according to the types of stimuli to which they respond. Armed with this basic information, we can now consider the pathways of somatic sensation.

PATHWAYS FOR PROPRIOCEPTION AND TACTILE SENSATION

As just discussed, the ascending tracts of the spinal cord can be divided into two major systems, the *posterior columns* and the *anterolateral columns*. Fibers that derive from receptors sensitive to tactile sensation and proprioception travel within the spinal cord in the dorsal columns. Figure 20–6 outlines the path that such fibers follow. Primary A-alpha and A-beta fibers enter the spinal cord; they then branch, with one collateral synapsing in the gray matter of the spinal cord, and the other entering the posterior column. Fibers carrying information from the legs comprise the medial part of the column, called the *fasciculus gracilis* (see Figure 20–5). Fibers from the chest and arms enter the lateral aspect of the posterior columns and form the *fasciculus cuneatis*. Both groups of posterior column fibers ascend to the

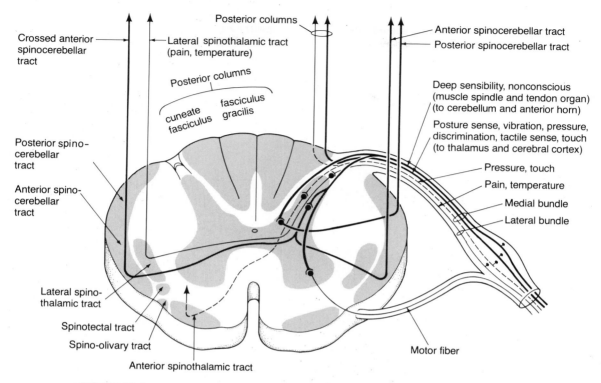

Crossed anterior spinocerebellar tract

Lateral spinothalamic tract (pain, temperature)

Posterior columns

Posterior columns

cuneate fasciculus   fasciculus gracilis

Anterior spinocerebellar tract

Posterior spinocerebellar tract

Deep sensibility, nonconscious (muscle spindle and tendon organ) (to cerebellum and anterior horn)

Posture sense, vibration, pressure, discrimination, tactile sense, touch (to thalamus and cerebral cortex)

Posterior spino-cerebellar tract

Anterior spino-cerebellar tract

Pressure, touch

Pain, temperature

Medial bundle

Lateral bundle

Lateral spino-thalamic tract

Spinotectal tract

Spino-olivary tract

Anterior spinothalamic tract

Motor fiber

FIGURE 20–5 A cross section of the spinal cord, showing the course of sensory fibers entering the cord at the dorsal horn. Fibers are shown entering the spinal cord through the dorsal root and either synapsing in the gray matter of the spinal cord and/or passing directly into an ascending tract. From Duus, P., *Topical Diagnosis in Neurology*, 2nd revised edition. Georg Thieme Verlag, Stuttgart, 1989. Reprinted by permission.

medulla, the part of the brain closest to the spinal cord, where they synapse on secondary neurons in the *gracile* and *cuneate* nuclei. Axons of these neurons ascend to the thalamus in a fiber tract called the *medial lemniscus*. In doing so, they cross from one side of the brain to the other, so that fibers from the left side of the body synapse on neurons in the right thalamus. You should recall that both the lateral and medial geniculate thalamic nuclei, the relay stations for the visual and auditory systems, also receive information from the contralateral side of the body. The thalamic nucleus receiving tactile and proprioceptive information via the medial lemniscus is called the *ventral posterior lateral nucleus*, or VPL. Tactile information from the face is processed in the nearby *ventral posterior medial nucleus*, or VPM.

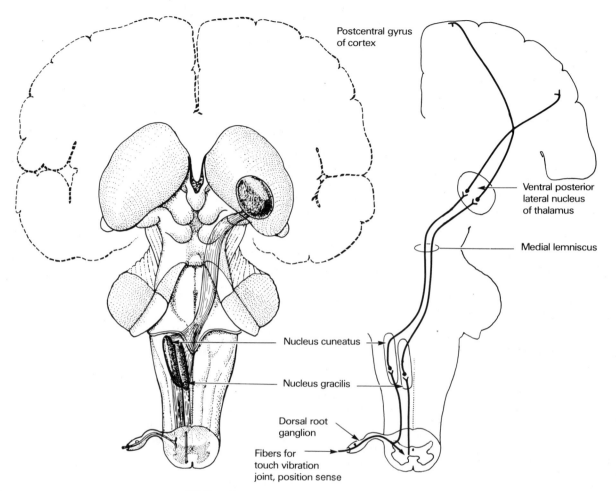

FIGURE 20-6   The course of the dorsal column—medial lemniscus sensory pathway, from receptors to the brain.

BOX 20-5

There are a number of diseases that selectively involve the posterior columns. Fortunately, the late complications of syphilis are much less common than in the days before penicillin; however, central nervous system involvement is still seen in patients who have not been adequately treated. *Tabes Dorsalis* is a form of neurosyphilis characterized by atrophy of the dorsal roots and posterior columns. In its advanced stages, patients with this disease have a markedly unsteady gait because of loss of position sense in the lower extremities. Patients may be able to stand with their eyes open, but, when they close their eyes, they will tend to

(continued)

(box continued)
topple over because of their loss of position sense. Similarly, they may be able to reach for an object fairly accurately under visual guidance, but will make wild flinging movements when their eyes are closed.

Vitamin B12 deficiency is another disease causing damage to the spinal cord. In this disease, peripheral nerves are involved as well, and the first sign may be progressive numbness, starting in the toes and fingertips and progressing toward the trunk. Loss of coordination due to lack of position sense is seen slightly later and is more prominent in the legs than the arms. Although the damage in the spinal cord is not completely limited to the dorsal columns, many of the early symptoms of this disease are due to damage of the spinal tract.

Thalamic fibers from VPL and VPM travel in a fiber tract called the *internal capsule* to the *primary sensory cortex* (S1), located in the *parietal lobe*. Figure 20–7 shows the location of primary sensory cortex on the lateral surface of the brain. Just posterior to S1 is an area that also responds to somatic sensory stimuli, called secondary sensory cortex (S2). This area does not receive direct thalamic input, but instead receives the output of cells from S1. Secondary sensory cortex is concerned with more complicated aspects of somatic perception, and lesions in this area have been shown to interfere with learning new tactile discriminations (Randolph & Semmes, 1974).

Primary sensory cortex has much in common with both primary auditory and primary visual cortex. First, tactile sense from the contralateral side of the body is represented in sensory cortex. Second, there is an orderly representation of one side of the body onto the surface of the brain. This projection of the body onto sensory cortex is called the *homunculus*, meaning little man (Figure 20–7). The first thing you will probably notice about the homunculus is that it looks like no human body you have ever seen. The face, lips, and hands are huge compared to the feet, legs, and trunk. This increased size of certain parts of the body corresponds to the increased tactile sensitivity of those areas as compared to other parts represented on smaller areas of cortex. You can make much finer sensory discriminations with your fingertips and lips than you can when stimuli are presented on your belly or legs.

BOX 20–6

The experimental data used to construct the homunculus in Figure 20–7 were obtained in a very interesting way. Wilder Penfield, a Canadian neurosurgeon, was a pioneer in surgical removal of epileptic foci in the brain as a treatment for intractable epilepsy. He performed surgery on patients who were anesthetized only with local anesthetic. Local anesthesia was used so that the patient could communicate and move voluntarily, allowing Dr. Penfield to

(continued)

(box continued)

avoid specific brain areas crucial for movement and speech. Since the brain itself has no specialized pain receptors, this was not unduly unpleasant for the patient.

Before removing a part of the brain he believed might be responsible for the patient's epileptic seizures, Dr. Penfield would gently stimulate that area with a mild electric shock. When he did this in areas of S1, patients would report various tactile sensations in particular areas on the contralateral side of the body. By stimulating systematically throughout S1, Penfield was able to generate a map of the projection of various parts of the body onto the brain.

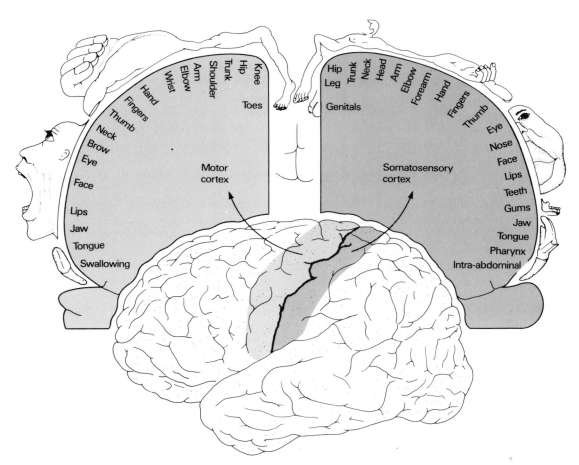

FIGURE 20–7   Human primary sensory cortex, A view of the surface of the brain, showing the location of motor and sensory cortex.

Human beings use their fingertips and hands to make most fine discriminations, so it makes sense that our sensory cortex should selectively emphasize sensory input from that part of our body. However, what about somatotopic maps from other animals for whom tactile information from the
forelimbs is not so important? Figure 20–8 displays what the homunculi
might look like for a rabbit, a cat, and a monkey. The most striking difference
between the cat, the rabbit, and the human is the lack of magnification of the
sensory input from the forelimb in the two lower animals. Instead, sensory
input from the face—especially the whiskers—is emphasized much more
than in human cortex. The homunculus for the monkey much more closely
approximates that of man, except that the hands still receive much less magnification.

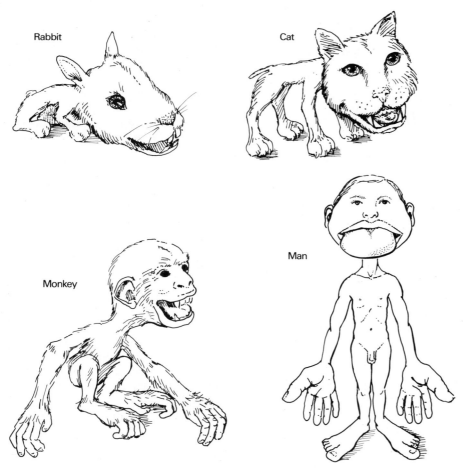

FIGURE 20-8   ''Homunculi'' for different types of animals.

The responses of single cells in primary sensory cortex have been studied in much the same way Hubel and Wiesel studied single cells in the visual system. In fact, recordings from single cortical neurons were made from sensory cortex considerably before single cells were studied in the visual cortex. Such recordings have in general verified the somatotopic organization that Penfield described. However, more detailed studies have shown that, instead of one homunculus, there are four distinct somatotopic maps in primary sensory cortex (Kaas, Merzenich, & Killackey, 1983). These maps correspond well to four areas of S1 that have been identified by anatomical methods. The areas have been creatively named 1, 2, 3a, and 3b by an anatomist named Brodmann, who divided the entire cortex into more than 40 separate areas (Brodmann, 1909). The maps are parallel to one another, which explains why Penfield (see preceding box) found only a single representation.

The four somatotopic maps differ from one another in the kind of stimuli that produce the best responses (Kaas, Merzenich, & Killackey, 1979). Cells in area 1 seem primarily sensitive to stimulation of rapidly adapting skin receptors, while those in area 2 respond best to deep pressure. Area 3a receives most of its input from muscle stretch receptors, while 3b responds to cutaneous stimulation of both transient and sustained types. This selectivity of different parts of cortex is not absolute; within any one map, cells can be found that respond to all modalities. However, it does demonstrate that the stimulus selectively of different receptor types is maintained throughout the somatic pathway.

The different functions of the four somatotopic maps in S1 were illustrated in an interesting way by Randolph and Semmes (1974). They made precise lesions in the cortices of monkeys, waited for the animals to recover, and then studied how differently placed lesions affected their behavior. Lesions in area 1 interfered with an animal's ability to make discriminations based on the texture of objects. In contrast, animals with lesions in area 2 could not accurately assess the sizes and shapes of objects. Lesions in area 3 prevented the monkeys from discriminating size, shape, or texture.

In addition to demonstrating the multiplicity of somatotopic maps in S1, single-cell recording techniques have provided more precise information about the response properties of individual cells. Cells in sensory cortex have receptive fields that are similar in many ways to those of cells in the visual system. They have well-defined receptive fields; that is, a given cell will respond only to stimulation of a circumscribed area of the body. They also exhibit spatial antagonism; stimulation of the central area of a cell's receptive field will result in excitation, while stimulation of the surrounding area will cause inhibition of the response (Mountcastle, 1957; Mountcastle & Darien-Smith, 1968). This center/surround organization is precisely analogous to that seen in retinal ganglion cells. Lateral antagonism in the somatic sensory system has the same function that it does in the visual system; it allows for enhanced discrimination between neighboring stimuli.

Receptive fields of cells in primary sensory cortex vary greatly in size.

Cells that respond to stimulation of the legs and trunk have receptive fields that are several square centimeters in area. In contrast, cells that respond to stimulation of the fingertips have receptive fields that are up to 100 times smaller. This variation in receptive field size correlates quite well with the relative magnification of the face and fingers on the homunculus in Figure 20–7. That is, cortical cells with the smallest receptive fields are those located in areas of the brain where the body surface is most magnified. Thus, both cortical magnification and variation in receptive field size combine to produce greater discriminative ability in the face and hands than in other parts of the body.

Some receptive fields have more complicated receptive fields than simple center/surround antagonism. Several groups of experimenters (Costanzo & Gardner, 1980; Hyvarinen & Poranen, 1978) have described cells that respond when an object is swept in a certain direction across the skin. However, when the object is moved in another direction, the cell responds either with inhibition or fails to respond at all. Figure 20–9 shows examples of responses of direction-specific neurons. The behavior of such cells should remind you of complex cells in visual cortex.

Another way in which visual and primary sensory cortex are similar is the overall way in which neurons are organized. Remember from Chapter 8 that

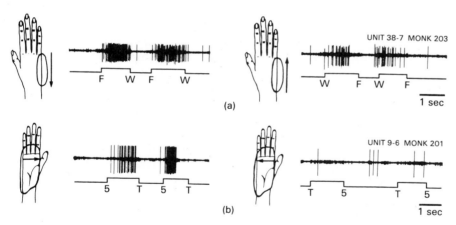

FIGURE 20-9   The direction sensitivity of two different neurons in primary sensory cortex. In (a), the receptive field of the cell is along the side of the hand; movement in either longitudinal direction evokes a response. The cell in (b) responds to movement in only one direction. From Costanzo, R. M., and E. P. Gardner (1980) A quantitative analysis of responses of direction sensitive neurons in somatosensory cortex of awake monkeys. *J. Neurophysiol.* 43: 1319–1341. Copyright 1980 by the American Physiological Society. Reprinted by permission.

visual cells were organized into columns; when Hubel and Wiesel advanced their electrodes through the cortex, they found that successive cells they encountered were similar both in their ocular dominance and in their preferred orientation. Similarly, S1 is also organized into discrete columns (Mountcastle, 1957; Kaas, Nelson, Sur, Lin, & Merzenich, 1979). If a given cortical cell close to the surface of the brain responds best to stimulation of rapidly adapting receptors, then the cells directly underneath will show the same selectivity. As one moves from one somatotopic map to another the relative widths of columns vary. For example, in area 1, columns of cells responsive to rapidly adapting receptors predominate, while in area 3a, columns of cells that respond to muscle stretch are relatively larger.

Perception of Shapes

We have been talking about proprioception as if feeling were a matter of passively allowing things to press against the skin. But feeling is an active process, in which the fingers are moved across the object, much as the eyes scan a visual scene. Just as the visual system must take account of the eye movements, so the proprioceptive system must "know" about (and perhaps make use of) the limb and finger movements.

Not coincidentally, it was one of the foremost theorists of visual perception, J. J. Gibson, who first noted the difference between passive and active feeling (Gibson, 1962). He asked subjects to determine the shapes of cookie cutters that were felt but not seen. The subjects did very well if allowed to run their hands across the shapes, but did poorly when the experimenter simply pressed the shapes against their hands.

We should note, however, that this difference may be due to the motion of the palpated shapes across the skin (Schwartz, Perey, & Azulay, 1975). Just as visual stimuli fade if they do not change (see Chapter 7), pressure stimuli undergo adaptation (Nafe & Wagoner, 1941). If the stimulus does not change, it eventually ceases to be sensed. If you place your hand in a bowl of water, you will experience another example of somatosensory adaptation. Very quickly, you will lose the awareness of your hand being surrounded by water that is likely to be of much different temperature than the air. The only place you will sense the difference is at the interface between air and water, perhaps because of small movements that continually change the location of the interface on your skin.

It is not surprising that there are interactions between proprioception and kinesthesis. There are also interactions between proprioception and vision. If you pick up two weights, you can judge that they weigh the same, or that one is heavier, with reasonable accuracy (remember Weber's Law, discussed in Chapter 2). However, if the two weights are of different sizes, your judgment will be affected. In general, you will judge the physically smaller of two equal weights to be heavier (Stevens & Rubin, 1970).

PAIN

The Anterolateral System

We have already seen that the receptors that respond to pain and temperature are distinct from those mediating other somatic sensations. This segregation is maintained within the spinal cord. The free nerve endings that are the receptors for pain and/or temperature transmit their responses to the cord along the smallest diameter primary afferent fibers, A-delta and C-fibers. These fibers enter the spinal cord via the dorsal root, and synapse on neurons within the gray matter of the spinal cord. Most of these second-order neurons send their axons across to the other side of the spinal cord, where they ascend to the brain as the anterolateral system. About 15% of these second-order neurons do not cross the midline but join the anterolateral system on the ipsilateral side.

Already, two important differences should be apparent between the anterolateral system and the dorsal column system. First, the axons in the dorsal columns are branches of primary afferent fibers themselves, while fibers in the anterolateral system are axons of second-order neurons. Second, while the dorsal columns consist of fibers that have not crossed the midline, most fibers in the anterolateral system have already crossed.

BOX 20–7

This second difference between the anterolateral and posterior column tracts is illustrated by a clinical picture seen after some types of spinal cord injuries. If either the right or left side of the spinal cord is damaged by trauma, a combination of deficits known as a *Brown-Sequard Syndrome* results. If, for example, the right side of the spinal cord is damaged, the right posterior columns obviously will be affected. This will produce a loss of touch and position sense on the right side of the body below the level of the injury. The anterolateral system on the right side of the cord will also be damaged; however, since this system has predominantly crossed, pain and temperature sensations will be reduced on the left side of the body, starting several spinal dermatomes below the site of the injury. This loss of pain and temperature on one side of the body, with loss of position sense and touch on the other side of the body, is an unfortunate but striking demonstration of the difference in spinal cord organization of the two somatic sensory pathways.

One other important difference between the two major somatic sensory systems is that, while the dorsal columns consist of a single fiber tract, the anterolateral system actually is composed of three distinct tracts. These different tracts mediate quite different types of pain perception. Remember our discussion of what happens when you accidentally stick yourself with a pin. The first feeling that you get will be a sensation of sharpness, or stinging. If you thought about it, you would probably classify that sensation as painful, but not particularly emotionally disturbing or even very unpleasant. Immediately thereafter, however, comes a more poorly localized burning pain that is much more disturbing than the initial sensation. The first sensation is called "fast pain" and is mediated by the *spinothalamic tract*, the largest fiber tract within the anterolateral system (see Figure 20–5). This tract receives its input from the relatively rapidly conducting A-delta fibers. Most spinothalamic fibers cross the midline of the spinal cord, and ascend to the thalamus (Figure 20–10). There they synapse in the same nucleus as did fibers from the posterior column system, the VPL nucleus. Cells from VPL that receive their input from the spinothalamic tract do not also respond to stimulation of the dorsal columns; the segregation of painful and tactile sensation is maintained within the thalamus. It is also maintained in S1, where the axons of VPL neurons project.

The other two fiber tracts within the anterolateral system are called the *spinoreticular* and *spinomesencephalic tracts*. Together, they mediate the sensation of temperature and burning pain previously described. Their primary input is from the much slower conducting C-fibers. While some second order neurons cross the midline like the spinothalamic tract, a much larger percentage remain on the ipsilateral side of the spinal cord during their ascent to the brainstem. Once reaching the brainstem, rather than synapsing directly in the thalamus, most fibers from the spinoreticular and spinomesencephalic tracts synapse in a poorly defined area called the *reticular formation*. This is a large area in the center of the brainstem extending from the medulla all the way to the thalamus. Within the reticular formation, many synapses are made; eventually, information about burning pain reaches the *central lateral* (CL) nucleus, an area of the thalamus that seems selectively pain sensitive (Giesler, Yezierski, Gerhart, & Willis, 1981). Axons of CL neurons project diffusely throughout the cortex, as well as to many areas of the brainstem.

When electrical recordings are made from single fibers in the anterolateral system, a number of classes of cells can be distinguished. Within the spinothalamic tract, the majority of fibers respond briskly to noxious thermal or mechanical stimuli, but not at all to nonpainful stimuli. These cells have been named "high threshold" (HT) cells. Another group responds to both innocuous and painful stimuli, and are called "wide dynamic range" (WDR) cells (Willis, 1981). Figure 20–11 shows a comparison of the responses of WDR and HT cells to a range of stimuli.

Cells in the spinothalamic tract can also be distinguished according to the size of their receptive fields. While most cells have quite discrete receptive fields, some cells in the spinothalamic tract have been found whose receptive fields extend to virtually the entire body surface (Giesler, Yezierski, Gerhart, & Willis, 1981). An example of one such cell is shown in Figure 20–12. Most of these cells respond only to noxious stimuli, and therefore can be classified as HT cells.

Within the VPL nucleus of the thalamus, the majority of cells seem to

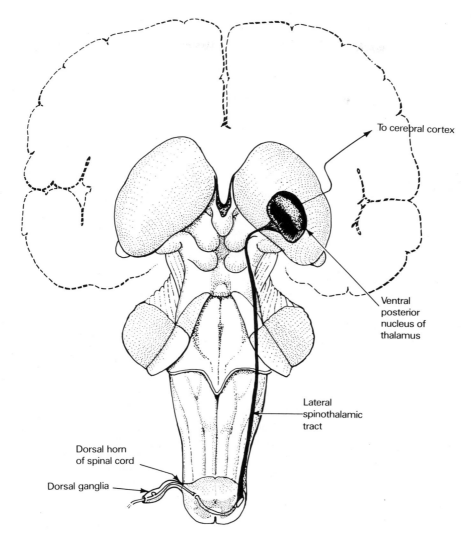

FIGURE 20-10 The lateral spinothalamic tract, from receptor to brain.

respond to tactile stimuli rather than nociceptive stimuli. However, some cells can be found that have responses similar to cells of the spinothalamic tract (Kenshalo, Giesler, Leonard, & Willis, 1980). Both WDR and HT cells have been found, with receptive field sizes that are quite similar to those of spinothalamic tract cells.

Nociceptive-specific cells have also been found in primary somatosensory cortex. Just as there are distinct columns of cells that respond to stimulation of rapidly adapting and slowly adapting tactile receptors, so there are columns of cells that respond selectively to nociceptive input (Lamour,

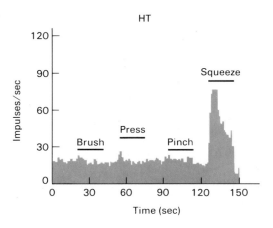
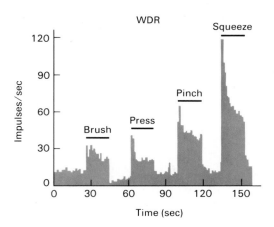

FIGURE 20-11 Responses of an HT and a WDR cell to different types of stimuli. The HT cell responds only minimally to all stimuli except a strong squeeze, to which it briskly reacts. The WDR cell responds with graded excitation to all stimuli, with response level increasing as strength of stimulation increases. From Willis, W. D. (1981) Ascending pathways from the dorsal horn. In *Spinal cord sensation: Sensory processing in the dorsal horn.* Brown, A. A., and M. Rethelyi (Eds) Edinburgh: Scottish Academic Press. Reprinted by permission.

Guilbark, & Willer, 1983). Within the nociceptive columns the majority of cells have response properties that are quite similar to nociceptive cells in the thalamus (Kenshalo & Isensee, 1983). However, in addition to cells with discrete, contralateral receptive fields, some cells have been found that have large, often bilateral receptive fields. It is interesting to consider what function such cells might have in the perception of pain. They are not likely to be useful in discriminating the precise location of the painful stimulus—cells with smaller receptive fields would do that job much better. Most of the cells with large receptive fields are WDR cells, so they are also not likely to help in determining the actual nature of a painful stimulus. Instead, these cells, as well as cells with large receptive fields in the thalamus, may be important in determining the affective or emotional response to painful stimuli, as well as in the central control of pain perception. As we shall see in the next section, the actual perception of a painful stimulus can be modulated greatly by a descending inhibitory system.

Central Inhibition of Pain Perception

As we have tried to make clear throughout this book, it is a general rule for all perceptual systems that one's perception of a given stimulus is not a direct copy of the stimulus. Instead, there is an often complex interaction between

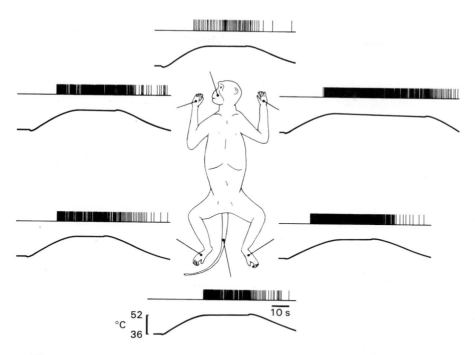

FIGURE 20-12 Responses of a spinothalamic tract neuron to stimulation of various locations on the monkey's body. A brisk response is generated by stimulation almost anywhere on the body surface. From Giesler, G. J., R. P. Yezierski, K. K. Gerhart, and W. D. Willis (1981) Spinothalamic tract neurons that project to medial and/or lateral thalamic nuclei: Evidence for a physiologically novel population of spinal cord neurons. *J. Neurophysiol.* 46: 1285–1308. Copyright 1981 by the American Physiological Society. Reprinted by permission.

the response of the peripheral receptors to a specific stimulus, the state of activation of neighboring receptors, and one's state of arousal or attention that determines the final percept. The color of a visual stimulus depends not only on the wavelength of the stimulus itself, but on the background as well. Similarly, a stimulus that is normally perceived as painful may feel quite different if other cutaneous receptors are stimulated simultaneously. This fact has been known for many years and underlies a number of methods, both ancient and modern, for reducing pain. The expression "bite the bullet" is a familiar one; it refers to times past when cowboys would bite on a bullet while an arrow was being removed. People realized that the perception of pain could be dulled, if only slightly, by the presence of a strong second stimulus.

BOX 20–8

A more modern example of how pain can be lessened by extraneous stimuli is the use of transcutaneous electrical stimulation in the treatment of chronic pain syndromes. A machine called a transepidermal nerve stimulation unit (TENS) provides low-level electrical current to the skin, usually close to the site of chronic pain. A number of studies have demonstrated that such stimulation significantly reduces the level of perceived pain (Warfield, Stein, & Frank, 1985; Hansson & Ekblom, 1983). This reduction in pain level often persists for hours after the TENS unit is turned off.

In 1965, Melzack and Wall proposed a theory of analgesia to account for these kinds of phenomena. In their model, both myelinated nonnociceptive fibers and unmyelinated C-fibers directly excite second order transmission cells. However, myelinated fibers also excite an interneuron within the dorsal horn, while unmyelinated pain fibers inhibit this same interneuron. Activity of the interneuron inhibits activity of the transmission cell. Thus, activity of the pain fiber alone will excite the transmission cell directly, and will act to inhibit the interneuron, also indirectly resulting in excitation. If the myelinated fiber is simultaneously stimulated, output of the transmission cell will be reduced through stimulation of the inhibitory interneuron. Thus, nonpainful stimulation will reduce the response of the transmission cell to nociceptive input. This theory has been dubbed the Gate Control hypothesis of analgesia.

The Gate Control theory easily explains the reduction in perceived pain produced by simultaneous, nonpainful cutaneous stimulation, such as that produced by TENS units (see previous box). More evidence in support of the theory comes from studies where myelinated sensory fibers are selectively inactivated. Under these conditions, noxious stimuli are perceived as more painful than when the myelinated fibers are functioning normally (Price, Hu, Dubner, & Gracely, 1977). The most direct explanation of this phenomenon is that activity of myelinated fibers exerts an inhibitory effect on pain transmission.

In addition to peripheral mechanisms of altering pain perception, the brain also exerts powerful descending influences to reduce pain under certain circumstances. This descending system can be demonstrated in a number of different ways. If one electrically stimulates particular areas within the brainstem, an analgesic effect will be produced (Hosobuchi, Adams, & Linchitz, 1977; Richardson & Akil, 1977). This phenomenon is called stimulation produced analgesia (SPA), and has proved to be useful in the treatment of patients with severe, intractable pain. Electrodes are surgically implanted into patients with this sort of pain, and small electric impulses are provided periodically throughout the day. Patients report a slow fading of their pain over several minutes after the onset of SPA, sometimes associated with a feeling of relaxation or well-being. Reactivity to nonpainful stimuli is preserved, and patients are able to perform normal intellectual functions.

The areas in the brain where SPA can be produced constitute a system for the central control of pain. Many experiments have been performed to map this system, which begins in the center of the brainstem just below the thalamus and extends downward to the medulla (Fields, 1987). The areas in which SPA is most effective have neurons whose axons project downward in the spinal cord and synapse in the dorsal horn onto or nearby to nociceptive primary afferents. Thus, it appears that SPA works by activating a preexisting system for pain control.

Another way in which scientists have studied the brain's ability to modulate the level of pain perception has been through the study of opiate analgesics. (Analgesia means the removal of pain.) Drugs such as heroin and morphine have been known for years to possess powerful analgesic properties. Over the last 20 years, a growing body of evidence has accumulated supporting the idea that this class of analgesics (called opiate analgesics because they are derived from the opium poppy) acts by exerting a specific excitatory effect on a class of brain receptors named opioid receptors. If one injects very small amounts of morphine into specific brain areas, a striking degree of analgesia is produced (Yaksh, 1978). Not coincidentally, the areas where morphine exerts its strongest effects are the same areas where electrical stimulation also produces analgesia. Both the analgesia produced by morphine and that produced by electrical stimulation can be abolished by pretreatment by naloxone, a drug with a chemical structure related to morphine (Akil, Mayer, & Liebeskind, 1976). Thus, the analgesia produced by either stimulus seems to result from stimulation of the same system in the brain.

Because of the specificity with which morphine and other opiates exert their effects, as well as the ability of drugs like naloxone to inhibit those effects, it was hypothesized that some neurons within the brain possessed receptors that were specifically sensitive to opioids. In fact, such receptors have recently been isolated, and have been found to be distributed in the brain in the same areas where electric stimulation produces analgesia (Snyder, 1980; Simon, Hiller, & Edelman, 1973). The ability of naloxone to inhibit the effects of morphine was found to be due to the fact that naloxone binds to opiate receptors without exciting them, thus rendering them inexcitable by opiate drugs.

Why should the brain possess receptors specifically for a class of drugs related to the opium poppy? The answer turns out to be quite simple; within the brain, there are endogenous substances, chemically related to opiate drugs, whose functions are to activate the brain's system for analgesia. The reason that opiate drugs are effective is that they are so similar to these endogenous chemicals. The first endogenous opiates to be discovered were called enkephalins (Hughes, Smith, Kosterlitz, Fothergill, Morgan, & Morris, 1975). Shortly thereafter, a different class of chemical, beta endorphin, derived from the hormone propiomelanocortin, was also found to stimulate opiate receptors (Herbert, Oates, Martens, Comb, & Rosen, 1983). More recently, over twenty different proteinlike substances have been isolated from brain tissue that are active at opiate receptor sites. Different subclasses of opiate receptors have also been isolated, each with slightly different actions when activated (Martin, 1984).

BOX 20–9

If pain makes sense because it forces us to deal with dangerous stimuli, why have an elaborate system to block it? Perhaps it is because the pain would interfere with other important activities even after we did all we could about the danger.

When an animal is stressed, it becomes less sensitive to painful stimuli. Maier, Drugan, and Grau (1982) showed that this effect was

greater when rats were subjected to painful shocks that they could not avoid than to pain that could be avoided (by running in a wheel).

This makes sense—if the pain cannot be avoided, hurting serves no purpose, but if the pain can be avoided, let it hurt so the animal will get away from it. This kind of pain alleviation is mediated by the opiate system.

To summarize, these data suggest that the brain possesses a descending system for modulating the perception of pain. This system can be directly activated by electrical stimulation of the central areas of the brainstem, or by use of morphinelike substances. The brain itself activates this system through a class of neurotransmitters called endogenous opiates. There are a number of situations where this descending system can be demonstrated. You have probably heard of the placebo effect, where a subject is given an inert "sugar pill" with some specific function ascribed to it, and subjectively experiences an improvement in symptoms. If such a placebo is given for the purpose of pain relief, subjects will report that their pain is decreased. However, if subjects are either pretreated with naloxone or given naloxone after the placebo, they will report an increase in their level of pain (Grevert, Albert, & Goldstein, 1983). Since naloxone's only known effect is to block the activity of the endogenous opiate system, the experiments just described suggest that placebos work by causing increased release of endogenous opiates within the brain to activate the brain's descending system of analgesia.

SUGGESTED READINGS

An excellent in-depth treatment of the sensory systems for touch and pain can be found in *Principles of Neural Science*, edited by E. R. Kandel and J. H. Schwartz (Elsivier, 1986). Chapters 23 through 26 discuss the structure and function of the somatosensory system from receptor to brain.

THE CHEMICAL SENSES: TASTE AND SMELL

21

INTRODUCTION

The senses of taste and smell provide us with a slightly different look at how the brain processes sensory information. The sensory systems we have discussed previously can be examined without having to refer to parts of the brain involved with nonsensory processing. While the information we receive from other senses certainly affects behavior, we have been able to discuss them in relative isolation. In contrast, both the gustatory and olfactory systems are intimately related to parts of the brain that mediate learning, as well as the primary drives of hunger and sex. As a consequence, when we discuss how chemical stimuli are processed, we will also have to consider their effects on specific behaviors.

Another difference between the chemical senses of taste and smell and the other sensory systems is that it is more difficult to describe the components of the stimulus important for our perception of it. The relevant aspects of a visual stimulus are its luminance, color, and spatial distribution—not surprising when a little bit about the physics of light is known. In contrast, philosophers and scientists have argued for centuries about what constitutes the primary qualities of smell and taste. The difficulty in defining what about the stimulus is important for sensation has had a great effect on how the chemical senses have been studied through the years.

TASTE (GUSTATION)

Anatomy of the Gustatory Pathway

Taste receptors are located primarily on the tongue, but are also found on the soft palate and other structures in the back of the throat. They are part of a sensory organ called a *taste bud*, which consists of about 50 receptor cells in close association with two other cell types called *supporting cells* and *basal cells*. Figure 21–1 shows a view of a taste bud—all three cell types are tightly arranged in a flasklike structure with a pore that opens onto the surface of the tongue; the receptor cells tend to be at the center of the taste bud while the supporting cells lie peripherally. At the tip of each receptor are small processes called microvilli extending through the opening pore and directly contacting the saliva in the mouth. Substances that produce taste stimulate the taste receptors by contacting the microvilli at the taste bud pore. Taste receptors have a life span of about 10 days, and are constantly being replaced by new receptors generated by mitotic division of the supporting cells (Pfaffman, 1978), and which migrate inward toward the center of the taste bud.

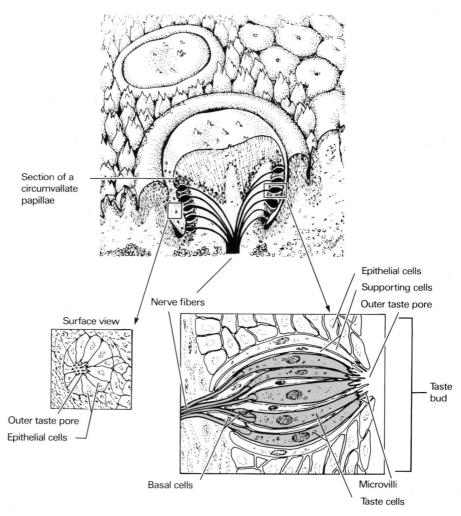

FIGURE 21-1 Schematic drawing of a taste bud within a circumvallate papillae. The top portion of the figure shows the location of the taste buds within the papillae, while the bottom figures show the taste bud itself.

Since taste receptors come from specialized epithelial cells (the supporting cells), they are not considered true neurons.

You may have noticed from personal experience that certain parts of the tongue are more sensitive to taste than others, so it is no surprise that taste buds are concentrated in specific areas. If you look at your own tongue in the mirror, you will notice that there are many small protruberances distributed along the edge. These are called papillae, and contain clusters of taste buds (see Figure 21–2). Fungiform papillae are the most numerous, and are found all along the edge of the tongue. Foliate and circumvallate papillae are found at the back of the tongue; the taste buds found in these papillae probably respond to different kinds of taste stimuli than those located in the fungiform papillae.

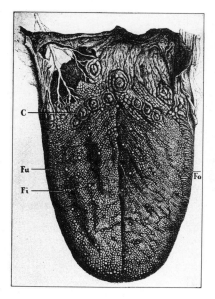
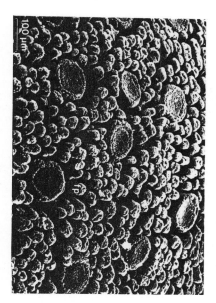

FIGURE 21–2   (a) Drawing of human tongue with different types of papillae. Those marked C are circumvallate, Fu are fungiform, Fi are filiform, and F o are F oliate. From Warren, H. C., and L. Carmichael, (1930) *Elements of Human Psychology*. Boston: Houghton Mifflin. (b) Scanning electron micrograph of the surface of a frog tongue with filiform papillae. From Graziadei, P., and R. S. Dehan (1971). The ultrastructure of frogs taste organs. *Acta Anat.* 80:563–603. New York: S. Karger AG, Basel. Reprinted by permission.

The receptor cells do not have axons of their own that carry taste information to the brain. Instead, they make synapses at the bottom of the taste bud with nerve fibers that project into the brainstem. A single nerve fiber will synapse with many individual taste receptors from an average of two different taste buds (Beidler, 1978). The taste fibers extend from the tongue and mouth areas to the brain as components of three large nerves, called the *facial, glossopharyngeal*, and *vagus* nerves. Fibers from all three nerves synapse in a part of the brainstem called the *solitary nucleus* (see Figure 21–3). From there, taste fibers travel in one of two directions. The majority of fibers ascend the brainstem to the *ventral posterior medial nucleus* (VPM) of the thalamus. Remember that the thalamus is the primary sensory relay station

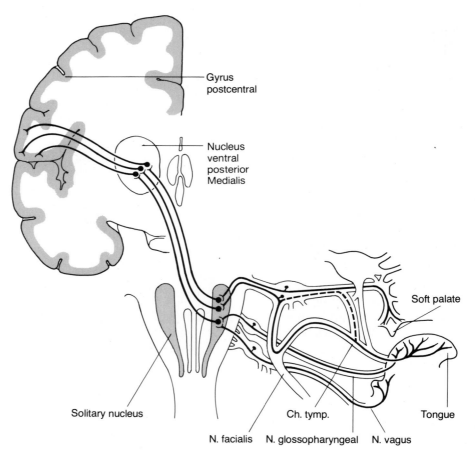

FIGURE 21-3   Diagram of the neuroanatomical pathway of taste fibers. Heavy lines show the paths most commonly seen. Most fibers travel from the chorda tympani (Ch. tymp.) to the facial nerve; other fibers travel in the vagus and glossopharyngeal nerves. From Brodal, A. (1981) *Neurological Anatomy*, 3rd Edition. New York: Oxford University Press. Reprinted by permission.

for all of the sensory systems we have discussed before. In fact, the VPM nucleus is also the sensory relay station for fibers from the somatosensory system that carry touch, pain, and temperature information from the face and mouth. Both fibers carrying taste information and fibers carrying somatosensory information travel from VPM to primary sensory cortex (S1). Not surprisingly, the area of sensory cortex sensitive to taste stimuli lies close to the area subserving touch, pain, and temperature sensations from the mouth and tongue.

BOX 21–1

The pathway just described is similar in many respects to the sensory pathways discussed for the visual, auditory, and somatosensory systems. There is an obligatory synapse at the thalamus, and from there, a monosynaptic relay to S1. However, some taste fibers from the solitary nucleus take an alternate route to the *amygdala* and *hypothalamus*, both of which are part of an area of the brain called the *limbic system* (Ricardo & Koh, 1978). This part of the brain has many complicated functions, but is particularly important for emotional responses and reward systems. One of the major differences between the chemical senses and the other sensory systems is the strong emotional responses that can be associated with gustatory and olfactory stimuli, so the fact that the sensory system for taste has a direct projection into this area is notable.

Psychophysics of Taste

In our discussions of the other sensory systems, it was possible to describe the basic qualities of the sensory stimulus that determined how the stimulus was perceived. For example, once we knew the frequency and intensity of a given auditory stimulus, the subjective perception could be fairly well predicted. What are the primary qualities for a gustatory stimulus? This question has been discussed since the time of Aristotle (384–322 B.C.), who proposed that there were seven basic taste qualities: sweet, bitter, sour, salty, astringent, pungent, and harsh (Bartoshuk, 1978). He felt that all other tastes could be produced by appropriate combinations of these qualities. The idea that combinations of primary sensory qualities could evoke seemingly different perceptions should be a familiar one; it is analogous to the theory of visual trichromacy discussed in Chapter 15.

The assumption that all tastes could be produced by a combination of a limited number of primary taste sensations has been accepted with little challenge since then, with arguments on this subject being devoted to what the primary taste qualities actually are. There has been consistent agreement that the qualities of sweet, sour, bitter, and salty represent primary modalities; however, the number and nature of other primary tastes has been vigorously debated. For example, Haller (1786) proposed that seven other qualities also required inclusion: rough, urinous, spirituous, aromatic, acrid, putrid, and insipid.

One of the first people to propose that all tastes could be produced by combinations of just four primaries was Kiesow (1896), a student of Wilhelm Wundt. He used sodium chloride (table salt), hydrochloric acid, sucrose, and quinine as stimuli that would produce pure sensations of salty, sour, sweet, and bitter. With combinations of these substances, he was able to produce a wide variety of different taste sensations. This observation was confirmed and extended by Henning (1927).

The hypothesis that taste quality is determined by the combined activity of four different channels that are each tuned to one of the four primary taste modalities is still viable today. Supporting this hypothesis is the fact that different areas of the tongue are selectively sensitive to different taste qualities. The tip of the tongue is quite sensitive to sweet stimuli but relatively insensitive to bitter and sour. The sides of the front part of the tongue are most responsive to salty stimuli (Pfaffmann, 1978), while sour is tasted best along the sides of the back part of the tongue. Bitter stimuli are tasted best on the back of the tongue and on the soft palate (Yamamoto & Kawamura, 1972). Most of the top surface of the tongue responds poorly to taste stimuli; this corresponds to the fact that there are very few taste buds on this part of the tongue.

Although there is much overlap, the different types of papillae seem to be preferentially sensitive to different stimuli. Figure 21–2(a) shows the approximate distribution of the different papillae on the human tongue. The fungiform papillae predominate along the circumference of the front part of the tongue. In this region are areas of sensitivity to sweet, salty, and sour stimuli, but bitter stimuli are not tasted well. The area along the surface of the back of the tongue, where bitter stimuli such as quinine are tasted best, is also the area where the circumvallate papillae predominate. Sour stimuli are tasted well over areas of the tongue that have a high density of any kind of papillae. Since the receptor cells of a given taste bud all have similar response characteristics, these data would suggest that different types of taste buds predominate in different types of papillae.

More evidence that taste is processed by four independent channels comes from experiments demonstrating that each of the four primary tastes can be adapted separately from each other. For example, subjects presented with a strong acid stimulus (for example, sour) for two minutes will become less sensitive to the taste of sour substances (Abrahams, Krakauer, & Dallenbach, 1937; Krakauer & Dallenbach, 1937; McBurney, Smith, & Shick, 1972). Similarly, adaptation to sugar reduces the sweetness of other sweet substances (McBurney, 1972), and chronic presentation of sodium chloride makes other salty stimuli seem less so (Smith & McBurney, 1969). This phenomenon is exactly analogous to adaptation in the visual system. For example, staring at a green object for several minutes will lower one's sensitivity to that color; because of the opponent processing of the human visual system, one will actually see a red afterimage after the object is removed. In the case of adaptation to a sour stimulus, the subject's taste threshold is raised both to restimulation by the same sour substance and to other sour tastes.

BOX 21-2 ∎

A similar phenomenon to taste adaptation is water taste. By appropriately combining primary taste stimuli, each of the four primary tastes can be perceived simply by drinking water (McBurney & Gent, 1979). Water taste is not as predictable as taste adaptation. If one adapts to a sweet stimulus, water will taste sour or bitter, while salt adaptation produces a similar sour/bitter taste. However, adapting to sour or bitter stimuli will produce a sweet water taste. Even more confusing, eating artichokes will make water taste sweet as well, even though there is no obvious bitter adapting taste (Bartoshuk, Lee, & Scarpolino, 1972).

Although the water tastes produced by adaptation to specific gustatory stimuli seem idiosyncratic, the evoked tastes combine additively with directly evoked tastes. Thus, if a sweet water taste is evoked by sour or bitter adapting stimuli, concurrent sweet stimuli will taste even sweeter (McBurney & Bartoshuk, 1973).

Another dramatic demonstration that different taste qualities are processed through independent channels comes from the use of taste-altering substances. If an extract from the plant *Gymnema sylvestre* is chewed, one selectively loses the capacity to appreciate sweet tastes. This is true whether sweetness is tested with sucrose or with an artificial sweetner such as saccharin. It is as if the activity from receptors sensitive to sweet tastes were completely abolished. This effect can also be demonstrated physiologically. Figure 21–4 shows the combined responses of many taste-sensitive nerve fibers to stimulation by the different primary tastes as well as saccharin. Before the administration of gymnemic acid, responses are seen to all substances tested; however, after the extract is painted on the tongue, the response to both sugar and saccharin is eliminated while the responses to sour, bitter, and salty stimuli are unchanged. This study demonstrates that the quality of sweet taste is processed independently from other taste qualities at an early point in the gustatory system. In addition, it shows that artificial sweet-tasting substances such as saccharin work by mimicking the effect of sugar at or near the level of the receptor.

The Physiology of Taste

Psychophysical studies have shown that taste sensations are carried in what seem to be independent channels. The responses of single taste receptors within the taste buds seem to provide a good explanation for this independence. The taste receptor, like other sensory receptor cells we have studied, has a negatively charged membrane potential in the resting state. When stimulated with the appropriate substance, it responds with a graded change in

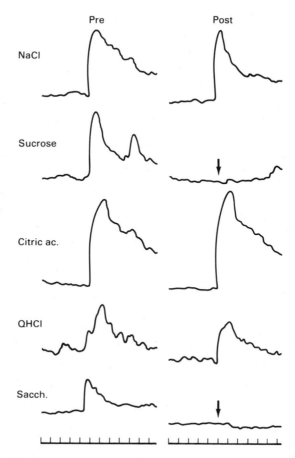

FIGURE 21-4 Summed responses of the chorda tympani to different taste stimuli, before and after administration of gymnemic acid. From Diamant, H., B. Oakley, L. Strom, C. Wells, and Y. Zotterman (1965) A comparison of neural and psychophysical responses to taste stimuli in man. *Acta Physiol. Scand.* 64:67–74. Reprinted by permission.

its level of polarization. Most commonly, receptor cells depolarize in response to a taste stimulus, but on occasion they can show a hyperpolarizing response (Ozeki & Sato, 1972). When the response of the receptor cell is one of depolarization, neurotransmitter substance within synaptic vesicles is released into the cleft between the receptor cell and the afferent sensory nerve fiber carrying taste information from the tongue to the brainstem. Each nerve fiber synapses on many taste receptors within a given taste bud, as well as from neighboring taste buds.

The response of the receptor cell to taste stimulation is called a generator potential, and is analogous to the generator potentials produced by hair cells in the cochlea or by rods and cones in the retina. As is true with the other receptors just mentioned, taste receptors do not generate action potentials; the strength of a response to a given stimulus is signaled by the amount of depolarization rather than by the frequency of action potentials being fired. In contrast, the afferent nerve fiber does fire action potentials, with the frequency of firing being related to the total amount of depolarization of all the receptor cells onto which it synapses.

Given all the psychophysical evidence suggesting that the four primary taste groups are processed in independent channels, one would expect that a given taste receptor would respond well to only one taste stimulus. However, when Kimura and Beidler (1961) first recorded from single taste receptor cells, they were surprised to find that most taste receptors were stimulated by at least two (and often more) of the basic taste qualities. Figure 21–5 shows the electrical responses of three taste receptor cells in the rat tongue to stimulation by salt, sugar, quinine, and acid. The first cell responds best to quinine, but also responds well to salt. The second cell responds almost equally to sugar, quinine, and acid but does not respond to salt. Sato (1973) studied the response properties of 109 taste receptor cells, and found that cells could respond to from 1 to 4 of the primary taste qualities.

The fact that most taste receptors respond to more than one taste quality raises problems for the contention that the four primary tastes are processed independently. For example, if a cell responds well to both sweet and salty stimuli, how will the brain know which is which? One possibility would be that it is the ensemble response of a large number of taste receptors that determines the resulting perception. Such a system would only work if sensitivity to the different taste qualities were distributed independently over the population of receptors. If, for example, salty and sweet were always linked together at the level of the receptor, there would be no way for the brain to somehow differentiate between them. However, if some cells responded to both salty and sweet tastes, but another cell responded only to sweet, the brain would be able to differentiate between the two stimuli.

Ozeki and Sato (1972) studied this question for rat taste receptor cells. They recorded from a large number of receptors, and determined the taste qualities to which each receptor responded. They found that the distribution of sensitivities to different taste types was independent; that is, there was no tendency for sensitivity to one primary taste quality to be linked to another. From these data, it seems most likely that there are individual taste receptor sites for each of the four primary taste qualities, and that these receptor sites are distributed randomly on the surface of taste receptor cells (Sato, 1980). Therefore, the hypothesis that there are four independent taste channels is consistent with the data just described.

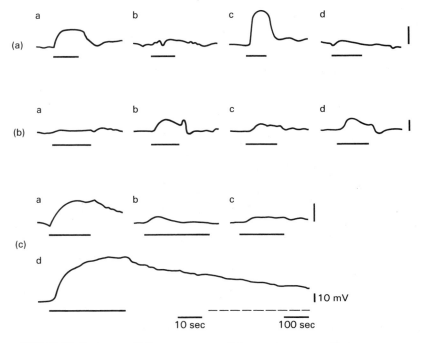

FIGURE 21-5 Intracellular responses of three gustatory cells in rat tongue to four different taste stimuli. For cells (a), (b), and (c), *a* represents the response to NaCl, *b* the response to sucrose, *c* the response to quinine, and *d* the response to HCl. From Ozeki, M., and M. Sato (1972) Responses of gustatory cells in the tongue of rat to stimuli representing four taste qualities. *Comp. Biochem. Physiol.* 41A:391–407. Copyright 1972 by Pergamon Press, Inc. Reprinted by permission.

BOX 21-3

Much recent work has focused on the intracellular events that result in depolarization of the receptor cell. It appears that different types of receptor cells use different mechanisms to produce depolarization, depending on the stimulus. Cells sensitive to sweet stimuli employ a series of second messengers; sweet substances cause an increase in cyclic AMP, which in turn activates a protein enzyme that acts to inactivate channels in the membrane permeable to potassium (Avenet, Hofmann, & Lindemann, 1988a; 1988b). The decrease in potassium conductance causes the cell to depolarize. Compare this to the transduction mechanism in rods and cones, in which an enzyme causes a decrease in a cyclic nucleotide

(continued)

(box continued)
(cyclic GMP), decreasing sodium conductance (see Box 5–5). To make things even more complicated, other investigators found that sweet stimuli caused depolarization of dog taste receptors by increasing membrane conductance to sodium (Simon, Labarca, & Robb, 1989). Thus, a single receptor cell may use two different ionic mechanisms to depolarize to a single type of stimulus.

Other taste receptors sensitive to bitter stimuli use an entirely different method of taste transduction. A subpopulation of rat taste receptor cells was found for which bitter stimuli caused an increase in intracellular calcium (Akabas, Dodd, & Al-Awqati, 1988). Stimulation with sweet stimuli did not cause this increase, which appeared to be a result of calcium release from endogenous storage sites rather than entry across the membrane. As a rise in intracellular calcium can produce transmitter release in the presynaptic terminals of axons, it is possible that in these cells, the critical factor for stimulus transduction is the change in calcium concentration rather than membrane depolarization.

The response characteristics of the nerve fibers onto which the receptor cells synapse are significantly more complicated than those of the receptors themselves. Like the receptor cells, single nerve fibers respond to more than one taste quality. Pfaffman (1941; 1955) was the first to record from single fibers in the *chorda tympani*, a segment of the cranial nerve that runs from the receptors in the tongue to the brainstem. He found that a given nerve fiber would respond best to one of the four primary taste qualities, but would usually respond to at least one other kind of taste stimulus. For a given stimulus type, the neuron would show an increased response as the concentration of the stimulus was increased. Figure 21–6 shows the responses to a single chorda tympani fiber that was most sensitive to salt in a wide variety of salt concentrations.

Pfaffman found that an individual nerve fiber was usually most sensitive to a single stimulus type, and he identified neurons as salt-best, sugar-best, and so on. He found that some cells responded almost solely to the stimulus type for which it was most sensitive, while others were more widely responsive. Figure 21–7 shows the concentration/response curves for two cells to different concentrations of all four stimulus types. The cell in the left half of the figure responds best to salt, but also responds well to increasing concentrations of both acid and sugar. In contrast the cell on the right responds best to sugar, only slightly to salt, and virtually not at all to bitter or sour stimuli.

Fibers coming from different parts of the tongue were also found to have different sensitivity profiles: not surprising since we have already noted that different parts of the tongue are differentially able to detect different taste qualities. Quinine-best neurons are rarely found coming from fungiform papillae on the front of the tongue, but are plentiful in the regions with foliate or circumvallate papillae (Frank, 1975). In the rat, sugar-best cells are rare

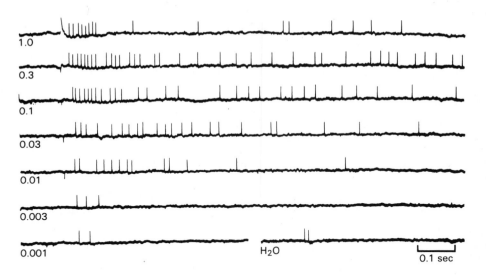

FIGURE 21-6   Responses of a single fiber in the rat gustatory nerve to NaCl solutions of increasing concentration. From Pfaffman, C. (1955) Gustatory nerve impulses in rat, cat, and rabbit. *J. Neurophysiol.* 18:429–440. Copyright 1955 by the American Physiological Society. Reprinted by permission.

coming from fungiform or circumvallate papillae, but are more common coming from foliate papillae. After recording from a range of nerve fibers coming from different areas of the tongue, Nowlis and Frank (1977) were able to determine stimulus profiles for four different cell types (see Figure 21–8). From the figure, it is clear that, when the four prototypic stimuli are used, it is possible to group the response characteristics of nerve fibers into four discrete groups.

The afferent nerve fibers just discussed travel to the brainstem where they have their synapses in the solitary nucleus. The cells in this region can also be characterized according to the primary taste quality to which they respond best. Scott, Yaxley, Sienkiewicz, and Rolls (1986) recorded from solitary nucleus cells in awake monkeys. They found that taste was *chemotopically* organized at this level of the brain, in the same way that touch is somatotopically organized and vision is retinotopically organized. In other words, certain brain areas were selectively sensitive to particular tastes. Posteriorly, or in the region within the nucleus closest to the spinal cord, cells were most responsive to sour stimuli. More anteriorly, sugar- and salt-sensitive cells predominated. Cells most sensitive to bitter tastes seemed to be distributed more generally.

Although Scott and others have been able to group cells in the brainstem

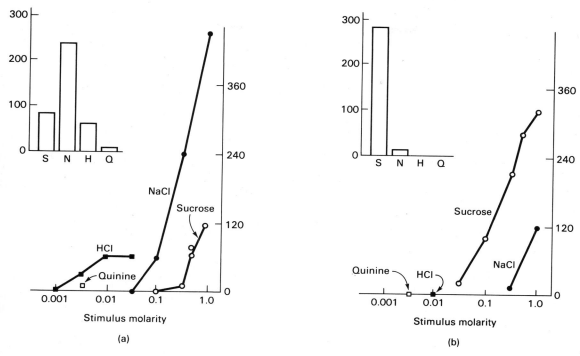

FIGURE 21-7   Responses of two different gustatory nerve fibers in the squirrel monkey to increasing concentrations of different stimuli. The relative
responsivity to different stimulus classes are shown in the histograms. From Pfaffman, C., M. Frank, L. Bartoshuk, and T. C. Snell
(1976) Coding gustatory information in the squirrel monkey chorda
tympani. In *Progress in Psychobiology and Physiological Psychology*, J. M. Sprague and A. N. Epstein (Eds) New York: Academic
Press. Reprinted by permission.

into discrete types according to which stimulus type they responded to best,
there seems to be much variability in the response patterns of these cells.
Smith, Van Buskirk, Travers, and Bieber (1983) recorded from cells in the
hamster *parabrachial nucleus*, the relay station in the brainstem just after
the solitary nucleus. He presented cells with an array of 18 different taste
stimuli. Although he could group cells into which primary stimulus they
were most sensitive to, there was much variability within a group. Figure
21–9 shows the responses of ten salt-sensitive cells to the 18 different stimuli; although there is a similarity to the general pattern of the responses, the
variability between individual cells is quite prominent. Instead of trying to
simply group cells by which single stimulus caused the best response, Smith
and colleagues performed a mathematical analysis that grouped cells by

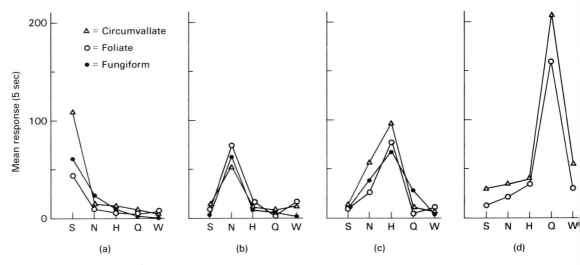

FIGURE 21-8   Response profiles of four different types of taste fibers in the hamster glossopharyngeal nerve. Responses to sucrose (S), salt (N), acid (H), and quinine (Q) are shown; within each class, nerve fibers have consistent response properties. From Nowlis, G. H., and M. Frank (1977) Qualities in hamster taste: Behavioral and neural evidence. In Sixth International Symposium on Olfaction and Taste. J. LeMagnen and P. Macleod, (Eds) London: Information Retrieval LTD, p. 241–248.

overall similarity of their responses to the entire array of stimuli. They found that cells could be grouped into three main clusters that could be roughly characterized as being most responsive to sweet, sour, and salty stimuli. Responsivity to bitter stimuli was present in many individual cells, but no clear group could be identified as being predominantly sensitive to bitter.

In summary, many taste phenomena can be accounted for by the hypothesis that taste is processed through four independent channels representing the four primary taste qualities. Cross-adaptation studies, the differing taste sensitivities over different tongue areas, and the results of studies in which different combinations of the primary taste stimuli are used to reproduce other tastes all provide support for this idea. Physiological studies also are roughly consistent, but show that single cells at many levels of the gustatory system will respond to more than one taste quality. The fact that taste sensitive neurons are so widely tuned means that the taste of a given stimulus cannot be signaled by the response of a single neuron or even an entire class of neurons, but instead is determined by comparing the responses of all classes of neurons to the same stimulus (Castellucci, 1986).

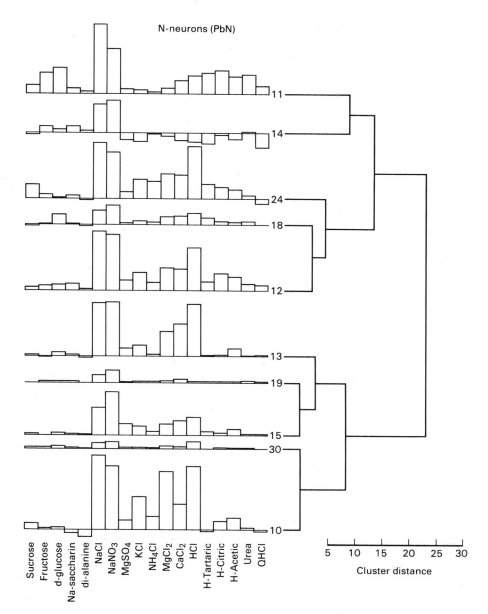

FIGURE 21-9   Responses of cells in the hamster parabrachial nucleus to each of 18 different stimuli. From Smith, D.V., R. L. Van Buskirk, J. B. Travers, and S. L. Bieber (1983) Gustatory neuron types in hamster brainstem. *J. Neurophysiol.* 50:522–540. Copyright 1983 by the American Physiological Society. Reprinted by permission.

Taste and Feeding

One of the differences between the gustatory system and the other sensory systems we have previously discussed is the close relationship of taste and behavior. Animals and human beings will modify their diets preferentially to include substances in which they are deficient. A good example of this is salt hunger—when salt depleted, animals will select a diet high in sodium, although this diet might not be selected when the animal is salt replete. This change in preferred diet results from the increased hedonistic value of salt in the deprived state (Scott & Mark, 1986); that is, the high salt diet tastes better when you are salt depleted. You can verify this phenomenon for yourself; after you have been exercising on a hot day, you may notice that you are using much more salt on your food than you would otherwise, and that salty foods such as potato chips are particularly tasty.

This effect has a physiological correlate at the level of the afferent taste fiber. Contreras and Frank (1979) recorded from single fibers of the chorda tympani of the rat under conditions of salt deprivation and repletion. They found that the fibers that were most salt sensitive under baseline conditions became significantly more sensitive to salt when the animal was deprived. Thus the increased tendency to eat a diet high in sodium may result from a change in the response properties of the receptors themselves.

Another example of how the gustatory system interacts with behavior is the phenomenon called conditioned taste aversion. If a novel taste stimulus is presented with a substance that produces significant gastrointestinal distress (that is, nausea and vomiting), the novel stimulus will acquire a strong negative association such that the animal will actively avoid foods with that taste (Garcia, Kimmeldorf, & Koelling, 1955). This effect is so strong that a single pairing of the novel stimulus with nausea will cause the animal to avoid that taste indefinitely. Taste aversion is another phenomenon about which you may have a subjective familiarity. Many people can recall a food that they once thought of quite fondly but that they now avoid because of a single episode of stomach upset, probably because of overeating! In this type of situation, the pleasurable associations that used to surround the taste of the food are replaced by less positive associations.

Is the conditioned taste aversion phenomenon a product of reinforcement systems outside the realm of the gustatory system, or do taste fibers themselves actually change their response characteristics to account for the change in hedonistic value of the stimulus? Chang and Scott (1984) asked this question by recording from neurons in the solitary nucleus of rats who had either been conditioned by the pairing of saccharin and nausea or had been exposed to saccharin without subsequent GI distress. They found that the response characteristics of the sweet-sensitive cells over a wide range of stimuli was altered so the response to saccharin more closely resembled the response to quinine (bitter) than to other sweet stimuli. Thus, the mechanism of conditioned taste aversion may be that the response of the gustatory system to the conditioned stimulus is altered so that it is more similar to the response of a naturally aversive stimulus.

The fact that single fibers in the gustatory system change their response properties under conditions of specific hungers or conditioned taste aversions implies that taste and mechanisms of reinforcement are intimately related in the brain. In fact, as we have discussed earlier, there is a direct connection between the gustatory system and the limbic system. Many experiments have been performed in which various components of limbic system have been surgically ablated and the effects of acquisition and retention of conditioned taste aversions and specific hungers have been studied. The integrity of both the hypothalamus and the amygdala appears to be necessary for the occurrence of conditioned taste aversion and specific hunger (Arthur, 1975; Mikulka, Freeman, & Lindstrom, 1977; Nachman & Ashe, 1974).

Flavor

So far, we have been discussing tastes—but we are really interested in the perception of flavor. Flavor depends not only on taste as determined by the responses of taste receptors, but on odor, color, texture, and other factors relating to general appearance. Texture is a somesthetic sensation, depending on the feel as the tongue touches the food, as well as on the pressure against the teeth and palate. Pity those who must have all food homogenized in a blender!

You will probably not be surprised to learn that odor contributes to flavor. Our ability to identify flavors is dramatically handicapped by eliminating odor perception (Mozel, Smith, Smith, Sullivan, & Swender, 1969). You know that you cannot really enjoy the flavor of food when you have a stuffed nose. You have probably also heard that with your nose pinched (and eyes shut) you can be given a piece of onion and think it is an apple. You can evaluate the contribution of odor in a less antisocial way by pinching your nose shut before a meal, and opening it partway through. Notice that when you open your nose it is not the odor that increases, it is the flavor. Adding an odorant to food generally seems to enhance its flavor, not its odor (Sekuler & Blake, 1985).

BOX 21-4

There is also a visual component to flavor that we do not usually think about. "Do you like green eggs and ham?" is a valid question asked in the children's classic by Dr. Seuss. Before white chocolate was familiar, its flavor was compared to that of ordinary brown chocolate in a psychophysical test. Blindfolded people found the samples of brown chocolate and white chocolate equally tasty, but without the blindfolds they rated the white samples less chocolately—although these were the same white chocolate samples that tasted fine when they were rated while wearing the blindfold (Duncker, 1939).

SMELL (OLFACTION)

While not as exquisitely sensitive as in some other animals, our sense of smell is nonetheless quite well developed. Smell is the phylogenetically oldest sensory system, and as such has some distinctive structural and functional characteristics. It is the only sensory system in which information reaches the neocortex without first passing through the thalamus—an obligate sensory relay station for all other senses.

Probably the most distinctive aspect of the olfactory system—at least for lower animals—is the relationship between odor and behavior. Odors act as stimuli for changes in hormone production, and as such have an effect on the timing of puberty, as well as the estrus cycle in rats and other rodents. In addition, certain odors are required for behaviors as diverse as sexual activity, suckling behavior in newborns, and selection of appropriate shelter (Halpern, 1987). The close relationship between odors and specific behaviors is a consequence of the connections the olfactory system makes with phylogenetically primitive portions of the brain.

The Search for Primary Odor Qualities

Just as was true for the sense of taste, the aspect of olfaction that most concerned early philosophers and scientists was how to describe and classify olfactory quality. Aristotle used exactly the same scheme for odors as he did for taste, except for the addition of an olfactory quality he called *fetid* (Cain, 1978). Although his actual classifications of taste and smell qualities were almost identical, Aristotle felt that taste was a sense much more amenable to logical description than was smell. Linnaeus (1752), whose major scientific contribution was in the classification of animal and plant species, also attempted to describe primary taste qualities. He grouped odors into seven classes: (1) aromatic, (2) fragrant, (3) ambrosial (musky), (4) alliaceous (garlicky), (5) hircine (goaty), (6) repulsive, and (7) nauseous (Cain, 1978). The Dutch physiologist Zwaardemaker (1895) proposed an updated version of this classification that was accepted until well into the twentieth century.

While these classification attempts were useful in that they provided a structure in which to discuss olfactory phenomena, they were based on introspection and personal experience rather than on experimental data. Henning (1916) was the first to try experimentally to define primary odors, and use different combinations of primary stimuli to produce other odors. He created an odor prism, with primary odors located at the corners (Figure 21–10). He proposed that all the odors lying along the edge between two corners resembled only the primaries located at those corners, while odors that were on a surface of the prism resembled more than two primary odors. This type of theory is similar in many ways to the trichromatic theory of color vision, as well as the theory of four primary taste stimuli. However, when experimental subjects were presented with a large variety of different odors, there was great variation in where on the prism each odor was placed, and Henning's theory eventually fell out of favor.

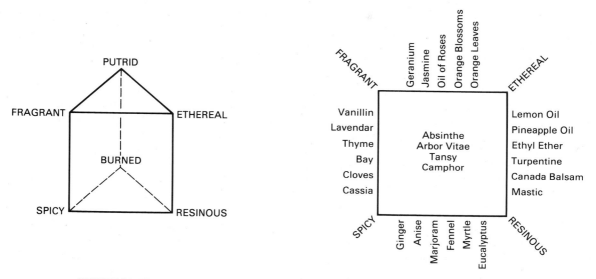

FIGURE 21-10 Hennings odor prism. After Woodworth, R. S. (1938).

More recently, attempts continue to be made to define primary odors. Amoore (1964) proposed that there were seven primary odor qualities, based on physicochemical properties of the stimulus. He thought that there were olfactory receptors corresponding to these seven primaries, with each receptor responding to a specific stimulus in proportion to how similar the physical structure of the stimulus molecule was to the primary for which the receptor was specifically tuned. Amoore presented subjects with a wide variety of different stimuli, and felt that all stimuli could be accounted for by appropriate combinations of his primaries. However, further studies showed that molecules with very similar structures generated quite different odors; in addition, different stimulus combinations produced odors that could not be predicted by combinations of the primary odors (Schiffman, 1974).

There is currently no accepted scheme for dividing odors into primary qualities, and it may be that the olfactory system is simply not designed in a way that allows for classification of odors in this manner. However, another line of research has recently revitalized the idea that there are indeed primary olfactory qualities. Studies of disorders of the sense of smell have led to the discovery of *specific anosmias*—that is, inability to smell very specific and restricted types of stimuli. These disorders are probably genetically based, with several dozen being demonstrated so far in human beings

(Amoore, 1971; 1982). The fact that some people are unable to smell a restricted range of stimuli suggests the possibility that they have an underlying abnormality in the receptor type specifically tuned to that stimulus type. With several dozen specific anosmias so far described, it may be that the number of primary taste qualities to which specific receptor types are tuned is far greater than what has been proposed in the theories of olfaction previously described.

Structure of the Olfactory System

Olfactory receptors are embedded in a portion of the nasal cavity called the *olfactory neuroepithelium*. Within this 2 to 5 square cm area there are about 6,000,000 receptors. Figure 21–11 schematically displays a portion of the neuroepithelial cell layer. The receptors are oriented perpendicularly to the epithelial surface, which is coated with a layer of mucus. Within the mucus are long cilia, connecting with the receptor tips. As is the case with taste receptors, the actual interaction between the sensory stimulus and the receptor occurs along the surface membrane of the terminal cilia. At the other end of the receptor, a thin nonmyelinated axon emerges, which joins with other fibers to form the olfactory nerve leading into the brain.

Also residing within the olfactory neuroepithelium are two other cell types, supporting cells and basal cells. Supporting cells are oriented in the

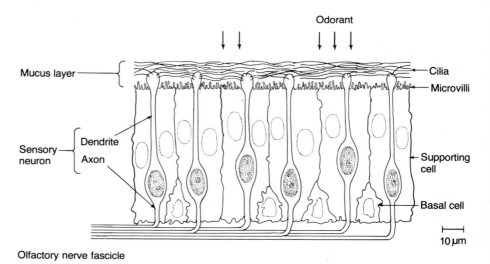

FIGURE 21–11   Drawing of the olfactory neuroepithelial layer. From Lancet, D. (1986) Vertebrate olfactory reception. Reproduced, with permission, from the *Annual Review of Neuroscience*, Volume 9, © 1986 by Annual Reviews Inc.

same direction as the receptors, but do not have cilia or axons. The basal cells lie close to the region of the receptor axons. Receptor cells have a normal life span of about 60 days, and new receptors are constantly being produced through differentiation of the basal cells. In many ways, this process is similar to what we have discussed for the gustatory system; however, olfactory receptors are different from taste receptors in two important ways. While taste receptors are modified epithelial cells without specialized neural structures, olfactory receptors are true neurons that possess axons projecting into the brain. In addition, as we shall discuss later, olfactory receptors respond to appropriate stimuli by generating action potentials, while taste receptors can only generate graded electrical potentials.

BOX 21-5

The axons of the olfactory receptors travel only a short distance, and synapse in the olfactory bulb (Figure 21-12). The anatomy of this structure has been extensively studied, and is remarkably similar in different species of animals. In many ways, it is analogous to the retina, with structural opportunities for convergence of information as well as lateral antagonism. Closest to the surface of the olfactory bulb, the axons of the olfactory receptors synapse in discrete areas called *glomeruli*. The dendrites of the *mitral*

cells, tufted cells, and *periglomerular cells* lie within the glomeruli; mitral and tufted cell axons extend out of the olfactory bulb while the periglomerular cells extend only from one glomerulus to another. Thus the periglomerular cells are in a position to mediate lateral interactions between glomeruli. Deeper within the olfactory bulb another class of nonprojection neurons called *granule cells* also appear to provide an opportunity for interactions between the output cells of neighboring glomeruli.

From the olfactory bulb, axons project to a number of different areas of the brain, including the amygdala, the *olfactory tubercle*, and *prepyriform cortex*. These areas are part of the limbic system, which we have talked about earlier in conjunction with the gustatory system; it is a phylogenetically old part of the brain concerned with reinforcement systems and primary drives, as well as many other things. From the limbic system, taste fibers finally project to the *medial dorsal nucleus* of the thalamus, and then to neocortex. This system is unique among the sensory systems in that the thalamus is not an obligate relay station before taste information reaches cortex, but instead receives information that has already been processed by cortical areas within the limbic system.

Physiology of Olfaction

At the receptor level, the processes involved in the initiation of olfaction are very similar to taste reception. Molecules that act as stimuli for smell become absorbed in the mucus layer just above the olfactory neuroepithelium. If a molecule is to excite a given receptor, it actually becomes attached to the

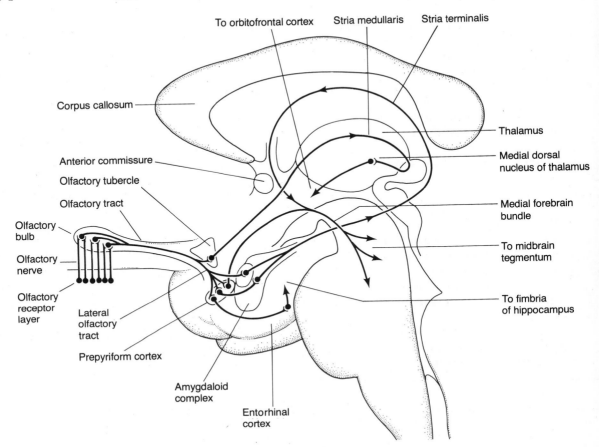

FIGURE 21-12 Schematic representation of the central olfactory pathways. Reprinted by permission of the publisher from "The chemical senses: Taste and smell" by Castellucci, V. G. In E. R. Kandel and J. H. Schwartz (Eds) *Principles of Neural Science*, 2nd Ed., pp. 409–425. Copyright 1985 by Elsevier Science Publishing Co., Inc.

membrane of the cilia of that receptor. At the point of attachment is a receptor protein, whose specific shape and electrical charge make it able to bind with molecules of some shapes but not others. Through a complex sequence of events within the receptor cell, binding of the stimulus molecule causes ion channels in the membrane to open, allowing sodium and potassium ions to flow into the cell (Lancet, 1986). The flow of positively charged ions into the receptor causes it to depolarize slightly—this is the generator potential seen in all receptors. As in other sensory systems, the generator potential is graded; the higher the concentration of stimulus molecules present in the mucus layer, the more molecules will bind with the receptor proteins on the receptor cell surface and the larger the generator potential will be.

At the other end of the receptor cell, near the axon hillock, is the area of the receptor where action potentials are produced. The number of action potentials generated in response to a specific stimulus depends on the size of the generator potential produced by that stimulus. In addition, the latency, or time from presentation of the stimulus to the observed response, depends on the concentration of the stimulus. A stimulus that produces a moderate-size response in the receptor axon may do so with a latency of about one second; however, if the stimulus is presented at a concentration 100 times less than the original stimulus, the response latency may increase to 30 seconds or more (Gesteland, 1978).

BOX 21-6

The process by which olfactory receptors depolarize in response to odorants is similar in many ways to taste transduction in taste receptor cells (see Box 21–3). Olfactory cells also make use of second messengers; when the appropriate stimulus binds to the receptor membrane, a specific protein—called guanosine triphosphate (GTP) binding protein—is activated (Pace, Hanski, Salomon, & Lancet, 1985; Sklar, Anholt, & Snyder, 1986). As in gustation, this results in an increase in intracellular cyclic AMP. Cyclic AMP in turn activates another protein that is responsible for opening ionic channels within the receptor membrane and causing depolarization (Nakamura & Gold, 1987). Using the techniques of molecular biology, the actual DNA sequence of the gene that produces the olfactory GTP binding protein has been determined (Jones & Reed, 1989).

An individual olfactory receptor will respond to a wide range of stimuli. Sicard and Holley (1984) recorded action potentials from a large number of receptor cell axons, in response to a standard set of 20 odors. They found that the responses to certain clusters of similar stimuli, such as camphors and aromatic compounds, seemed to be grouped within certain cells. However, the response characteristics of most cells were quite broad, and they were unable to define specific groups of receptors. The results therefore do not provide clear evidence that there are a relatively small number of receptor types, but instead suggest that the population of receptor types is significantly larger than in other sensory systems.

Recordings of cells in the olfactory bulb also demonstrate a number of interesting properties. Cells in the olfactory bulb respond to a wide range of different stimuli, but have certain odors to which they respond better than others. There is also a variety of responses that cells may make; some cells respond with a burst of action potentials at stimulus onset, stimulus removal, or both (Shibuya, Ai, & Takagi, 1962). Inhibition also plays a role in the responses seen at this level; while most responses to stimuli involve an increase in the number of action potentials produced, some cells inhibit their firing in response to certain odors (Matthews, 1972). In a manner suggestive of the response properties of retinal ganglion cells, some olfactory bulb neurons will respond with excitation to some odors and inhibition to others (Mancia, von Baumgarten, & Green, 1962).

Within the olfactory bulb, different odors seem to stimulate different populations of glomeruli (Shepherd, 1985). Benson et al. (1985) stimulated rats with specific odors, using an anatomical technique in which activated neurons could be labeled with a radioactive dye. They found that entire glomeruli were uniformly activated by certain stimuli, although a neighboring glomerulus may not be excited at all. Thus, cells within a given glomerulus all have the same response characteristics to different odors.

In our discussion of the structure of the olfactory bulb, we noted that the periglomerular cells provided the potential for communication between glomeruli. The fact that neighboring glomeruli have distinctly different responses to different olfactory stimuli raises the question of whether there is a lateral inhibitory network between the glomeruli that acts to sharpen the response properties of the different glomeruli. To test this, Wilson and Leon (1987) recorded from cells within the olfactory bulb in the rat, marking the position of each cell from which they recorded. They found that, if a given cell was strongly excited by a certain olfactory stimulus, they could predict that other surrounding cells at distances that would place them in neighboring glomeruli would be inhibited by that stimulus. From these data, they concluded that an inhibitory network existed between glomeruli.

From the olfactory bulb, fibers enter the complicated circuitry of the limbic system, and from there to thalamus and frontal cortex. The responses of cells to olfactory stimuli in these areas vary greatly; cells in the limbic system will respond to olfactory stimuli as well to many other stimuli that are not smell related. The segment of the olfactory pathway projecting to medial thalamus and then to cortex may be specifically involved in learning behaviors based on olfactory cues. Slotnick and Kaneko (1981) trained rats to perform a discrimination task based either on a visual or olfactory cue. After the rats had learned the task, a small lesion was placed in either the medial dorsal nucleus of the thalamus or in the amygdala. The experimenters found that neither lesion affected performance on the task based on visual discrimination. However, destruction of the medial thalamus severely disrupted performance of the olfactory discrimination task, while the lesion in the amygdala did not affect the task. Thus, the thalamocortical portion of the olfactory system seems to have a function in olfactory learning not shared by the limbic system.

PHEROMONES

One consequence of the olfactory system's close interconnections with the limbic system is the role that odors have in modulating sexual behavior and other primary drives such as aggression and shelter seeking. It has been known for many years that animals secrete or excrete substances whose odor affects the behavior of other members of the same species. These substances are called *pheromones*. Two kinds of pheromones have been described. Primary pheromones act by altering the release of specific hormones within the target animal, and so affect behavior by inducing estrus, stimulating the occurrence of puberty, and so on. Releasing or signaling pheromones probably act by providing a method of chemical communication to affect behaviors relating to aggression, maternal infant interactions, aggregation, and other social behaviors (Halpern, 1987). As they do not act via hormonal manipulation, the response to releasing pheromones is much faster than to primary pheromones.

Some examples may help to illustrate the action of primary and releasing pheromones. If female rats are all housed together, none of them will go into estrus (the time in their reproductive cycle when they are fertile and receptive to sexual advances by the male). This is called the Lee-Boot effect, and is due to an increase in circulating prolactin blood levels. Rats whose estrus cycles are suppressed by group housing will go into estrus if a male rat is introduced into the group. That this is mediated by an olfactory stimulus is demonstrated by the fact that the induction of estrus can also be produced by odors from male urine. When various female hormones are measured, it is found that male urine odors stimulate a surge in luteinizing hormone (LH), which in turn induces estrus (Halpern, 1987).

Similar effects can be demonstrated in human beings. McClintock (1971) asked young women in a dormitory to record the dates of their menstrual periods over a year's time. By the end of the year, roommates were very likely to be having their periods at the same time. Women who did not live in such close proximity with each other were less likely to have their menstrual cycles linked. Although the specific chemical was not isolated in this study, it is very likely that this effect is mediated by a primary pheromone.

BOX 21–7

There are many other examples that demonstrate that the sense of smell in human beings is more sensitive than we might think. One study demonstrated the ability of humans to recognize gender from odors. A group of subjects was each asked to wear an undershirt for 24 hours (and to forgo deodorant, soap, and perfume for both the day of the experiment and the day before). The shirts were then placed in bags, and the subjects were each presented with three bags to smell. First, each was asked which of the three shirts was his or her own—75% chose correctly. They were then asked to pick which of two shirts was worn by a male—again 75% were correct (Russell, 1976). In a related study, 6-week-old infants were able to recognize a pad worn in its own mother's breast, rather than one worn by a stranger. This is apparently not inborn, for the performances of 2-week-old babies were random (Russell, 1976).

Pheromones also act as clues that allow the initiation of certain behaviors. Odors from female hamsters are necessary for the male to initiate mating behavior. Specific substances are necessary for specific behaviors to occur.

For example, female hamster vaginal secretions have both a volatile and a nonvolatile component. The volatile component seems to contain the pheromone responsible for attracting the male hamster to the vicinity of the female, while the nonvolatile component is associated with the pheromone that stimulates mounting behavior (O'Connell & Meredith, 1984). By either eliminating the volatile component of the vaginal secretions or reducing the olfactory response to it by damaging the olfactory responses, male hamsters will be less proficient at locating a responsive female by chemical cues; however, mounting behavior was not abolished if the nonvolatile component was still present.

Many of the effects of pheromones are mediated by the structures of the olfactory system that we have just discussed. However, olfactory stimuli are also processed via a closely related parallel system called the *vomeronasal system*. Receptors lie in a separate part of the nasal cavity called *Jacobson's organ*, and their axons synapse within the *accessory olfactory bulb*, which lies quite close to the primary olfactory bulb. From the accessory olfactory bulb, fibers extend to the same limbic structures as do primary olfactory bulb fibers. Damage to the vomeronasal system may have specific alterations in the response of animals to specific pheromones, without affecting responses to other olfactory stimuli. For example, damage to the vomeronasal system does not affect the attraction of male hamsters by the pheromone in volatile vaginal secretions, but the response to the nonvolatile secretions (initiation of mounting behavior) is reduced (O'Connell & Meredith, 1984). Similarly, an intact vomeronasal system is required both for the suppression of estrus in group-housed rats and for the induction of estrus by male odor (Reynolds & Keverne, 1979; Johns, Feder, Komisaruk, & Mayer, 1978—in Halpern, 1987).

SUGGESTED READINGS

An excellent detailed discussion about the mechanism underlying taste and learned taste aversions can be found in a review by T. R. Scott and G. P. Mark called "Feeding and taste" in *Progress in Neurobiology*, Vol. 27, pages 293–317 (1986). More information about pheromes and the anatomic substrate for pheromone action is offered in a review by M. Halpern "The organization and function of the vomeronasal system," in *Ann. Rev. Neurosci.* Vol. 10, pages 325–362 (1987).

Chapter 32 in E. R. Kandel and J. H. Schwartz' *Principles of Neural Science* (Elsivier, 1986) provides a very readable discussion about the anatomy and physiology of the gustatory and olfactory systems.

APPENDIX

Perception and sensation are a part of the branch of psychology known as experimental psychology—they are vulnerable to research by the experimental method. The data are often presented graphically and sometimes mathematically. At times, a point we wish to make in this book can only be understood by understanding the graphic or mathematical presentation of data. We all get a little rusty in those areas, so we are providing this appendix to review the basic ideas necessary to understand graphs and equations. We also are including material on logarithms and trigonometric functions, which may not be familiar, but which may be useful to read over when they are encountered in the text.

GRAPHS AND EQUATIONS

When there is a relation between two things, we like to be able to express it so that others may understand what it is. In this book, we are often dealing with such relations; there are those between the energy of a stimulus and how bright or loud it seems, between the energy of a stimulus and how much effect it has on a particular nerve cell, between the size of a stimulus and how far away it seems to be, and so forth.

Let us consider another more familiar relation. There is a relation between how much beer we drink in a pub and how much we owe at the end of the evening. This can serve as an illustration for how we express relations between two things.

Suppose that you go to a pub where the beer is delivered by a metered pump at your table (like the pumps in a gas station that read out exactly how much gas they delivered). Suppose there is a cover charge of $1 to go in, and you fill your glass from the pump at your table as often as you like. Beer costs 10¢ per ounce; when you leave, they read the pump to see how much you took, multiply by 10¢, add the dollar cover charge, and that is your bill.

We can draw a picture of what your bill would be depending on how much you drink (Figure A–1). Such a picture is called a *graph*. There are two axes: the horizontal axis (called the *x*-axis) represents the amount drunk, the vertical axis (called the *y*-axis) represents how much you pay. The farther to the right you go, the more you have consumed; the higher up you go (on the graph), the more you pay. Of course, there is a relationship between the two (the more you drink, the more you pay), which we can represent by a curve on the graph.

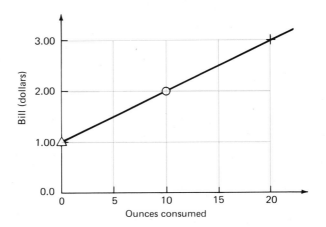

FIGURE A–1   Graphical representation of the bill in a pub versus the number of ounces of beer consumed. The three symbols represent the three cases discussed; the line corresponds to Equation (A–1).

Suppose you are a teetotaler. You drink no beer and pay only the $1 cover; on the graph in Figure A–1, your evening plots as the triangle (0 oz consumed, $1 charge). If you drank 10 oz, you would pay $2 (10 times 10¢ is $1, plus $1 cover); you would plot the circle on Figure A–1 (10 oz, $2; we would say the *abscissa* is 10, and the *ordinate* is 2). If you drank 20 oz, your bill would be $3 (cross), and so on. If we marked a point for every possible amount consumed, every one of the points would fall on the solid line drawn through the three symbols. That line represents the relationship between amount consumed and amount paid. If arithmetic had never been invented, the pub could post a graph like Figure A–1 as a price list. You would go to the *x*-axis, find the amount you drank, move up to the line, and read off the amount of the bill as the ordinate.

Restaurants don't post graphs of their rate of charging, because it is simpler to spell out the charges. In fact, we sort of did this in telling you how to compute a bill, but in a wordy way. There is a second way to express this relation: write an *equation*. An equation is a shorthand way of saying the rule we spelled out. It uses several symbols to represent longer phrases. For example, + and − , which you know from arithmetic, stand for the words "added to" and "reduced by." Letters are assigned the roles of the things being related; in this example we could say that x represents the amount drunk and y represents the bill. We need one more essential symbol: = is read "equals," and it means that the stuff to the left of it is equal to (or worth as much as) the stuff on the right. We can now write the equation for charges in the pub; it reads

$$y = 1.00 + 0.10x \tag{A-1}$$

(The 0.10 written next to the x means multiply x by 0.10.) Equation (A–1) can be read as "the bill (in dollars) is equal to \$1 plus \$0.10 times the number of ounces consumed."

Equation (A–1) is the equation of the line in Figure A–1; both the equation and the graph say the same thing. The equation is neater in that it takes less room and can be used with as much precision as you wish. The graph cannot be read to great accuracy, but it gives a good overall picture of what is going on. You can see at a glance that you pay more the more you drink, that the minimum bill is \$1, and that your total bill is less per ounce if you drink more.

Equations are easy to manipulate once you get the hang of it, giving results that are equivalent but look different. As long as you do the same thing to both sides, the statement remains true. For example,

$$10y = 10.0 + x \tag{A-2}$$

is also true. Ten times your bill is \$10 plus \$1 per oz. You can also rearrange terms without affecting the truth:

$$y = 0.1x + 1.00 \tag{A-3}$$

(you pay 10¢ an oz plus \$1).

Equation (A–3) is in a standard form for the equation of a straight line:

$$y = mx + b \tag{A-4}$$

(in Equation (A–3) $m = 0.1$ and $b = 1.00$). In this form, m is the slope of the line (\$ per ounce) and b is the y-intercept (\$1 is the value where the line hits the y-axis, which is where $x = 0$). Any straight line on a graph can be represented in this form.

Of course, not all lines are straight, and not all equations are so simple. There is, however, a correspondence between equations and curves on graphs: every equation can be drawn on a graph, and every curve on a graph can be represented (at least approximately) by an equation.

Consider a slightly harder equation:

$$y = x^2 \tag{A-5}$$

This equation says that y is given by the square of x. Let us plot this equation as a curve on a graph in Figure A–2. If $x = 0$, $x^2 = 0$, y is 0; this point is where the two axes meet, which is called the *origin*. It is shown as a triangle in Figure A–2. If $x = 1$, 1^2 also is 1 ($1 \times 1 = 1$), so $y = 1$; the point where $x = 1$

and $y = 1$ is plotted with a circle. When $x = 2$, $y = 2^2 = 2 \times 2 = 4$. The point at which $x = 2$ and $y = 4$ is shown by a cross. When $x = 3$, $y = x^2 = 3^2 = 3 \times 3 = 9$ (tilted triangle), which is nearly off the top of the picture. Although we have run out of space for larger values, we can indicate what y would be for any small value of x; the solid curve is the one that corresponds to Equation (A–5).

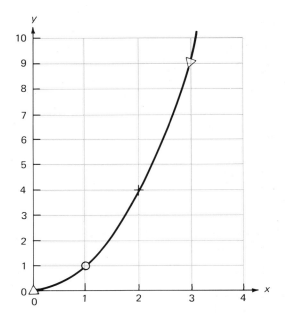

FIGURE A-2 Graphic representation of the equation $y = x^2$ (Equation A–5). The four symbols correspond to points discussed.

LOGARITHMS

When we plotted Figure A–2, we ran out of space before getting very far into the graph. We could help things by shrinking the y-axis so that fewer inches would be eaten up by large numbers, but then we would squeeze down all the details in the small numbers. For example, the ordinate in Figure A–3 is 1/10 the scale of that in Figure A–2, which lets us get about three times as far out on the x-axis, but makes it hard to see what is happening when x takes the small values seen in Figure A–2. A better way to handle the problem of rapidly growing numbers is to use a logarithmic scale. Many of the figures in this book are on logarithmic scales.

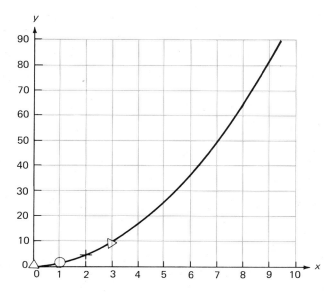

FIGURE A-3 Another graph of the equation $y = x^2$, on a compressed vertical scale.

First, what is a *logarithm*? A logarithm is the exponent to which 10 must be raised to give a particular number. (10 is only one possible base for logarithms, but it is the only one we use in this book.) The equation

$$y = \log(x) \tag{A-6}$$

reads "y is (or equals) the power to which 10 must be raised to give x." (The short form "log" means logarithm and will be used from here on.) We could say this another way:

$$10^y = x \tag{A-7}$$

or

$$10^{\log(x)} = x \tag{A-8}$$

Equation (A-8) tells us how to take the "antilog": to find the number given its logarithm, take 10 to the power $\log(x)$.

Now let us consider some properties of exponents of 10 (or of any number, for that matter). An exponent tells how many times to multiply a number by itself:

$$10^1 = 10 \tag{A-9}$$

$$10^2 = 10 \times 10 = 100 \tag{A-10}$$

$$10^3 = 10 \times 10 \times 10 = 1000 \tag{A-11}$$

$$10^4 = 10 \times 10 \times 10 \times 10 = 10,000 \tag{A-12}$$

This gives us a way to prepare a table of logs. Look at Equation (A–9), and compare it to (A–8); it is the same equation with numbers written in. So log x is 1 when x is 10; we can write log 10 = 1. Similarly, Equation (A–10) tells us that log 100 = 2, and we can write a table based on Equations (A–8) to (A–12):

$$\log 10 = 1$$

$$\log 100 = 2$$

$$\log 1000 = 3$$

$$\log 10,000 = 4$$

and so forth. Notice how slowly the logs grow as compared to the increases in the sizes of the numbers.

BOX A–1

Let us consider what happens when we multiply powers of 10. Look at Equations (A–9) and (A–10); suppose we multiply them—we get

$$10^1 \times 10^2 = (10 \times 10 \times 10) = 10^3$$
$$= 10^{1+2} \qquad (A–13)$$

In fact, it is a general rule that when we multiply 10^a times 10^b we get 10 raised to the *sum* of the two powers:

$$10^a \times 10^b = 10^{a+b'} \qquad (A–14)$$

Now consider what that means for logs. If $x = 10^a$, $a = \log x$; also $y = 10^b$, and $b = \log y$. Let us further set $z = 10^{a+b}$ so that $a + b = \log z$. Now, we can substitute x, y, and z for the things they represent in Equation (A–14) and get

$$xy = z \qquad (A–15)$$

We are allowed to do the same thing to both sides of an equation, and it will still be true. So we can take the log of both sides of Equation (A–15), and get

$$\log (xy) = \log z \qquad (A–16)$$

Log $z = a + b$, which is log x + log y; putting

this in place of log z on the right side of (A–16) gives a very important result:

$$\log (xy) = \log x + \log y \qquad (A–17)$$

In words, the log of the product of two numbers is the sum of the log of each. Adding logs is equivalent to multiplication.

If adding logs is equivalent to multiplication, subtracting must be equivalent to division. We can see this from Equation (A–17). Subtract log y from both sides of the equation (we are allowed to do the same thing to both sides):

$$\log (xy) - \log y = \log x + \log y - \log y$$

$$\log (xy) - \log y = \log x \qquad (A–18)$$

If log $x = \log (xy) - \log y$, it must be equivalent to log $(x\,y/y)$ which is log x.

This fact lets us expand our log table. Log 10 = 1; if we subtract log 10 from log 10 we get 0, which is equivalent to dividing 10 by 10 (=1):

$$\log 10 - \log 10 = 1 - 1$$

$$\log (10/10) = 1 - 1$$

(continued)

(box continued)

$$\log 1 = 0$$

We can go further:

$$\log 1 - \log 10 = 0 - 1$$

$$\log (1/10) = -1$$

We can see that negative logs correspond to fractions.

$$\log (1/100) = -2$$

$$\log (1/1000) = -3$$

So far, all our logs have been integers (whole numbers). How can we deal with logs that are fractions? What would be the power to which 10 is raised to give, say, 2? To understand this, we must delve further into the rules for powers of numbers.

Suppose we multiply a log by some number. For example, what is 2 times the log of x?

$$2 \log x = \log x + \log x \qquad \text{(A–19)}$$

Addition of logs is equivalent to multiplication (Equation A–17):

$$\log x + \log x = \log (xx) = \log (x^2) \qquad \text{(A–20)}$$

Similarly,

$$3 \log x = \log (xxx) = \log x^3 \qquad \text{(A–21)}$$

In short, multiplication of a log is equivalent to raising a number to a power:

$$n \log x = \log x^n \qquad \text{(A–22)}$$

But suppose n is not a whole number. Say n is a fraction:

$$n = 1/m \qquad \text{(A–23)}$$

then we know that

$$1/m \log x = \log x^{1/m} \qquad \text{(A–24)}$$

We also know then that

$$m(1/m) \log x = m\log x^{(1/m)} = \log x \qquad \text{(A–25)}$$

In other words

$$(x^{1/m})^m = x \qquad \text{(A–26)}$$

so $x^{1/m}$ must be the mth root of x. For example, if m is $1/2$, that means square root, for the square root squared is the original number.

This result lets us find values for fractional logarithms. For example, take the square root:

$$10^{1/2} = \sqrt{10} = 3.16228$$

so

$$\log 3.16228 = 0.5$$

We can multiply by 10 by adding 1 (if you don't see why, review the table based on Equation A–8 and the result in Equation A–17):

$$\log 31.6228 = 1.5$$

and so forth.

It turns out that

$$10^{0.3} = 2$$

or

$$\log 2 = 0.3$$

Then we know that log 4 must be 0.6, either by doubling log 2 ($2^2 = 4$) or by adding log 2 to log 2 ($2 \times 2 = 4$). With no further information, you should be able to find that

$$\log 8 = 0.9$$

$$\log 80 = 1.9$$

$$\log 400 = 2.6$$

$$\log 0.2 = -0.7$$

and a large number of other results.

Summary of Logarithms

We can summarize rules for manipulating logs (derived in the preceding box) with two statements:

1. *Addition of logs corresponds to multiplication of numbers* (Equation A–17). You can find the product of two numbers by finding the log of each (from a log table), adding the two logs, and finding the number corresponding to the sum (in the table). Similarly, subtraction corresponds to division.
2. *Multiplying a log by a number corresponds to raising to a power* (Equation A–22). Twice the log of a number is the sum of the log and itself; from 1. above, that corresponds to the number times itself, or the number squared (raised to the power 2).

Now that we "know" what logs are, and have some idea of the values they take, let us draw the picture corresponding to them. Figure A–4 shows the function of "log x" versus x. (That is, we have plotted $y = \log x$.) As we said before, the log of 1 is 0, so the curve crosses the x-axis at $x = 1$ ($y = \log 1 = 0$).

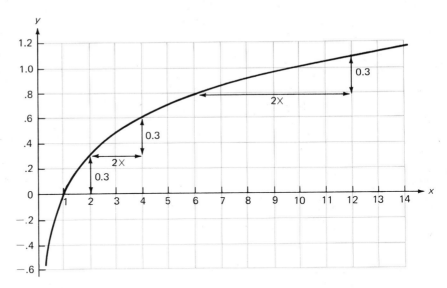

FIGURE A–4   A graph of the function $y = \log x$. The vertical arrows indicate a difference in height of 0.3, which occurs for each doubling of the x-axis.

For values of x less than 1 (fractions) log x is negative; it is below the x-axis. As x becomes larger than 1, log x also increases. It does not, however, increase nearly as rapidly as x. When x is 10, log x is 1—but log x does not reach a value of 2 until x is 100. The value of log x increases by the same amount (same difference) for constant ratios of x; there is the same 0.3 difference in height of the curve when x changes by a factor of 2 whether x goes from 1 to 2, from 2 to 4, or from 6 to 12 (indicated on the figure). The same 0.3 difference in height would be found where x goes from 100 to 200, or from 1024 to 2048, or from 79,020 to 158,040.

Log Axes

The point of learning about logarithms is that we use log scales on the axes of many of our graphs. A log scale simply means the numbers along the axis are placed in positions corresponding to their logs. In Figures A–1 to A–4, the numbers along all the scales were placed in the same way as the inches are marked on a ruler; this is called a *linear* scale. Each number is placed at a position as far from the origin as the number itself says it is. You could simply place a ruler along a line and use its scale (inches or mm) instead of buying graph paper; there is the same distance between 0 and 1 as between 1 and 2, or 2 and 3, or 100 and 101.

A log scale is one in which the distance from the origin to a number is the log of the number. Thus 10 is one unit farther from the origin than 1, 100 is one unit farther than 10, and so forth. Graph paper can be purchased already ruled in this way; it is called *log paper.*

Figure A–5 shows a sheet of log paper in which only the x-axis is ruled as a log scale. Notice the wide space between 1 and 2 and the progressively narrower spaces between 2 and 3, 3 and 4, and so on until the space between 9 and 10 is small. In fact, the space between 10 and 20 is as small as the space between 1 and 2—because they are in the same ratio and therefore the same distance apart on a log scale. The y-axis on this paper is the same linear scale we are already familiar with. Graph paper of this type, on which one axis is logarithmic and one is linear, is called *semilog paper.*

We have plotted the function $y = \log x$ on the semilog paper of Figure A–5; this is the same function plotted on linear paper in Figure A–4. We can verify that the same points appear: $\log x$ is 0 at $x = 1$, $\log x$ is 1 at $x = 10$, $\log x$ is negative for x less than 1, and so on. The curve we saw in Figure A–4 plots a straight line on semilog paper, however. Plotting on a log scale squeezed it to the left and straightened it out.

To see why the function $y = \log x$ plots as a straight line on semilog paper, think about what we are doing. The numbers on the x-axis are placed according to their logs; when we find a number (x) on the x-axis, we are at the position $\log x$. We are really plotting versus $\log x$—and what are we plotting versus $\log x$? Why, $\log x$! Figure A–5 shows $\log x$ versus $\log x$—naturally the two are always equal, and we are plotting the straight line $y = x$. To make this point clearer, we have written the values of $\log x$ under some of the x's on the x-axis; these numbers line up in the ordinary linear (ruler) scale way. If you look only at the $\log x$ scale, you can easily see that we are plotting each number versus itself.

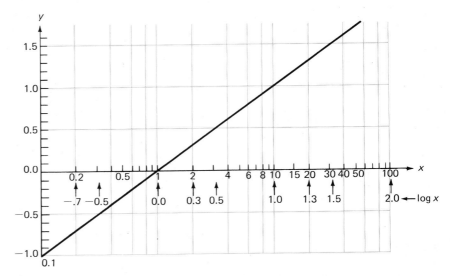

FIGURE A–5   The function $y = \log x$ plotted on semilog paper. Numbers on the x-axis are spaced according to their logs. Logs of the numbers on the x-axis are indicated beneath them, showing regular spacing.

An even more interesting thing happens when we use graph paper on which both axes are ruled as log scales. Such paper, available in the campus bookstore, is called *log-log paper* (also known as double-log paper, or full-log paper). A sample is shown in Figure A–6. The scales on log-log paper are just like the log scale on semilog paper—it is just that both of them are that way. Now when we find a point y corresponding to x, we are plotting $\log y$ versus $\log x$.

What happens if we plot an equation such as Equation (A–5) on log-log paper? (Equation A–5 said $y = x^2$). We have done so on Figure A–6. When x is 1, y is also 1 (circle). When x is 2, y is 4 (cross); when x is 3, y is 9 (triangle). These points, which fell on an upward curve in Figures A–2 and A–3, fall on a straight line on the log-log plot. In fact, the Equation (A–5) is the straight line on this plot shown by the solid line.

We can explain why this equation gives us a straight line by reviewing what we said about logs. If we take logs of both sides of Equation (A–5) (which does not change its validity),

$$\log y = \log x^2 \tag{A–27}$$

From Equation (A–22) we can rewrite this equation as

$$\log y = 2 \log x \tag{A–28}$$

Now remember that log y is the thing we plot on the y-axis (using the linear scale to the left), and log x is what we are plotting linearly on the x-axis

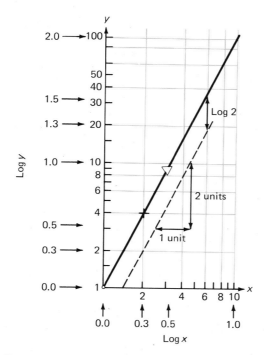

FIGURE A-6   The functions $y = x^2$ (solid line) and $y = 1/2\, x^2$ (dashed line) on log-log coordinates. Three of the points plotted on Figure A–2 are indicated by the same symbols as in that figure. Logs of numbers along the y-axis and x-axis are indicated.

(linear scale below). If we call log $y = Y$ and let $X = \log x$, Equation (A–27) reads

$$Y = 2\,X \tag{A–29}$$

which is the equation of a straight line on the actual linear scales. In fact, it is a straight line with a slope of 2; there is a 2-log unit increase in height for every log unit across.

This result is quite general: if an equation of the form

$$y = a\,x^n \tag{A–30}$$

is plotted on log-log coordinates, it will plot as a straight line with a slope of n. This is true whether n is larger than 1 or fractional, positive or negative. (A negative n, as in the case of a negative power of 10, means 1 divided by the number to that power.)

Equation (A–30) introduced another quantity: a. Now, a is a multiplier, which was unity (1) in Equation (A–5). If a is not 1, it will change the position of the line. For example, if $a = 1/2$, Equation (A–5) would read

$$y = 1/2 \, x^2 \qquad\qquad\qquad\qquad\text{(A–31)}$$

and every y would be 1/2 as large as it was. In an equation such as (A–4), plotted on linear paper, a would represent a change in slope—here we are plotting on log paper, and the effect is quite different. On Figure A–6 we have plotted Equation (A–31) with a dashed line. (When $x = 1$, $y = 1/2$; when $x = 2$, $y = 4/2 = 2$; when $x = 3$, $y = 9/2 = 4.5$. You should find and verify these points on the figure.) The effect is that the line has *shifted* down a constant amount—that amount is the log of 2. We have divided every value of y by 2, therefore we subtract the log of 2. We can express this idea a little more mathematically by taking logs of both sides of Equation (A–31):

$$\log y = \log (1/2 \, x^2) \qquad\qquad\qquad\text{(A–32)}$$

The log of a product is the sum of the logs, so

$$\log y = \log x^2 + \log 1/2 \qquad\qquad\qquad\text{(A–33)}$$

We also note that the log of 1 divided by a number is minus the log of the number (if you prefer, you could have started by saying $\log y = \log x^2/2$ and noting that the log of a ratio is the difference of the logs)

$$\log y = \log x^2 - \log 2 \qquad\qquad\qquad\text{(A–34)}$$

and with the exponentiation rule (A–22)

$$\log y = 2 \log x - \log 2 \qquad\qquad\qquad\text{(A–35)}$$

On the linear scale, with $X = \log x$ and $Y = \log y$

$$Y = 2X - \log 2 \qquad\qquad\qquad\qquad\text{(A–36)}$$

which is the equation of a straight line just like Equation (A–4). The y intercept, $-\log 2$, represents a shift downward of the curve by log 2 (which is 0.3).

The important point to gain from the preceding discussion is this: *multiplication (or division) on a log axis has the effect of shifting the curve by a constant amount*. Multiplication of x shifts the curve to the left or right; multiplication of y shifts it up or down. (With a straight line, you cannot say whether it shifted down or to the right—other functions are less forgiving.) The shifting of a curve along a logarithmic axis when the parameter plotted on that axis is multiplied by some factor is quite general. It is also true on semilogarithmic plots, a useful fact to remember when looking at plots of response versus log (intensity).

NORMAL PROBABILITY AXES

Other axes have been designed that convert specific nonlinear functions into straight lines, just as log axes convert power functions into straight lines. Of particular value in the study of sensory and perceptual systems is *normal probability paper*. The probability axis is spaced so that equal standard deviations (*z* scores) are equally spaced. As a result, a cumulative normal distribution (the integral of the normal distribution) plots as a straight line.

Probability axes are commonly used when plotting psychometric functions. As explained in Box A–2, we may view the probability of detection curve (such as in Figure 2–1[b]) as the integral of an underlying normal distribution representing the probability of the threshold taking any particular value. On linear paper, such as in Figure 2–1b, the function is an ogive. Replotted on probability paper, it becomes a straight line, as shown in Figure A–7.

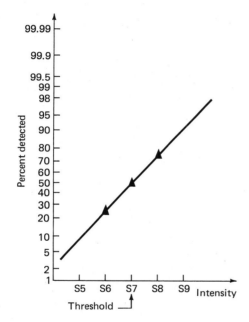

FIGURE A–7 Data of Table 2–1 plotted on normal probability paper. The ogive of Figure 2–1(b) appears as a straight line. Notice that the stimuli for which the subject scores 100% (or 0%) cannot be plotted on this figure, as they are off the paper.

BOX A–2

Notice that only three of the "data" points in Table 2–1 appear in the plot in Figure A–7. 0% and 100% are an infinite number of standard deviations below and above the mean, respectively, and so are off the bottom and top of the paper. The axes shown range from 1% to 99.99%. To obtain 99.99% would require one "no" in 10,000 trials! With a finite number of

(continued)

(box continued)
trials, you can only estimate the percentages. For example, with only four trials, you can obtain 50% (2 "no"s) or 75% (1 "no"). There is no way to obtain 90% even if that is the "true" value, for you cannot have 3.6 "yesses." If all four responses were "yes," you would not know that the next was not going to be a "no," or whether the "true" value is 75.0001%, 90%, or 99.999%. Thus, perfect scores (all "yes" or all "no") cannot be plotted on probability axes.

The value of using probability paper is that it is far easier to draw a straight line than a curve. The exact curve in Figure 2–1(b) would be hard to determine or to draw, but the straight line in Figure A–7 is easily drawn with just a ruler. We are reasonably good at seeing how to place a straight line among a spattering of points. If more precision or objectivity is desired, it is straightforward to perform a simple linear regression (on the coordinates of the probability plot, not the raw numbers). The threshold can then be determined by where the line intersects 50% detection.

Normal probability paper is also useful for receiver operatic characteristic (ROC) curves, like that in Figure 2–9. Since the underlying distributions of noise and signal + noise are assumed to be normal distributions (Figure 2–8), the use of normal probability axes makes sense. In this application, both the x-axis and the y-axis are probability axes. Plotted this way, the ROC curves become straight lines. If the standard deviations of the noise and the signal + noise distributions are equal (as in the example in Figures 2–8 and 2–9), the line will have a slope of unity (be parallel to the diagonal), and d' can be determined from the line's distance from the diagonal. If the standard deviations are not equal, the ROC curve will still be a straight line, but its slope will not be unity. This is a simple way to demonstrate that the assumption of equal standard deviations is not valid in a particular case.

SINES AND COSINES

The sinusoids and sine functions we are talking about are the same ones that plagued you in trigonometry. This relationship is shown by Figure A–8. Consider a clock with only one hand, and say that hand is 1.0 unit long. Let us ask for the height of the pointer end of the hand (relative to the pivot) as a function of the angular position of the hand. Start at 12:00 o'clock (0°); the hand is vertical, as high as it can be, at a height of 1.0 (its length). As time passes the angle θ increases, and the pointer gets lower and lower. At 3:00 o'clock the hand is horizontal, having moved 90°, and the height is 0.0. Then, the pointer drops below the pivot, and the height becomes increasingly negative, until 6:00 o'clock when the hand is again vertical (180°). This time the pointer is as far below the pivot as it can be, at -1.0. As the hand moves around to the left, it again rises, until at 9:00 o'clock (270°) it is horizontal, and the height is again 0.0. The height then becomes more positive as the hand returns to its starting point (12:00 o'clock, which is both 0° and 360°). The same picture repeats as many times as the hand goes around. We have traced just over 2 cycles of sinusoid, as a function of the angle, θ; if the hand rotates at a constant speed (as clocks are supposed to), we could just as well label the x-axis with the time at which that angle was achieved.

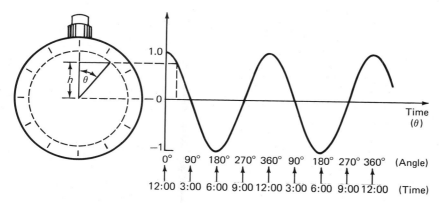

FIGURE A-8   One-handed clock, showing how the height of the pointer end of the hand traces a cosine function in time. Cosine function shown to the right.

The particular sinusoidal function we have traced is a *cosine*; that this is the same kind of cosine encountered in trigonometry may be seen from the small triangle sketched in the clock face. This triangle shows how we could find the height (h) when the hand is at the angle θ shown. It is a right triangle; the hypotenuse is the hand, and the height is the side adjacent to the angle θ. The definition of a cosine is that it is the ratio of the adjacent side of a right triangle to the hypotenuse, or

$$\cos\theta = h/\text{hypotenuse}$$

As the hypotenuse is 1.0, $h = \cos\theta$ is the function shown.

Now compare the cosine function in Figure A–8 with the sine function at the top of Figure A–9. The only difference between them is that they start at different places. If we place the 0° point of the cosine at the leftmost measurement point for the wavelength λ in Figure A–9, the two would superimpose perfectly. This shift is called a difference in *phase*; there is a 90° phase shift between the sine wave and the cosine wave. That is,

$$\cos\theta = \sin(\theta + 90°)$$

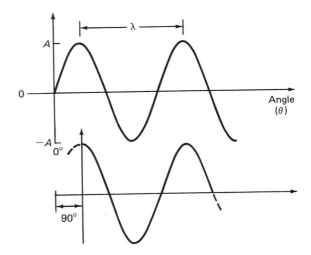

FIGURE A-9 Sine function (top), indicating that it is the same as the cosine function (below) shifted by 90°.

In fact, we could derive the sine wave (rather than cosine) from the clock by asking for the excursion of the pointer along the direction at 90° to vertical (that is, horizontal). At 0° the horizontal excursion is 0.0—the pointer is neither right nor left of center. At 90° it is at the maximum rightmost (positive) excursion; at 180° it is back to zero, and so forth. The horizontal excursion is given by the unlabeled side of the triangle drawn into the clock, the side opposite the angle θ. Recall that the sine is defined as the ratio of the opposite side of a right triangle to the hypotenuse.

REFERENCES

Abrahams, H., Krakaver, D., & Dallenbach, K. (1937). Gustatory adaptation to salt. *Am. J. Psychol., 49,* 462–469.

Abramov, I. (1968). Further analyses of the responses of LGN cells. *J. Opt. Soc. Am., 58,* 574–579.

Adams, A. J., & Afanador, A. J. (1971). Ganglion cell receptive field organization at different levels of light adaptation. *Am. J. Optom., 48,* 889–896.

Adey, W. R., & Noda, H. (1973). Influence of eye movements on geniculo-striate excitability in the cat. *J. Physiol., 235,* 805–821.

Adrian, E. D., & Zotterman, T. (1926). The impulses produced by sensory nerve endings. II. The response of a single end-organ. *J. Physiol., 61,* 151–171.

Akabas, M. H., Dodd, J., & Al-Awqati, Q. (1988). A bitter substance induces a rise in intracellular calcium in a subpopulation of rat taste cells. *Science, 242,* 1047–1050.

Akil, H., Mayer, D. J., & Liebeskind, J. C. (1976). Antagonism of stimulation produced analgesia by naloxone, a narcotic antagonist. *Science, 191,* 961–962.

Albrecht, D. G., & DeValois, R. L. (1981). Striate cortex responses to periodic patterns with and without the fundamental harmonics. *J. Physiol., 319,* 497–514.

Albrecht, D. G., DeValois, R. L., & Thorell, L. G. (1980). Visual cortical neurons: Are bars or gratings the optimal stimuli?, *Science, 207,* 88–90.

Amoore, J. E. (1964). Current status of the steric theory of odor. *Ann. N.Y. Acad. Sci., 116,* 457–476.

Amoore, J. E. (1971). Olfactory genetics and anosmia. In L. M. Beidler (Ed.), *Handbook of sensory physiology, Vol. 4: Chemical senses: Olfaction* (pp. 245–256). Berlin: Springer-Verlag.

Amoore, J. E. (1982). Odor theory and odor classification. In E. T. Theimer (Ed.), *Fragrance chemistry—The science of the sense of smell* (pp. 27–76). New York: Academic Press.

Andersen, R. A., Essick, G. K., & Siegel, R. M. (1985). Encoding of spatial location by posterior parietal neurons, *Science, 230,* 456–458.

Arend, L. E., & Goldstein, R. (1987). Simultaneous constancy, lightness, and brightness. *J. Opt. Soc. Amer., A 4,* 2281–2285.

Arthur, J. B. (1975). Taste aversion learning is impaired by interpolated amygdaloid stimulation but not by post training amygdaloid stimulation. *Behav. Biol., 13,* 369–376.

Atkinson, J., & Campbell, F. W. (1974). The effect of phase on the perception of compound gratings. *Vision Res., 14,* 159–162.

Attneave, F. (1954). Some informational aspects of visual perception. *Psych. Rev., 61,* 183–193.

Attneave, F. (1957). Physical determinants of the judged complexity of shapes. *J. Exper. Psychol., 53,* 221–227.

Attneave, F. (1959). *Applications of information theory to psychology.* New York: Holt, Rinehart & Winston.

Attneave, F. (1962). Perception and related areas. In S. Koch (Ed.), *Psychology: A study of a science, Vol. 4* (pp. 619–659). New York: McGraw-Hill.

Attneave, F. (1971). Multistability in perception. *Sci. Am., 225,* 62–72.

Attwell, D., & Wilson, M. (1980). Behaviour of the rod network in the tiger salamander retina mediated by membrane properties of individual rods. *J. Physiol., 309,* 287–315.

Aubert, H. (1886). Die bewegungsemp-findung. *Arch. ges. Physiol., 39,* 347–370.

Avenet, P., Hofmann, F., & Lindemann, B. (1988a). Signalling in taste receptor cells: cAMP dependent protein kinase causes depolarization by closure of 44 pS k-channels. *Comp. Biochem. Physiol. (A), 90,* 681–685.

Avenet, P., Hofmann, F., & Lindemann, B. (1988b). Transduction in taste receptor cells requires cAMP dependent protein kinase. *Nature, 331,* 351–354.

Badcock, D. R. (1984a). Spatial phase or luminance profile discrimination? *Vision Res., 24,* 613–623.

Badcock, D. R. (1984b). How do we discriminate relative spatial phase? *Vision Res., 24,* 1847–1854.

Baker, H. D., & Rushton, W. A. H. (1965). The rod-sensitive pigment in normal cones. *J. Physiol., 176,* 56–72.

Balkema, G. W., & Bunt-Milam, A. H. (1982). Cone outer segment shedding in the goldfish retina characterized with the ^{3}H-fucose technique. *Investig. Ophthal. & Vis. Sci., 23,* 319–331.

Barlow, H. B. (1953). Summation and inhibition in the frog's retina. *J. Physiol., 119,* 69–88.

Barlow, H. B. (1964). Dark adaptation: A new hypothesis. *Vision Res., 4,* 47–58.

Barlow, H. B. (1977). Performance, perception, dark-light, and gain boxes. *Neurosci. Res. Program Bull., 15,* 394–397.

Barlow, H. B., Blakemore, C., & Pettigrew, J. D. (1967). The neural mechanisms of binocular depth discrimination. *J. Physiol., 193,* 327–342.

Barlow, H. B., FitzHugh, R., & Kuffler, S. W. (1957). Dark adaptation, absolute threshold, and purkinje shift in single units of the cat's retina. *J. Physiol., 137,* 327–337.

Barlow, H. B., & Hill, R. M. (1963). Selective sensitivity to direction of movement in ganglion cells of the rabbit retina. *Science, 139,* 412–414.

Barlow, H. B., Hill, R. M., & Levick, W. R. (1964). Retinal ganglion cells responding selectively to direction and speed of image motion in the rabbit. *J. Physiol., 173,* 377–407.

Barlow, H. B., & Levick, W. R. (1969). Changes in the maintained discharge with adaptation level in the cat retina. *J. Physiol., 202,* 699–718.

Barlow, H. B., Narasimhan, R., & Rosenfeld, A. (1972). Visual pattern analysis in machine and animals. *Science, 177,* 567–574.

Barlow, H. B., & Reeves, B. C. (1979). The versatility and absolute efficiency of detecting mirror symmetry in random dot displays. *Vision Res., 19,* 783–793.

Bartley, S. H. (1938). Subjective brightness in relation to flash rate and the light-dark ratio. *J. Exp. Psychol., 23,* 313–319.

Bartoshuk, L. M., Lee, C-H, & Scarpolino, R. (1972). Sweet taste of water induced by artichoke. *Science, 178,* 988–990.

Bartoshuk, L. M. (1978). In E. C. Carterette & M. P. Friedman (Eds.) *Handbook of perception, Vol. VIA: Tasting and smelling,* (pp. 3–18). New York: Academic Press.

Batteau, D. W. (1967). The role of the pinna in human localization. *Proc. R. Soc. Lond. Ser. B., 168,* 158–180.

Baylor, D. A., & Hodgkin, A. L. (1974). Changes in time scale and sensitivity in turtle photoreceptors. *J. Physiol., 242,* 729–758.

Baylor, D. A., Fuortes, M. G. F., & O'Bryan, P. M. (1971). Receptive fields of cones in the retina of the turtle. *J. Physiol., 214,* 265–294.

Baylor, D. A., Nunn, B. J., & Schnapf, J. L. (1984). The photocurrent, noise and spectral sensitivity of rods of the monkey. *Macaca Fascicularis. J. Physiol., 357,* 575–607.

Baxter, W. T., & Dow, B. M. (1989). Horizontal organization of orientation-sensitive cells in primate visual cortex. *Biol. Cybern., 61,* 171–182.

Beck, J. (1966). Effect of orientation and of shape similarity on perceptual grouping. *Percept. Psychophys., 1,* 300–302.

Beck, J. (1972). Similarity groupings and peripheral discriminability under uncertainty. *Am. J. Psychol., 85,* 1–20.

Beck, J., & Gibson, J. J. (1955). The relation of apparent shape to apparent slant in the perception of objects. *J. Exp. Psychol., 50,* 125–133.

Beidler, L. M. (1978). Biophysics and Chemistry of Taste. In E. C. Carterette & M. P. Friedman (Eds.) *Handbook of perception, Vol. VIA: Tasting and smelling,* (pp. 21–49). New York: Academic Press.

von Békésy, G. (1928). Zur theorie des horens; die schwingungsform der basilarmembran. *Phys. Z., 29,* 793–810.

von Békésy, G. (1942). Uber die schwingungen

der schneckentrennwand beim praparet und ohrenmodell. *Akust. Z., 7,* 173–186.

von Békésy, G. (1947). The variation of phase along the basilar membrane with sinusoidal vibrations. *J. Acoust. Soc. Am., 19,* 452–460.

von Békésy, G. (1960). *Experiments in Hearing,* E. G. Wever (Ed.). New York: McGraw-Hill.

von Békésy, G. (1961). Concerning the fundamental component of periodic pulse patterns and modulated vibrations observed on the cochlear model with nerve supply. *J. Acoust. Soc. Am., 33,* 888–896.

Benimoff, N. I., Schneider, S., & Hood, D. C. (1982). Interactions between rod and cone channels above threshold: a test of various models. *Vision Res., 22,* 1133–1140.

Benson, T. E., Burd, G. D., Green, C. A., Pedersen, P. E., Landis, D. M. D., & Shepherd, G. M. (1985). High resolution 2-deoxyglucose autoradiography in quick-frozen slabs of neonatal rat olfactory bulb. *Brain Res. 339,* 67–78.

Berardi, N., Bisti, S., Cattaneo, A., Fiorentini, A., & Maffei, L. (1982). Correlation between the preferred orientation and spatial frequency of neurones in visual areas 17 and 18 of the cat. *J. Physiol., 323,* 603–618.

Berenberg, R. A., Shefner, J. M., & Sabol, J. (1987). Quantitative assessment of position sense at the ankle: A functional approach. *Neurology, 37,* 89–94.

Bergen, J. R., & Adelson, E. H. (1988). Early vision and texture perception. *Nature, 333,* 363–364.

Berlin, B., & Kay, P. (1969). *Basic color terms, their universality and evolution.* Berkeley, Calif.: University of California Press.

Berman, N., & Cynader, M. (1972). Comparison of receptive-field organization of the superior colliculus in siamese and normal cats. *J. Physiol, 224,* 363–389.

Berman, P. W., & Leibowitz, H. W. (1965). Some effects of contour on simultaneous brightness contrast. *J. Exp. Psychol., 69,* 251–256.

Bernstein, I. H., Fisicaro, S. A., & Fox, J. A. (1976). Metacontrast suppression and criterion content: A discriminant function analysis. *Percept. Psychophys., 20,* 198–204.

Berrien, F. K. (1946). The effects of noise. *Psych. Bull., 43,* 141–161.

Bhatia, B. (1975). Minimum separable as a function of speed of a moving object. *Vision Res., 15,* 23–33.

Bien, B. (1988). The promise of neural networks. *Amer. Scientist, 776,* 561–564.

Billone, M., & Raynor, S. (1973). Transmission of radial shear forces to cochlear hair cells. *J. Acoust. Soc. Am., 54,* 1143–1156.

Bisti, S., Maffei, L., & Piccolino, M. (1974). Visuovestibular interactions in the cat superior colliculus. *J. Neurophysiol., 37,* 146–155.

Bishop, P. O., Coombs, J. S., & Henry, H. B. (1971). Responses to visual contours; spatio-temporal aspects of excitation in the receptive fields of simple striate neurones. *J. Physiol., 219,* 625–657.

Blake, R., & Camisa, J. (1978). Is binocular vision always monocular? *Science, 200,* 1497–1499.

Blake, R., & Cormack, R. H. (1979). Psychophysical evidence for a monocular visual cortex in stereoblind humans. *Science, 203,* 274–275.

Blake, R., & Hirsch, H. V. B. (1975). Deficits in binocular depth perception in cats after alternating monocular deprivation. *Science, 190,* 1114–1116.

Blakemore, C., & Campbell, F. W. (1969). On the existence of neurones in the human visual system selectively sensitive to the orientation and size of retinal images. *J. Physiol., 203,* 237–260.

Blakemore, C., & Cooper, G. F. (1970). Development of the brain depends on the visual environment. *Nature, 228,* 477–478.

Blakemore, C., & Sutton, P. (1969). Size adaptation: A new aftereffect. *Science, 166,* 245–247.

Blakemore, C., & Van Sluyters, R. C. (1974). Reversal of the physiological effects of monocular deprivation in kittens: Further evidence for a sensitive period. *J. Physiol., 237,* 195–216.

Blakemore, C., & Van Sluyters, R. C. (1975). Innate and environmental factors in the development of the kitten's visual cortex. *J. Physiol., 248,* 663–716.

Blasdel, G. G., & Salama, G. (1986). Voltage-sensitive dyes reveal a modular organization in monkey striate cortex. *Nature, 321,* 579–585.

Blough, D. S. (1955). Method for tracing dark adaptation in the pigeon. *Science, 121,* 703–704.

Bok, D. (1985). Retinal photoreceptor-pigment epithelium interactions. *Investig. Ophthal. & Vis. Sci., 26,* 1659–1694.

Bonds, A. B. (1989). Role of inhibition in the specification of orientation selectivity of cells in the cat striate cortex. *Visual Neurosci, 2,* 41–55.

Boring, E. G. (1930). A new ambiguous figure. *Am. J. Psychol., 42,* 444–445.

Boring, E. G. (1942). *Sensation and Perception in the History of Experimental Psychology.* New York: Appleton-Century-Crofts.

Boring, E. G., Langfeld, H. S., & Weld, H. P. (1948). *Foundations of psychology.* New York: Wiley.

Borresen, C. R., & Lichte, W. H. (1962). Shape constancy: Dependence upon stimulus familiarity. *J. Exp. Psychol., 63,* 91–97.

Bowling, D. B., & Wieniawa-Narkiewicz, E. (1986). The distribution of on- and off-centre X- and Y-like cells in the A layers of the cat's lateral geniculate nucleus. *J. Physiol., 375,* 561–572.

Boycott, B. B., & Dowling, J. E. (1969). Organization of the primate retina: Light microscopy. *Philos. Trans. R. Soc. Lond., 255,* 109–184.

Boycott, B. B., Dowling, J. E., Fisher, S. K., Kolb, H., & Laties, A. M. (1975). Interplexiform cells of the mammalian retina and their comparison with catecholamine-containing retinal cells. *Proc. R. Soc. Lond., 191,* 353–368.

Boycott, B. B., & Wässle, H. (1974). The morphological types of ganglion cells of the domestic cat's retina. *J. Physiol., 240,* 397–419.

Boyd, I. A., & Davey, M. R. (1968). *Composition of peripheral nerves.* Edinburgh: E. and S. Livingstone, Ltd.

Boynton, R. M. (1988). Color vision. *Ann. Rev. Psychol., 39,* 69–100.

Boynton, R. M., & Gordon, J. (1965). Bezold-Brücke hue shift measured by color-naming technique. *J. Opt. Soc. Am., 55,* 78–86.

Boynton, R. M., & Montag, E. (1988). Categorical color names. *Proc. Int. Soc. for Eye Res., 5,* 154.

Braddick, O. (1988). Contours revealed by concealment. *Nature, 333,* 803–804.

Bradley, A., Switkes, E., & DeValois, K. (1988). Orientation and spatial frequency selectivity of adaptation to color and luminance gratings. *Vision Res., 28,* 841–856.

Brauner, J. D., & Lit, A. (1976). The Pulfrich effect, simple reaction time, and intensity discrimination. *Am. J. Psychol., 89,* 105–114.

Breitmeyer, B. G., & Ganz, L. (1976). Implications of sustained and transient channels for theories of visual pattern masking, saccadic suppression, and information processing. *Psychol. Rev., 83,* 1–36.

Brigell, M., & Uhlarik, J. (1980). Bending the parallels of the Poggendorff figure. *Bull. Psychonom. Soc., 16,* 1–4.

Brill, M. H., & West, G. (1986). Chromatic adaptation and color constancy: A possible dichotomy. *COLOR Res. and Applic., 11,* 196–204.

Brin, K. P., & Ripps, H. (1977). Rhodopsin photoproducts and rod sensitivity in the skate retina. *J. Gen. Physiol., 69,* 97–120.

Brindley, G. S., & Merton, P. A. (1960). The absence of position sense in the human eye. *J. Physiol., 153,* 127–130.

Brodmann, K. (1909). *Vergleichende lokalisationslehre der grosshirnrinde in ihren prinzipien dargestellt auf grund des zellenbaues.* Leipzig: Barth.

Brooke, R. N. L., Downer, J. C., & Powell, T. P. S. (1965). Centrifugal fibres to the retina in the monkey and cat. *Nature, 207,* 1365–1367.

Brosgole, L., & Whalen, P. (1967). The effect of meaning on the allocation of visually induced movement. *Percept. Psychophys., 2,* 275–277.

Brown, C. M. (1984). Computer vision and natural constraints. *Science, 224,* 1299–1305.

Brown, J. E., & Pinto, L. H. (1974). Ionic mechanism for the photoreceptor potential of the retina of *Bufo marinus. J. Physiol., 236,* 575–591.

Brown, J. F. (1931). The visual perception of velocity. *Psychologische forschung, 14,* 199–232. Reprinted in *Readings in the study of visually perceived movement,* I. M. Spigel (Ed.). New York: Harper and Row, 1965.

Brown, J. L. (1965). The structure of the visual system. In C. H. Graham (Ed.), *Vision and Visual Perception,* (pp. 39–59). New York: Wiley.

Brown, K. T., Watanabe, K., & Murakami, M. (1965). The early and late receptor potentials of monkey cones and rods. *Cold Spring Harbor Symp. Quant. Biol., 30,* 457–482.

Brown, P. K., & Wald, G. (1964). Visual pigment in single rods and cones of the human retina. *Science, 144,* 45–52.

Brownell, W. E., Bader, C. R., Bertrand, D., & Ribaupierre, Y. de (1985). Evoked mechanical responses of isolated cochlear outer hair cells. *Science, 227,* 194–196.

Bruce, C., Desimone, R., & Gross, C. G. (1981).

Visual properties of neurons in a polysensory area in superior temporal sulcus of the macaque. *J. Neurophysiol., 46,* 369–384.

Bruell, J. H., & Albee, G. W. (1955). Notes toward a motor theory of visual egocentric localization. *Psychol. Rev., 62,* 391–399.

Brugge, J. F., & Merzenich, M. M. (1973). Responses of neurones in auditory cortex of macaque monkey to monaural and binaural stimulation. *J. Neurophysiol., 36,* 1138–1158.

Burbeck, C. A. (1987). Position and spatial frequency in large-scale localization judgments. *Vision Res., 27,* 417–427.

Burdick, C. K., & Miller, J. D. (1975). Speech perception by the chinchilla: Discrimination of sustained /a/ and /i/. *J. Acoust. Soc. Am., 58,* 415–427.

Burgess, P. R., & Perl, E. R. (1973). Cutaneous mechanoreceptors and nociceptors. In A. Iggo (Ed.), *Handbook of sensory physiology, Vol. 2. Somatosensory System.* Heidelberg: Springer-Verlag.

Burgess, P. R., Wei, J. Y., Clark, F. J., & Simon, J. (1982). Signalling of kinesthetic information by peripheral sensory receptors. *Ann Rev. Neurosci., 5,* 171–187.

Burke, W., & Sefton, A. J. (1966). Discharge patterns of principle cells and inhibitory interneurons in lateral geniculate nucleus of rat. *J. Physiol., 187,* 201–212.

Burkhardt, D. A., & Berntson, G. G. (1972). Light adaptation and excitation: Lateral spread of signals within frog retina. *Vision Res., 12,* 1095–1111.

Burr, D. C. (1987). Implications of the Craik-O'Brien illusion for brightness perception. *Vision Res., 27,* 1903–1913.

Bushnell, M. C., Goldberg, M. E., & Robinson, D. L. (1981). Behavioral enhancement of visual responses in monkey cerebral cortex. I. Modulation in posterior parietal cortex related to selective visual attention. *J. Neurophysiol., 46,* 755–772.

Cain, W. S. (1978). History of research on smell. In E. C. Carterette & M. P. Friedman (Eds.) *Handbook of perception, Vol. VIA: Tasting and smelling* (pp. 197–243). New York: Academic Press.

Campbell, F. W. (1974). The transmission of spatial information through the visual system. In F. O. Schmitt and F. G. Worden (Eds.), *The Neurosciences/Third Study Program.* (pp. 95–103). Cambridge, Mass.: MIT Press.

Campbell, F. W., & Robson, J. G. (1968). Application of Fourier analysis to the visibility of gratings. *J. Physiol., 197,* 551–566.

Campbell, F. W., & Wurtz, R. H. (1978). Saccadic omission: Why we do not see a grey-out during a saccadic eye movement. *Vision Res., 18,* 1297–1303.

Campbell, F. W., Howell, E. R., & Johnstone, J. R. (1978). A comparison of threshold and suprathreshold appearance of gratings with components in the low and high spatial frequency range. *J. Physiol., 284,* 193–201.

Carl, J. W., & Hall, C. F. (1972). The application of filtered transforms to the general classification problem. *IEEE Trans. on Computers, C-21,* 785–790.

Castelloci, V. F. (1986). The chemical senses: Taste and smell. In E. R. Kandel, & J. H. Schwartz (Eds.) *Principles of Neural Science,* 2nd edition, (pp: 409–428). New York: Elsivier.

Cavanagh, P., Tyler, C. W., & Favreau, O. E. (1984). Perceived velocity of moving chromatic gratings. *J. Opt. Soc. Amer. A, 1,* 893–899.

Chalupa, L. M., & Rhoades, R. W. (1977). Responses of visual, somatosensory, and auditory neurones in the golden hamster's superior colliculus. *J. Physiol., 270,* 595–626.

Chan, R. Y., & Naka, K. -I. (1976). The amacrine cell. *Vision Res., 16,* 1119–1129.

Chang, F- C. T., & Scott, T. R. (1984). Conditioned taste aversions modify neural responses in the rat nucleus tractus solitaripus. *J. Neurosci. 4,* 1850–1862.

Chase, R., & Kalil, R. E. (1972). Suppression of visual evoked responses to flashes and pattern shifting during voluntary saccades. *Vision Res., 12,* 215–220.

Cherry, C. (1953). Some experiments on the recognition of speech, with one and with two ears. *J. Acoust. Soc. Am., 25,* 975–979.

Churchland, P. S., & Sejnowski, T. J. (1988). Perspectives on cognitive neuroscience. *Science, 242,* 741–745.

Cicerone, C. M., & Green, D. G. (1980). Dark adaptation within the receptive field centre of rat retinal ganglion cells. *J. Physiol., 301,* 535–548.

Clarke, P. G. H., Donaldson, I. M. L., & Whitteridge, D. (1976). Binocular mechanisms in cortical areas I and II of the sheep. *J. Physiol., 256,* 509–526.

Cleland, B. G., & Enroth-Cugell, C. (1968). Quantitative aspects of sensitivity and summation in the cat retina. *J. Physiol., 198*, 17–38.

Cleland, B. G., Dubin, M. W., & Levick, W. R. (1971). Sustained and transient neurones in the cat's retina and lateral geniculate nucleus. *J. Physiol., 217*, 473–496.

Cleland, B. G., & Lee, B. B. (1985). A comparison of visual responses of cat lateral geniculate nucleus neurones with those of ganglion cells afferent to them. *J. Physiol., 369*, 249–268.

Cleland, B. G., & Levick, W. R. (1974). Brisk and sluggish concentrically organized ganglion cells in the cat's retina. *J. Physiol., 240*, 421–456.

Cleland, B. G., Levick, W. R., & Sanderson, K. J. (1973). Properties of sustained and transient ganglion cells in the cat retina. *J. Physiol., 228*, 649–680.

Cleland, B. G., Levick, W. R., & Wässle, H. (1975). Physiological identification of a morphological class of cat retinal ganglion cells. *J. Physiol., 248*, 151–171.

Coleman, P. D., Flood, D. G., Whitehead, M. C., & Emerson, R. C. (1981). Spatial sampling by dendritic trees in visual cortex. *Brain Res., 214*, 1–21.

Contreras, R., & Frank, M. (1979). Sodium deprivation alters neural responses to gustatory stimuli. *J. Gen. Physiol., 73*, 569–594.

Costanzo, R. M., & Gardner, E. P. (1980). A quantitative analysis of responses of direction sensitive neurons in somatosensory cortex of awake monkeys. *J. Neurophysiol., 43*, 1319–1341.

Cooper, F. S., Delattre, P. C., Liberman, A. M., Borst, J. M., & Gerstman, L. J. (1952). Some experiments on the perception of synthetic speech sounds. *J. Acoust. Soc. Am., 24*, 597–606.

Copenhagen, D. R., & Owen, W. G. (1980). Current-voltage relations in the rod photoreceptor network of the turtle retina. *J. Physiol. 308*, 159–184.

Coren, S. (1972). Subjective contours and apparent depth. *Psychol. Rev., 79*, 359–367.

Coren, S., & Girgus, J. S. (1973). Visual spatial illusions: Many explanations. *Science, 179*, 503–504.

Coren, S., & Komoda, M. K. (1973). Apparent lightness as a function of perceived direction of incident illumination. *Am. J. Psychol., 86*, 345–349.

Coren, S., Porac, C., & Ward, L. M. (1979). *Sensation and perception*. New York: Academic Press.

Corey, D. P., & Hudspeth, A. J. (1979). Ionic basis of the receptor potential in a vertebrate hair cell. *Nature, 281*, 675–677.

Corey, D. P., & Hudspeth, A. J. (1983). Kinetics of the receptor current in bullfrog saccular hair cells. *J. Neurosci., 3*, 962–976.

Cornsweet, T. N. (1970). *Visual perception*. New York: Academic Press.

Crouch, J. E., & McClintic, J. R. (1971). *Human Anatomy and Physiology*. New York: Wiley.

Cusick, C. G., & Kaas, J. H. (1988). Cortical connections of area 18 and dorsolateral visual cortex in squirrel monkeys. *Visual Neurosci., 1*, 211–237.

Cutting, J. E., & Eimas, P. D. (1975). Phonetic feature analyzers and the processing of speech in infants. In: J. F. Kavanagh & J. E. Cutting (Eds.), *The role of speech in language* (pp. 127–148). Cambridge, Mass.: MIT Press.

Cutting, J. E., & Rosner, B. S. (1974). Categories and boundaries in speech and music. *Percept. Psychophys., 20*, 55–60.

Cynader, M., Berman, N., & Hein, A. (1973). Cats reared in stroboscopic illumination: Effects on receptive fields in visual cortex. *Proc. Natl. Acad. Sci., 70*, 1353–1354.

Cynader, M., & Chernenko, G. (1976). Abolition of directional sensitivity in the visual cortex of the cat. *Science, 193*, 504–505.

Cynader, M., & Regan, D. (1982). Neurons in cat visual cortex tuned to the direction of motion in depth: Effect of positional disparity. *Vision Res., 22*, 967–982.

Dacheux, R. F., & Miller, R. F. (1976). Photoreceptor-bipolar cell transmission in the perfused retina eyecup of the mudpuppy. *Science, 191*, 963–964.

Dallenbach, K. M. (1951). A puzzle picture with a new element of concealment. *Am. J. Psychol., 64*, 431–433.

Dallos, P., & Harris, D. (1978). Properties of auditory nerve responses in absence of outer hair cells. *J. Neurophysiol., 41*, 365–383.

Dallos, P., Santos-Sacchi, J., & Flock, A. (1982). Intracellular recordings from cochlear outer hair cells. *Science, 218*, 582–584.

Damasio, A. R. (1981). Central achromatopsia. *Neurology, 31*, 920–921.

Damasio, A. R. (1985). Disorders of complex visual processing: Agnosias, achromatopsia, Balint's Syndrome, and related difficulties of orientation and construction. In Mesulam, M. M. (Ed.) *Principles of behavioral neurology*, Philadelphia: F. A. Davis.

Damasio, A. R., & Benton, A. L. (1979). Impairment of hand movements under visual guidance. *Neurology, 29,* 170–178.

Daniel, P. M., & Whitteridge, D. (1961). The representation of the visual field on the cerebral cortex of monkeys. *J. Physiol., 159,* 203–221.

Darwin, C. J. (1975). On the dynamic use of prosody in speech perception. In A. Cohen and S. G. Nooteboom (Eds.) *Structure and process in speech perception* (pp. 178–193). New York: Springer-Verlag.

Daugman, J. G. (1984). Spatial visual channels in the Fourier plane. *Vision Res., 24,* 891–910.

Davis, H., Benton, R. W., Lorell, W. P., Fernandez, C., Golstein, R., Katsuki, T., Legouix, J. P., McAliffe, D. R., & Taksaki, I. (1953). Acoustic trauma in the guinea pig. *J. Acoust. Soc. Am., 25,* 1180–1189.

Davis, H., & Silverman, S. R. (1970). *Hearing and Deafness.* New York: Holt, Rinehart, & Winston.

Daw, N. W. (1968). Colour coded ganglion cells in the goldfish retina: Extension of their receptive field properties by means of new stimuli. *J. Physiol., 197,* 567–592.

Daw, N. W., & Wyatt, H. J. (1976). Kittens reared in a unidirectional environment: Evidence for a critical period. *J. Physiol., 257,* 155–170.

Dawson, W. W., & Perez, J. M. (1973). Unusual retinal cells in the dolphin eye. *Science, 181,* 747–749.

Day, R. H. (1965). Inappropriate constancy explanation of spatial distortions. *Nature, 207,* 891–893.

Delattre, P. C., Liberman, A. M., & Cooper, F. S. (1955). Acoustic loci and transitional cues for consonants. *J. Acoust. Soc. Am., 27,* 769–773.

DeMonasterio, F. M., Gouras, P., & Tolhurst, D. J. (1975). Trichromatic colour opponency in ganglion cells of the rhesus monkey retina. *J. Physiol., 251,* 197–216.

DeMonasterio, F. M., & Schein, S. J. (1982). Spectral bandwidths of color-opponent cells of geniculocortical pathway of macaque monkeys. *J. Neurophysiol., 47,* 214–224.

Derrington, A. M., & Badcock, D. R. (1985). The low level motion system has both chromatic and luminance inputs. *Vision Res., 25,* 1879–1884.

Desimone, R., Schein, S. J., Moran, J., & Un-gerleider, L. G. (1985). Contour, color and shape analysis beyond the striate cortex. *Vision Res., 25,* 441–452.

Desmedt, J. E. (1960). Neurophysiological mechanisms controlling acoustic input. In G. L. Rasmussen and W. F. Windle (Eds.), *Neural mechanisms of the auditory and vestibular systems.* Springfield, Ill.: Charles C Thomas.

DeValois, K. (1977). Independence of black and white: Phase-specific adaptation. *Vision Res., 17,* 209–215.

DeValois, K. K., DeValois, R. L., & Yund, E. W. (1979). Responses of striate cortex cells to grating and checkerboard patterns. *J. Physiol., 291,* 483–505.

DeValois, K. K., & Tootell, R. B. H. (1983). Spatial-frequency-specific inhibition in cat striate cortex cells. *J. Physiol., 336,* 359–376.

DeValois, R. L. (1978). Spatial processing of luminance and color information. *Invest. Ophthalmol. 17,* 834–835.

DeValois, R. L., Abramov, I., & Jacobs, G. H. (1966). Analysis of response patterns of LGN cells. *J. Opt. Soc. Am., 56,* 966–977.

DeValois, R. L., Albrecht, D. G., & Thorell, L. G. (1982). Spatial frequency selectivity of cells in macaque visual cortex. *Vision Res., 22,* 545–559.

DeValois, R. L., & DeValois, K. K. (1988). *Spatial Vision.* New York: Oxford University Press.

DeValois, R. L., Morgan, H. C., Polson, M. C., Mead, W. R., & Hull, E. M. (1974). Psychophysical studies of monkey vision. I. Macaque luminosity and color vision tests. *Vision Res., 14,* 53–67.

DeValois, R. L., Yund, E. W., & Hepler, N. (1982). The orientation and direction selectivity of cells in macaque visual cortex. *Vision Res., 22,* 531–544.

DeYoe, E. A., & Van Essen, D. C. (1988). Concurrent processing streams in monkey visual cortex. *Trends in Neurosci., 11,* 219–226.

Diamant, H., Oakley, B., Strom, L., Wells, C., & Zotterman, Y. (1965). A comparison of neural and psychophysical responses to taste stimuli in man. *Acta Physiol. Scand., 64,* 67–74.

Djamgoz, M. B. A., Reynolds, S. H., Rowe, J. S., & Ruddock, K. H. (1981). Control of retinal S-potentials in dark adapted and bleached retina. *Vision Res., 21,* 1581–1584.

Dorman, M. F., Raphael, L. J., & Liberman, A. M. (1979). Some experiments on the sound of silence in phonetic perception. *J. Acoust. Soc. Am., 65,* 1518–1532.

Dowling, J. E. (1965). Foveal receptors of the monkey retina: Fine structure. *Science, 147,* 57–59.

Dowling, J. E. (1967). The organization of vertebrate visual receptors. In J. M. Allen (Ed.), *Molecular organization and biological function* pp. 186–210. New York: Harper & Row.

Dowling, J. E. (1968). Synaptic organization of the frog retina: An electron microscopic analysis comparing the retinas of frogs and primates. *Proc. R. Soc. Lond. Ser. B., 170,* 205–228.

Dowling, J. E. (1970). Organization of vertebrate retinas. *Invest. Ophthalmol., 9,* 655–680.

Dowling, J. E. (1977). Receptoral and network mechanisms of visual adaptation. *Neurosci. Res. Prog. Bull., 15,* 397–407.

Dowling, J. E. (1978). How the retina "sees." *Invest. Ophthalmol., 17,* 832–834.

Dowling, J. E., & Boycott, B. B. (1965). Neural connections of the retina: Fine structure of the inner plexiform layer. *Cold Spring Harbor Symp. Quant. Biol., 30,* 393–402.

Dowling, J. E., & Boycott, B. B. (1966). Organization of the primate retina: Electron microscopy. *Proc. R. Soc. Lond. Ser. B., 166,* 80–111.

Dowling, J. E., & Cowan, W. M. (1966). An electron microscopic study of normal and degenerating centrifugal fiber terminals in the pigeon retina. *Z. Zellforsch. Mikrosk. Anat., 71,* 14–28.

Dowling, J. E., & Ehinger, B. (1975). Synaptic organization of the amine-containing interplexiform cells of the goldfish and cebus monkey retinas. *Science, 188,* 270–273.

Dowling, J. E., & Ehinger, B. (1978a). The interplexiform cell system. I. Synapses of the dopaminergic neurons of the goldfish retina. *Proc. R. Soc. Lond. Ser. B., 201,* 7–26.

Dowling, J. E., & Ehinger, B. (1978b). Synaptic organization of the dopaminergic neurons in the rabbit retina. *J. Comp. Neurol., 180,* 203–220.

Dowling, J. E., & Ripps, H. (1972). Adaptation in skate photoreceptors. *J. Gen. Physiol., 60,* 698–719.

Dowling, J. E., & Ripps, H. (1976). Potassium and retinal sensitivity. *Brain Res., 107,* 617–622.

Draper, S. W. (1978). The Penrose triangle and a family of related figures. *Perception, 7,* 283–296.

Dreher, B. (1972). Hypercomplex cells in the cat's visual cortex. *Invest. Ophthalmol., 11,* 355–356.

Dreher, B., Fukada, Y., & Rodieck, R. W. (1976). Identification, classification and anatomical segregation of cells with X-like and Y-like properties in the lateral geniculate nucleus of old-world primates. *J. Physiol., 258,* 433–452.

Drum, B. (1982). Summation of rod and cone responses at absolute threshold. *Vision Res., 22,* 823–826.

Dubin, M. W. (1970). The inner plexiform layer of the vertebrate retina: A quantitative and comparative electron microscopic analysis. *J. Comp. Neurol., 140,* 479–506.

Dubin, M. W., & Cleland, B. G. (1977). Organization of visual inputs to interneurons of the lateral geniculate nucleus of the cat. *J. Neurophysiol., 40,* 410–427.

Duclaux, R., & Kenshalo, D. R. (1980). Response characteristics of cutaneous warm receptors in the monkey. *J. Neurophysiol., 43,* 1–15.

Duncker, K. (1939). The influence of past experience upon perceptual properties. *Am. J. Psychol., 52,* 255–265.

Dursteler, M. R., & Wurtz, R. H. (1988). Pursuit and optokinetic deficits following chemical lesions of cortical areas MT and MST. *J. Neurophysiol., 60,* 940–965.

Easter, S. S. Jr. (1968a). Excitation in the goldfish retina: Evidence for a non-linear intensity code. *J. Physiol., 195,* 253–271.

Easter, S. S. Jr. (1968b). Adaptation in the goldfish retina. *J. Physiol., 195,* 273–281.

Ebrey, T. G., & Honig, B. (1977). New wavelength-dependent visual pigment nomograms. *Vision Res., 17,* 147–151.

Edelman, G. M. (1987). *Neural Darwinism: The theory of neuronal group selection.* New York: Basic Books.

Edelstyn, N. M. J., & Hammond, P. (1988). Relationship between cortical lamination and texture sensitivity in complex neurones of the striate cortex in cats. *J. Comp. Neurol., 278,* 397–404.

Egan, J. P., & Hake, H. W. (1950). On the masking pattern of a simple auditory stimulus. *J. Acoust. Soc. Am., 22,* 622–630.

Ehinger, B., Falck, B., & Laties, A. M. (1969). Adrenergic neurons in teleost retina. *Z. Zellforsch, 97,* 285–297.

Eimas, P. D., & Corbit, J. D. (1973). Selective adaptation of linguistic feature detectors. *Cognit. Psychol., 4*, 99–109.

Eimas, P. D., Cooper, W. E., & Corbit, J. D. (1973). Some properties of linguistic feature detectors. *Percept. Psychophys., 13*, 247–252.

Ejima, Y., & Takahashi, S. (1988). Illusory contours induced by isoluminant chromatic patterns. *Vision Res., 28*, 1367–1377.

Ekman, G. (1964). Is the power law a special case of Fechner's law? *Perceptual and Motor Skills, 19*, 730.

Eliasof, S., Barnes, S., & Werblin, F. (1987). The interaction of ionic currents mediating single spike activity in retinal amcrine cells of the tiger salamander. *J. Neurosci., 7*, 3512–3524.

Enoch, J. M. (1963). Optical properties of the retinal receptors. *J. Opt. Soc. Am., 53*, 71–85.

Enroth, C. (1952). The mechanism of flicker and fusion studied on single retinal elements in the dark-adapted eye of the cat. *Acta. Physiol. Scand., 27*, (Suppl. 100), 1–67.

Enroth-Cugell, C., & Pinto, L. H. (1970). Algebraic summation of centre and surround inputs to retinal ganglion cells of the cat. *Nature, 226*, 458–459.

Enroth-Cugell, C., & Robson, J. G. (1966). The contrast sensitivity of retinal ganglion cells of the cat. *J. Physiol., 187*, 517–552.

Enroth-Cugell, C., & Shapley, R. M. (1973). Flux, not retinal illumination, is what cat retinal ganglion cells really care about. *J. Physiol., 233*, 311–326.

Epstein, W. (1965). Nonrelational judgments of size and distance. *Am. J. Psychol., 78*, 120–123.

Epstein, W., & Baratz, S. S. (1964). Relative size in isolation as a stimulus for relative perceived distance. *J. Exp. Psychol., 67*, 507–513.

Evans, E. F. (1975). The sharpening of cochlear frequency selectivity in the normal and abnormal cochlea. *Audiology, 14*, 419–422.

Evans, J. A., Hood, D. C., & Holtzman, E. (1978). Differential effects of cobalt ions on rod and cone synaptic activity in the isolated frog retina. *Vision Res., 18*, 145–151.

Eysel, U. T., Muche, T., & Worgotter, F. (1988). Lateral interactions at direction-selective striate neurones in the cat demonstrated by local cortical inactivation. *J. Physiol., 399*, 657–675.

Fahle, M. (1982). Binocular rivalry: Suppression depends on orientation and spatial frequency. *Vision Res., 22*, 787–800.

Fain, G. L. (1975). Quantum sensitivity of rods in the toad retina. *Science, 187*, 838–841.

Famiglietti, E. V. Jr., & Kolb, H. (1976). Structural basis for ON- and OFF-center responses in retinal ganglion cells. *Science, 194*, 193–195.

Farber, D. B., Brown, B. M., & Lolley, R. N. (1978). Cyclic GMP: Proposed role in visual cell function. *Vision Res., 18*, 497–499.

Ferster, D. (1988). Spatially opponent excitation and inhibition in simple cells of the cat visual cortex. *J. Neurosci., 8*, 1172–1180.

Ferster, D., & Koch, C. (1987). Neuronal connections underlying orientation selectivity in cat visual cortex. *Trends in Neurosci., 10*, 487–492.

Fesenko, E. E., Kolesnikov, S. S., & Lyubarsky, A. L. (1985). Induction by cyclic GMP of cationic conductance in plasma membrane of retinal rod outer segment. *Nature, 313*, 310–313.

Festinger, L., & Easton, A. M. (1974). Inferences about the efferent system based on a perceptual illusion produced by eye movements. *Psychol. Rev., 18*, 44–58.

Fields, H. L. (1987). *Pain.* New York: McGraw Hill.

Fillenbaum, S., Schiffman, H. R., & Butcher, J. (1965). Perceptions of off-size versions of a familiar object under conditions of rich information. *J. Exp. Psychol., 69*, 298–303.

Fischler, H., Frei, E., Spira, D., & Rubinstein, M. (1967). Dynamic response of middle ear structures. *J. Acoust. Soc. Am., 41*, 1220–1231.

Fisher, G. H. (1970). An experimental and theoretical appraisal of the perspective and size-constancy theories of illusions. *Q. J. Exp. Psychol., 22*, 631–652.

Fisher, L. J. (1979). Interplexiform cell of the mouse retina: A Golgi demonstration. *Invest. Ophthalmol., 18*, 521–523.

Fitzgerald, H. E. (1968). Autonomic pupillary reflex activity during early infancy and its relation to social and non-social visual stimuli. *Dissertation Abstracts, 28*, 3896B–3897B.

Flaming, D. G., & Brown, K. T. (1979). Effects of calcium on the intensity-response curve of toad rods. *Nature, 278*, 852–853.

Fodor, J. A., & Bever, T. G. (1965). The psychological reality of linguistic segments. *J. Verb. Learn. Verb. Behav., 4*, 414–420.

Frank, M. (1975). Response patterns of rat glossopharyngeal taste neurons. In D. A. Denton & J. P. Coghlan (Eds.), *Olfaction and taste V* pp. 59–64. New York: Academic Press.

Freed, M. A., Smith, R. G., & Sterling, P. (1987). Rod bipolar array in the cat retina: Pattern of input from rods and GABA-accumulating amacrine cells. *J. Comp. Neurol., 266,* 445–455.

Freedman, S. J., & Fisher, H. G. (1968). The role of the pinna in auditory localization. In S. J. Freedman (Ed.), *Neuropsychology of spatially oriented behavior* (pp. 135–152). Pacific Grove, Calif.: Brooks/Cole.

Frishkopf, L. S., & Goldstein, M. H. (1963). Responses to acoustic stimuli from single units in the eighth nerve of the bullfrog. *J. Acoust. Soc. Am., 35,* 1219–1228.

Frishman, L. J., & Levine, M. W. (1983). Statistics of the maintained discharge of cat retinal ganglion cells. *J. Physiol., 339,* 475–494.

Frishman, L. J., Schweitzer-Tong, D. E., & Goldstein, E. B. (1983). Velocity tuning of cells in dorsal lateral geniculate nucleus and retina of the cat. *J. Neurophysiol., 50,* 1393–1414.

Frishman, L. J., Sieving, P. A., & Steinberg, R. H. (1988). Contributions to the electroretinogram of currents originating in proximal retina. *Visual Neurosci., 1,* 307–315.

Frost, B. J., & Nakayama, K. (1983). Single visual neurons code opposing motion independent of direction. *Science, 220,* 744–745.

Frumkes, T. E., & Temme, L. A. (1977). Rod-cone interaction in human scotopic vision. II. Cones-influence rod increment thresholds. *Vision Res., 17,* 673–679.

Fukada, Y. (1971). Receptive field organization of cat optic nerve fibers with special reference to conduction velocity. *Vision Res., 11,* 209–226.

Fukada, Y., & Saito, H. (1972). Phasic and tonic cells in the cat's lateral geniculate nucleus. *Tohoku J. Exp. Med., 106,* 209–210.

Fukuda, Y., & Stone, J. (1974). Retinal distribution and central projections of Y-, X-, and W-cells of the cat's retina. *J. Neurophysiol., 37,* 749–772.

Fuster, J. M., & Jervey, J. P. (1981). Inferotemporal neurons distinguish and retain behaviorally relevant features of visual stimuli. *Science, 212,* 952–955.

Gallego, A. (1971). Horizontal and amacrine cells in the mammal's retina. *Vision Res. Suppl., 3,* 33–50.

Galletti, C., Battaglini, P. P., & Aicardi, G. (1988). 'Real motion' cells in visual area V2 of behaving macaque monkeys. *Exp. Brain Res., 69,* 279–288.

Ganz, L. (1966). Mechanism of figural after-effects. *Psychol. Bull., 73,* 128–150.

Garcia, J., Kimmeldorf, D. J., & Koelling, F. A. (1955). Conditional aversion to saccharin resulting from exposure to gamma radiation. *Science, 122,* 157–158.

Garey, L. J., & Powell, T. P. S. (1971). An experimental study of the termination of the lateral geniculo-cortical pathway in the cat and monkey. *Proc. R. Soc. Lond. Ser. B., 179,* 41–63.

Garner, W. R. (1947). The effect of frequency spectrum on temporal integration of energy in the ear. *J. Acoust. Soc. Am., 19,* 808–815.

Gässler, G. (1954). Über die hörschwelle für schallereignisse mit verschieden breitem frequenzspektrum. *Acustica, 4,* 408–414.

Gelb, A. (1929). Die 'Farbenkonstanz' der Sehdinge. *Handb. Norm. Pathol. Physiol., 12,* 594–678.

Geldard, F. A. (1972). *The human senses,* 2nd Ed. New York: Wiley.

Georgopoulos, A. P., Lurito, J. T., Petrides, M., Schwartz, A. B., & Massey, J. T. (1989). Mental rotation of the neuronal population vector. *Science, 243,* 234–236.

Geschwind, N. (1972). Language and the brain. *Sci. Am., 226,* 76–83.

Geschwind, N. (1979). Specializations of the human brain. In *The Brain* pp. 108–117. San Francisco: W. H. Freeman.

Gesteland, R. C. (1978). The neural code: integration neural mechanisms. In E. C. Carterette & M. P. Friedman (Eds.). *Handbook of Perception, Vol. VIA: Tasting and Smelling* (pp. 259–276). New York: Academic Press.

Gibson, E. J. (1970). The development of perception as an adaptive process. *Am Sci., 58,* 98–107.

Gibson, E. J., Gibson, J. J., Smith, O. W., & Flock, H. (1959). Motor parallax as a determinant of perceived depth. *J. Exp. Psychol., 58,* 40–51.

Gibson, J. J. (1937). Adaptation, after-effect and contrast in the perception of tilted lines. II. Simultaneous contrast and the areal restriction of the after-effect. *J. Exp. Psychol., 20,* 553–569.

Gibson, J. J. (1950). *The perception of the visual world.* Boston: Houghton Mifflin.

Gibson, J. J. (1966). *The senses considered as perceptual systems.* Boston: Houghton Mifflin.

Gibson, J. J. (1968). What gives rise to the perception of motion? *Psychol. Rev., 75,* 335–346.

Gibson, J. J. (1962). Observations on active touch. *Psych. Rev., 69,* 477–491.

Giesler, G. J., Yezierski, R. P., Gerhart, K. K., & Willis, W. D. (1981). Spinothalamic tract neurons that project to medial and/or lateral thalamic nuclei: Evidence for a physiologically novel population of spinal cord neurons. *J. Neurophysiol., 46,* 1285–1308.

Gilbert, C. D. (1977). Laminar differences in receptive field properties of cells in cat primary visual cortex. *J. Physiol., 268,* 391–421.

Gilbert, C. D. (1983). Microcircuitry of the visual cortex. *Ann. Rev. Neurosci., 6,* 217–247.

Gilbert, C. D., & Wiesel, T. N. (1985). Intrinsic connectivity and receptive field properties in visual cortex. *Vision Res., 25,* 365–374.

Gilchrist, A. L. (1977). Perceived lightness depends on perceived spatial arrangement. *Science, 195,* 185–187.

Ginsburg, A. P. (1975). Is the illusory triangle physical or imaginary? *Nature, 257,* 219–220.

Glezer, V. D., Cooperman, A. M., Ivanov, V. A., & Tsherbach, T. A., (1976). An investigation of spatial frequency characteristics of the complex receptive fields in the visual cortex of the cat. *Vision Res., 16,* 789–797.

Gogel, W. C. (1970). The adjacency principle and three-dimensional visual illusions. *Psychon. Monogr. Suppl., 3,* 153–169.

Gogel, W. C. (1976). An indirect method of measuring perceived distance from familiar size. *Percept. Psychophys., 20,* 419–429.

Gogel, W. C., & Sturm, R. D. (1972). A comparison of accomodative and fusional convergence as cues to distance. *Percept. Psychophys., 11,* 166–168.

Gold, G. H., & Dowling, J. E. (1979). Photoreceptor coupling in retina of the toad, *Bufo Marinus.* I. Anatomy. *J. Neurophysiol., 42,* 292–310.

Goldstein, E. B. (1979). Rotation of objects in pictures viewed at an angle: Evidence for different properties of two types of pictorial space. *J. Exp. Psychol.: Human Percept. & Perf., 5,* 78–87.

Goldstein, M. H. Jr. (1974). The auditory periphery. In V. B. Mountcastle (Ed.), *Medical physiology,* 13th Ed. St. Louis: C. V. Mosby.

Goldwater, B. C. (1972). Psychological significance of pupillary movements. *Psychol. Bull., 77,* 340–355.

Gombrich, E. H. (1961). *Art and illusion,* 2nd Ed. Princeton, N.J.: Princeton University Press.

Gordon, J., & Abramov, I. (1977). Color vision in the peripheral retina. II. Hue and saturation. *J. Opt. Soc. Am., 67,* 202–207.

Gosline, C. J., MacLeod, D. I. A., & Rushton, W. A. H. (1973). Rod dark-adaptation measured above the cone threshold. *J. Physiol., 234,* 27P–28P.

Gouras, P. (1968). Identification of cone mechanisms in monkey ganglion cells. *J. Physiol., 199,* 533–547.

Grabowski, S. R., & Pak, W. L. (1975). Intracellular recordings of rod responses during dark adaptation. *J. Physiol., 247,* 363–391.

Graham, C. H. (1965). Some fundamental data. In C. H. Graham (Ed.), *Vision and visual perception.* pp. 68–80. New York: Wiley.

Graham, C. H., & Bartlett, N. R. (1939). The relation of size of stimulus and intensity in the human eye. II. Intensity thresholds for red and violet light. *J. Exp. Psychol., 24,* 574–587.

Graham, N. (1979). Does the brain perform a Fourier analysis of the visual scene? *Trends Neurosci., 2,* 207–208.

Graham, N., & Nachmias, J. (1971). Detection of grating patterns containing two spatial frequencies: A comparison of single-channel and multiple-channel models. *Vision Res., 11,* 251–259.

Granit, R. (1977). *The purposive brain.* Cambridge, Mass.: MIT Press.

Granit, R., Holmberg, T., & Zewi, M. (1938). On the mode of action of visual purple on the rod cell. *J. Physiol., 94,* 430–440.

Green, M., Corwin, T., & Zemon, V. (1976). A comparison of Fourier analysis and feature analysis in pattern-specific color aftereffects. *Science, 192,* 147–148.

Green, D. G., Dowling, J. E., Siegel, T. M., & Ripps, H. (1975). Retinal mechanisms of visual adaptation in the skate. *J. Gen. Physiol., 65,* 483–502.

Green, M., & Odom, J. V. (1986). Correspondence

matching in apparent motion: Evidence for three-dimensional spatial representation. *Science, 233,* 1427–1429.

Greenberg, D. P. (1989). Light reflection models for computer graphics. *Science, 244,* 166–173.

Greenlee, M. W., & Magnussen, S. (1988). Interactions among spatial-frequency and orientation channels adapted concurrently. *Vision Res. 28,* 1303–1309.

Greenwood, D. D., & Maruyama, N. (1965). Excitatory and inhibitory response areas of auditory neurons in the cochlear nucleus. *J. Neurophysiol., 28,* 863–892.

Gregory, R. L. (1970). *The intelligent eye.* New York: McGraw-Hill.

Gregory, R. L. (1978). *Eye and brain,* 3rd Ed. New York: McGraw-Hill.

Gregory, R. L., & Harris, J. P. (1975). Illusion destruction by appropriate scaling. *Perception, 4,* 203–220.

Gregory, R. L., & Harris, J. P. (1984). Real and apparent movement nulled. *Nature, 307,* 729–730.

Gregory, R. L., & Wallace, J. G. (1963). Recovery from early blindness: A case study. *Quart. J. Exper. Psychol.* (Monograph suppl. 2.) Heffers: Cambridge.

Grevert, P., Albert, L. H., & Goldstein, A. (1983). Partial antagonism of placebo analgesia by naloxone. *Pain, 14,* 129–143.

Grigg, P., Cinerman, G. A., & Riley, L. H. (1973). Joint position sense after total hip replacement. *J. Bone and Joint Surgery, 55A,* 1016–1025.

von Grunau, M., & Frost, B. J. (1983). Double-opponent-process mechanism underlying RF-structure of directionally specific cells of cat lateral suprasylvian visual area. *Exp. Brain Res., 49,* 84–92.

Grüsser, O.J., & Creutzfeldt, O. (1957). Eine neurophysiologische Grundlage des Brücke-Bartley-Effektes: Maxima der Impulsfrequenz retinaler und corticaler Neurone bei Flimmerlicht mittlerer Frequenzen. *Pfluegers Arch., 263,* 668–681.

Gulick, W. L. (1971). *Hearing: Physiology and psychophysics.* New York: Oxford University Press.

Gulick, W. L., Gescheider, G. A., & Frisina, R. D. (1989). *Hearing: Physiological acoustics, neural coding, and psychoacoustics.* New York: Oxford University Press.

Guyton, A. C. (1987). *Basic neuroscience: Anatomy and physiology.* Philadelphia: Saunders.

Haber, L. H., Moore, B. D., & Willis, W. D. (1982). Electrophysiological response properties of spinoreticular neurons in the monkey. *J. Comp. Neurol., 207,* 75–84.

Hahn, H., Kuckulies, G., & Bissar, A. (1940). Eine systematische untersuchung der geshmacksschwellen II. *Zeitschrift fur Sinnesphysiologie, 68,* 185–260.

Halasz, N., & Shepherd, G. M. (1983). Neurochemistry of the vertebrate olfactory bulb. *Neurosci., 10,* 579–619.

Halle, M., & Stevens, K. N. (1959). Analysis by synthesis. In W. Wathen-Dunn and L. E. Woods (Eds.), *Proceedings of the seminar on speech compression and processing.* AFCRC-TR-59-198. Vol. II. Washington, D.C.: U.S. Air Force.

Haller, A. von. *First Lines of Physiology* (1966). New York: Johnson Reprint Corp. (originally published 1786).

Halpern, M. (1987). The Organization and function of the vomeronasal system. *Ann. Rev. Neurosci., 10,* 325–362.

Hamalainen, H., Vartiainen, M., Karvanen, L., & Jarvilehto, T. (1982). Paradoxical heat sensations during moderate cooling of the skin. *Brain Res., 251,* 77–81.

Hammond, P., & Mouat, G. S. V. (1988). Neural correlates of motion after-effects in cat striate cortical neurones: Interocular transfer. *Exp. Brain Res., 72,* 21–28.

Hammond, P., Mouat, G. S. V., & Smith, A. T. (1988). Neural correlates of motion after-effects in cat striate cortical neurones: Monocular adaptation. *Exp. Brain Res., 72,* 1–20.

Hansson, P., & Ekblom, A. (1983). Transcutaneous electrical nerve stimulation (TENS) as compared to placebo TENS for the relief of acute oro-facial pain. *Pain, 15,* 157–165.

Harmon, L. D., & Julesz, B. (1973). Masking in visual recognition: Effects of two-dimensional filtered noise. *Science, 180,* 1194–1197.

Harris, J. D. (1952). Pitch discrimination. *J. Acoust. Soc. Am., 24,* 750–755.

Harris, J. D., Sergeant, R. L. (1971). Monaural/binaural minimum audible angles for a moving sound source. *J. Speech Hear. Res., 14,* 618–629.

Hartline, H. K. (1938). The response of single optic nerve fibers of the vertebrate eye to illumination of the retina. *Am J. Physiol., 121,* 400–415.

Hartline, H. K. (1949). Inhibition of activity of visual receptors by illuminating nearby retinal areas in the *Limulus* eye. *Fed. Proc., 8,* 69.

Hartline, H. K., & Ratliff, F. (1957). Inhibitory interaction of receptor units in the eye of *Limulus. J. Gen. Physiol., 40,* 357–376.

Hartline, H. K., Wagner, H. G., & MacNichol, E. F. (1952). The peripheral origin of nervous activity in the visual system. *Cold Spring Harbor Symp. Quant. Biol., 17,* 125–141.

Hartline, H. K., Wagner, H. G., & Ratliff, F. (1956). Inhibition in the eye of *Limulus. J. Gen. Physiol., 39,* 651–673.

Harvey, L. O. Jr., & Michon, J. A. (1974). Detectability of relative motion as a function of exposure duration, angular separation, and background. *J. Exp. Psychol., 103,* 317–325.

Hastorf, A. H., & Way, K. S. (1952). Apparent size with and without distance cues. *J. Gen. Psychol., 47,* 181–188.

Hata, Y., Tsumoto, T., Sata, H., Hagihara, K., & Tamura, H. (1988). Inhibition contributes to orientation selectivity in visual cortex of cat. *Nature, 336,* 815–817.

Haynes, L. W., & Yau, K.-W. (1985). Cyclic GMP-sensitive conductance in outer segment membranes of catfish cones. *Nature, 317,* 61–64.

Hebb, D. O. (1949). *The organization of behavior.* New York: Wiley.

Hecht, S. (1937). Rods, cones, and the chemical basis of vision. *Physiol. Rev., 17,* 239–290.

Hecht, S., Haig, C., & Chase, A. M. (1937). The influence of light adaptation on subsequent dark adaptation of the eye. *J. Gen. Physiol., 20,* 831–850.

Hecht, S., Shlaer, S., & Pirenne, M. H. (1942). Energy, quanta, and vision. *J. Gen. Physiol., 25,* 819–840.

Hedden, W. L., & Dowling, J. E. (1978). The interplexiform cell system. II. Effects of dopamine on goldfish retinal neurons. *Proc. R. Soc. Lond. Ser. B., 201,* 27–55.

Heffner, H. E., & Heffner, R. S. (1984). Temporal lobe lesions and perception of species-specific vocalizations by macaques. *Science, 226,* 75–76.

Heggelund, P. (1981). Receptive field organization of complex cells in cat striate cortex. *Exp. Brain Res., 42,* 99–107.

Heinemann, E. G. (1955). Simultaneous brightness induction as a function of inducing and test field luminance. *J. Exp. Psychol., 50,* 89–96.

Heinemann, E. G., Tulving, E., & Nachmias, J. (1959). The effect of oculomotor adjustments on apparent size. *Am. J. Psychol., 72,* 32–45.

Heller, A. First lines of physiology. New York: Johnson Reprint Corp. (1966). (Originally published, Edinburgh: Charles Eliot, 1786.)

von Helmholtz, H. C. F. (1924). *Physiological Optics,* Vol. II, trans. J. Southall. Rochester, N.Y.: Optical Society of America.

von Helmholtz, H. (1866). *Treatise on physiological optics,* Vol. III, J. P. C. Southall (Ed.) (translated from the 3rd German edition). New York: Dover, 1962.

von Henning, H. (1927). Psychologische studien am geshmackssinn. In: E. Abderhalden (Ed.), *Handbuch der biologischen Arbeitsmethoden.* Berlin: Urban and Schwarzenberg.

Helson, H. (1948). Adaptation level as a basis for a quantitative theory of frames of reference. *Psychol. Rev., 55,* 297–313.

Helson, H. (1964). Current trends and issues in adaptation level theory. *Am. Psychol., 19,* 26–28.

Hemilä, S. (1977). Background adaptation in the rods of the frog's retina. *J. Physiol., 265,* 721–741.

Henneman, R. H. (1935). A photometric study of the perception of object color. *Arch. Psychol., 27,* 5–88.

Henning, H. (1916). *Der Geruch.* Leipzig: Barth.

Herbert, E., Oates, E., Martens, G., Comb, & Rosen, M. (1983). Generation of diversity and evolution of opioid peptides. *Cold Spring Harbor Symp. Quant. Biol., 48, pt. 1,* 375–384.

Hess, C., & Pretori, H. (1894). Messende Untersuchungen über die Gesetzmassigkeit des sumultanen Heligkeits-Contrastes. *Arch. Ophthalmol., 40,* 1–24.

Hess, E. H. (1965). Attitude and pupil size. *Sci. Am., 212,* 46–54.

Hess, E. H., & Polt, J. M. (1960). Pupil size as related to interest value of visual stimuli. *Science, 132,* 349–350.

Hess, E. H., & Polt, J. M. (1964). Pupil size in relation to mental activity during simple problem-solving. *Science, 140,* 1190–1192.

von der Heydt, R., & Peterhans, E. (1989). Mechanisms of contour perception in monkey visual cortex. I. Lines of pattern discontinuity. *J. Neurosci., 9*, 1731–1748.

von der Heydt, R., Peterhans, E., & Baumgartner, G. (1984). Illusory contours and cortical neuron responses. *Science, 224*, 1260–1262.

Hirsch, H. V. B., & Spinelli, D. N. (1970). Visual experience modifies distribution of horizontally and vertically oriented receptive fields in cats. *Science, 168*, 869–871.

Hochberg, J. E. (1971a). Perception. I. Color and shape. In J. W. Kling & L. A. Riggs (Eds.), *Woodworth and Schlosberg's experimental psychology*, 3rd Ed. (pp. 395–474). New York: Holt, Rinehart & Winston.

Hochberg, J. E. (1971b). Perception. II. Space and movement. In J. W. Kling & L. A. Riggs (Eds.), *Woodworth and Schlosberg's experimental psychology*, 3rd Ed. (pp. 475–530). New York: Holt, Rinehart, and Winston.

Hochberg, J. E., & Beck, J. (1954). Apparent spatial arrangement and perceived brightness. *J. Exp. Psychol., 47*, 263–266.

Hochberg, J. E., & McAlister, E. (1953). A quantitative approach to figural "goodness." *J. Exp. Psychol., 46*, 361–364.

Hochberg, J. E., & Silverstein, A. (1956). A quantitative index of stimulus similarity: Proximity vs. difference in brightness. *Am. J. Psychol., 69*, 456–458.

Hochstein, S., & Shapley, R. M. (1976). Linear and nonlinear spatial subunits in Y cat retinal ganglion cells. *J. Physiol., 262*, 265–284.

Hodgkin, A. L., & Huxley, A. F. (1952). A quantitative description of membrane current and its application to conduction and excitation in nerve. *J. Physiol., 117*, 500–544.

Hoffmann, K.-P., & Stone, J. (1971). Conduction velocity of afferents to cat visual cortex: A correlation with cortical receptive field properties. *Brain Res., 32*, 460–466.

Holway, A. H., & Boring, E. G. (1940). The moon illusion and the angle of regard. *Am. J. Psychol., 53*, 509–516.

Holway, A. H., & Boring, E. G. (1941). Determinants of apparent visual size with distance variant. *Am J. Psychol., 54*, 21–37.

Hood, D. C. (1978). Psychophysical and physiological tests of proposed physiological mechanisms of light adaptation. In J. C. Armington, J. Krauskopf, &

B. R. Wooten (Eds.), *Visual psychophysics and physiology* (pp. 141–155). Academic Press.

Hood, J. D. (1972). Fundamentals of identification of sensorineural hearing loss. *Sound, 6*, 21–26.

Hosobuchi, Y., Adams, J. E., & Linchitz, R. (1977). Pain relief by electrical stimulation of the central grey matter in humans and its reversal by naloxone. *Science, 197*, 183–186.

Howard, I. P., & Templeton, W. B., (1966). *Human spatial orientation*. New York: Wiley.

Hubbard, A. E., & Mountain, D. C. (1983). Alternating current delivered into the scala media alters sound pressure at the eardrum. *Science, 222*, 510–512.

Hubel, D. H., & Livingstone, M. S. (1983). Blobs and color vision. *Can. J. Physiol. and Pharmacol., 61*, 1433–1441.

Hubel, D. H., & Livingstone, M. S. (1987). Segregation of form, color, and stereopsis in primate area 18. *J. Neurosci., 7*, 3378–3415.

Hubel, D. H., & Wiesel, T. N. (1959). Receptive fields of single neurones in the cat's striate cortex. *J. Physiol., 148*, 574–591.

Hubel, D. H., & Wiesel, T. N. (1961). Integrative action in the cat's lateral geniculate body. *J. Physiol., 155*, 385–398.

Hubel, D. H., & Wiesel, T. N. (1962). Receptive fields, binocular interaction and functional architecture in the cat's visual cortex. *J. Physiol., 160*, 106–154.

Hubel, D. H., & Wiesel, T. N. (1963). Receptive fields of cells in striate cortex of very young visually inexperienced kittens. *J. Neurophysiol., 26*, 994–1002.

Hubel, D. H., & Wiesel, T. N. (1965a). Receptive fields and functional architecture in two non-striate visual areas (18 and 19) of the cat. *J. Neurophysiol., 28*, 229–289.

Hubel, D. H., & Wiesel, T. N. (1965b). Binocular interaction in striate cortex of kittens reared with artificial squint. *J. Neurophysiol., 28*, 1041–1059.

Hubel, D. H., & Wiesel, T. N. (1968). Receptive fields and functional architecture of monkey striate cortex. *J. Physiol., 195*, 215–243.

Hubel, D. H., & Wiesel, T. N. (1970). Stereoscopic vision in macaque monkey. *Nature, 225*, 41–42.

Hubel, D. H., & Wiesel, T. N. (1972). Laminar and columnar distribution of geniculocortical fibers in the macaque monkey. *J. Comp. Neurol., 146,* 421–450.

Hubel, D. H., & Wiesel, T. N. (1974a). Sequence regularity and geometry of orientation columns in the monkey striate cortex. *J. Comp. Neurol., 158,* 267–294.

Hubel, D. H., & Wiesel, T. N. (1974b). Uniformity of monkey striate cortex: A parallel relationship between field size, scatter, and magnification factor. *J. Comp. Neurol., 158,* 295–306.

Hubel, D. H., & Wiesel, T. N. (1977). Functional architecture of macaque monkey visual cortex. *Proc. R. Soc. Lond. Ser. B., 198,* 1–59.

Hubel, D. H., Wiesel, T. N., & LeVay, S. (1977). Plasticity of ocular dominance columns in monkey striate cortex. *Philos. Trans. R. Soc. Lond., 278,* 377–409.

Hubel, D. H., Wiesel, T. N., & Stryker, M. P. (1978). Anatomical demonstration of orientation columns in macaque monkey. *J. Comp. Neurol., 177,* 361–380.

Hudspeth, A. J. (1982). Extracellular current flow and the site of transduction by vertebrate hair cells. *J. Neurosci., 2,* 1–10.

Hudspeth, A. J. (1985). The cellular basis of hearing: The biophysics of hair cells. *Science, 230,* 745–752.

Huggins, A. W. F. (1964). Distortion of the temporal pattern of speech: Interruption and alternation. *J. Acoust. Soc. Am., 36,* 1055–1064.

Hughes, G. W., & Maffei, L. (1965). On the origin of the dark discharge of retinal ganglion cells. *Arch. Ital. Biol., 103,* 45–59.

Hughes, G. W., & Maffei, L. (1966). Retinal ganglion cell response to sinusoidal light stimulation. *J. Neurophysiol., 29,* 333–352.

Hughes, J., Smith, T. W., Kosterlitz, H. W., Fothergill, L. A., Morgan, B. A., & Morris, H. R. (1975). Identification of two related pentapeptides from the brain with potent agonist activity. *Nature, 258,* 577–579.

Hurvich, L. M., & Jameson, D. (1955). Some quantitative aspects of an opponent colors theory. II. Brightness, saturation and hue in normal and dichromatic vision. *J. Opt. Soc. Am., 45,* 602–616.

Hurvich, L. M., & Jameson, D. (1957). An opponent-process theory of color vision. *Psychol. Rev., 64,* 384–404.

Hyvarinen, J., & Poranen, A. (1978). Movement sensitive and direction and orientation selective cutaneous receptive fields in the hand area of the post central gyrus in monkeys. *J. Physiol. (Lond.), 283,* 523–537.

Imig, T. J., Ruggero, M. A., Kitzes, L. M., Javel, E., & Brugge, J. F. (1977). Organization of auditory cortex in the owl monkey *(Aotus trivirgatus). J. Comp. Neurol., 171,* 111–128.

Ingle, D. (1985). The goldfish is a retinex animal. *Science, 227,* 651–654.

Ingling, C. R. Jr. (1977). The spectral sensitivity of the opponent-color channels. *Vision Res., 17,* 1083–1090.

Ingling, C. R. Jr., & Tsou, B. H.-P. (1977). Orthogonal combination of the three visual channels. *Vision Res., 17,* 1075–1083.

Ingling, C. R. Jr., Lewis, A. L., Loose, D. R., & Myers, K. J. (1977). Cones change rod sensitivity. *Vision Res., 17,* 555–563.

International Commission on Illumination. (1932). *Proceedings of the eighth session.* Cambridge: Cambridge University Press.

Ittelson, W. H. (1968). *The Ames demonstrations in perception.* New York: Hefner.

Ittelson, W. H., & Kilpatrick, F. P. (1951). Experiments in perception. *Sci. Am., 185,* 50–55.

Iwai, E. (1985). Neuropsychological basis of pattern vision in macaque monkeys. *Vision Res., 25,* 425–439.

Jahoda, G. (1966). Geometric illusions and environment: A study in Ghana. *Br. J. Psychol., 57,* 193–199.

Jakiela, H. G., Enroth-Cugell, C., & Shapley, R. (1976). Adaptation and dynamics in X-cells and Y-cells of the cat retina. *Exp. Brain Res., 24,* 335–342.

Jameson, D., & Hurvich, L. M. (1961). Complexities of perceived brightness. *Science, 133,* 174–179.

Jáñez, L. (1984). Visual grouping without low spatial frequencies. *Vision Res., 24,* 271–274.

Jerger, J. F. (1957). Auditory adaptation. *J. Acoust. Soc. Am., 29,* 357–363.

Johansson, R. S., & Vallbo, A. B. (1983). Tactile sensory coding in the glabrous skin of the human hand. *Trends Neurosci., 6,* 27–32.

Johns, M. A., Feder, H. H., Komisaruk, B. R., & Mayer, A. D. (1978). Urine-induced reflex ovulation in anovulatory rats may be a vomeronasal effect. *Nature, 272*, 446–448.

Johnston, J. C., & McClelland, J. L. (1974). Perception of letters in words: Seek not and ye shall find. *Science, 184*, 1192–1194.

Johnstone, B. M., Taylor, K. J., & Boyle, A. J. (1970). Mechanics of guinea pig cochlea. *J. Acoust. Soc. Am., 47*, 504–509.

Jones, D. T., & Reed, R. R. (1989). G olf: An olfactory neuron specific G protein involved in odorant signal transduction. *Science, 244*, 790–795.

Jones, J. P., & Palmer, L. A. (1987). An evaluation of the two-dimensional Gabor filter model of simple receptive fields in cat cortex. *J. Neurophysiol., 58*, 1233–1258.

Judd, D. B. (1951). Basic correlates of the visual stimulus. In S. S. Stevens (Ed.), *Handbook of experimental psychology*. (pp. 811–867), New York: Wiley.

Julesz, B. (1964). Binocular depth perception without familiarity cues. *Science, 145*, 356–362.

Julesz, B. (1971). *Foundations of Cyclopean Perception*. Chicago: University of Chicago Press.

Julesz, B. (1974). Cooperative phenomena in binocular depth perception. *Amer. Scientist, 62*, 32–43.

Julesz, B. (1981). Textons, the elements of texture perception, and their interactions. *Nature, 290*, 91–97.

Julesz, B., & Krose, B. (1988). Visual texture perception: Features and spatial filters. *Nature, 333*, 302–303.

Kaas, J. H., Merzenich, M. M., & Killackey, H. P. (1983). The reorganization of somatic sensory cortex following peripheral nerve damage in adult and developing mammals. *Ann. Rev. Neurosci., 6*, 325–336.

Kaas, J. H., Nelson, R. J., Sur, M., Lin, C.-S., & Merzenich, M. M. (1979). Multiple representations of the body within the primary somatosensory cortex of primates. *Science, 204*, 521–523.

Kahneman, D., & Beatty, J. (1967). Pupillary responses in a pitch discrimination task. *Percept. Psychophys., 2*, 101–105.

Kahneman, D., & Pearler, W. S. (1969). Incentive effects and pupillary changes in association learning. *J. Exp. Psychol., 79*, 312–318.

Kaiser, P. K. (1967). Perceived shape and its dependency on perceived slant. *J. Exper. Psychol., 75*, 345–353.

Kaneko, A. (1971). Electrical connections between horizontal cells in the dogfish retina. *J. Physiol., 213*, 95–105.

Kaneko, A., & Hashimoto, H. (1969). Electrophysiological study of single neurons in the inner nuclear layer of the carp retina. *Vision Res., 9*, 37–55.

Kaneko, A., & Shimazaki, H. (1975). Effects of external ions on the synaptic transmission from photoreceptors to horizontal cells in the carp retina. *J. Physiol., 252*, 509–522.

Kanisza, G. (1979). *Organization in vision: Essays on gestalt perception*. New York: Praeger.

Kaplan, E., Marcus, S., & So, Y. T. (1979). Effects of dark adaptation on spatial and temporal properties of receptive fields in cat lateral geniculate nucleus. *J. Physiol., 294*, 561–580.

Kaplan, E., & Shapley, R. M. (1982). X and Y cells in the lateral geniculate nucleus of macaque monkeys. *J. Physiol., 330*, 125–143.

Kardos, L. (1934). Ding und Schatten. *Z. Psychol. Ergebnisse, 23*.

Kato, H., Bishop, P. O., & Orban, G. A. (1978). Hypercomplex and simple/complex classifications in cat striate cortex. *J. Neurophysiol., 41*, 1071–1095.

Katsuki, Y. (1961). Neural mechanisms of auditory sensations in cat. In W. A. Rosenblith (Ed.), *Sensory communication* (pp. 561–583). Cambridge, Mass.: MIT Press.

Katz, B. (1950) Depolarization of sensory terminals and the initiation of impulses in the muscle spindle. *J. Physiol., 111*, 261–282.

Kaufman, L. (1974). *Sight and mind*. New York: Oxford University Press.

Kaufman, L., & Rock, I. (1962). The moon illusion. I. *Science, 136*, 953–961.

Kayama, Y. (1985). Ascending, descending and local control of neuronal activity in the rat lateral geniculate nucleus. *Vision Res., 25*, 339–347.

Kelly, D. H. (1976). Pattern detection and the two-dimensional Fourier transform: Flickering checkerboards and chromatic mechanisms. *Vision Res., 16*, 277–287.

Kenkel, F. (1913). Untersuchungen über den Zusammenhang Zwischen Erscheinungsgrösse und

Erscheinungsbewegung bei einigen sogenannten optischen Täuschungen. *Z. Psychol., 67,* 358–449.

Kennedy, J. M. (1980). Blind people recognizing and making haptic pictures. In W. Schiff and E. Foulke (Ed.), *The perception of pictures* (pp. 305–331). Cambridge: Cambridge University Press.

Kenshalo, D. R., & Duclaux, R. (1977). Response properties of cutaneous cold receptors in the monkey. *J. Neurophysiol., 40,* 319–332.

Kenshalo, D. R., Giesler, G. J., Leonard, R. B., & Willis, B. D. (1980). Responses of neurons in primate ventral posterior lateral nucleus to noxious stimuli. *J. Neurophysiol., 43,* 1594–1614.

Kenshalo, D. R., & Isensee, O. (1983). Responses of primate S1 cortical neurons to noxious stimuli. *J. Neurophysiol., 50,* 1479–1496.

Khanna, S. M., & Leonard, D. G. B. (1982). Basilar membrane tuning in the cat cochlea. *Science, 215,* 303–304.

Kiang, N. Y.-S. (1968). A survey of recent developments in the study of auditory physiology. *Ann. Otol. Rhinol. Laryngol., 77,* 656–675.

Kiang, N. Y.-S., Moxon, E. C., & Levine, R. A. (1970). Auditory nerve activity in cats with normal and abnormal cochleas. In G. E. Wostenholme and J. Knight (Eds.), *Sensorineural hearing loss* (pp. 241–273). London: Churchill.

Kiang, N. Y.-S., Pfeiffer, R. R., Warr, W. B., & Bakus, A. S. (1965). Stimulus coding in the cochlear nucleus. *Ann. Otol. Rhinol. Laryngol., 74,* 463–485.

Kiang, N. Y.-S., Watanabe, T., Thomas, E. C., & Clark, L. F. (1962). Stimulus coding in the cat's auditory nerve. *Ann. Otol. Rhinol. Laryngol., 71,* 1009–1026.

Kiang, N. Y.-S., Rho, J. M., Northrop, C. C., Liberman, M. C., & Ryugo, D. K. (1982). Hair-cell innervation by spiral ganglion cells in adult cats. *Science, 217,* 175–177.

Kiesow, F. (1896). Beitrage zur physiologischen psychologie des geschmackssinnes. *Philosophische Studien., 12,* 255–278.

Kimura, D. (1973). The asymmetry of the human brain. *Sci. Am., 228,* 70–78.

Kimura, K., & Beidler, L. M. (1961). Microelectrode study of taste receptors of rat and hamster. *J. Cell. Comp. Physiol., 187,* 131–140.

Klein, A. B. (1936). *Colour cinematography.* London: Chapman & Hall.

Kleinschmidt, J., & Dowling, J. E. (1975). Intracellular recordings from gecko photoreceptors during light and dark adaptation. *J. Gen. Physiol., 66,* 617–648.

Klumpp, R. G., & Eady, H. R. (1956). Some measurements of interaural time difference thresholds. *J. Acoust. Soc. Amer., 28,* 859–860.

Knudsen, E. I. (1983). Early auditory experience aligns the auditory map of space in the optic tectum of the barn owl. *Science, 222,* 939–942.

Knudsen, E. I. (1988). Early blindness results in a degraded auditory map of space in the optic tectum of the barn owl. *Proc. Natl. Acad. Sci., 85,* 6211–6214.

Knudsen, E. I., & Konishi, M. (1978). Center-surround organization of auditory receptive fields in the owl. *Science, 202,* 778–780.

Knudsen, E. I., Konishi, M., & Pettigrew, J. D. (1977). Receptive fields of auditory neurons in the owl. *Science, 198,* 1278–1280.

Koenig, W., Dunn, H. K., & Lacy, L. Y. (1946). The sound spectrograph. *J. Acoust. Soc. Am., 17,* 19–49.

Koffka, K. (1935). *Principles of gestalt psychology.* New York: Harcourt Brace.

Köhler, W., & Wallach, H. (1944). Figural aftereffect, an investigation of visual processes. *Proc. Am. Philos. Soc., 88,* 269–357.

Kolata, G. (1985). What causes nearsightedness? *Science, 229,* 1249–1250.

Kolb, B., & Whishaw, I. Q. (1985). *Fundamentals of human neuropsychology* (2nd Ed.). New York: Freeman.

Kolb, H. (1974). The connections between horizontal cells and photoreceptors in the retina of the cat: Electron microscopy of Golgi preparations. *J. Comp. Neurol., 155,* 1–14.

Kolb, H., & Nelson, R. (1981). Amacrine cells of the cat retina. *Vision Res., 21,* 1625–1633.

Kolb, H., Nelson, R., & Mariani, A. (1981). Amacrine cells, bipolar cells and ganglion cells of the cat retina: A Golgi study. *Vision Res., 21,* 1081–1114.

Kolers, P. A., & von Grünau, M. (1975). Visual construction of color is digital. *Science, 187,* 757–759.

Kolers, P. A., & von Grünau, M. (1976). Shape and color in apparent motion. *Vision Res., 16,* 329–335.

Kolers, P. A., & Pomerantz, J. R. (1971). Figural change in apparent motion. *J. Exp. Psychol., 87,* 99–108.

Komatsu, H., & Wurtz, R. H. (1988a). Relation of cortical areas MT and MST to pursuit eye movements. I. Localization and visual properties of neurons. *J. Neurophysiol., 60,* 580–603.

Komatsu, H., & Wurtz, R. H. (1988b). Relation of cortical areas *MT* and *MST* to pursuit eye movements. III. Interaction with full-field visual stimulation. *J. Neurophysiol., 60,* 621–643.

Komatsu, Y., Nakajima, S., Toyama, K., & Fetz, E. E. (1988). Intracortical connectivity revealed by spike-triggered averaging in slice preparations of cat visual cortex. *Brain Res., 442,* 359–362.

Komoda, M. K., & Ono, H. (1974). Oculomotor adjustments and size-distance perception. *Percept. Psychophys., 15,* 353–360.

Korte, A. (1915). Kinematoskopische Untersuchungen. *Z. Psychol., 72,* 193–296.

Krakavaer, D., & Dallenbach, K. (1937). Gustatory adaptation to sweet, sour and bitter. *Am. J. Psychol., 49,* 469–475.

Krubitzer, L. A., & Kaas, J. H. (1989). Cortical integration of parallel pathways in the visual system of primates. *Brain Res., 478,* 161–165.

Kuffler, S. W. (1953). Discharge patterns and functional organization of mammalian retina. *J. Neurophysiol., 16,* 37–68.

Kuffler, S. W., & Nicholls, J. G. (1976). *From neuron to brain.* Sunderland, Mass.: Sinauer Associates.

Kuhl, P. K., & Meltzoff, A. N. (1982). The bimodal perception of speech in infancy. *Science, 218,* 1138–1140.

Kuhl, P. K., & Miller, J. D. (1975). Speech perception by the chinchilla: Voiced-voiceless distinction in alveolar plosive consonants. *Science, 190,* 69–72.

Kuwada, S., Yin, T. C. T., & Wickesberg, R. E. (1979). Response of cat inferior colliculus neurons to binaural beat stimuli: Possible mechanisms for sound localization. *Science, 206,* 586–588.

Ladefoged, P., DeClerk, J., Lindau, M., & Papcun, G. (1972). An auditory motor theory of speech production. *UCLA Phonetics Lab. Working Papers in Phonetics, 22,* 48–76.

Lamb, T. (1986). Transduction in vertebrate photoreceptors: The roles of cyclic GMP and calcium. *Trends in Neurosci.,* May 1986, 224–228.

Lamb, T. D., McNaughton, P. A., & Yau, K.-W. (1981). Spatial spread of activation and background desensitization in toad rod outer segments. *J. Physiol., 319,* 463–496.

LaMotte, R. H., Thalhammer, J. G., Torebjork, H. E., & Robinson, C. J. (1982). Peripheral neural mechanisms of cutaneous hyperalgesia following mild injury by heat. *J. Neurosci., 2,* 765–781.

Lamour, Y., Guilbark, G., & Willer, J. C. (1983). Rat somatosensory (Sm1) cortex: II. Laminar and columnar organization of noxious and non-noxious inputs. *Exp. Brain Res., 49,* 46–54.

Lancet, D. (1986). Vertebrate olfactory reception. *Ann. Rev. Neurosci., 9,* 329–355.

Land, E. H. (1986). Recent advances in retinex theory. *Vision Res., 26,* 7–21.

Land, E. H., & McCann, J. J. (1971). Lightness and retinex theory. *J. Opt. Soc. Amer., 61,* 1–11.

Langdon, J. (1951). The perception of a changing shape. *Q. J. Exp. Psychol., 3,* 157–165.

Langner, G., Bonke, D., & Scheich, H. (1981). Neuronal discrimination of natural and synthetic vowels in field L of trained mynah birds. *Exp. Brain Res., 43,* 11–24.

Lasater, E. M., & Lam, D. M. K. (1984). The identification and some functions of GABAergic neurons in the distal catfish retina. *Vision Res., 24,* 497–506.

Laties, A. M., & Liebman, P. A. (1970). Cones of living amphibian eye: Selective staining. *Science, 168,* 1475–1477.

Lee, B. B., Elepfandt, A., & Virsu, V. (1981). Phase of responses to sinusoidal gratings of simple cells in cat striate cortex. *J. Neurophysiol., 45,* 818–828.

Leeper, R. W. (1935). A study of a neglected portion of the field of learning: The development of sensory organization. *J. Genet. Psychol., 46,* 41–75.

Le Grand, T. (1957). *Light, colour, and vision,* trans. R. Hunt, T. Walsh, & F. Hunt. New York: Wiley.

Lehiste, I. (1976). Suprasegmental features of speech. In N. J. Lass (Ed.), *Contemporary issues in experimental phonetics* (pp. 225–239). New York: Academic Press.

Lehky, S. R., & Sejnowski, T. J. (1988). Network model of shape-from-shading: Neural function arises from both receptive and projective fields. *Nature, 333,* 452–454.

Lehmkuhle, S. W., & Fox, R. (1975). Effect of binocular rivalry suppression on the motion after-effect. *Vision Res., 15*, 855–859.

Lehmkuhle, S., & Fox, R. (1980). Effect of depth separation on metacontrast masking. *J. Exper. Psychol.: Human Percept. & Perform., 6*, 605–621.

Leibowitz, H. W. (1955a). The relation between rate threshold for the perception of movement and luminance for various durations of exposure. *J. Exp. Psychol., 49*, 209–214.

Leibowitz, H. W. (1955b). Effect of reference lines on the discrimination of movement. *J. Opt. Soc. Am., 45*, 829–830.

Leibowitz, H. W. (1971). Sensory, learned, and cognitive mechanisms of size perception. *Ann. N.Y. Acad. Sci., 188*, 47–62.

Leibowitz, H. W., & Gwozdecki, J. (1967). The magnitude of the Poggendorff illusion as a function of age. *Child Devel., 38*, 573–580.

Leibowitz, H. W., Johnson, C. A., & Isabelle, E. (1972). Peripheral motion detection and refractive error. *Science, 177*, 1207–1208.

Leicester, J., & Stone, J. (1967). Ganglion, amacrine, and horizontal cells of the cat's retina. *Vision Res., 7*, 695–705.

Lennie, P. (1980). Parallel visual pathways: a review. *Vision Res., 20*, 561–594.

Lennie, P., & D'Zmura, M. (1988). Mechanisms of color vision. *CRC Critical Rev. in Neurobiol., 3*, 333–401.

Lettvin, J. Y., Maturana, H. R., McCulloch, W. S., & Pitts, W. H. (1959). What the frog's eye tells the frog's brain. *Proc. Inst. Radio Engineers, 47*, 1940–1951.

Leventhal, A. G., Rodieck, R. W., & Dreher, B. (1981). Retinal ganglion cell classes in the old world monkey: Morphology and central projections. *Science, 213*, 1139–1142.

Levick, W. R. (1967). Receptive fields and trigger features of ganglion cells of the rabbits retina. *J. Physiol., 188*, 285–307.

Levick, W. R., Kirk, D. L., & Wagner, H. G. (1981). Neurophysiological tracing of a projection from temporal retina to contralateral visual cortex of the cat. *Vision Res., 21*, 1677–1679.

Levine, J. D., Gordon, N. C., & Fields, H. L. (1978). The mechanism of placebo analgesia. *Lancet, 2*, 654–657.

Levine, M. W., & Abramov, I. (1975). An analysis of spatial summation in the receptive fields of goldfish retinal ganglion cells. *Vision Res., 15*, 777–789.

Levine, M. W., & Frishman, L. J. (1984). Interactions between rod and cone channels: A model that includes inhibition. *Vision Res., 24*, 513–516.

Levine, M. W., Frishman, L. J., & Enroth-Cugell, C. (1987). Interactions between the rod and the cone pathways in the cat retina. *Vision Res., 27*, 1093–1104.

Levine, M. W., Saleh, E. J., & Yarnold, P. R. (1988). Statistical properties of the maintained discharge of chemically isolated ganglion cells in goldfish retina. *Visual Neurosci., 1*, 31–46.

Levine, M. W., & Shefner, J. M. (1975). Independence of "on" and "off" responses of retinal ganglion cells. *Science, 190*, 1215–1217.

Levine, M. W., & Shefner, J. M. (1977). Variability in ganglion cell firing patterns; implications for separate "on" and "off" processes. *Vision Res., 17*, 765–777.

Levine, M. W., & Troy, J. B. (1986). The variability of the maintained discharge of cat dorsal lateral geniculate cells. *J. Physiol., 375*, 339–359.

Levine, M. W., & Zimmerman, R. P. (1988). Evidence for local circuits within the receptive fields of retinal ganglion cells in goldfish. *Visual Neurosci., 1*, 377–385.

Levinson, E., & Sekuler, R. (1975). The independence of channels in human vision selective for direction of movement. *J. Physiol., 250*, 347–366.

Liberman, A. M. (1957). Some results of research on speech perception. *J. Acoust. Soc. Am., 29*, 117–123.

Liberman, A. M. (1982). On finding that speech is special. *Amer. Psychol., 37*, 148–167.

Liberman, A. M., Cooper, F. S., Shankweiler, D. S., & Studdert-Kennedy, M. (1967). Perception of the speech code. *Psychol. Rev., 74*, 431–461.

Liberman, A. M., Delattre, P. C., & Cooper, F. S. (1952). The role of selected stimulus variables in the perception of the unvoiced stop consonants. *Am. J. Psychol., 65*, 497–516.

Liberman, A. M., Delattre, P. C., Gerstman, L. J., & Cooper, F. S. (1956). Tempo of frequency change as a cue for distinguishing classes of speech sounds. *J. Exp. Psychol., 52*, 127–137.

Liberman, A. M., Harris, K. S., Eimas, P. D.,

Lisker, L., & Bastian, J. (1961). An effect of learning on speech perception: Discrimination of durations of silence with and without phonemic significance. *Lang. Speech, 4*, 175–195.

Liberman, A. M., Harris, K. S., Hoffman, H. S., & Griffith, B. C. (1957). Discrimination of speech sounds within and across phoneme boundaries. *J. Exp. Psychol., 54*, 358–368.

Liberman, A. M., Ingemann, F., Lisker, L., Delattre, P., & Cooper, F. S. (1959). Minimal rules for synthesizing speech. *J. Acoust. Soc. Am., 31*, 1490–1499.

Liberman, A. M., & Mattingly, I. G. (1989). A specialization for speech perception. *Science, 243*, 489–494.

Liberman, A. M., & Studdert-Kennedy, M. (1978). Phonetic perception. In R. Held, H. W. Liebowitz, & H. L. Teuber (Eds.), *Handbook of sensory physiology* Vol. VIII. (pp. 143–178). Berlin: Springer-Verlag.

Lichten, W., & Lurie, S. (1950). A new technique for the study of perceived size. *Am. J. Psychol., 63*, 280–282.

Licklider, J. C. R. (1956). Auditory frequency analysis. In C. Cherry (Ed.), *Information theory*. New York: Academic Press.

Lieberman, P. (1977). *Speech physiology and acoustic phonetics: An introduction*. New York: Macmillan.

Liebman, P. A., & Pugh Jr., E. N. (1979). The control of phosphodiesterase in rod disk membranes: Kinetics, possible mechanisms and significance for vision. *Vision Res., 19*, 375–380.

Lindsay, P. H., & Norman, D. A. (1977). *Human Information Processing: An Introduction to Psychology*. New York: Academic Press.

Livingstone, M. S., & Hubel, D. H. (1987a). Connections between layer 4B of area 17 and the thick cytochrome oxidase stripes of area 18 in the squirrel monkey. *J. Neurosci., 7*, 3371–3377.

Livingstone, M. S., & Hubel, D. H. (1987b). Psychophysical evidence for separate channels for the perception of form, color, movement, and depth. *J. Neurosci., 7*, 3461–3468.

Livingstone, M. S., & Hubel, D. H. (1988). Segregation of form, color, movement, and depth: Anatomy, physiology, and perception. *Science, 240*, 740–749.

Loewenfeld, I. E. (1968). Comment on Hess' findings. *Sur. Opthathalmol., 11*, 293–294.

Long, R. R. (1977). Sensitivity of cutaneous cold fibers to noxious heat: paradoxical cold discharge. *J. Neurophysiol., 40*, 489–502.

Lowel, S., Bischof, H.-J., Leutenecker, B., & Singer, W. (1988). Topographic relations between ocular dominance and orientation columns in the cat striate cortex. *Exp. Brain Res., 71*, 33–46.

Lowenstein, W. R., & Mendelson, M. (1965). Components of receptor adaptation in a Pacinian Corpuscle. *J. Physiol. (Lond.), 177*, 377–397.

Lu, C., & Fender, D. H. (1972). The interaction of color and luminance in stereoscopic vision. *Investig. Ophthal., 11*, 482–490.

Lund, N. J., & MacKay, D. M. (1983). Sleep and the McCollough effect. *Vision Res., 23*, 903–906.

Lynch, J. C., Mountcastle, V. B., Talbot, W. H., & Yin, T. C. T. (1977). Parietal lobe mechanisms for directed visual attention. *J. Neurophysiol., 40*, 362–389.

Lysakowski, A., Standage, G. P., & Benevento, L. A. (1988). An investigation of collateral projections of the dorsal lateral geniculate nucleus and other subcortical structures to cortical areas V1 and V4 in the macaque monkey: A double label retrograde tracer study. *Exp. Brain Res., 69*, 651–661.

MacKay, D. M. (1967). Ways of looking at perception. In W. Watheu-Dunn (Ed.), *Models for the perception of speech and visual form*. Cambridge, Mass.: MIT Press.

Maffei, L., & Fiorentini, A. (1973). The visual cortex as a spatial frequency analyzer. *Vision Res., 13*, 1255–1267.

Maffei, L., & Fiorentini, A. (1976). The unresponsive regions of visual cortical receptive fields. *Vision Res., 16*, 1131–1139.

Maffei, L., & Fiorentini, A. (1977). Spatial frequency rows in the striate visual cortex. *Vision Res., 17*, 257–264.

Maguire, G., Lukasiewicz, P., & Werblin, F. (1989). Amacrine cell interactions underlying the response to change in the tiger salamander retina. *J. Neurosci., 9*, 726–735.

Maier, S. F., Drugan, R. C., & Grau, J. W. (1982). Controllability, coping behavior, and stress-induced analgesia in the rat. *Pain, 12*, 47–56.

Makous, W., & Boothe, R. (1974). Cones block signals from rods. *Vision Res., 14*, 285–294.

Malchow, R. P., & Yazulla, S. (1986). Separation and light adaptation of rod and cone signals in the retina of the goldfish. *Vision Res., 26*, 1655–1666.

Mancia, M., von Baumgarten, R., & Green, J. D. (1962). Response patterns of olfactory bulb neurons. *Arch. Ital. Biol., 100*, 449–462.

Marc, R. E., & Sperling, H. G. (1976). Color receptor identities of goldfish cones. *Science, 191*, 487–489.

Marchiafava, P. L., & Torre, V. (1978). The responses of amacrine cells to light and intracellularly applied currents. *J. Physiol., 276*, 83–102.

Marks, W. B. (1965). Visual pigments of single goldfish cones. *J. Physiol., 178*, 14–32.

Marks, W. B., Dobelle, W. H., & MacNichol, Jr., E. F. (1964). Visual pigments of single primate cones. *Science, 143*, 1181–1183.

Marler, P. (1975). On the origin of speech from animal sounds. In J. F. Kavanagh & J. E. Cutting (Eds.), *The role of speech in language* (pp. 11–37). Cambridge, Mass.: MIT Press.

Marr, D. (1976). Early processing of visual information. *Phil. Trans. Roy. Soc. Lond. B, 275*, 483–524.

Marr, D. (1982). *Vision*. San Francisco: W. H. Freeman.

Marrocco, R. T., & Li, R. H. (1977). Monkey superior colliculus: Properties of single cells and their afferent inputs. *J. Neurophysiol., 40*, 844–860.

Martin, K. A. C. (1988a). The lateral geniculate nucleus strikes back. *Trends in Neurosci., 11*, 192–194.

Martin, K. A. C. (1988b). From enzymes to visual perception: A bridge too far? *Trends in Neurosci., 11*, 380–387.

Martin, W. R. (1984). Pharmacology of opioids. *Pharmacol. Rev., 35*, 283–323.

Masland, R. H., & Tauchi, M. (1986). The cholinergic amacrine cell. *Trends in Neurosci.*, May, 1986, 218–223.

Massaro, D. W., & Anderson, N. H. (1970). A test of a perspective theory of geometrical illusions. *Am. J. Psychol., 83*, 567–575.

Massey, S. C., & Redburn, D. A. (1987). Transmitter circuits in the vertebrate retina. *Progress in Neurobiol., 28*, 55–96.

Mathews, D. (1972). Response patterns of single neurons in the tortoise olfactory epithelium and olfactory bulb. *J. Gen. Physiol., 60*, 166–180.

Matin, E., Clymer, A. B., & Matin, L. (1972). Metacontrast and saccadic suppression. *Science, 178*, 179–181.

Matin, L., & MacKinnon, G. E. (1964). Autokinetic movement: Selective manipulation of directional components by image stabilization. *Science, 143*, 147–148.

Matthews, B. H. C. (1933). Nerve endings in mammalian muscle. *J. Physiol., 78*, 1–53.

Matthews, H. R., Murphy, R. L. W., Fain, G. L., & Lamb, T. D. (1988). Photoreceptor light adaptation is mediated by cytoplasmic calcium concentration. *Nature, 334*, 67–69.

Matthews, G., & Watanabe, S.-I. (1987). Properties of ion channels closed by light and opened by guanosine 3′, 5′-cyclic monophosphate in toad retinal rods. *J. Physiol., 389*, 691–715.

Mattingly, I. G., Liberman, A. M., Syrdal, A. K., & Halwes, T. (1971). Discrimination in speech and nonspeech modes. *Cognit. Psychol., 2*, 131–157.

Maunsell, J. H. R., & Newsome, W. T. (1987). Visual processing in monkey extrastriate cortex. *Ann. Rev. Neurosci., 10*, 363–401.

Mavilya, M. (1972). Spontaneous vocalization and babbling in hearing-impaired infants. In C. G. M. Fant (ed.), *International symposium in speech communication ability and profound deafness* (pp. 163–171). Washington, D. C.: Alexander Graham Bell Association for the Deaf.

May, J. G., & Matteson, H. H. (1976). Spatial frequency-contingent color aftereffects. *Science, 192*, 145–147.

McBurney, D. H. (1972). Gustatory cross-adaptation between sweet tasting compounds. *Perception and Psychophysics, 11*, 225–227.

McBurney, D. H., & Bartoshuk, L. M. (1973). Interactions between stimuli with different taste qualities. *Physiology and Behavior, 10*, 249–252.

McBurney, D. H., & Gent, J. F. (1979). On the nature of taste qualities. *Psych. Bull., 86*, 151–167.

McBurney, D. H., Smith, D. V., & Shick, T. R. (1972). Gustatory cross-adaptation: Sourness and bitterness. *Perception and Psychophysics, 11*, 228–232.

McClintock, M. K. (1971). Menstrual synchrony and suppression. *Nature, 229*, 244–245.

McClurkin, J. W., & Marrocco, R. T. (1984). Visual cortical input alters spatial tuning in monkey lateral geniculate nucleus cells. *J. Physiol., 348*, 135–152.

McCollough, C. (1965). Color adaptation of edge detectors in the human visual system. *Science, 149,* 1115–1116.

McGuire, B. A., Stevens, J. K., & Sterling, P. (1986). Microcircuitry of beta ganglion cells in cat retina. *J. Neurosci., 6,* 907–918.

McGurk, H., & MacDonald, J. (1976). Hearing lips and seeing voices. *Nature, 264,* 746–748.

Melzack, R., & Wall, P. D. (1965). Pain mechanisms: A new theory. *Science, 150,* 971–979.

Melzack, R., & Wall, P. D. (1982). *The challenge of pain.* New York: Basic Books.

Mershon, D. H., & Gogel, W. C. (1970). Effect of stereoscopic cues on perceived whiteness. *Am. J. Psychol., 83,* 55–67.

Merzenich, M. M., Knight, P. L., & Roth, G. L. (1975). Representation of cochlea within primary auditory cortex in the cat. *J. Neurophysiol., 38,* 231–249.

Métin, C., & Frost, D. O. (1989). Visual responses of neurons in somatosensory cortex of hamsters with experimentally induced retinal projections to somatosensory thalamus. *Proc. Natl. Acad. Sci., 86,* 357–361.

Michael, C. R. (1972). Functional organization of cells in superior colliculus of the ground squirrel. *J. Neurophysiol., 35,* 833–846.

Michael, C. R. (1973). Opponent-color and opponent-contrast cells in the lateral geniculate nucleus of the ground squirrel. *J. Neurophysiol., 36,* 536–550.

Michael, C. R. (1979). Color-sensitive hypercomplex cells in monkey striate cortex. *J. Neurophysiol., 42,* 726–744.

Michael, C. R. (1981). Columnar organization of color cells in monkey's striate cortex. *J. Neurophysiol., 46,* 587–604.

Michael, C. R. (1985). Laminar segregation of color cells in the monkey's striate cortex. *Vision Res., 25,* 415–423.

Michael, C. R. (1988). Retinal afferent arborization patterns, dendritic field orientations, and the segregation of function in the lateral geniculate nucleus of the monkey. *Proc. Natl. Acad. Sci., 85,* 4914–4918.

Mikulka, P. J., Freeman, F. G., & Lidstrom, P. (1977). The effect of training technique and amygdala lesions on the acquisition and retention of taste aversion. *Behav. Biol., 19,* 509–517.

Miles, F. A., & Fuller, J. H. (1975). Visual tracking and the primate flocculus. *Science, 189,* 1000–1002.

Miller, G. A., Heise, G. A., & Lichten, W. (1951). The intelligibility of speech as a function of the context of the test materials. *J. Exp. Psychol., 41,* 329–335.

Miller, J. L., & Eimas, P. D. (1977). Studies on the perception of place and manner of articulation: A comparison of the labial-alveolar and nasal-stop distinctions. *J. Acoust. Soc. Am., 61,* 835–845.

Miller, J. W., & Bartley, S. H. (1954). A study of object shape as influenced by instrumental magnification. *J. Gen. Psychol., 50,* 141–146.

Miller, R. F., & Dacheux, R. F. (1976). Synaptic organization and ionic basis of on and off channels in mudpuppy retina. I. Intracellular analysis of chloride-sensitive electrogenic properties of receptors, horizontal cells, bipolar cells, and amacrine cells. *J. Gen. Physiol., 67,* 639–659.

Miller, R. F., & Slaughter, M. M. (1986). Excitatory amino acid receptors of the retina: Diversity of subtypes and conductance mechanisms. *Trends in Neurosci.,* May, 1986, 211–218.

Mills, A. W. (1972). Auditory localization. In J. V. Tobias (Ed.), *Foundations of modern auditory theory.* Vol. II. (p. 301). New York: Academic Press.

Minsky, M., & Papert, S. (1969). *Perceptrons.* Cambridge, Mass.: MIT. Press.

Mitchell, D. E., Reardon, J., & Muir, D. W. (1975). Interocular transfer of the motion after-effect in normal and stereoblind observers. *Exp. Brain Res., 22,* 163–173.

Moberg, E. (1983). The role of cutaneous afferents in position sense, kinesthesia, and motor function of the hand. *Brain., 106,* 1–19.

Mohler, C. W., & Wurtz, R. H. (1977). Role of striate cortex and superior colliculus in visual guidance of saccadic eye movements in monkeys. *J. Neurophysiol., 40,* 74–94.

Moore, B. C. J. (1977). *Psychology of hearing.* Baltimore: University Park Press.

Morrell, F. (1972). Integrative properties of parastriate neurons. In A. G. Karczmar & J. C. Eccles (Eds.), *Brain and human behavior* (pp. 259–289). Heidelberg: Springer-Verlag.

Morse, P. A., & Snowden, C. T. (1975). An investigation of categorical speech discrimination by rhesus monkeys. *Percept. Psychophys., 17,* 9–16.

Mountcastle, V. B. (1957). Modality and topographic properties of single neurons of cat's somatic sensory cortex. *J. Neurophysiol., 20,* 408–434.

Mountcastle, V. B., & Darien-Smith, I. (1968). Neural mechanisms in somesthesia. In V. B. Mountcastle (Ed.) *Medical Physiology: Vol. II.* (pp. 1372–1423). St. Louis: Mosby.

Movshon, J. A. (1975). The velocity tuning of single units in cat striate cortex. *J. Physiol., 249,* 445–468.

Movshon, J. A., Thompson, I. D., & Tolhurst, D. J. (1978a). Spatial summation in the receptive fields of simple cells in the cat's striate cortex. *J. Physiol., 283,* 53–77.

Movshon, J. A., Thompson, I. D., & Tolhurst, D. J. (1987b). Receptive field organization of complex cells in the cat's striate cortex. *J. Physiol., 283,* 79–99.

Mozell, M. M., Smith, B. P., Smith, P. E., Sullivan, R. L., & Swender, P. (1969). Nasal chemoreception in flavor identification. *Arch. Otolaryng., 90,* 367–373.

Mullen, K. T., & Baker, C. L., Jr. (1985). A motion aftereffect from an isoluminant stimulus. *Vision Res., 25,* 685–688.

Müller, F., Wässle, H., & Voigt, T. (1988). Pharmacological modulation of the rod pathway in the cat retina. *J. Neurophysiol., 59,* 1657–1672.

Murakami, M., & Shimoda, Y. (1977). Identification of amacrine and ganglion cells in the carp retina. *J. Physiol., 264,* 801–818.

Murch, G. M. (1976). Classical conditioning of the McCollough effect: Temporal parameters. *Vision Res., 16,* 615–619.

Myerson, J., Manis, P. B., Meizin, F. M., & Allman, J. M. (1977). Magnification in striate cortex and retinal ganglion cell layer of owl monkey: A quantitative comparison. *Science, 198,* 855–857.

Nachman, M., & Ashe, J. (1974). Effects of basolateral amygdala lesions on neophobia, learned taste aversions, and sodium appetite in rats. *J. Comp. Physiol. Psychol., 87,* 622–643.

Nafe, J. P., & Wagoner, K. S. (1941). The nature of sensory adaptation. *J. Gen. Psych., 25,* 295–321.

Naka, K.-I. (1977). Functional organization of catfish retina. *J. Neurophysiol., 40,* 26–43.

Naka, K.-I., & Rushton, W. A. H. (1966). S-potentials from colour units in the retina of fish (*Cyprinidae*). *J. Physiol., 185,* 536–555.

Nakamura, T., & Gold, G. H. (1987). A cyclic nucleotide gated conductance in olfactory receptory cilia. *Nature, 325,* 442–444.

Nakatani, K., & Yau, K.-W. (1988). Calcium and light adaptation in retinal rods and cones. *Nature, 334,* 69–72.

Nathans, J., Piantanida, T. P., Eddy, R. L., Shows, T. B., & Hogness, D. S. (1986). Molecular genetics of inherited variation in human color vision. *Science, 232,* 203–210.

Nathans, J., Thomas, D., & Hogness, D. S. (1986). Molecular genetics of human color vision: The genes encoding blue, green, and red pigments. *Science, 232,* 193–202.

Nawrot, M., & Blake, R. (1989). Neural integration of information specifying structure from stereopsis and motion. *Science, 244,* 716–718.

Neff, W. D. (1961). Neural mechanisms of auditory discrimination. In W. A. Rosenblith (Ed.), *Sensory communication* (pp. 259–275). Cambridge, Mass.: MIT Press.

Neff, W. D., Casseday, J. H. (1977). Effects of unilateral ablation of auditory cortex on monaural cat's ability to localize sound. *J. Neurophysiol., 40,* 44–52.

Neisser, U. (1967). *Cognitive psychology.* New York: Appleton-Century-Crofts.

Nelson, D. A., & Marler, P. (1989). Categorical perception of a natural stimulus continuum: Birdsong. *Science, 244,* 976–978.

Nelson, J. I., Kato, H., & Bishop, P. O. (1977). Discrimination of orientation and position disparities by binocularly activated neurons in cat striate cortex. *J. Neurophysiol., 40,* 260–283.

Nelson, R. (1982). AII amacrine cells quicken time course of rod signals in the cat retina. *J. Neurophysiol., 47,* 928–947.

Nelson, R., & Kolb, H. (1983). Synaptic patterns and response properties of bipolar and ganglion cells in the cat retina. *Vision Res., 23,* 1183–1195.

Nelson, R., Lützow, A. V., Kolb, H., & Gouras, P. (1975). Horizontal cells in cat retina with independent dendritic systems. *Science, 189,* 137–139.

Nelson, T. M., & Bartley, S. H. (1956). The perception of form in an unstructured field. *J. Gen. Psychol., 54,* 57–63.

Nelson, T. M., Bartley, S. H., & Bourassa, C. (1961). The effect of areal characteristics of targets upon shape-slant invariance. *J. Psychol., 52,* 479–490.

Newsome, W. T., & Pare, E. B. (1988). A selective impairment of motion perception following lesions of the middle temporal visual area (MT). *J. Neurosci., 8,* 2201–2211.

Newsome, W. T., Wurtz, R. H., & Komatsu, H. (1988). Relation of cortical areas MT and MST to pursuit eye movements. II. Differentiation of retinal from extraretinal inputs. *J. Neurophysiol., 60,* 604–619.

Newton, I. (1704). *Optics.* 1st Ed. London: W. Innys.

Noda, H. (1975). Discharges in relay cells of the lateral geniculate nucleus of the cat during spontaneous eye movements in light and darkness. *J. Physiol., 250,* 579–595.

Norcia, A. M., Sutter, E. E., & Tyler, C. W. (1985). Electrophysiological evidence for the existence of coarse and fine disparity mechanisms in human. *Vision Res., 25,* 1603–1611.

Normann, R. A., & Werblin, F. S. (1974). Control of retinal sensitivity I. Light and dark adaptation of vertebrate rods and cones. *J. Gen. Physiol., 63,* 37–61.

Northmore, D. P. M., & Muntz, W. R. A. (1974). Effects of stimulus size on spectral sensitivity in a fish. *(Scardinus erythrophthalmus),* measured with a classical conditioning paradigm. *Vision Res., 14,* 503–514.

Norton, T. T. (1974). Receptive field properties of superior colliculus cells and development of visual behavior in kittens. *J. Neurophysiol., 37,* 674–689.

Nothdurft, H. C., & Lee, B. B. (1982). Responses to coloured patterns in the macaque lateral geniculate nucleus: Pattern processing in single neurones. *Exp. Brain Res., 48,* 43–54.

Nowlis, G. H., & Frank, M. (1977). Qualities in hamster taste: Behavioral and neural evidence. In LeMagnen, J., & MacLeod, P. (Eds.) *Sixth international symposium on olfaction and taste* (pp. 241–248). London: Information Retrieval LTD.

Ochs, A. L. (1979). Is Fourier analysis performed by the visual system or by the visual investigator. *J. Opt. Soc. Am., 69,* 95–98.

O'Connell, R. J., & Meredith, M. (1984). Effects of volatile and nonvolatile chemical signals on male sex behaviors mediated by the main and accessory olfactory system. *Behav. Neurosci., 98,* 1083–1093.

Ojemann, G., & Mateer, C. (1979). Human language cortex: Localization of memory, syntax, and sequential motor-phoneme identification systems. *Science, 205,* 1401–1403.

Ono, H. (1969). Apparent distance as a function of familiar size. *J. Exp. Psychol., 79,* 109–115.

Osgood, C. E., & Heyer, A. W. (1951). A new interpretation of figural after-effects. *Psychol. Rev., 59,* 98–118.

Østerberg, G. (1935). Topography of the layer of rods and cones in the human retina. *Acta Ophthalmol. Suppl., 6,* 1–103.

Otis, C. S., Cerf, J. A., & Thomas, G. (1957). Conditioned inhibition of respiration and heartrate in the goldfish. *Science, 126,* 263–264.

Ozeki, M., & Sato, M. (1972). Responses of gustatory cells in the tongue of rat to stimuli representing four taste qualities. *Comp. Biochem. Physiol., 41A,* 391–407.

Pace, U., Hanski, E., Salomon, Y., & Lancet, D. (1985). Odorant-sensitive adenylate cyclase may mediate olfactory reception. *Nature, 316,* 255–258.

Pantev, C., Hoke, M., Lütkenhöner, B., & Lehnertz, K. (1989). Tonotopic organization of the auditory cortex: Pitch versus frequency representation. *Science, 246,* 486–488.

Pantle, A. (1970). Adaptation to pattern spatial frequency; effects on visual movement sensitivity in humans. *J. Opt. Soc. Am., 60,* 1120–1124.

Pantle, A., & Sekuler, R. (1969). Contrast response of human visual mechanisms sensitive to orientation and direction of motion. *Vision Res., 9,* 397–406.

Park, J. N., & Michaelson, G. J. (1974). Direct judgments under different size-information conditions. *Percept. Psychophys., 15,* 57–60.

Pastore, R. E., Ahroon, W. A., Baffrito, K. J., Friedman, C., Pulea, J. S., & Fink, E. A. (1977). Common factor model of categorical perception. *J. Exp. Psych.: Hum. Percept. Perf., 3,* 686–696.

Pearler, W. S., & McLaughlin, J. P. (1967). The question of stimulus content and pupil size. *Psychonomic Science, 8,* 505–506.

Peichl, L., & Wässle, H. (1981). Morphological identification of on- and off-centre brisk transient

(Y) cells in cat retina. *Proc. Roy. Soc. Lond. B, 212*, 139–156.

Peichl, L., & Wässle, H. (1983). The structural correlate of the receptive field centre of β ganglion cells in the cat retina. *J. Physiol., 341*, 309–324.

Penfield, W., & Rasmussen, T. (1950). *The cerebral cortex of man. A clinical study of localization of function.* New York: MacMillan.

Penn, R., & Hagins, W. A. (1972). Kinetics of the photocurrent of retinal rods. *Biophysics J., 12*, 1073–1094.

Penrose, L. S., & Penrose, R. (1958). Impossible objects: A special type of illusion. *Br. J. Psychol., 49*, 31–33.

Pepperberg, D. R., Brown, P. K., Lurie, M., & Dowling, J. E. (1978). Visual pigment and photoreceptor sensitivity in the isolated skate retina. *J. Gen. Physiol., 71*, 369–396.

Perrett, D. I., Rolls, E. T., & Caan, W. (1982). Visual neurones responsive to faces in the monkey temporal cortex. *Exp. Brain Res., 47*, 329–342.

Peterhans, E., & von der Heydt, R. (1989). Mechanisms of contour perception in monkey visual cortex. II. Contours bridging gaps. *J. Neurosci., 9*, 1749–1763.

Peterson, G. E., & Barney, H. L. (1952). Control methods used in a study of the vowels. *J. Acoust. Soc. Am., 24*, 175–184.

Petry, S., & McShane, R. C. (1988). Subjective contours to the second power. *Investig. Ophthal. and Visual Sci., 29* (Suppl.), 401.

Petry, S., & Siegel, S. (1989). Parametric analysis of subjective contours. *Investig. Ophthal. and Visual Sci., 30* (Suppl.), 254.

Pettigrew, J. D., & Konishi, M. (1976). Neurons selective for orientation and binocular disparity in the visual walst of the barn owl *(Tyto alba)*. *Science, 193*, 675–678.

Pfaffmann, C. (1941). Gustatory afferent impulses. *J. Cell. Comp. Physiol., 17*, 243–258.

Pfaffmann, C. (1955). Gustatory nerve impulses in rat, cat, and rabbit. *J. Neurophysiol., 18*, 429–440.

Pfaffman, C. (1978). Neurophysiological mechanisms of taste. *Am. J. Clin. Nutr., 31*, 1058–1067.

Pfaffman, C. (1978). The vertebrate phylogeny, neural code, and integrative processes of taste. In E. C. Carterette & M. P. Friedman (Eds.), *Handbook of perception, Vol. 6A: Tasting and smelling* (pp. 51–123). New York: Academic Press.

Piantanida, T. (1988). The molecular genetics of color vision and color blindness. *Trends in Genet., 4*, 319–323.

Pickles, J. O., Comis, S. D., & Osborne, M. P. (1984). Cross-links between stereocilia in the guinea pig organ of Corti, and their possible relation to sensory transduction. *Hearing Res., 15*, 103–112.

Pitblado, C. B., & Kaufman, L. (1967). On classifying the visual illusions. In L. Kaufman (Ed.), *Contour descriptor properties of visual shape.* Sperry Rand Research Center Report SRRC-CR 67-43, (pp. 32–53). Cited by L. Kaufman (1974). *Sight and mind.* New York: Oxford University Press.

Poggio, G. F., & Fischer, B. (1977). Binocular interaction and depth sensitivity in striate and prestriate cortex of behaving rhesus monkey. *J. Neurophysiol., 40*, 1392–1405.

Poggio, G. F., Gonzalez, F., & Krause, F. (1988). Stereoscopic mechanisms in monkey visual cortex: Binocular correlation and disparity selectivity. *J. Neurosci., 8*, 4531–4550.

Poggio, G. F., Motter, B. C., Squatrito, S., & Trotter, Y. (1985). Responses of neurons in visual cortex (V1 and V2) of the alert macaque to dynamic random-dot stereograms. *Vision Res., 25*, 397–406.

Poggio, G. F., & Talbot, W. H. (1981). Mechanisms of static and dynamic steropsis in foveal cortex of the rhesus monkey. *J. Physiol., 315*, 469–492.

Poizner, H. (1981). Visual and "phonetic" coding of movement: Evidence from American sign language. *Science, 212*, 691–693.

Pokorny, J., & Smith, V. C. (1977). Evaluation of single-pigment shift model of anomolous trichromacy. *J. Opt. Soc. Am., 67*, 1196–1209.

Pollen, D. A., Andrews, B. W., & Feldon, S. E. (1978). Spatial frequency selectivity of periodic complex cells in the visual cortex of the cat. *Vision Res., 18*, 665–682.

Pollen, D. A., & Ronner, S. F. (1975). Periodic excitability changes across the receptive fields of complex cells in the striate and parastriate cortex of the cat. *J. Physiol., 245*, 667–697.

Pollen, D. A., & Ronner, S. F. (1981). Phase relationships between adjacent simple cells in visual cortex. *Science, 212*, 1409–1411.

Pollen, D. A., & Ronner, S. F. (1982). Spatial computation performed by simple and complex cells in the visual cortex of the cat. *Vision Res., 22,* 101–118.

Pollen, D. A., Gaska, J. P., & Jacobson, L. D. (1988). Responses of simple and complex cells to compound sine-wave gratings. *Vision Res., 28,* 25–39.

Polyak, S. (1957). *The vertebrate visual system,* H. Klüver (Ed.). Chicago: University of Chicago Press.

Porat, M., & Zeevi, Y. Y. (1989). Localized texture processing in vision: Analysis and synthesis in Gaborian space. *IEEE Trans. Biomed. Engineering, 36,* 115–128.

Postman, L., & Egan, J. P. (1949). *Experimental psychology.* New York: Harper & Row.

Price, D. D., Hu, J. W., Dubner, R., & Gracely, R. H. (1977). Peripheral suppression of first pain and central summation of second pain evoked by noxious heat pulses. *Pain, 3,* 57–68.

Price, D. D., Hayes, R. L., Ruda, M. A., & Dubner, R. (1978). Spatial and temporal transformations of input to spinothalamic tract neurons and their relation to somatic sensations. *J. Neurophysiol., 41,* 933–947.

Priestly, J. (1772). *The history and present state of discoveries relating to vision, light, and colours.* London: J. Johnson.

Puckett, J. de W., & Steinman, R. M. (1969). Tracking eye movements with and without saccadic correction. *Vision Res., 9,* 295–303.

Pugh, E., & Altman, J. (1988). A role for calcium in adaptation. *Nature, 334,* 16–17.

Purkinje, J. E. (1825). *Neue Beiträge zur Kenntniss des Sehens in subjectiver Hinsicht.* 108–110. Cited by E. G. Boring (1942). *Sensation and perception in the history of experimental psychology.* New York: Appleton-Century-Crofts, pp. 177–178.

Randolph, M., & Semmes, J. (1974). Behavioral consequences of selective subtotal ablations in the post central gyrus of Maccaca mulatta. *Brain Res., 70,* 55–70.

Ratliff, F. (1976). On the psychophysiological bases of universal color terms. *Proc. Am. Philos. Soc., 120,* 311–330.

Ratliff, F. (1984). Why Mach Bands are not seen at the edges of a step. *Vision Res., 24,* 163–165.

Ratliff, F., & Sirovich, L. (1978). Equivalence classes of visual stimuli. *Vision Res., 18,* 845–851.

Ratliff, F., Knight, B. W., & Graham, N. (1969). On tuning and amplification by lateral inhibition. *Proc. Natl. Acad. Sci., 62,* 733–740.

Reger, S. N. (1960). Effect of middle ear muscle action on certain psychological measurements. *Ann. Otol. Rhinol. Laryngol., 69,* 1179–1198.

Repp, B. H., Liberman, A. M., Eccardt, T., & Pesetsky, D. (1978). Perceptual integration of acoustic cues for stop, fricative, and affricative manner. *J. Exp. Psychol., Hum. Percept. Perform., 4,* 621–637.

Restle, F. (1970). Moon illusion explained on the basis of relative size. *Science, 167,* 1092–1096.

Reynolds, G. S., & Stevens, S. S. (1960). Binaural summation of loudness. *J. Acoust. Soc. Am., 32,* 1337–1344.

Reynolds, J., & Keverne, E. B. (1979). The accessory olfactory system and its role in the pheromonally mediated suppression of oestrus in grouped mice. *J. Reprod. Fert., 57,* 31–35.

Ricardo, J. A., & Koh, E. T. (1978). Anatomical evidence of direct projections from the nucleus of the solitary tract to the hypothalamus, amygdala, and other forebrain structures in the rat. *Brain Res., 153,* 1–26.

Richards, W. (1973). Visual processing in scotomata. *Exp. Brain Res., 17,* 333–347.

Richardson, D. E., & Akil, H. (1977). Pain reduction by electrical brain stimulation in man. *J. Neurosurg., 47,* 178–183.

Richter, A., & Simon, E. J. (1974). Electrical responses of double cones in the turtle retina. *J. Physiol., 242,* 673–683.

Riggs, L. A., (1973). Curvature as a feature of pattern vision. *Science, 181,* 1070–1072.

Riggs, L. A., Merton, D. A., & Morton, H. B. (1974). Suppression of visual phosphenes during saccadic eye movements. *Vision Res., 14,* 997–1011.

Ritter, M. (1977). Effect of disparity and viewing distance on perceived depth. *Percept. Psychophys., 22,* 400–407.

Robinson, D. L., Goldberg, M. E., & Stanson, G. B. (1978). Parietal association cortex in the primate: Sensory mechanisms and behavioral modulations. *J. Neurophysiol., 41,* 910–932.

Robson, J. G., Tolhurst, D. J., Freeman, R. D., & Ohzawa, I. (1988). Simple cells in the visual cortex of the cat can be narrowly tuned for spatial frequency. *Visual Neurosci., 1,* 415–419.

Rock, I. (1974). The perception of disoriented figures. *Sci. Am., 230*, 78–85.

Rock, I. (1975). *An introduction to perception.* New York: Macmillan.

Rock, I. (1984). *Perception.* New York: Scientific American Books.

Rock, I., & Brosgole, L. (1964). Grouping based on phenomenal proximity. *J. Exp. Psychol., 67*, 531–538.

Rock, I., & Kaufman, L. (1962). The moon illusion. II. *Science, 136*, 1023–1031.

Rock, I., & McDermott, W. (1964). The perception of visual angle. *Acta Psychol., 22*, 119–134.

Rodieck, R. W. (1967). Maintained activity in cat retinal ganglion cells. *J. Neurophysiol., 30*, 1043–1071.

Rodieck, R. W. (1973). *The vertebrate retina.* San Francisco: W. H. Freeman.

Rodieck, R. W. (1979). Visual pathways. *Ann. Rev. Neurosci., 2*, 193–225.

Rodieck, R. W., & Stone, J. (1965). Analysis of receptive fields of cat retinal ganglion cells. *J. Neurophysiol., 28*, 833–849.

Rodman, H. R., & Albright, T. D. (1989). Single-unit analysis of pattern-motion selective properties in the middle temporal visual area (MT). *Exp. Brain Res., 75*, 53–64.

Rose, D. (1977). Responses of single units in cat visual cortex to moving bars as a function of bar length. *J. Physiol., 271*, 1–23.

Rose, J. E., Brugge, J. F., Anderson, D. J., & Hind, J. E. (1968). Patterns of activity in single auditory nerve fibers of the squirrel monkey. In A. V. S. deReuck & J. Knight (Eds.), *Hearing mechanisms in vertebrates.* (pp. 144–157). London: Churchill.

Rose, J. E., Galambos, R., & Hughes, J. R. (1959). Microelectrode studies of the cochlear nuclei of the cat. *Johns Hopkins Hosp. Bull., 104*, 211–251.

Rose, J. E., Hind, J. E., Anderson, D. J., & Brugge, J. F. (1971). Some effects of stimulus intensity on response of auditory nerve fibers in the squirrel monkey. *J. Neurophysiol., 34*, 685–699.

Rushton, W. A. H. (1961a). Rhodopsin measurement and dark adaptation in a subject deficient in cone vision. *J. Physiol., 156*, 193–205.

Rushton, W. A. H. (1961b). Peripheral coding in the nervous system. In W. R. Rosenblith (Ed.), *Sensory communication* (pp. 169–181). Cambridge: MIT. Press.

Rushton, W. A. H. (1965). *The Ferrier Lecture, 1962.* Visual Adaptation. *Proc. Soc. Lond. Ser. B., 162*, 20–46.

Rushton, W. A. H., & Westheimer, G. (1962). The effect upon the rod threshold of bleaching neighbouring rods. *J. Physiol., 164*, 318–329.

Russell, M. J. (1976). Human olfactory communication. *Nature, 260*, 520–522.

Ryan, A., & Dallos, P. (1975). Absence of cochlear outer hair cells: Effect on behavioral auditory threshold. *Nature, 253*, 44–46.

Sagi, D., & Julesz, B. (1985). "Where" and "what" in vision. *Science, 228*, 1217–1219.

Saito, T., Kujiraoka, T., & Yonaha, T. (1983). Connections between photoreceptors and horseradish peroxidase-injected bipolar cells in the carp retina. *Vision Res., 23*, 353–362.

Saito, H.-A., Shimahara, T., & Fukada, Y. (1970). Four types of responses to light and dark spot stimuli on the cat optic nerve. *Tohoku J. Exp. Med., 102*, 127–133.

Sakata, H., Shibutani, H., & Kawano, K. (1980). Spatial properties of visual fixation neurons in posterior parietal association cortex of the monkey. *J. Neurophysiol., 43*, 1654–1672.

Samuel, A. G., & Newport, E. L. (1979). Adaptation of speech by nonspeech: Evidence for complex acoustic cue detectors. *J. Exp. Psychol. Hum. Percept. Perform., 5*, 563–578.

Sandell, J. H., & Schiller, P. H. (1982). Effect of cooling area 18 on striate cortex cells in the squirrel monkey. *J. Neurophysiol., 48*, 38–48.

Sandel, T. T., Teas, D. C., Fedderson, W. E., & Jeffress, L. A. (1955). Localization of sound from single and paired sources. *J. Acoust. Soc. Am., 27*, 842–852.

Sanderson, K. J., Bishop, P. O., & Darien-Smith, I. (1971). The properties of the binocular receptive fields of lateral geniculate neurons. *Exp. Brain Res., 13*, 178–207.

Sato, M. (1973). Gustatory receptor mechanism in mammals. *Adv. Biophys., 4*, 103–152.

Sato, T. (1980). Recent advances in the physiology of taste cells. *Prog. Neurobiol., 14*, 25–67.

Scharf, B. (1961). Complex sounds and critical bands. *Psychol. Bull., 58*, 205–217.

Scharf, B. (1970). Critical bands. In J. V. Tobias (Ed.), *Foundations of modern auditory theory*, Vol. 1. (pp. 157–202). New York: Academic Press.

Schatz, C. (1954). The role of context in the perception of stops. *Language, 30,* 47–56.

Schein, S. J., Marrocco, R. T., & DeMonasterio, F. M. (1982). Is there a high concentration of color-selective cells in area V4 of monkey visual cortex? *J. Neurophysiol., 47,* 193–213.

Schellart, N. A. M., & Spekreijse, H. (1973). Origin of the stochastic nature of ganglion cell activity in isolated goldfish retina. *Vision Res., 13,* 337–347.

Schiffman, H. R. (1967). Size estimation of familiar objects under informative and reduced conditions of viewing. *Am. J. Psychol., 80,* 229–235.

Schiffman, H. R. (1976). *Sensation and perception: An integrated approach.* New York: Wiley.

Schiffman, S. S. (1974). Physicochemical correlates of olfactory quality. *Science, 185,* 112–117.

Schiller, P. H., Finlay, B. L., & Volman, S. F. (1976a). Quantitative studies of single-cell properties in monkey striate cortex. I. Spatiotemporal organization of receptive fields. *J. Neurophysiol., 39,* 1288–1319.

Schiller, P. H., Finlay, B. L., & Volman, S. F. (1976b). Quantitative studies of single-cell properties in monkey striate cortex. III. Spatial frequency. *J. Neurophysiol., 39,* 1334–1351.

Schiller, P. H., & Malpeli, J. G. (1978). Functional specificity of lateral geniculate nucleus laminae of the rhesus monkey. *J. Neurophysiol., 41,* 788–797.

Schnapf, J. L., Kraft, T. W., Nunn, B. J., & Baylor, D. A. (1988). Spectral sensitivity of primate photoreceptors. *Visual Neurosci., 1,* 255–261.

Schneider, B., Moraglia, G., & Jepson, A. (1989). Binocular unmasking: An analog to binaural unmasking? *Science, 243,* 1479–1481.

Schneider, B., Parker, S., Ostrosky, D., Stein, D., & Kanow, G. (1974). A scale for the psychological magnitude of number. *Percept. Psychophys., 16,* 43–46.

Schneider, G. E. (1969). Two visual systems. *Science, 163,* 895–902.

Scholes, J. H. (1975). Colour receptors, and their connexions in the retina of a cyprinid fish. *Phil. Trans. R. Soc. Lond. Ser. B., 270,* 61–118.

Schouten, J. F., Ritsma, R. J., & Cardozo, B. L. (1962). Pitch of the residue. *J. Acoust. Soc. Am., 34,* 1418–1424.

Schumann, F. (1904). Einige Beobachtungen über die Zusammenfassung von Gesichlseindrücken zu Einheiten. *Psychol. Studies, 1,* 1–32.

Schwartz, A. S., Perey, A. J., & Azulay, A. (1975). Further analysis of active and passive touch in pattern discrimination. *Bull. Psychon. Soc., 6,* 7–9.

Schwartz, E. A. (1975). Cones excite rods in the retina of the turtle. *J. Physiol., 246,* 639–651.

Schwartz, E. A. (1976). Electrical properties of the rod syncytium in the retina of the turtle. *J. Physiol., 257,* 379–406.

Scott, T. R., & Mark, G. P. (1986). Feeding and taste. *Prog. Neurobiol., 27,* 293–331.

Scott, T. R., Yaxley, S., Sienkiewicz, Z. J., & Rolls, E. T. (1986). Gustatory responses in the nucleus tractus solitarius of the alert cynomolgus monkey. *J. Neurophysiol., 55,* 182–200.

Seashore, C. E. (1938). *Psychology of music.* New York: McGraw-Hill.

Segall, M. H., Campbell, D. T., & Herskovits, M. J. (1963). Cultural differences in the perception of geometric illusions. *Science, 139,* 769–771.

Sejnowski, T. J., Koch, C., & Churchland, P. S. (1988). Computational neuroscience. *Science, 241,* 1299–1306.

Sekuler, R., & Blake, R. (1985). *Perception.* New York: Knopf.

Sekuler, R., & Ganz, L. (1963). After-effect of seen motion with stabilized retinal image. *Science, 139,* 419–420.

Selfridge, O. G. (1959). Pandemonium: A paradigm for learning. In D. V. Blake & A. M. Uttley (Eds.), *Symposium on the mechanization of thought processes.* (pp. 511–529). London: H. M. Stationery Office.

Selfridge, O. G., & Neisser, U. (1960). Pattern recognition by machine. *Sci. Am., 203*(2), 60–68.

Shapley, R. (1986). The importance of contrast for the activity of single neurons, the VEP and perception. *Vision Res., 26,* 45–61.

Shapley, R., & Enroth-Cugell, C. (1984). Visual adaptation and retinal gain controls. *Prog. in Retinal Res., 3,* 263–346.

Shapley, R., & Hochstein, S. (1975). Visual spatial summation in two classes of geniculate cells. *Nature, 256,* 411–413.

Shapley, R., & Lennie, P. (1985). Spatial frequency analysis in the visual system. *Ann. Rev. Neurosci., 8,* 547–583.

Shapley, R., & Perry, V. H. (1986). Cat and monkey retinal ganglion cells and their visual functional roles. *Trends in Neurosci.*, May, 1986, 229–235.

Shechter, S., Hochstein, S., & Hillman, P. (1988). Shape similarity and distance disparity as apparent motion correspondence cues. *Vision Res., 28,* 1013–1021.

Shefner, J. M., & Levine, M. W. (1976). A psychophysical demonstration of goldfish trichromacy. *Vision Res., 16,* 671–673.

Shefner, J. M., & Levine, M. W. (1977). Interactions between rod and cone systems in the goldfish retina. *Science, 198,* 750–753.

Shepard, R. N., & Judd, S. A. (1976). Perceptual illusion of rotation of three-dimensional objects. *Science, 191,* 952–954.

Shepard, R. N., & Metzler, J. (1971). Mental rotation of three-dimensional objects. *Science, 171,* 701–703.

Shepherd, G. M. (1979). *The synaptic organization of the brain.* New York: Oxford University Press.

Shepherd, G. M. (1985). The olfactory system: The uses of neural space for a nonspatial modality. *Prog. Clin. Biol. Res., 176,* 99–114.

Sherman, S. M. (1979). The functional significance of X and Y cells in normal and visually deprived cats. *Trends Neurosci., 2,* 192–195.

Sherman, S. M., Wilson, J. R., Kaas, J. H., & Webb, S. V. (1976). X- and Y-cells in the dorsal lateral geniculate nucleus of the owl monkey *(Aotus trivirgatus). Science, 192,* 475–477.

Sherrington, C. S. (1918). Observations on the sensual role of the proprioceptive nerve supply of the extrinsic ocular muscles. *Brain, 41,* 332–343.

Shibuya, T., Ai, N., & Takagi, S. (1962). Response types of single cells in the olfactory bulb. *Proc. Japan Acad., 38,* 231–233.

Sicard, G., & Holley, A. (1984). Receptor cell responses to odorants: Similarities and differences among odorants. *Brain Res., 292,* 283–296.

Sigel, C., & Nachmias, J. (1975). A re-evaluation of curvature-specific chromatic after-effects. *Vision Res., 15,* 829–836.

Sillito, A. M., Salt, T. E., & Kemp, J. A. (1985). Modulatory and inhibitory processes in the visual cortex. *Vision Res., 25,* 375–381.

Sillito, A. M., & Versiani, V. (1977). The contribution of excitatory and inhibitory inputs to the length

preference of hypercomplex cells in layers II and III of the cats striate cortex. *J. Physiol., 273,* 775–790.

Simon, E. J., Hiller, J. M., & Edelman, I. (1973). Stereospecific binding of the potent narcotic analgesic (3H) etorphine to rat-brain homogenate. *Proc. Natl. Acad. Sci. (USA), 70,* 1947–1949.

Simon, S. A., Labarca, P., Robb, R. (1989). Activation by saccharides of a cation selective pathway on canine lingual epithelium. *Am. J. Physiol., 256,* R394–402.

Simpson, J. J., & Graf, W. (1985). The selection of reference frames by nature and its investigators. In B. Jones & M. Jones (Eds.), *Adaptive Mechanisms in Gaze Control: Facts and Theories* (pp. 3–16). Elsevier Science Publishers.

Singer, W. (1977). Control of thalamic transmission by corticofugal and ascending reticular pathways in the visual system. *Physiol. Rev., 57,* 386–420.

Sivian, L. J., & White, S. D. (1933). On minimum audible sound fields. *J. Acoust. Soc. Am., 4,* 288–321.

Sklar, P. B., Anholt, R. R., & Snyder, S. H. (1986). The odorant sensitive adenylate cyclase of olfactory receptor cells. *J. Biol. Chem., 261,* 15538–15543.

Slotnik, B. M., & Kaneko, N. (1981). Role of mediodorsal thalamus nucleus in olfactory discrimination in rats. *Science, 214,* 91–92.

Small, A. M. (1973). Psychoacoustics. In F. D. Minifie, T. J. Hixon, & F. Williams (Eds)., *Normal aspects of speech, hearing and language* (pp. 343–421). Englewood Cliffs, N.J.: Prentice Hall.

Smith, D. V., & McBurney, D. H. (1969). Gustatory cross adaptation: Does a single mechanism code the salty taste? *J. Exper. Psychol., 80,* 101–105.

Smith, D. V., Van Buskirk, R. L., Travers, J. B., & Bieber, S. L. (1983). Gustatory neuron types in hamster brainstem. *J. Neurophysiol., 50,* 522–540.

Smith, V. C., Pokorny, J., & Starr, S. J. (1976). Variability of color mixture data—I. Interobserver variability in the unit coordinates. *Vision Res., 16,* 1087–1094.

Snyder, S. H. (1980). Brain peptides as neurotransmitters. *Science, 209,* 976–983.

So, Y. T., & Shapley, R. M. (1981). Spatial tuning of cells in and around lateral geniculate nucleus of the cat: X and Y relay cells and perigeniculate interneurons. *J. Neurophysiol., 45,* 107–120.

Sokoloff, L. (1975). Influence of functional activity

on local cerebral utilization. In D. H. Ingvar & N. A. Lassen (Eds.), *Brain work. The coupling of function, metabolism and blood flow in the brain* (pp. 385–388). New York: Academic Press.

Solomon, S. J., Pasik, T., & Pasik, P. (1981). Extrageniculostriate vision in the monkey. VIII. Critical structures for spatial localization. *Exp. Brain Res., 44,* 259–270.

Sparks, D. L., & Porter, J. D. (1983). Spatial localization of saccade targets. II. Activity of superior colliculus neurons preceding compensatory saccades. *J. Neurophysiol., 49,* 64–74.

Spitzer, H., Desimone, R., & Moran, J. (1988). Increased attention enhances both behavioral and neuronal performance. *Science, 240,* 338–340.

Spitzer, H., & Hochstein, S. (1985). A complex-cell receptive-field model. *J. Neurophysiol., 53,* 1266–1286.

Spoehr, K. T., & Lehmkuhle, S. W. (1982). *Visual Information Processing.* San Francisco: W. H. Freeman.

Spoendlin, H. (1970). Structural basis of peripheral frequency analysis. In R. Plomp & G. F. Smoorenburg, *Frequency analysis and periodicity detection in hearing.* Leiden Sijthoff: pp. 2–36.

Stanford, L. R. (1987). X-cells in the cat retina: Relationships between the morphology and physiology of a class of cat retinal ganglion cells. *J. Neurophysiol., 58,* 940–964.

Stein, B. E., Magalhães-Castro, B., & Kruger, L. (1975). Superior colliculus: Visuotopic-somatic overlap. *Science, 189,* 224–226.

Stell, W. K. (1967). The structure and relationships of horizontal cells and photoreceptor-bipolar synaptic complexes in goldfish retina. *Am. J. Anat., 121,* 401–424.

Stell, W. K. (1975). Horizontal cell axons and axon terminals in goldfish retina. *J. Comp. Neurol., 159,* 503–520.

Stell, W. K., Ishida, A. T., & Lightfoot, D. O. (1977). Structural basis for on- and off-center responses in retinal bipolar cells. *Science, 198,* 1269–1271.

Stenson, H. H. (1966). The physical factor structure of random forms and their judged complexity. *Percept. Psychophys., 1,* 303–310.

Sterling, P. (1983). Microcircuitry of the cat retina. *Ann. Rev. Neurosci., 6,* 149–185.

Stevens, C. F. (1984). Biophysical studies of ion channels. *Science, 225,* 1346–1350.

Stevens, J. C., & Rubin, L. L. (1970). Psychophysical scales of apparent heaviness and the size-weight illusion. *Percept. and Psychophys., 8,* 225–230.

Stevens, J. K., Emerson, R. C., Gerstein, G. L., Kallos, T., Neufeld, G. R., Nichols, C. W., & Rosenquist, A. C. (1976). Paralysis of the awake human: Visual perceptions. *Vision Res., 16,* 93–98.

Stevens, K. N. (1973). Potential role of property detectors in the perception of consonants. *Q. Prog. Rep. Res. Lab. Electronics MIT, 110,* 155–168.

Stevens, S. S. (1956). The direct estimation of sensory magnitudes: Loudness. *Am. J. Psychol., 69,* 1–25.

Stevens, S. S. (1957). On the psychophysical law. *Psychol. Rev., 64,* 153–181.

Stevens, S. S. (1962). The surprising simplicity of sensory metrics. *Am. Psychol., 17,* 29–39.

Stevens, S. S. (1972). Perceived level of noise by Mark VII and decibels (E). *J. Acoust. Soc. Am., 51,* 575–601.

Stevens, S. S., & Davis, H. (1938). *Hearing.* New York: Wiley.

Stevens, S. S., & Newman, E. B. (1934). The localization of pure tones. *Proc. Natl. Acad. Sci., 20,* 593–596.

Stevens, S. S., & Volkmann, J. (1940). The relation of pitch to frequency, a revised scale. *Am. J. Psychol., 53,* 329–353.

Stiles, W. S., & Crawford, B. H. (1933). The luminous efficiency of rays entering the eye pupil at different points. *Proc. R. Soc. Lond. Ser. B., 112,* 428–450.

Stone, J., Dreher, B., & Leventhal, A. (1979). Hierarchical and parallel mechanisms in the organization of visual cortex. *Brain Res. Rev., 1,* 345–394.

Stone, J., & Freeman Jr., R. B. (1971). Conduction velocity groups in the cat's optic nerve classified according to their retinal origin. *Exp. Brain Res., 13,* 489–497.

Stone, J., & Fukuda, Y. (1974). Properties of cat retinal ganglion cells: A comparison of W-cells with X- and Y-cells. *J. Neurophysiol., 37,* 722–748.

Stone, J., & Hoffmann, K.-P. (1971). Conduction velocity as a parameter in the organisation of the afferent relay in the cat's lateral geniculate nucleus. *Brain Res., 32,* 454–459.

Stone, J., & Hoffmann, K.-P. (1972). Very slow-conducting ganglion cells in the cat's retina: A major, new functional type? *Brain Res., 43*, 610–616.

Strelioff, D., Sitko, S. T., & Honrubia, V. (1976). Role of inner and outer hair cells in neural excitation. *Trans. Am. Acad. Ophthalmol. Otolaryngol. 82*, 322–326.

Stromeyer, C. F. (1974). Curvature detectors in human vision? *Science, 184*, 1199–1200.

Stromeyer, C. F., Lange, A. F., & Ganz, L. (1973). Spatial frequency phase effects in human vision. *Vision Res., 13*, 2345–2360.

Stromeyer, C. F., & Klein, S. (1974). Spatial frequency channels in human vision as asymmetric (edge) mechanisms. *Vision Res., 14*, 1409–1420.

Studdert-Kennedy, M. (1976). Speech perception. In N. J. Lass (Ed.), *Contemporary issues in experimental phonetics* (pp. 243–293). New York: Academic Press.

Studdert-Kennedy, M., & Shankweiler, D. (1970). Hemispheric specialization for speech perception. *J. Acoust. Soc. Am., 48*, 579–594.

Suga, N., & Manabe, T. (1982). Neural basis of amplitude-spectrum representation in auditory cortex of the mustached bat. *J. Neurophysiol., 47*, 225–255.

Suga, N., O'Neill, W. E., & Manabe, T. (1979). Harmonic-sensitive neurons in the auditory cortex of the mustache bat. *Science, 203*, 270–274.

Sullivan, D. G., & Georgeson, M. A. (1977). The missing fundamental illusion: Variation of spatio-temporal characteristics with dark adaptation. *Vision Res., 17*, 977–981.

Sur, M., Garraghty, P. E., & Roe, A. W. (1988). Experimentally induced visual projections into auditory thalamus and cortex. *Science, 242*, 1437–1441.

Sur, M., & Sherman, S. M. (1982). Linear and nonlinear W-cells in C-laminae of the cat's lateral geniculate nucleus. *J. Neurophysiol., 47*, 869–884.

Sutherland, N. S. (1973). Object recognition. In E. C. Carterette & M. P. Friedman (Eds.), *Handbook of perception, Volume III: Biology of perceptual systems.* (pp. 157–185). New York: Academic Press.

Swets, J. A., Tanner Jr., W. P., & Birdsall, T. G. (1961). Decision processes in perception. *Psychol. Rev., 68*, 301–340.

Tachibana, M., & Kaneko, A. (1988). Retinal bipolar cells receive negative feedback input from GABAergic amacrine cells. *Visual Neurosci., 1*, 297–305.

Tanaka, K. (1985). Organization of geniculate inputs to visual cortical cells in the cat. *Vision Res., 25*, 357–364.

Tangney, J., Weisstein, N., & Berbaum, K. (1979). Masking independent of both separation and spatial frequency. *Vision Res., 19*, 817–823.

Teeven, R. C., & Birney, R. C. (1961). *Color vision.* Princeton, N.J.: Van Nostrand.

Teller, D. Y. (1984). Linking propositions. *Vision Res., 24*, 1233–1246.

Thouless, R. H. (1931). Phenomenal regression to the real object. *Br. J. Psychol., 21*, 339–359.

Timney, B. N., & Muir, D. W. (1976). Orientation anisotrophy: Incidence and magnitude in Caucasian and Chinese subjects. *Science, 193*, 699–701.

Tolhurst, D. J. (1973). Separate channels for the analysis of the shape and the movement of a moving visual stimulus. *J. Physiol., 231*, 385–402.

Tolhurst, D. J., & Thompson, I. D. (1982). Organization of neurones preferring similar spatial frequencies in cat striate cortex. *Exp. Brain Res., 48*, 217–227.

Tomita, T. (1970). Electrical activity of vertebrate photoreceptors. *Q. Rev. Biophys., 3*, 179–222.

Tomita, T., Kaneko, A., Murakami, M., & Pautler, E. L. (1967). Spectral response curves of single cones in the carp. *Vision Res., 7*, 519–531.

Tong, L., & Green, D. G. (1977). Adaptation pools and excitation receptive fields of rat retinal ganglion cells. *Vision Res., 17*, 1233–1236.

Tong, Y. C., Dowell, R. C., Blamey, P. J., & Clark, G. M. (1983). Two-component hearing sensations produced by two-electrode stimulation in the cochlea of a deaf patient. *Science, 219*, 993–994.

Tonndorf, J., & Khanna, S. M. (1970). The role of the tympanic membrane in middle ear transmission. *Ann. Otol. Rhinol. Laryngol., 79*, 743–753.

Tootell, R. B. H., Hamilton, S. L., & Switkes, E. (1988). Functional anatomy of macaque striate cortex. IV. Contrast and magno-parvo streams. *J. Neurosci., 8*, 1594–1609.

Tootell, R. B., Silverman, M. S., & DeValois, R. L. (1981). Spatial frequency columns in primary visual cortex. *Science, 214*, 813–815.

Tootell, R. B. H., Silverman, M. S., Hamilton, S. L., DeValois, R. L., & Switkes, E. (1988). Functional anatomy of macaque striate cortex. III. Color. *J. Neurosci., 8*, 1569–1593.

Toyoda, J.-I. (1973). Membrane resistance changes underlying the bipolar cell response in the carp retina. *Vision Res., 13*, 283–294.

Toyoda, J.-I., Hashimoto, H., & Ohtsu, K. (1973). Bipolar-amacrine transmission in the carp retina. *Vision Res., 13*, 295–307.

Toyoda, J.-I., Kujiraoka, T. (1982). Analyses of bipolar cell responses elicited by polarization of horizontal cells. *J. Gen. Physiol., 79*, 131–145.

Trezona, P. W. (1970). Rod participation in the "blue" mechanism and its effect upon colour matching. *Vision Res., 10*, 317–332.

Ts'o, D. Y., & Gilbert, C. D. (1988). The organization of chromatic and spatial interactions in the primate striate cortex. *J. Neurosci., 8*, 1712–1727.

Turvey, M. T. (1973). On peripheral and central processes in vision: Inferences from an information processing analysis of masking with patterned stimuli. *Psychol. Rev., 80*, 1–52.

Tynan, P., & Sekuler, R. (1975). Moving visual phantoms: A new contour completion effect. *Science, 188*, 951–952.

Uhr, L. (1973). *Pattern recognition, learning, and thought*. Englewood Cliffs, N.J.: Prentice Hall.

Ullman, S. (1986). Artificial intelligence and the brain: Computational studies of the visual system. *Ann. Rev. Neurosci., 9*, 1–26.

Updyke, B. V. (1974). Characteristics of unit responses in superior colliculus of the Cebus monkey. *J. Neurophysiol., 37*, 896–909.

Van Essen, D. C. (1979). Visual areas of the mammalian cerebral cortex. *Ann. Rev. Neurosci., 2*, 227–263.

Vaney, D. I. (1986). Morphological identification of serotonin-accumulating neurons in the living retina. *Science, 233*, 444–446.

Vitz, P. C., & Todd, T. C. (1971). A model of the perception of simple geometric figures. *Psychol. Rev., 78*, 207–228.

Waite, H., & Massaro, D. W. (1970). Test of Gregory's constancy scaling explanation of the Müller-Lyer illusion. *Nature, 227*, 733–734.

Wald, G. (1945). Human vision and the spectrum. *Science, 101*, 653–658.

Wald, G., & Brown, P. K. (1965). Human color vision and color blindness. *Cold Spring Harbor Symp. Quant. Biol., 30*, 345–359.

Wald, G., Brown, P. K., & Smith, P. H. (1955). Iodopsin. *J. Gen. Physiol., 38*, 623–681.

Wallach, H. (1948). Brightness constancy and the nature of achromatic colors. *J. Exp. Psychol., 38*, 310–324.

Wallach, H. (1959). The perception of motion. *Sci. Am., 201*, 55–60.

Wallach, H. (1963). The perception of neutral colors. *Sci. Am., 208*, 107–116.

Wallach, H. (1987). Perceiving a stable environment when one moves. *Ann. Rev. Psychol., 38*, 1–27.

Wallach, H., & Austin, P. (1954). Recognition and the localization of visual traces. *Am. J. Psychol., 57*, 338–340.

Wallach, H., & O'Connell, D. N. (1953). The kinetic depth effect. *J. Exp. Psychol., 45*, 205–217.

Wallach, H., O'Connell, D. N., & Neisser, U. (1953). The memory effect of visual perception of three-dimensional form. *J. Exp. Psychol., 45*, 360–368.

Walliser, K. (1969a). Zusammenhange zwischen dem schallreiz und der periodentonhohe. *Acustica, 21*, 319–328.

Walliser, K. (1969b). Zur unterschiedsschwell der periodentonhohe. *Acustica, 21*, 329–336.

Walls, G. L. (1967). *The vertebrate eye and its adaptive radiation*. New York: Hafner.

Walters, J. W., & Harwerth, R. S. (1978). The mechanism of brightness enhancement. *Vision Res., 18*, 777–779.

Warfield, C. A., Stein, J. M., & Frank, H. A. (1985). The effect of transcutaneous electrical nerve stimulation on pain after thoracotomy. *Ann. Thorac. Surg., 39*, 462–465.

Warren, R. M. (1970). Elimination of biases in loudness judgments for tones. *J. Acoust. Soc. Am., 48*, 1397–1403.

Warren, R. M. (1981). Measurement of sensory intensity. *Behav. and Brain Sci., 4*, 175–223.

Wasserman, G. S., Felsten, G., & Easland, G. S. (1979). The psychophysical function: Harmonizing Fechner and Stevens. *Science, 204*, 85–87.

Wässle, H., Boycott, B. B., & Illing, R. B. (1981). Morphology and mosaic of on- and off-beta cells in the cat retina and some functional considerations. *Proc. Roy. Soc. Lond. B., 212*, 177–195.

Wässle, H., Peichl, L., & Boycott, B. B. (1981). Morphology and topology of on- and off-alpha cells in the cat retina. *Proc. Roy. Soc. Lond. B, 212,* 157–175.

Watson, A. B., & Robson, J. G. (1981). Discrimination at threshold: Labelled detectors in human vision. *Vision Res., 21,* 1115–1122.

Watt, R. J., & Morgan, M. J. (1983). The recognition and representation of edge blur: Evidence for spatial primitives in human vision. *Vision Res., 23,* 1465–1477.

Weiler, R., & Marchiafava, P. L. (1981). Physiological and morphological study of the inner plexiform layer in the turtle retina. *Vision Res., 21,* 1635–1638.

Weiss, A. D. (1963). Auditory perception in relation to age. In J. E. Birren, R. N. Butler, S. W. Greenhouse, L. Sokoloff, & M. Tarrow (Eds.), *Human aging.* PHS Publ. No. 986. Washington, D.C.: U.S. Department of Health, Education, and Welfare.

Weiss, T. F. (1964). A model for firing patterns at auditory nerve fibers. Research Laboratory in Electronics Technical Report No. 418. Cambridge, Mass.: MIT Press.

Weiss, T. F. (1966). A model of the peripheral auditory system. *Kybernetik, 3,* 153–175.

Weiss, T. F. (1982). Bidirectional transduction in vertebrate hair cells: A mechanism for coupling mechanical and electrical processes. *Hearing Res., 7,* 353–360.

Weisstein, N. (1968). A Rashevsky-Landahl neural net: Simulation of metacontrast. *Psychol. Rev., 75,* 494–521.

Weisstein, N. (1970). Neural symbolic activity: A psychophysical measure. *Science, 168,* 1489–1491.

Weisstein, N., & Harris, C. S. (1974). Visual detection of line segments: An object superiority effect. *Science, 186,* 752–755.

Weisstein, N., Maguire, W., & Berbaum, K. (1977). A phantom-motion after-effect. *Science, 198,* 955–957.

Weisstein, N., Harris, C. S., Berbaum, K., Tangney, J., & Williams, A. (1977). Contrast reduction by small localized stimuli: Extensive spatial spread of above-threshold orientation-selective masking. *Vision Res., 17,* 341–350.

Werblin, F. S. (1971). Adaptation in a vertebrate retina. Intracellular recordings in *Necturus. J. Neurophysiol., 34,* 228–241.

Werblin, F. S. (1974). Control of retinal sensitivity.

II. Lateral interactions at the outer plexiform layer. *J. Gen. Physiol., 63,* 62–87.

Werblin, F. S. (1977). Regenerative amacrine cell depolarization and formation of on-off ganglion cell response. *J. Physiol., 264,* 767–785.

Werblin, F. S., & Dowling, J. E. (1969). Organization of the retina of the mudpuppy, *Necturus maculosus.* II. Intracellular recording. *J. Neurophysiol., 32,* 339–355.

Werker, J. F. (1989). Becoming a native listener. *Amer. Scient., 77,* 54–59.

Werner, H. (1935). Studies on contour. *Am. J. Psychol., 47,* 40–64.

Wertheimer, M. (1912). Experimentelle studien über des Sehen von Bewegung. *Z. Psychol., 61,* 161–265.

Wertheimer, M. (1923). Untersuchungen zur Lehre von der Gestalt. II. *Psychol. Forsch., 5,* 301–350. Abridged and translated by M. Wertheimer in *Readings in Perception,* Beardsley & Wertheimer (Eds.). New York: Van Nostrand, 1958.

Westheimer, G. H. (1975). The eye. In V. B. Mountcastle (Ed.), *Medical physiology,* Vol. I, 13th Ed. St. Louis: C. V. Mosby, pp. 440–457.

Wever, E. G. (1949). *Theory of Hearing.* New York: Wiley.

Wever, E. G., & Bray, C. W. (1930). Present possibilities for auditory theory. *Psychol. Rev., 37,* 365–380.

Wever, E. G., & Bray, C. W. (1937). The perception of low tones and the resonance-volley theory. *J. Psychol., 3,* 101–114.

Wever, E. G., & Lawrence, M. (1954). *Physiological acoustics.* Princeton, N.J.: Princeton University Press.

Whalen, D. H., & Liberman, A. M. (1987). Speech perception takes precedence over nonspeech perception. *Science, 237,* 169–171.

Whitehorn, D., & Burgess, P. R. (1973). Changes in polarization of central branches of myelinated mechanoreceptor and nociceptor fibers during noxious and innocuous stimulation of the skin. *J. Neurophysiol., 36,* 226–237.

Whitfield, I. C., & Evans, E. F. (1965). Responses of auditory cortical neurons to stimuli of changing frequency. *J. Neurophysiol., 28,* 655–672.

Whitten, D. N., & Brown, K. T. (1973). Photopic suppression of monkeys' rod receptor potential, apparently by a cone-initiated lateral inhibition. *Vision Res., 13*, 1629–1658.

Wiesel, T. N., & Hubel, D. H. (1963). Single-cell responses in striate cortex of kittens deprived of vision in one eye. *J. Neurophysiol., 26*, 1003–1017.

Wiesel, T. N., & Hubel, D. H. (1965). Comparison of the effects of unilateral and bilateral eye closure on cortical unit responses in kittens. *J. Neurophysiol., 28*, 1029–1040.

Wiesel, T. N., & Hubel, D. H. (1966). Spatial and chromatic interactions in the lateral geniculate body of the rhesus monkey. *J. Neurophysiol., 29*, 1115–1156.

Wiesel, T. N., & Hubel, D. H. (1974). Ordered arrangement of orientation columns in monkeys lacking visual experience. *J. Comp. Neurol., 158*, 307–318.

Williams, D. R., & MacLeod, D. I. A. (1979). Interchangeable backgrounds for cone after-images. *Vision Res., 19*, 867–877.

Williams, D. W., Wilson, H. R., & Cowan, J. D. (1982). Localized effects of spatial-frequency adaptation. *J. Opt. Soc. Amer., 72*, 878–887.

Willis, W. D. (1981). Ascending pathways from the dorsal horn. In A. B. Brown & M. Rethely (Eds.) *Spinal cord sensation: Sensory processing in the dorsal horn.* Edinburgh: Scottish Academic Press.

Willis, W. D. (1985). Pain pathways in the primate. In M. J. Correia & A. A. Perachio (Eds.), *Contemporary sensory neurobiology.* New York: Alan R. Liss, Inc.

Wilson, D. A., & Leon, M. (1987). Evidence of lateral synaptic interactions in olfactory bulb output cell responses to odors. *Brain Res., 417*, 175–180.

Wilson, M. E., & Cragg, B. G. (1967). Projections from the lateral geniculate nucleus in the cat and monkey. *J. Anat., 101*, 677–692.

Wilson, H. R., McFarlane, D. K., & Phillips, G. C. (1983). Spatial frequency tuning of orientation selective units estimated by oblique masking. *Vision Res., 23*, 873–882.

Witkovsky, P. (1971). Synapses made by myelinated fibers running to teleost and elasmobranch retinas. *J. Comp. Neurol., 142*, 205–222.

Wollberg, Z., & Newman, J. D. (1972). Auditory cortex of squirrel monkey: Response patterns of single cells to species-specific vocalizations. *Science, 175*, 212–214.

Wong, E., & Weisstein, N. (1982). A new perceptual context-superiority effect: Line segments are more visible against a figure than against a ground. *Science, 218*, 587–589.

Wong-Riley, M. T. T. (1979). Changes in the visual system of monocularly sutured or enucleated cats demonstrable with cytochrome oxidase histochemistry. *Brain Res., 171*, 11–28.

Woodmansee, J. J. Jr. (1965). An evaluation of pupil response as a measure of attitude toward Negroes. *Doctoral dissertation, University of Colorado.*

Woodruff, M. L., Bownds, D., Green, S. H., Morrisey, J. L., & Shedlovsky, A. (1977). Guanosine 3′, 5′-cyclic monophosphate and the in vitro physiology of frog photoreceptor membranes. *J. Gen. Physiol., 69*, 667–679.

Wooten, B. R., & Werner, J. S. (1979). Short-wave cone input to the red-green opponent channel. *Vision Res., 19*, 1053–1054.

Wright, W. D. (1952). The characteristics of tritanopia. *J. Opt. Soc. Am., 42*, 509–521.

Wurtz, R. H., & Goldberg, M. E. (1971). Superior colliculus cell responses related to eye movements in awake monkeys. *Science, 171*, 82–84.

Wurtz, R. H., & Mohler, C. W. (1976). Organization of monkey superior colliculus: Enhanced visual response of superficial cell layers. *J. Neurophysiol., 39*, 745–765.

Yaksh, T. L. (1978). Narcotic analgesics: CNS sites and mechanisms of action as revealed by intracerebral injection techniques. *Pain, 4*, 299–359.

Yamamoto, T., & Kawamura, Y. (1972). Gustatory responses from circumvallate and foliate papillae of the rat. *Journal of the Physiological Society of Japan, 34*, 83–84.

Yau, K.-W., & Nakatani, K. (1984). Cation selectivity of light-sensitive conductance in retinal rods. *Nature, 309*, 352–354.

Yoshikami, S., & Hagins, W. A. (1971). Ionic basis of dark current and photocurrent of retinal rods. *Biophys. J., 10*, 60a.

Yoshikami, S., Robinson, W. E., & Hagins, W. A. (1974). Topology of the outer segment membranes of retinal rods and cones revealed by fluorescent probe. *Science, 185*, 1176–1179.

Young, R. W. (1978). The daily rhythm of shedding and degradation of rod and cone outer segment membranes in the chick retina. *Invest. Ophthalmol., 17*, 105–116.

Zahs, K. R., & Stryker, M. P. (1988). Segregation of ON and OFF afferents to ferret visual cortex. *J. Neurophysiol., 59,* 1410–1429.

Zeigler, H. P., & Leibowitz, H. (1957). Apparent visual size as a function of distance for children and adults. *Am. J. Psychol., 70,* 106–109.

Zeki, S. (1973). Color coding in rhesus monkey prestriate cortex. *Brain Res., 53,* 422–427.

Zeki, S. M. (1974). Functional organization of a visual area in the posterior bank of the superior temporal sulcus of the rhesus monkey. *J. Physiol., 236,* 549–573.

Zeki, S. (1983a). The distribution of wavelength and orientation selective cells in different areas of monkey visual cortex. *Proc. Roy. Soc. B, 217,* 449–470.

Zeki, S. (1983b). Colour coding in the cerebral cortex: The responses of wavelength-selective and colour-coded cells in monkey visual cortex to changes in wavelength composition. *Neurosci., 9,* 767–781.

Zeki, S., & Shipp, S. (1988). The functional logic of cortical connections. *Nature, 335,* 311–317.

Zimbardo, P. G., Andersen, S. M., & Kabat, L. G. (1981). Induced hearing deficit generates experimental paranoia. *Science, 212,* 1529–1531.

Zurif, E. B. (1980). Language mechanisms: A neuropsychological perspective. *Amer. Scient., 68,* 305–311.

Zwaardemaker, H. (1895). *Die Physiologie des Geruchs.* Leipzig: Engelmann.

Zwicker, E., & Feldtkeller, R. (1956). *Das Ohr als Nachrichtenempfänger.* Stuttgart: S. Hirzel Verlag.

Zwicker, E., Flottorp, G., & Stevens, S. S. (1957). Critical bandwidth in loudness summation. *J. Acoust. Soc. Am., 29,* 548–557.

Zwislocki, J. J. (1981). Sound analysis in the ear: A history of discoveries. *Amer. Scient. 69,* 184–192.

Author Index

GLOSSDEX

2AFC *See* Two alternative forced choice

4AFC *See* Four alternative forced choice

2¹/₂D sketch Hypothetical viewer-centered representation of space generated as input for the full three-dimensional representation, 321

Abscissa Horizontal position on a graph, **600**

Absolute threshold Minimum detectable amount of stimulation, **8**, 15; auditory, 26, 486–487. *See also* Minimum audible field, Minimum audible pressure; visual, 24–25, 144–149. *See also* Dark adaptation, Spectral sensitivity

Absorbance spectrum Curve relating percentage of light absorbed by a pigment to the wavelength of the light (also called *absorption spectrum* or *percentage absorption*), 101, 141, 144, 405, 410, 411, 413

Accommodation Process of focusing the eye on objects at varying distances, 75–**78**, 306–307. *See also* Ciliary muscles, Lens

Achromatopsia Inability to see colors, due to damage in higher cortex, **201**

Acoustic reflex Reflex protecting the ear from intense sounds by contraction of the stapedius and tensor tympani muscles, 445

Action potential Electrical event by which a neuron can transmit information for long distances along its axon, **42**–49, 50, 52, 56–57, 63, 115, 546, 595

Active transport Energy-requiring process by which Na⁺ is pumped out of a nerve cell and K⁺ is pumped in, **47**

Acuity Ability to discern fine details, **81**, 93, 220, 267, 417

Adaptation Changing sensitivity to accommodate different levels of stimulation, 139–158, 430, 448–449, 495, 538, 564, 578–579. *See also* Dark adaptation, Light adaptation

Adaptation level Theory that perceived lightness is judged relative to mean luminance in the entire scene, **329**, 335

Adapting pool Local region of retina in which all neurons adapt as a unit, 154–155

Additive color mixture Superposition of two or more colored lights, 390–394. *See also* Metameric match

Afferent Nerve fiber carrying sensory information to the central nervous system, 552–553, 555–556

Aftereffect Altered perception due to previously presented stimuli, 261, 269, 579. *See also* Figural aftereffect, McCullough effect, Movement aftereffect

Afterimages Images of a stimulus seen after the physical stimulus is extinguished, **156**–157, 343. *See also* Emmert's law; negative, **157**, 417; positive, **156**–157

Albedo *See* Reflectance

All-or-none principle Principle stating that all action potentials are of the same size, regardless of the strength of the stimulus that produced them, **44**

Amacrine cells Laterally conducting cells of the inner plexiform layer of the retina, **90**, 108–110, 112, 113

Ambiguous figure A pattern that can be interpreted in either of two ways, **284**, 285–286. *See also* Reversible figure

Ames demonstrations 290–291, 345–346. *See also* Illusion, Trapezoidal window

Analgesia The reduction of pain, 568–572

Analysis-by-synthesis Model of perception in which an internal representation is built by making perceptual hypotheses, 281, 540

Anamorphic art Pictures that can be seen "correctly" only if viewed with a specific distortion, 362–363

Annulus Ring-shaped visual stimulus, **104**

Anomalous trichromat Trichromat with an abnormal visual pigment in one cone type, **412**

Anosmia Inability to sense odors, **591**

Anterior chamber Front chamber of the eye, between cornea and iris, **73**

Anterolateral columns Columns at the sides of the spinal cord, mediating pain sensations, **556**, 565–566. *See also* Spinomesencephalic tract, Spinothalamic tract

Apex Top of the cochlea, farthest from the oval window, **446**, 456

Apparent movement Impression of movement given by stationary stimuli, **365**, 374. *See also* Autokinetic effect, Movement aftereffect, Pulfrich effect, Stroboscopic movement

Aqueous humor Fluid in the anterior chamber of the eye, **73**

Articulation Formation of speech sounds by the vocal apparatus, 516–518

Artificial intelligence Computer models of perceptual systems, 253–258, 301. *See also* Parallel distributed processing

Ascending series Method of limits in which threshold is approached from below, **10**

Astigmatism Defect of the eye in which focus is different for stimuli of different orientations, **81**

Auditory cortex Portion of temporal lobe devoted to the auditory sense, 451–452, 469–471, 503, 537

Auditory fatigue Loss in sensitivity following an intense auditory stimulus, 493–494

Auditory localization Ability to discern the position of a sound source in space, 433, 442, 502–510. *See also* Auditory receptive fields, Cone of confusion, Monaural cues

Auditory nerve Fibers that convey information from the cochlea to the brainstem, 449–450, 453, 464, 472–475, 491–492

Auditory receptive field Area of space to which an auditory neuron is tuned, 503–504, 505

Autokinetic effect Apparent random motion of a small stimulus in a large, blank field, **377**

Axon Long extension that carries output information from a neuron, **35**, 38–49, 546, 552, 595

Axon terminal End of the axon furthest from the cell body, where it is presynaptic to other cells, **35**, 53–57

Azimuth Lateral position, **506**–510

Balint's syndrome Disorder of perception in which patient has difficulty integrating parts of the visual scene, **202**

Bandwidth Range of frequencies represented in a stimulus (can also mean range to which a system is sensitive), **495–497**

Base Part of cochlea nearest the oval window, 456

Basilar membrane Major membrane of the cochlea, separating the cochlear duct from the scala tympani, **446**, 455–463, 468–469, 481, 487, 492–493, 498, 501. *See also* Envelope, Place theory, Resonance curve, Telephone theory

Beats Periodic changes in loudness of a sound consisting of two tones of similar frequency, 480–481, 521

Beta movement Stroboscopic movement of a stimulus from one position to another (also called *optimal movement*), **379**. *See also* Stroboscopic movement

Bezold-Brücke hue shift Change in hue of a light as its intensity is changed, **26**

Binaural cues Cues to the position of a sound source requiring the use of both ears, **505**; head movements, 508–509; intensity differences, 506–507; timing differences, 507–508

Binocular cues Cues to depth or distance based on binocular disparity, **297**, 311–320. *See also* Binocular disparity, Convergence

Binocular disparity Difference between the images on the two retinae due to differences in depth, 198, **313–319**

Binocular interaction Combination of signals from the two eyes, 180, 320–321

Binocular rivalry Condition in which dichoptic stimuli conflict, so only one may be seen at a time, 319–320, 370

Bipolar cells Retinal cells that conduct signals from the outer plexiform layer to the inner plexiform layer, **90**, 103, 107, 108–109, 110, 111

Blind spot Optic disc, where there are no receptors, **75**, 76, 77

Blobs Areas of dark cytochrome oxidase staining in V1, where cells sensitive to wavelength are found (also called *puffs*), **188**–189, 196–197, 424, 430

Bloch's law Trade-off between intensity and duration of equally detectable lights, **26**

Blocking agent Drug that prevents a transmitter from having its effect at a synapse, **57**

Bottom-up processing *See* Top-down processing

Brightness Apparent amount of

light emanating from an object, **326–337**, 420

Brightness enhancement Increased brightness of a flickering light, 336–337

Broca's area Region in frontal cortex of the left hemisphere of the brain that is essential for the production of speech, **543**

CFF *See* Critical fusion frequency

CIE *See* Commission Internationale de l'Éclairage

CIE color diagram Color space defined by the CIE, **400–404**, 414–417, 418

CL *See* Central lateral nucleus

CSF *See* Contrast sensitivity function

Camouflage *See* Masking, simultaneous

Cataract Condition in which the lens of the eye becomes opaque, **73–74**, 79, 282

Cell assembly Groupings of neurons hypothesized to "learn" by strengthening synaptic connections, 282. *See also* Parallel distributed processing

Central lateral nucleus (CL) Nucleus of the thalamus that serves as a pain relay, **566**

Centrifugal fibers Efferent fibers from the central nervous system to the peripheral sense organs, **91**, 453. *See also* Feedback

Channels Hypothetical visual detectors of different spatial frequencies and/or orientations, **226–231**, 237–247, 269, 371

Characteristic frequency Frequency to which an auditory nerve fiber is most sensitive, **464**, 493

Choroid Layer of the eye that lies between the sclera and pigment epithelium, **74**

Chromophore Active portion of a visual pigment, **95**

Ciliary muscles Muscles that control state of visual accommodation, **74**. *See also* Accommodation

Closure Gestalt principle stating that people tend to see figures as enclosed wholes, **265**

Cochlea Spiral structure of the inner ear containing the Organ of Corti, **445**. *See also* Basilar membrane, Hair cells, Organ of Corti

Cochlear duct Middle chamber of the cochlea, containing the endolymph (also call *scala media*), **446**

Cochlear microphonic Gross potential reflecting the activity of auditory hair cells, **60**

Cochlear nucleus First relay station for auditory nerve fibers entering the brainstem, **450**, 465–467

Cognitive learning 282–283

Color aftereffects Apparent color of a black-and-white stimulus as a result of inspection of a colored pattern, 242–244. *See also* McCullough effect

Color blindness Condition in which certain color discriminations cannot be made (more properly called *color defects*), 412–417. *See also* Achromatopsia, Anomalous trichromat, Dichromacy, Monochromacy

Color constancy Tendency for the color of an object to be perceived as the same regardless of the spectral composition of the light illuminating it, **428**, 429–430. *See also* Lightness constancy

Color matching *See* Metameric match

Color naming Psychophysical technique in which the subject assigns names to lights of various wavelengths, 419

Color perception 428–431. *See also* Additive color mixture, Color naming, Metameric matching, Opponent process theory, Saturation, Subtractive color mixture, Surface color, Trichromatic theory

Color space Geometric representation of the facts of color mixing, **399–404**. *See also* CIE color diagram

Columns, cortical Organization of cortex such that cells with similar properties are found in vertical columns, **184**, 564. *See also* Hypercolumns, Ocular dominance columns, Orientation columns

Columns, spinal Collections of axons running along the length of the spinal cord, carrying information toward (or from) the brain. *See* Anterolateral columns, Posterior columns

Commission Internationale de l'Éclairage (CIE) International commission that defined standards of light and color, **401**. *See also* CIE color diagram

Common fate Gestalt principle stating that items moving in the same direction at the same speed are grouped together, 264, 309

Complementary colors Pairs of lights that when added together yield white, **418**

Complex cells Type of cell in the visual cortex that does not select for position of a stimulus within its receptive field, 174–176, 177–179, 244–245, 372

Complex sounds Sounds containing more than one frequency component, 436, 438–440, 480–482, 495–501, 508

Complexity Measure of information content in a figure, 267–268

Concentric cells Cells in visual cortex with circular receptive fields having center/surround organization, 178

Conditioned taste aversion Acquired distaste for a flavor as a result of association with illness, 588–589

Cone Receptor cell in the retina that operates in relatively high luminance (photopic) conditions, 91–100, 148–149, 151, 154. *See also* Cone pigments

Cone of confusion Locus of points in space that would produce the same timing or intensity differences if a sound source were located at any of them, 508–509

Cone pigments Photopigments in the cones, 101–102; in color blindness, 412; spectral sensitivities of, 410, 411, 413, 426

Confusion loci Lines on the CIE color diagram representing colors that appear alike to a dichromat, 414–417

Conjugate eye movements Shifts of gaze in which both eyes move in the same direction, 85–86

Consonants Low energy speech sounds, 515, 517–518, 526, 527–532; fricative, **518**; glide, **518**; lateral, **518**; nasal, **518**; plosive, **517**, 527–529, 538; unvoiced, **517**, 527–529,538; voiced, **517**, 530–532

Constant stimuli, method of Psychophysical method in which intensity varies randomly from presentation to presentation, **12**, 15

Context in motion detection, 381–382; in speech perception, 529, 535; in vision, *see* Set

Continuity Gestalt principle stating that parts group to form a single entity, **264**–265

Contralateral On the opposite side of the body, **160**, 192–194, 565

Contrast Difference between the brightest and the dimmest parts of a pattern, **19**, 107, 109, 120, 152, 153, 213, 302, 319, 331, 333–335. *See also* Rayleigh contrast, Weber contrast

Contrast sensitivity Inverse of the contrast required for detection of a pattern, 167, **221–225**, 227–229

Contrast sensitivity function (CSF) Curve relating contrast sensitivity to spatial frequency of the stimulus, **221**–223, 227–229, 237–239

Control of pupil size 80–82

Convergence Disjunctive eye movement in which the eyes turn inward, **86**, 311–313

Cornea Clear front surface of the eye through which light enters, **73**, 75

Cornsweet illusion Alternative name for Craik-O'Brien illusion. *See* Craik-O'Brien illusion

Corpus callosum Band of axons interconnecting the two hemispheres of the brain, **160**

Corridor illusion Illusion of size due to distance, 343–345, 347. *See also* Illusion

Cortex Outer layers or "rind" of the brain. *See* Auditory cortex, Mediotemporal cortex, V2, V3, V4, Visual area I, S1

Corti's arch Rigid triangle of cells within the organ of Corti, **447**

Craik-O'Brien illusion Illusion of uniform brightness in a region in which luminance changes gradually, 123, 125, 223–224, 253, 279. *See also* Missing fundamental illusion

Criterion Intensity sufficient to prompt a decision that the stimulus was present, **12**, 29–32, 143

Critical band Range of frequencies within which stimuli interact, **497**; auditory, 495–499; spatial frequency, **232–236**

Critical fusion frequency (CFF) Frequency at which a flickering light appears steady, **337**

Cross-modal interactions Interactions between the senses, 564, 570, 589

Cross-modal matching Psychophysical scaling method in which the subject matches apparent intensities across two sensory modalities, **22**

Cultural differences in perception 283

Cuneatis *See* Posterior columns

Current Flow of charged particles in an electrical circuit, **36**

Cutaneous receptors *See* Tactile sensation

Cyclic AMP Nucleotide involved in the transduction process in chemical sensory receptors, 582, 595

Cyclic GMP Nucleotide involved in the transduction process in visual receptors, **98**

Cytochrome oxidase Enzyme involved in energy production in cells, **188**. *See also* Blobs, Thick stripes, Thin stripes

d′ Detectability of a stimulus, in signal detection theory, **28**–31

DL Difference limen. *See* Difference threshold

Dark adaptation Gradual lowering of visual threshold with time in the dark, 144, **145**, 146. *See also* Adaptation, Photochromatic interval, Photopic system, Purkinje shift, Scotopic system

Decibel (Db) Logarithmic intensity scale, used particularly to express amplitude of sound waves, **437**–438, 445, 490

Decremental conduction *See* Electrotonic conduction

Demons Hypothetical detectors and decision-makers in Pandemonium model. *See* Pandemonium

Dendrite Portion of a neuron specialized for receiving neural inputs, **35**

Depolarization For a nerve cell, becoming less polarized (more positive) inside, **40**, **448**, **582**, **595**

Depth of field Extent to which an object can move in distance from a lens and still be in reasonable focus, **82**

Depth perception Perception of the distances of objects from the observer, **297–323**, **336**

Dermatome Area of the body innervated by a single spinal root, **554–555**

Descending pathways *See* Centrifugal fibers

Descending series Method of limits in which the threshold is approached from above, **10**. *See also* Method of limits

Deuteranope Dichromat lacking the medium wavelength-sensitive pigment, **412**, **415–417**

Development of cortical neurons **191–195**, **505**. *See also* Phonemic boundaries

Dichoptic presentation Presentation of independent stimuli to each eye, **312**, **319**

Dichromacy Form of color blindness in which only two color mechanisms are functional, **406–408**, **412–417**. *See also* Deuteranope, Protanope, Tritanope

Difference threshold Smallest detectable difference between two stimuli, the just noticeable difference (also called *jnd* or *ΔI*), **15**, **477–478**, **536**

Diffusion Force tending to make freely moving particles spread out so their concentration is constant throughout a container, **39**

Diopter Measure of the strength of a lens: one over the focal length in meters, **71**

Diplopia Double vision, **86**, **315**

Direct scaling *See* Magnitude estimation

Direction selective cells *See* Motion detectors

Discs Photopigment-rich membrane packets in outer segments of photoreceptors. *See* Outer segment, Shedding

Disjunctive eye movement Shift of gaze such that the eyes move in opposite directions, **86**

Disparity *See* Binocular disparity

Distal stimulus Actual object being perceived, **281**, **338–339**, **356**, **540**

Doppler shift Change in pitch of a sound source moving relative to the observer, **510**

Dorsal root ganglion Collection of cell bodies of afferents to the spinal cord, **553–554**

Double opponent field Type of visual receptive field in which the antagonistic center and surround each exhibit spectral opponency, **424**

Dyad Synaptic complex in the inner plexiform layer of the retina, **108**, **109**

EPSP *See* Excitatory postsynaptic potential

ERG *See* Electroretinogram

Eardrum *See* Tympanic membrane

Efferent Fiber carrying information from the central nervous system to the periphery. *See* Centrifugal fibers, Gamma motorneurons

Ehrenstein illusion Illusion of shape, **348**. *See also* Illusion

Electromagnetic radiation Form of energy of which visible light is a portion, **65–67**, **387–389**

Electroretinogram (ERG) Gross potential reflecting the activity of retinal neurons, **60**, **155**, **158**

Electrotonic conduction Passive spread of electrical signal within a cell, **39**, **40**, **41**, **42**, **48**, **97**, **115**

Emmert's law Relationship between apparent size of an afterimage and the distance to the surface against which it is seen, **343**

Emmetrope Person whose eye is correctly focused at infinity when unaccommodated, **78**

Endolymph Potassium-rich fluid in the cochlear duct, **446**, **448**

End-stopped Selective for the length of a stimulus. *See* Hypercomplex cells

Enkephalins Endogenous neurotransmitters chemically related to opioids, **571–572**

Envelope Maximum displacement of the basilar membrane during a sustained sound as a function of position along the membrane, **458–460**

Equilibrium potential Voltage difference across a permeable membrane when there is no net movement of ions, **39**

Equiluminant Differing in color but not in luminance (also called *isoluminant*), **203–206**, **273**, **310**, **349**, **383–384**, **406**

Excitatory postsynaptic potential (EPSP) Depolarization caused by transmitter released from a presynaptic cell, **56**, **57**

Extracellular space Fluid-filled space surrounding the cells, 37, 38, 61

Extraocular muscles Muscles that move the eye, **73**, 82–86, 377

Eye-head movement system System that follows a moving stimulus with eye and head movements, **365**, 373–378

Eye movement 82–84, 350. *See also* Extraocular muscles, Inflow theory, Outflow theory, Saccadic movement, Smooth pursuit movement

Eyeshine Light reflected from the back of the eye that appears to come from the pupil, 88

FAE *See* Figural aftereffect

Far point Most distant point for which a myopic eye can produce a sharp image on the retina, 79

Farsightedness *See* Hypermetropia

Feature detectors Cells sensitive to specific aspects of the stimulus display, 128–130, **180–181**, 250, 253, 538, 542

Feedback Process by which "higher" centers affect their inputs. 91, 166, 196, 453

Field adaptation That component of visual adaptation due to neural processes, **154–156**

Figural aftereffect (FAE) Change in perception of a figure caused by inspection of another pattern, **239–240**, 261. *See also* Movement aftereffect

Figure Central object attended to in a scene, 268–272

Flavor 589. *See also* Conditioned taste aversion

Flicker Rapid flashing of a light, 149–150, 336, 391

Focal length Measure of the strength of a lens: the distance from lens to focal point, 70–72

Focal point Point at which a lens focuses parallel light rays, 71

Forced choice Psychophysical method in which a subject must decide which of several alternatives contained the stimulus, **12**. *See also* Four alternative forced choice, Two alternative forced choice

Formant Frequency band emphasized by the vocal apparatus in voiced phonemes, **524–532**

Four alternative forced choice (4AFC) Psychophysical method in which the subject chooses which of four windows holds the stimulus, **13**, 14, 15

Fourier transform Mathematical procedure for approximating a function as a sum of sinusoids, **210–217**, 226–231, 247, 441, 463

Fovea Region in central retina specialized for fine detail discrimination, **75**, 93, 126, 147, 188, 373. *See also* Acuity, Cones

Frame of reference Visual frame of orientation or position of a figure, 276–277, 381–382

Frequency Number of complete vibrations per unit time, **66**, 210–211, 435

Frontal plane projection Projection of a visual scene upon a plane in front of the eyes, like a photograph, **356–357**

Fundamental frequency Lowest frequency component of a complex waveform, **215**, 229, 267, 481

Fuse Combine dichoptic views into a single, coherent image, **316**

Gamma motorneuron Fiber that causes contraction of the muscle spindle fibers, **549**

Ganglion cells Output cells of the retina whose axons form the optic nerve, 90–91, 110–113, 115–119, 128–137, 155, 161, 244–245, 331, 367, 422–423; orientation selective, **130**–131; special types of, 128–130, 367, 422; W-cells, 136, **137**, 171; X-cells, 131–137, 166, 167, 175; Y-cells, 131–137, 166, 171, 175, 177, 337

Gate control theory Theory that pain signals are modulated by other stimuli, 570

Generator potential Slow potential produced within a receptor cell in response to a stimulus, **50–52**, 98, 448, 546, 582–583, 595

Generic recognition Recognition of the general class an object is in, rather than its specific identity, **201**

Gestalt psychology School of psychology that emphasizes properties of figures that transcend their components, **259–272**. *See also* Closure, Common fate, Continuity, Figure, Ground, Prägnanz, Proximity, Similarity, Symmetry

Glabrous skin Smooth or hairless skin, **549–550**

Glia Non-neural cells providing support and nourishment for neurons, **48**, 87

Glomeruli Synaptic regions in the olfactory bulb, **593**

Golgi tendon organ *See* Tendon organs

Gracilis *See* Posterior columns

Gradient Gradual change in luminance, from light gray to dark gray, **333–335**

Grating Visual pattern of alternating light and dark bars. *See* Sinusoidal grating, Square wave, Triangle wave

Gross potential Voltage due to the summed activity of a large number of neurons, **60**. *See also* Cochlear microphonic, Electroretinogram

Ground Remainder of a scene after figure has been segregated, 268–272

Gustation 577–579, 588–589. *See also* Conditioned taste aversion, Flavor

Gymnema sylvestre Plant whose extract depresses sensitivity to sweetness, **579**

Hair cells Receptor cells in the organ of Corti, 447–449, 453, 468, 469

Harmonics High frequency multiples of the fundamental frequency, 215, 229–230, 267, 440

Helicotrema Connection between the scala tympani and scala vestibuli in the cochlea, **446**

Hemianopia Scotoma affecting one side of the visual field, **160**–161, 201

Hering illusion Illusion of shape, 347. *See also* Illusion

Hermann grid Illusion in which dark patches appear in the intersections of white stripes, **125**, 127

Hertz (Hz) Measure of frequency of a sound wave, equal to one cycle per second, **435**

Hierarchical model Model in which information flows from receptors to higher centers only. *See* Pandemonium, Top-down processing

Horizontal cells Laterally conducting cells of the outer plexiform layer of the retina, **90**, 103, 106–107

Homunculus Representation of the surface of the body on the somatosensory cortex, **559**–561

Horopter Surface representing all points that may be simultaneously viewed with no binocular disparity, **315**–316

Hue Essential color of a light, **389**

Hypercolumn Collection of orientation or ocular dominance columns representing all orientations or ocular dominances in a visual area, **187**–191

Hypercomplex cells Types of cells in the visual cortex that have the property of selecting for length of a bar of light (more commonly called *end-stopped* cells, which may be either simple or complex), 175–178

Hypermetropia Farsightedness, 79–80

Hyperpolarization For a nerve cell, becoming more polarized (more negative) inside, 54, 97

IPA *See* International Phonetic Association

IPSP *See* Inhibitory postsynaptic potential

Illuminance Photometric unit of light striking a surface, **68**

Illusion Stimulus that leads to erroneous perception, 285–294, 343–355, 377–378, 564. *See also* Ambiguous figure, Autokinetic effect, Craik-O'Brien illusion, Hermann grid, Impossible figure, Mach bands, Movement aftereffect, Pulfrich effect, Reversible figures, Staircase illusion

Image-retina system Perceptual system that responds to movement of an image across the retina, **365**, 366–373

Imaginary lights Colors that contain a negative component, **403**

Impossible figure Drawing of an object that cannot actually exist as depicted, **292**–294

Induced movement Apparent motion of a stimulus caused by motion of nearby stimuli, **382**

Inferior colliculus Midbrain nucleus in the auditory pathway, **450**, 504, 505

Inferotemporal cortex Cortex in the temporal lobe of the brain concerned with identification of visual stimuli, 200–201

Inflow theory Theory that eye positions are monitored by receptors in the extraocular muscles, **374**

Inhibitory postsynaptic potential (IPSP) Hyperpolarization caused by transmitter released from a presynaptic cell, 56, 57

Inner ear Fluid-filled part of the ear, **440**, 445–449. *See also* Basilar membrane, Cochlea, Hair cells, Organ of Corti

Inner nuclear layer Layer of the retina containing cell bodies of horizontal cells, bipolar cells, amacrine cells, and interplexiform cells, **90**

Interblob regions Areas of the upper layers of V1 cortex between the cytochrome oxidase blobs, **188**, 196–197

Internal capsule Fibers from thalamus to somatosensory cortex, **559**

International Phonetic Association (IPA) Organization that devised an alphabet for representing speech sounds (phonetic alphabet), 515. *See also* Vowel quadrilateral

Interplexiform cells Cells in the retina that conduct signals from the inner plexiform layer to the outer plexiform layer, **91**, 111

Interposition Occlusion of a distant object by a nearer object, a cue to depth, 299–300

Inter-spike interval histogram Histogram of times between successive action potentials fired by a neuron, **473**–474

Intracellular space The fluid-filled volume inside a cell, 37, 38, 61

Iodopsin The first cone pigment to be isolated chemically, **101**

Ion An atom with too few or too many electrons, giving it an electrical charge, **36–39**, **46–47**, **55**, **98**, **448**, **582**, **595**; calcium = Ca^{++}; chloride = Cl^-; potassium = K^+; sodium = Na^+

Ipsilateral On the same side of the body, **160**, **192–194**

Iris Smooth muscle ring controlling size of the pupil, the colored part of the eye, **73**. *See also* Pupil

Irradiance Radiometric measure of light striking a surface, **68**

Isochronal threshold Threshold for motion measured for a constant duration stimulus, **366**

Isointensity contour Plot of responses of an auditory nerve fiber to various frequencies, **463**

Isoluminance *See* Equiluminance

Isomerization Change in configuration of a visual pigment chromophore that has absorbed a photon of light, **96**

jnd Just noticeable difference. *See* Difference threshold

Jastrow illusion Illusion of size, **349**. *See also* Illusion

KDE *See* Kinetic depth effect

Kinetic depth effect (KDE) Depth impression produced by moving a two-dimensional stimulus, **310**

Kinetic optical occlusion Successive eclipsing of objects by a moving object, a cue to depth, **383**

Korte's laws Relationships among intensity, timing, and spatial configuration of stimuli that produce stroboscopic motion, **379–380**

LGN *See* Lateral geniculate nucleus

Landolt C Test of acuity, **267**

Lateral antagonism Process by which responses in one region in a receptive field oppose the responses from another area (often called *lateral inhibition*), **119–127**, **222–224**, **331**, **465–467**, **498**, **504**, **562**. *See also* Craik-O'Brien illusion, Hermann grid, Lightness constancy, Mach bands, Simultaneous contrast, Staircase illusion

Lateral geniculate nucleus (LGN) Part of the thalamus that relays visual signals to the cortex, **163–168**, **422**, **427**, **430**. *See also* Magnocellular system, Parvocellular system, Principal cells

Lateral inhibition Older term for lateral antagonism, still generally used in sensory systems other than vision. *See* Lateral antagonism

Law of specific nerve energies Principle that firing of sensory nerves is interpreted as a stimulus of the appropriate modality, **50**

Lens Optical component that produces an image of an object, **69–73**; of the eye, **73**, **75–80**, **81**. *See also* Accommodation, Cataract, Focal length

Lens equation Relationship between focal length of a lens and object and image distances, **71–72**

Light adaptation Decrease in sensitivity with increases in ambient light, **151–153**. *See also* Adaptation, Photopic system, Weber's law

Lightness Apparent whiteness or grayness of an object, **271–272**, **326–337**

Lightness constancy Tendency to judge surface color as the

same despite changes in illumination, **326–337**

Limen *See* Threshold

Limits, method of *See* Method of limits

Limulus polyphemus Horseshoe crab, **84**, **128**

Locus Frequency defining one end of the transition of a formant in speech, **529–532**, **539**

Logarithm (log) Exponent to which 10 is raised to give a particular number; usually referred to as a *log*, **602–610**

Log law Fechner's logarithmic relationship between stimulus intensity and apparent magnitude: $S = c \cdot \log(I)$, **19**, **23**

Loudness Apparent magnitude of sound, **481**, **485–502**

Luminance Photometric measure of light emitted or reflected by an area of surface, **68**

Luminous flux Photometric unit of total light emitted by a source, **68**

MAA *See* Minimum audible angle

MAE *See* Movement aftereffect

MAF *See* Minimum audible field

MAP *See* Minimum audible pressure

MT *See* Mediotemporal cortex

MTF *See* Modulation transfer function

Mach bands Illusory light and dark bands produced at the transition from a uniformly illuminated area to a gradient, **120**, **122**, **123**

Macula lutea Pigmented central region of the retina containing the fovea, **75**

Magnitude estimation Psychophysical scaling method in which the subject assigns numbers according to the apparent magnitudes of the stimuli, **20**

Magnitude production Psychophysical scaling method in which the subject sets a stimulus intensity so the apparent magnitude is at a preassigned level, **20**

Magnocellular system Visual processing stream that starts with the large cells of the deep layers of the LGN, **166**–168, 169, 183, 195–198, 201–206, 225, 247, 273, 310, 322, 349, 383

Maintained discharge Ongoing activity of a sensory neuron in the absence of any change in stimulation, **115**, 117

Masking Obscuring a stimulus by presenting another stimulus, 123, **231**–236, 278–281; auditory, **498**–501; backward, **231**–233, 269, 278–280, 376. *See also* Metacontrast; forward, **231**; simultaneous, **231**, 233–236, 278. *See also* Camouflage

McCullough effect Color aftereffect, **242**–243

Medial geniculate nucleus Part of the thalamus that relays auditory signals to temporal cortex, **450**

Medial lemniscus Somatosensory tract from spinal cord to thalamus, **557**

Mediotemporal cortex (MT) Visual area in the magnocellular stream, also known as *V5*, that analyzes movement, orientation, and position, **198**, 201–202, 372–373, 376, 383

Meissner corpuscle Somatosensory receptor, **549**–550

Mel A scale that measures pitch, **476**

Merkel cells Somatosensory receptor cells, **549**–550

Metacontrast Backward masking in which the mask is spatially separate from the test, **280**. *See also* Masking, backward

Metameric match Two colored

stimuli that look alike but have different spectra, 398–399

Metathetic continuum Variable for which a larger numerical value does not imply a greater quantity, **16**

Methods, psychophysical *See* Constant stimuli, Forced choice, Method of limits, Magnitude estimation, Magnitude production

Method of adjustment Method of limits in which the subject controls the stimulus intensity, 9, 14

Method of limits Psychophysical methods in which intensity is varied until threshold is reached, **8**. *See also* Ascending series, Descending series, Method of adjustment

Microelectrode Small electrode that can be placed inside or near single cells, **61**, 62, 63

Micromanipulator Device for the precise positioning of a microelectrode, **62**

Micropipette A kind of microelectrode made of glass, **62**

Microspectrophotometer Instrument that measures the absorption spectrum of single photoreceptors, **410**

Middle ear Air-filled chamber containing the ossicles, **440**, 443–445. *See also* Ossicles, Stapedius, Tensor tympani

Minimum audible angle (MAA) Smallest detectable movement of a sound source in space, **510**

Minimum audible field (MAF) Absolute auditory threshold measured using loudspeakers, **486**

Minimum audible pressure (MAP) Absolute auditory threshold measured using headphones, **486**

Missing fundamental illusion Illusion that the fundamental frequency is still present when only its harmonics are present, **225**. *See*

also Craik-O'Brien illusion; auditory, 481

Modulation transfer function (MTF) Plot of magnitude of responses of a system as a function of frequency, **218**–221

Monaural cues Cues to the location of a sound source that require only one ear, 509–510. *See also* Doppler shift

Mondrian Abstract complex visual pattern used to test color constancy, **332**–334, 430

Monochromacy Condition of complete color blindness in which only one visual pigment is functional, 404, **405**, 406, 417

Monochromatic light Light consisting of only one wavelength, **387**

Monochromator Instrument that delivers nearly monochromatic light, **390**

Monocular cues Cues to depth that require only one eye, **297**, 298–311. *See also* Movement cues, Pictorial cues

Moon illusion Illusion that the horizon moon is larger than the zenith moon, **352**–355

Motion detectors Cells that respond best to stimuli that are moving, often in a preferred direction, 128, 131, 171, 175, 202, 242, 367–368, 369–373, 563

Motion parallax Relative movement of objects at different distances, a cue to depth, 297, **307**–309, 383

Motor theory of speech perception Theory that speech sounds are perceived according to an analysis-by-synthesis model, 538–542

Movement aftereffect (MAE) Impression of motion resulting from previous inspection of a moving target, **368**–371, 384

Movement cues Depth cues derived from motion, 307. *See also* Kinetic depth effect, Motion parallax

Müller-Lyer illusion   Illusion of length of lines, 349–352. *See also* Illusion

Muscle spindle   Stretch receptive organ in voluntary muscles, 50–51, 548–549

Myelin   Part of a glial cell that wraps around axons, speeding conduction of action potentials, **48**, 49, 552

Myopia   Nearsightedness, **79**

Nanometer (nm)   Measure of length; 1 nm = 10^{-9} meter, **387**

Nasal retina   Half of the retina nearest the nose, **160**

Near point   Closest distance at which the lens can project a focused image on the retina, 78–80

Nearsightedness   *See* Myopia

Necker cube   Reversible figure, **287–289**, 290

Necturus   A salamander, the mud puppy, **104**

Negative light   Use of a primary in a metameric match such that it is added to the light being matched, 398–399

Nerve spike   *See* Action potential

Neuron   Cell that is the basic unit of the nervous system, 35

Neurotransmitter   *See* Transmitter

Neutral point   Monochromatic light that a dichromat confuses with white, **408**, 415, 416

Nociception   Sense of pain, **545**, 551–553. *See also* Pain perception

Nodes of Ranvier   Gaps in the myelin sheath, 49

Noise   Random variation in a sensory channel, 27

Normal probability paper   Axes on which the integral of a normal distribution plots as a straight line, 610–612

Notational space   Unstructured field used for ambiguous figures and the primal sketch, 6, 34, 64, 208, 386, 454, 484, 512

Nystagmus   Rapid back-and-forth eye movement, **84**

Oblique muscles   Type of extraocular muscle, **82**

Occipital cortex   Part of the brain near the back of the head, containing mainly visual processing areas, **159**. *See also* Visual area I, V2, V3

Ocular dominance   Classification of cortical cells according to how strongly they are driven by each eye, **185**, 192–194

Ocular dominance columns   Slab-like groups of cells in visual cortex that are all driven primarily by the same eye, 185–188, 191

Odor prism   System for representing the classification of odorants, 591

OFF-center cell   Cell that produces an OFF response to the presentation of light in the center of its receptive field, **110**, 117, 168

OFF response   Response in which increased activity or depolarization occurs at offset of the stimulus (and decreased activity or hyperpolarization usually occurs at onset), **117**, 120, 157

Offset response   Response to the termination of a stimulus, **108**, 110, 117

Ogive   Continuously increasing ''S''-shaped curve, 9

Olfaction   The sense of smell, 590–596, 597

Olfactory bulb   Part of the brain where olfactory receptors first synapse, **593–595**

Olfactory neuroepithelium   The olfactory sensory organ, **592**

Ommatidium   Single facet of a compound eye, **84**

ON-OFF response   Response in which there is increased activity or depolarization at both onset and offset of the stimulus, **110**, 117

ON-center cell   Cell that produces an ON response to the presentation of light in the center of its receptive field, **110**, 117, 168

ON response   Response in which increased activity or depolarization occurs at onset of the stimulus (and decreased activity or hyperpolarization usually occurs at offset), **117**, 120

Onset response   Response to the initiation of a stimulus, **108**, 110, 117, 118

Opiate analgesics   Narcotics derived from the opium poppy, used as pain killers, 571–572

Opponent-process theory   Theory stating that the three fundamental color processes represent trade-offs in red/green, yellow/blue, and black/white systems, 419–421

Opsin   Large protein portion of a visual pigment molecule, **95**

Optic chiasm   Intersection of the optic nerves, **160**

Optic disc   Region where the optic nerve fibers leave the eyeball, also called the *blind spot*, **75**, 93

Optic nerves   Bundles of ganglion cell axons connecting the eyes and brain, **91**, 190

Optic radiation   Bundles of axons of LGN principal cells connecting the LGN to the visual cortex, **165**

Optics   Study of the reflection and refraction of light, 69–73, 79–80

Orbison illusion   Illusion of shape, **348**. *See also* Illusion

Ordinate Vertical position (height) of a point on a graph, **600**

Organ of Corti Primary auditory receptor structure on the basilar membrane of the cochlea, **447**, 449. *See also* Basilar membrane, Hair cells

Orientation columns Slab-like groups of cells in the visual cortex, all of which possess the same optimal stimulus orientation preference, 183, **184–185**, 191, 194

Orientation of figures Angle at which complex visual patterns are viewed, 275–277

Oscilloscope Device for displaying voltage as a function of time, **59**

Ossicles Three small bones in the inner ear: the malleus ("hammer"), incus ("anvil"), and stapes ("stirrup"), **443–444**

Outer ear External sound-gathering portion of the ear, **440**, 441–443. *See also* Pinna, Tympanic membrane

Outer nuclear layer Layer of the retina containing the cell bodies of rods and cones, **90**

Outer segment Part of the visual receptors that contains the visual pigment, **91**, 97. *See also* Shedding

Outflow theory Theory that positions (of eyes or limbs) are monitored by noting the signals sent to the muscles, **374–376**, 546–547

Oval window Soft opening through which the stapes affects the fluid of the cochlea, **443**

PDP *See* Parallel distributed processing

PSTH *See* Peri-stimulus time histogram

Pacinian corpuscle Somatosensory receptor, **549**

Pain perception 565–572. *See also* Nociception

Pale stripes Areas of minimal cytochrome oxidase staining in V2, part of the parvocellular stream, **196**, 424

Pandemonium Hierarchical, parallel-processing model for pattern recognition, 255–257

Panum's fusion area Space near enough to the horopter for binocular images to be fused, **316**. *See also* Horopter

Papillae Protuberances on the tongue containing the taste buds, **575**, 578, 583–584

Parallel distributed processing (PDP) Model of neural network capable of learning, used in artificial intelligence, 255, **257–258**

Parallel processing Principle that neurons work in parallel to process various aspects of a stimulus, 167, 355

Parietal cortex *See* Posterior parietal cortex (visual), Somatosensory cortex

Parvocellular system Visual processing stream that starts with the small cells of the LGN, **166–168**, 169, 183, 188, 195–198, 200–201, 203–206, 236, 247, 427

Pattern playback Machine that converts painted "spectrograms" into sound (also called *vocoder*), **526–532**

Pattern recognition 251–259

Penumbra Lighter peripheral portion of a shadow. *See* Shadows

Perception The interpretation of sensory information to give an internal representation of the world, 1, 249–251

Perceptual hypothesis Subconscious "guess" about the nature of a distal stimulus, **281–294**, 339, 351, 513, 535, 540

Perilymph Fluid in the scala vestibuli and scala tympani of the cochlea, **446**, 448

Period Time or space required for one cycle of a repeating waveform. *See* Frequency, Fundamental frequency, Spatial frequency

Periodicity pitch Phenomenon that the pitch of a complex tone is determined by the fundamental common to the harmonics, even if the fundamental is omitted, **481–482**. *See also* Missing fundamental illusion

Peri-stimulus time histogram (PSTH) Plot of firing rate of a neuron versus time relative to stimulation, **117**

Perspective Projection of a three-dimensional world onto a two-dimensional surface, **303–304**, 344–348

Phantom grating Illusory grating seen in a blank area flanked by moving gratings, 371

Phantom limb Perception of motion of an amputated limb, 547

Phase Relative position (in time or space) of two or more sinusoids, **210–211**, 230, 246, 436, 475, 480, 507–508

Phasic response *See* Transient response

Phi movement Illusion of movement without apparent displacement (also called *pure movement*), 379. *See also* Stroboscopic movement

Pheromones Odorants that affect behavior, **596–598**

Phon Unit of loudness based on comparisons to a 1000 Hz tone, **488**

Phoneme Basic unit of speech sounds, **515–537**

Phonemic boundary Transition point for two acoustic stimuli heard as different phonemes, **536**, 537

Phonetic differences Differences in speech sounds that do not imply differences in meaning, **515**

Photochromatic interval Range of luminances between absolute threshold and the threshold for detecting colors, **150**

Photometric units Units of photometry, **68**

Photometry Measurement of light according to its effectiveness for human vision, **68**

Photon A quantum (particle) of light, **66**, **67**, **100**, **387**

Photopic system Cone-mediated visual system used in bright lighting, **68**, **145–151**

Photopigment *See* Pigment, visual

Pictorial cues Depth cues that can be presented in a stationary, two-dimensional display, **297**. *See also* Interposition, Perspective, Texture

Pictures of pictures **361–362**

Pigment, visual Chemical in the outer segments of receptors that absorbs light, **95–97**, **101–102**. *See also* Cone pigments, Iodopsin, Porphyropsin, Retinal, Rhodopsin

Pigment epithelium Darkly colored layer of cells behind the retina, **74**, **87–88**, **97**

Pinna Outer funnel-like part of the ear, **441–442**

Pitch Psychological aspect of sound related mainly to the fundamental frequency, **435**, **470–471**, **476–480**, **482**. *See also* Periodicity pitch, Pitch shift

Pitch shift Change in pitch of a tone with changes in amplitude, **479**, **480**

Place theory Theory that different positions along the basilar membrane are sensitive to different frequencies, **455**, **456–464**. *See also* Traveling wave

Plateau spiral Inducing figure for movement aftereffect, **368**

Plexiform layers Synaptic layers in the retina, **88**; inner (layer nearest the ganglion cells), **88**, **90**, **108–110**; outer (layer nearest the receptors), **88**, **90**, **102–107**

Poggendorf illusion Illusion of alignment, **273–275**. *See also* Illusion

Ponzo illusion Illusion of size due to distance, **344–345**, **347**. *See also* Illusion

Porphyropsin Photopigment found in rods of certain cold-blooded animals, **101**

Posterior columns The cuneate fasciculus and fasciculus gracilis, columns of the spinal cord mediating proprioception and the tactile sense, **556**

Posterior parietal cortex Cortex in parietal lobe of the brain concerned with the location of visual stimuli, **202–203**

Postsynaptic potential Potential difference caused by release of a transmitter at a synapse, **56**. *See also* Excitatory postsynaptic potential, Inhibitory postsynaptic potential

Potential difference Voltage difference, **36**

Power law Psychophysical relationship stating that apparent magnitude is proportional to stimulus magnitude raised to an exponent: $S = k \cdot I^n$, **20**, **21**, **489–490**

Prägnanz Gestalt principle stating that features group to form "good" figures, **264–268**, **299**

Preattentive process A process that works automatically, without conscious effort, **263**

Presbycusis Loss of sensitivity for higher frequency sounds with advancing age (also called *presbyacusia*), **487**, **526**

Presbyopia Decrease in accommodative ability with advancing age, **78**, **79**, **80**. *See also* Accommodation

Primal sketch Basic sketch made from features, **321**

Primary colors, additive Three colored lights that can be added to match any other light; usually taken as red, green, and blue, **398**, **403–404**, **408–409**. *See also* Metameric match

Principal cell Type of cell in the LGN that projects to the visual cortex (also called *relay cell*), **177**

Prisms, inverting Device to invert the visual image, **74–75**

Propagation of action potentials **47–49**

Proprioception Sense of position of the body and limbs, **545**, **546–549**

Prosodic element Qualitative aspect of relatively large segments of speech (also called *suprasegmental features*), **534**

Prosopagnosia Condition in which patient is unable to recognize subtle visual distinctions, such as recognizing faces, **201**

Protanope Dichromat lacking the long wavelength-sensitive pigment, **412**, **415–416**

Prothetic continuum Variable for which larger values imply a greater quantity, **16**

Proximal stimulus Stimulus pattern at the receptors, such as the image on the retina, **281**, **338–339**

Proximity Gestalt principle stating that nearby items are grouped together, **260–261**

Psychometric function Plot of percentage detection or score as a function of stimulus strength, **9**, 11, 12

Psychophysics Study of the capability of an organism to detect, quantify, or identify a stimulus, **7** *ff. See also* Constant stimuli, Forced choice, Method of limits, Signal detection theory

Pulfrich effect Apparent motion in depth of a moving object viewed with a filter placed before one eye, **383**

Pupil Central opening of the iris, **73**, 80–82

Purity, colorimetric Relative amount of monochromatic light in a mixture with white light, **387**, 390

Purkinje shift Difference in spectral sensitivity between the photopic and scotopic states, 146–147

Quantum of light *See* Photon

RL Reiz limen. *See* Absolute threshold

ROC curve *See* Receiver operating characteristic curve

Radiance Radiometric measure of light emitted or reflected by an area of surface, **68**

Radiant flux Radiometric measure of total light emitted by a source, **67**

Radiometric measures Measures of the energy of light, 67, **68**

Random dot stereogram Stereogram in which each separate image is a jumble of randomly placed dots, **317**–318, 322. *See also* Stereogram

Rayleigh contrast Ratio of modulation amplitude to mean light level, **213**, 229–236

Receiver operating characteristic curve (ROC curve) Plot of percentage "hits" versus percent-age "false alarms" in a signal detection experiment, **29**–32

Receptive field Area in which stimulation leads to response of a particular sensory neuron; auditory, 503–505; somatosensory, 563–564, 566; visual, **106**, 118–119, 171, 171–174, 177–178

Receptors Neurons sensitive to stimulus energy, **49**–53, 546, 580–583, 593, 595; auditory, *See* Hair cells; visual, **88**, 91–102. *See also* Cone, Rod

Rectus muscles Type of extraocular muscles, **82**

Redundancy Repeated or over-represented information, **253**

Reflectance Percentage of light incident on an object that is reflected by it (also called *albedo*), **326**

Refraction Changing the direction of light rays as with a lens or prism, **69**

Refractory period Period of time following an action potential during which the cell cannot produce another action potential, **47**

Regression to the real Tendency to correct for tilt when perceiving shapes, **357**–359

Reissner's membrane Partition between scala vestibuli and the cochlear duct, **446**

Relay cell *See* Principal cell

Resistance Electrical property of impeding the flow of current in a circuit, **36**

Resonance curve Relationship between frequency of a sound and amplitude of vibration of a point on the basilar membrane, **460**–462

Resting membrane potential Voltage difference between the inside and the outside of a neuron at rest, **37**–39

Retina Thin layer of neural tissue lining the back of the eye, **74**, 75, 88–137; anatomy of, 88–91. *See also* Amacrine cells, Bipolar cells, Cone, Fovea, Ganglion cells, Horizontal cells, Inner nuclear layer, Interplexiform cells, Optic disc, Outer nuclear layer, Plexiform layers, Rod

Retinal Vitamin A derivative found in visual pigments, **96**. *See also* Chromophore

Retinex Theory of color processing and color constancy, **332**–335

Reversible figure A pattern in which figure and ground may exchange roles, 269, **286**–289, 335. *See also* Necker cube

Rhodopsin The visual pigment found in the rods of mammals and some other animals, **101**, 141, 147, 405. *See also* Chromophore, Opsin

Ricco's law Trade-off between area of stimulus and stimulus strength for small spots of light that are equally detectable, **25**

Rivalry *See* Binocular rivalry

Rod Receptor cell in the retina that is sensitive in low luminance (scotopic) conditions, **91**–102, 147–149, 151, 417

Round window Pressure-release of the scala tympani in the cochlea, **446**

Ruffini ending Somatosensory receptor, **549**

S1 Primary somatosensory cortex. *See* Primary somatosensory cortex

SDLB *See* Simultaneous dichotic loudness balance

Saccadic movement Abrupt eye movement to a new fixation point, 86, 375

Saccadic suppression Temporary insensitivity of the visual sys-

geniculate nucleus, Medial geniculate nucleus, Ventral posterior lateral nucleus, Ventral posterior medial nucleus

Thick stripes   Areas of dark cytochrome oxidase staining in V2, part of the magnocellular stream, **196**

Thin stripes   Areas of dark cytochrome oxidase staining in V2, containing cells with wavelength selectivity, **196**, 424, 430

Threshold   Minimal perceptible quantity, 8, 143, 145; for action potential, 45. *See also* Absolute threshold, Difference threshold, Isochronal threshold

Timbre   Quality of sound imparted by harmonics and other high frequencies, **440**, 476

Tones   Sounds represented by single sinusoids, **435**, 476–480, 485–495, 506–507, 510

Tonic response   *See* Sustained response

Tonotopic map   Systematic relationship between location of cells in the brain and the sound frequencies to which they are most sensitive, **452**, 469–471

Top-down processing   Concept that "higher" centers modulate and guide the processing done in the "lower" centers, **258**–259

Transient response   Type of response that is only present immediately following a change in the stimulus (also called a *phasic response*), **108**, 133, 137, 551. *See also* ON-OFF response

Transition   Rapid shift in the frequency of a formant, **529**–532, 536–538, 539

Transmission curve   Characteristic of a filter expressed by percentage transmission as a function of wavelength, **394**

Transmitter   Chemical substance used in neuronal communication at synapses, **53**, 57–58, 99, 109

Trapezoidal window   Demonstration of shape constancy, 290–292. *See also* Ames demonstrations, Illusion

Traveling wave   Pattern of vibration of the basilar membrane in which waves move from base to apex, with a maximum amplitude at a position determined by the sound frequency, **456**–460. *See also* Place theory

Triad   Synaptic complex in the receptor invaginations of the retina, **102**

Triangle wave   Pattern of a series of uniform increases and decreases, **216**, 219

Trichromacy   Normal human condition of having three color systems, and so requiring three primaries to match any light, **408**–409, 412

Trichromatic theory   Theory that the existence of three additive primary colors indicates three broad fundamental color systems, 409–412

Tritanope   Dichromat lacking the short wavelength-sensitive pigment, **412**, 415

Two alternative forced choice (2AFC)   Psychophysical method in which the subject chooses in which of two possibilities the stimulus lies, **13**, 32

Tympanic membrane   Membrane at end of outer ear canal that vibrates in response to sound (also called the *eardrum*), **442**, 443, 486

Umbra   Dark central portion of a shadow. *See* Shadows

Unique colors   Colors that seem psychologically "pure"; specifically red, yellow, green, and blue, **419**

Univariance   Principle that individual receptors cannot signal the wavelength of the light they have absorbed, 149, **405**

Unstructured field   Visual display lacking cues to size or distance, **342**

V1   *See* Visual area 1

V2   Secondary visual cortex, **159**, 196–197, 199–200

V3   Area of visual cortex in the magnocellular stream, 196–197

V4   Area of visual cortex in the parvocellular stream, 196–198, 200–201, 430, 431

V5   *See* Mediotemporal cortex

VPL   *See* Ventral posterior lateral nucleus

VPM   *See* Ventral posterior medial nucleus

Ventral posterior lateral nucleus   Nucleus of the thalamus that relays tactile and proprioceptive information about the body to the cortex, **557**, 567

Ventral posterior medial nucleus   Nucleus of the thalamus that relays taste information, as well as tactile and proprioceptive information about the face, to the cortex, **557**, 576–577

Vertebrate eye   73–82

Visual angle   Angle of view subtended by an object, **337**–343

Visual area I   Primary visual cortex (also called *striate cortex*, *V1*), **159**, 168–182, 183–191, 198–199, 246. *See also* Complex cells, Hypercolumns, Hypercomplex cells, Magnocellular system, Ocular dominance columns, Orientation columns, Parvocellular system, Simple cells

Visual pigment   *See* Chromophore, Cone pigment, Iodopsin, Porphyropsin, Retinal, Rhodopsin

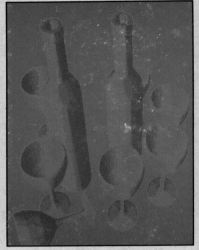
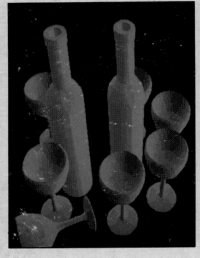
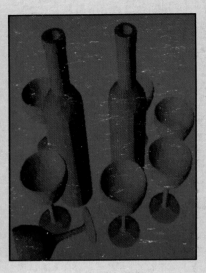

Color Plate A. See page 205

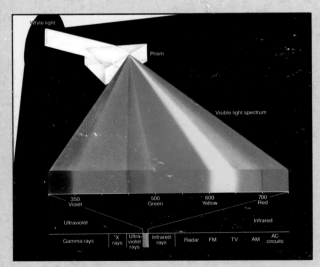

Color Plate E. See page 388

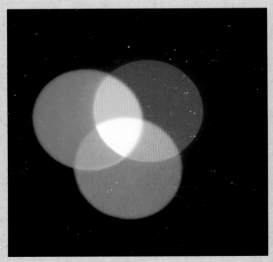

Color Plate F. See page 392